Neurobiology of TRP Channels

Neurobiology of TRP Channels

Editor: Alessandra Crooks

AMERICAN
MEDICAL PUBLISHERS
www.americanmedicalpublishers.com

AMERICAN
MEDICAL PUBLISHERS
www.americanmedicalpublishers.com

Cataloging-in-Publication Data

Neurobiology of TRP channels / edited by Alessandra Crooks.
p. cm.
Includes bibliographical references and index.
ISBN 979-8-88740-302-1
1. TRP channels. 2. Neurobiology. 3. Membrane proteins. 4. Ion channels. 5. Biochemistry.
6. Neurology. I. Crooks, Alessandra.
QP552.T77 N48 2023
572.696--dc23

American Medical Publishers,
41 Flatbush Avenue,
1st Floor, New York,
NY 11217, USA

ISBN 979-8-88740-302-1 (Hardback)

Contents

Preface

This book has been a concerted effort by a group of academicians, researchers and scientists, who have contributed their research works for the realization of the book. This book has materialized in the wake of emerging advancements and innovations in this field. Therefore, the need of the hour was to compile all the required researches and disseminate the knowledge to a broad spectrum of people comprising of students, researchers and specialists of the field.

Transient receptor potential (TRP) channels refer to a group of ion channels located on the plasma membrane of animal cell types. These channels play an important role in the regulation of basic cellular processes and have implications in the initiation of various forms of cancer. Various functions are regulated by TRP channels, which include homeostasis, mechanical sensations, cardiovascular regulation, lysosomal function, cell proliferation and growth. Mutations in TRP channels are associated with several diseases like skeletal dysplasia, kidney disorders and neurodegenerative disorders. Furthermore, TRP channels are implicated in neurologic disorders, like lysosomal storage disorder, neuropathic pain, mucolipidosis type IV and cell injury caused due to cerebral ischemia. In the nervous system, TRP channels are responsible for excitotoxic cell death caused due to anoxia, receptor signaling and neurite outgrowth. This book is a valuable compilation of topics, ranging from the basic to the most complex advancements in the study of TRP channels. It strives to provide a fair idea about this discipline and to help develop a better understanding of the latest advances within this field. This book includes contributions of experts and scientists which will provide innovative insights into this field.

At the end of the preface, I would like to thank the authors for their brilliant chapters and the publisher for guiding us all-through the making of the book till its final stage. Also, I would like to thank my family for providing the support and encouragement throughout my academic career and research projects.

Editor

1

Transient Receptor Potential Channels as an Emerging Target for the Treatment of Parkinson's Disease: An Insight into Role of Pharmacological Interventions

Bhupesh Vaidya and Shyam Sunder Sharma*

Department of Pharmacology and Toxicology, National Institute of Pharmaceutical Education and Research (NIPER), Mohali, India

Correspondence:
Shyam Sunder Sharma
sssharma@niper.ac.in

Parkinson's disease (PD) is a neurodegenerative disorder characterized by the symptoms of motor deficits and cognitive decline. There are a number of therapeutics available for the treatment of PD, but most of them suffer from serious side effects such as bradykinesia, dyskinesia and on-off effect. Therefore, despite the availability of these pharmacological agents, PD patients continue to have an inferior quality of life. This has warranted a need to look for alternate strategies and molecular targets. Recent evidence suggests the Transient Receptor Potential (TRP) channels could be a potential target for the management of motor and non-motor symptoms of PD. Though still in the preclinical stages, agents targeting these channels have shown immense potential in the attenuation of behavioral deficits and signaling pathways. In addition, these channels are known to be involved in the regulation of ionic homeostasis, which is disrupted in PD. Moreover, activation or inhibition of many of the TRP channels by calcium and oxidative stress has also raised the possibility of their paramount involvement in affecting the other molecular mechanisms associated with PD pathology. However, due to the paucity of information available and lack of specificity, none of these agents have gone into clinical trials for PD treatment. Considering their interaction with oxidative stress, apoptosis and excitotoxicity, TRP channels could be considered as a potential future target for the treatment of PD.

Keywords: Parkinson's disease, TRP channels, TRPM2, TRPV1, TRPC1

INTRODUCTION

Parkinson's disease (PD) is a neurodegenerative condition characterized mainly by the loss of dopaminergic neurons in regions of the basal ganglia. It is the second most prevalent form of neurodegenerative disorder and stands next to Alzheimer's disease (AD) in terms of number of individuals affected across the globe (Parkinson's News Today, 2020). There are a number of therapeutics (Levodopa, Dopamine (D2) receptor agonists, monoamine oxidase B inhibitors, catechol-*o*-methyl transferase inhibitors, Adenosine 2A antagonists) approved for the treatment of PD. However, most of them provide only symptomatic relief. Also, currently available drugs show severe side effects and require frequent dosing resulting in low patient compliance of these medications. This has warranted a search for new mechanisms as well as molecular targets which could be utilized for the development of drug candidates in PD (Kumar et al., 2009; Uppalapati et al., 2014; Das and Sharma, 2015; Zhen and Chu, 2020). There are a number of *in vitro* and *in vivo* models which have been used for the therapeutic screening of pharmacological agents targeting these new molecular targets in PD. PD models include administration of neurotoxins such as 1-methyl-4-phenyl-1,2,3,6-tetrahydropyridine (MPTP), 1-methyl-4-phenylpyridinium (MPP^+), rotenone, 6-hydroxydopmaine (6-OHDA) and alpha-synuclein pro-fibrils to induce dopaminergic neuronal death in the substantia nigra and the striatum. In addition, transgenic mice (knock-in and knock-out) are available for induction of PD. Pathophysiology of PD is complex and multi-factorial. Studies done using these preclinical models as well as PD patients have pointed out at the involvement of Ca^{2+} overload and oxidative stress in PD pathology. Cumulative evidence in recent times has demonstrated a major contribution of Transient Receptor Potential (TRP) channels toward Ca^{2+} mediated excitotoxicity and oxidative stress-induced dopaminergic neuronal death in PD. In total, 28 members of the TRP family have been discovered in mammals which are activated in response to diverse physiological stimuli (Zheng, 2013; Samanta et al., 2018). However, most of these members are non-selective cation channels which are responsible for the influx of monovalent and divalent ions, including Ca^{2+} into the cell. Oxidative stress and reactive oxygen species (ROS) have also been postulated to play a role in mechanisms involving activation and inhibition of these TRP channels (Adhya and Sharma, 2019; Akyuva and Naziroglu, 2020). These properties make them an attractive target for the treatment of neurodegenerative conditions, including PD (Thapak et al., 2020c). As a result, last few decades have seen enormous progress in the field of TRP research, and many of the TRP channel modulators like AMG571, MK-2295 and AZD1386 (TRPV1 antagonists) have even managed to progress to the clinical trials for the treatment of pain disorders (Kaneko and Szallasi, 2014). However, further analysis of these TRP channel modulators has exposed their dark side with side effects raging form hyperthermia and to reduced noxious perception to heat (Gavva, 2009; Kaneko and Szallasi, 2014). Thus, most of these studies had to be terminated owing to the risk of scalding injuries to the patients. Keeping in mind the crucial role of these channels, it is now expected that detailed structure-activity relationships and pharmacophore studies would help to improve their safety and efficacy and ensure the translational success of TRP channel modulators in PD.

In this review, we have provided a detailed account of preclinical evidence suggesting the vital involvement of TRP channels in PD and how their knowledge may help researchers in this field gain in-depth insight about these channels. Additionally, a number of upcoming drug candidates targeting TRP channels have also been discussed.

TRP FAMILY

TRP family of ion channels was first discovered in 1969 when some of the drosophila fly mutants turned blind in response to bright light (Cosens and Manning, 1969). This identification was followed by a series of biochemical, electrophysiological and molecular studies which led to the characterization of the TRP channel family. It is now well established that these channels are evolutionarily conserved across species and are found in most cells, tissues, and organisms. Subsequently, a total of 28 members belonging to 6 subfamilies were identified in mammals which include TRPV (Vanilloid), TRPM (Melastatin), TRPC (Canonical), TRPML (Mucolipin), TRPA (Ankyrin), and TRPP (Polycystic) (Li, 2017). Besides, other families, such as TRPY and TRPN were also identified in the non-mammalian species. Amongst these, TRPY is the most distant relative which is only present in yeast. It plays a role in the release of Ca^{2+} from the vacuoles when exposed to hyperosmotic conditions (Denis and Cyert, 2002; Venkatachalam and Montell, 2007). TRPN has also been reported but only in a limited number of vertebrates such as xenopus and zebrafish, where it serves as the mechanosensitive channel for performing the normal physiological function (Hardie, 2007). However, these channels bear little relevance to human disease and hence have not been discussed in greater detail. Structurally all the TRP channels form six transmembrane helixes with both the N and C terminal located within the cytoplasm. These channels are activated in response to a diverse range of physiological and sensory stimuli which include mechanical, thermal, electrical and chemical cues (Steinberg et al., 2014). Therefore, these TRP channels are involved in the sensation of touch, vision, olfaction, temperature and nociception (Voets et al., 2005). Moreover, these TRPs exhibit a widespread expression in the brain areas involved in pathophysiology of PD, making them a very relevant molecular target for the discovery of new drugs to treat PD (**Table 1**). The detailed role of TRP channels has been discussed in the further sections.

CONTRIBUTION OF TRP CHANNELS TO PD

TRPV Involvement in PD

TRPV channels are abundantly expressed in several areas of the brain. Although different members of the TRPV subfamily perform a very diverse physiological role, all of these have modest permeability toward Ca^{2+}. It makes them important for various central nervous system (CNS) functions, including learning and memory (Thapak et al., 2020a). It has therefore been reported that any change in the expression of TRPV channels contributes toward CNS disease pathologies such as AD, PD, cerebral ischemia, depression and anxiety (Bashiri et al., 2018; Thapak et al., 2020c).

Amongst the members of the TRPV family, TRPV1/4/5 have been studied for their involvement in PD pathology. TRPV1 is expressed in the regions, striatum and substantia nigra, which are known to be affected in PD (Musella et al., 2009; Nam et al., 2015). However, its role remains controversial pertaining to modulation of different downstream signaling pathways by it. Though an upregulation of TRPV1 has been reported by several authors in different PD models, both agonists and antagonists targeting

TABLE 1 | Expression of the different TRP channels in the regions involved in the pathophysiology of PD.

S No.	TRP channel	Substantia nigra pars compacta	Striatum	Subthalamic nuclei	Substantia nigra pars reticulata	References
1	TRPV1[c]	+	+	+	nd	Roberts et al., 2004; Musella et al., 2009; Nam et al., 2015
2	TRPV2*[nk]	nd	+	nd	nd	Kunert-Keil et al., 2006; Shibasaki et al., 2013
3	TRPV3[nk]	+	+	nd	nd	Xu et al., 2002; Guatteo et al., 2005
4	TRPV4[rd]	+	+	nd	nd	Guatteo et al., 2005; Tjaša et al., 2016
5	TRPV5*[nk]	nd	nd	nd	+	Kumar et al., 2017
6	TRPV6[nk]	+	+	nd	+	Lehen'kyi et al., 2012
7	TRPM1[nk]	nd	nd	nd	nd	Fonfria et al., 2006
8	TRPM2[id]	+	+	+	+	Fonfria et al., 2005; Lee et al., 2013; Yu et al., 2014
9	TRPM3*[nk]	nd	nd	nd	nd	Lee et al., 2003
10	TRPM4[nk]	+	+	nd	nd	Mrejeru et al., 2011; Chen et al., 2019
11	TRPM5*[nk]	nd	nd	nd	nd	Kunert-Keil et al., 2006
12	TRPM6*[nk]	nd	nd	nd	nd	Kunert-Keil et al., 2006
13	TRPM7[id]	+	+	nd	nd	Fonfria et al., 2005; Yu et al., 2014
14	TRPM8[nk]	+	nd	nd	nd	Ordás et al., 2019
15	TRPC1[rd]	+	+	+	+	Martorana et al., 2006; Sun et al., 2017
16	TRPC2[nk]	nd	nd	nd	nd	
17	TRPC3[rd]	+	+	+	+	Chung et al., 2007
18	TRPC4[nc]	+	+	+	+	Chung et al., 2007
19	TRPC5[nc]	+	+	+	+	Chung et al., 2007
20	TRPC6[nc]	+	+	+	+	Chung et al., 2007
21	TRPC7[nk]	+	+	+	+	Chung et al., 2007
22	TRPML1*[nk]	nd	nd	nd	nd	Anglade et al., 1997; Dong et al., 2008; Grimm et al., 2012
23	TRPML2[nk]	nd	nd	nd	nd	
24	TRPML3[nk]	nd	nd	nd	nd	
25	TRPA1[nk]	nd	+	nd	nd	Bodkin et al., 2014
26	TRPP1[nk]	nd	nd	nd	nd	
27	TRPP2[nk]	nd	nd	nd	nd	
28	TRPP3[nk]	nd	nd	nd	nd	

*+Expression is this region has been determined. [nd]Expression in this region has not yet been determined. *Expression in basal ganglia has been characterized but individual distribution within basal ganglia has not been reported in much detail. [c]There is a controversy related to whether the expression is increased or reduced in PD. [nk]Change of expression in PD has not yet been studied. [id]Expression is known to be increased in PD. [rd]Expression is known to be reduced in PD. [nc]No change of expression in PD.*

these have been successful in alleviating symptoms of disease in the preclinical stages (**Figure 1**) (Nam et al., 2015; Li et al., 2019).

Studies related to other TRPV channels like TRPV4/5 have also been carried out but remain rather limited. Expression of TRPV4 was downregulated in SNpc and striatum of rats after 6-OHDA administration suggesting a possible correlation between TRPV4 expression and neuronal death (Tjaša et al., 2016). Similarly, there is not much data to support the involvement of TRPV5 channels in PD. However, a transcriptome analysis suggested its possible role in the regulation of the pathophysiological hallmarks of PD in 6-OHDA treated rats (Li et al., 2019). Nevertheless, the lack of enough data and the absence of any pharmacological study targeting these channels have denied them a concrete claim as a possible drug target for PD.

TRPM Involvement in PD

TRPM channel subfamily has been extensively explored for its potential involvement in pathophysiology of several neurodegenerative disorders including PD (Ostapchenko et al., 2015; Sun et al., 2018b; Thapak et al., 2020b). It has been reported that the members of the TRPM subfamily lead to an influx of monovalent and divalent cations inside the cell which might serve as a contributing factor for the excitotoxicity mediated neuronal death (Adhya and Sharma, 2019).

Amongst these, TRPM2 channels have gained importance for their involvement in several mechanisms related to neuronal death. These channels are activated in response to oxidative stress and adenosine diphosphate ribose (ADPR), both of which are increased in PD. Though the permeability ratio of TRPM2 for Ca^{2+} to Na^{+} (PCa:PNa) is nearly 0.7 indicating a higher permeability for Na^{+}, a substantial Ca^{2+} influx also takes place because of the longer opening time of TRPM2 channels (Belrose and Jackson, 2018). The increased Ca^{2+} levels as a result of TRPM2 activation lead to excitotoxicity and contribute toward the aggravation of the underlying PD pathology.

Apart from TRPM2, TRPM7 has also been investigated for its involvement in PD. Genetic variants of TRPM7 have been

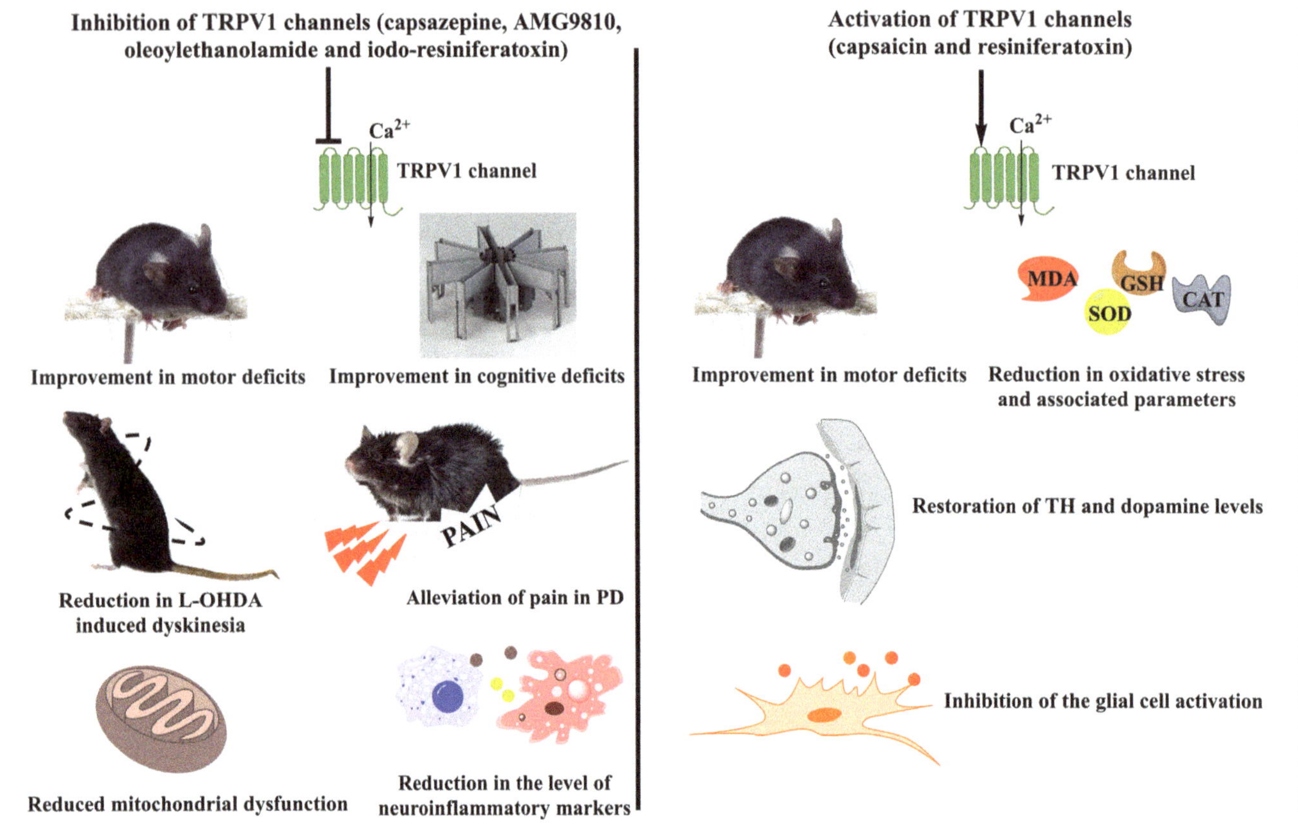

FIGURE 1 | Controversial role of TRPV1 channels in PD. A number of TRPV1 modulators have been tested for their beneficial effects in PD. Different agents working either via TRPV1 inhibition or TRPV1 activation have been studied for the mitigation of PD symptoms in preclinical models. Inhibition of TRPV1 led to an improvement in the motor and cognitive deficits of PD accompanied by reduced mitochondrial dysfunction and decreased levels of inflammatory mediators. Moreover, TRPV1 inhibitors also showed a reduction in the 6-OHDA induced dyskinesias and provided relief from pain which is one of the major non-motor symptoms of PD. On the other hand, TRPV1 activation had similar effects on improvement of motor coordination. It also reduced the levels of oxidative stress and led to the restoration of the tyrosine hydroxylase and dopamine levels. Furthermore, a significant reduction in the microglial activation was also observed after the administration of TRPV1 activators. TRPV1, Transient Receptor Potential Vanilloid 1; PD, Parkinson's disease; 6-OHDA, 6-hydroxydopamine; TH, Tyrosine hydroxylase; MDA, Malondialdehyde; SOD, superoxide dismutase; GSH, glutathione; CAT, catalase.

linked to the ionic dyshomeostasis, mitochondrial dysfunction, inflammation and increased oxidative stress, all of which led to its identification as a candidate susceptibility gene for familial PD (Hermosura et al., 2005; Hermosura and Garruto, 2007). In addition, PC-12 cells exposed to 6-OHDA also showed an increased expression of TRPM7, which was reduced after overexpression of miR-22. Furthermore, miR-22 overexpression also protected from the effects of TRPM7 upregulation by inhibition of apoptosis, reduction of ROS and improved cell viability (Yang et al., 2016). Despite these findings, there are other controversial reports which have observed neuroprotective effects of the TRPM7 mediated Mg^{2+} influx in the MPP^{+} based *in vitro* model (Shindo et al., 2015). Hence, more studies with selective TRPM7 modulators are required to conclusively elucidate the role of these channels in PD.

TRPM8 is another candidate belonging to the TRPM subfamily which has been identified as a risk factor for pain in PD (Williams et al., 2020). Pain is a frequently occurring non-motor symptom, which has been reported in about 86% of the PD patients (Beiske et al., 2009; Skogar and Lokk, 2016). Therefore, strategies targeting TRPM8 channels could be utilized in future for the management of pain in PD patients.

In totality, these findings suggest that TRPM channels are critical molecular players for neuronal death in PD (**Figure 2**). However, the dearth of information related to their signaling pathways has largely limited the development of selective modulators for these channels in the PD models.

TRPC Involvement in PD

TRPC subfamily has a widespread distribution in the CNS. It was also shown to exhibit high expression in the areas of SNpc and striatum, both of which are involved in the pathophysiology of PD (Sukumaran et al., 2017). As a result, different members of the TRPC subfamily have been investigated for their potential involvement in PD. TRPC1 was the first member of the TRPC subfamily to be identified in mammals. It is localized to the dendritic processes and co-expressed with tyrosine hydroxylase (TH) in the dopaminergic neurons of the SNpc (Martorana et al., 2006). This pointed out at the physiological relevance of TRPC1 channels in the dopaminergic

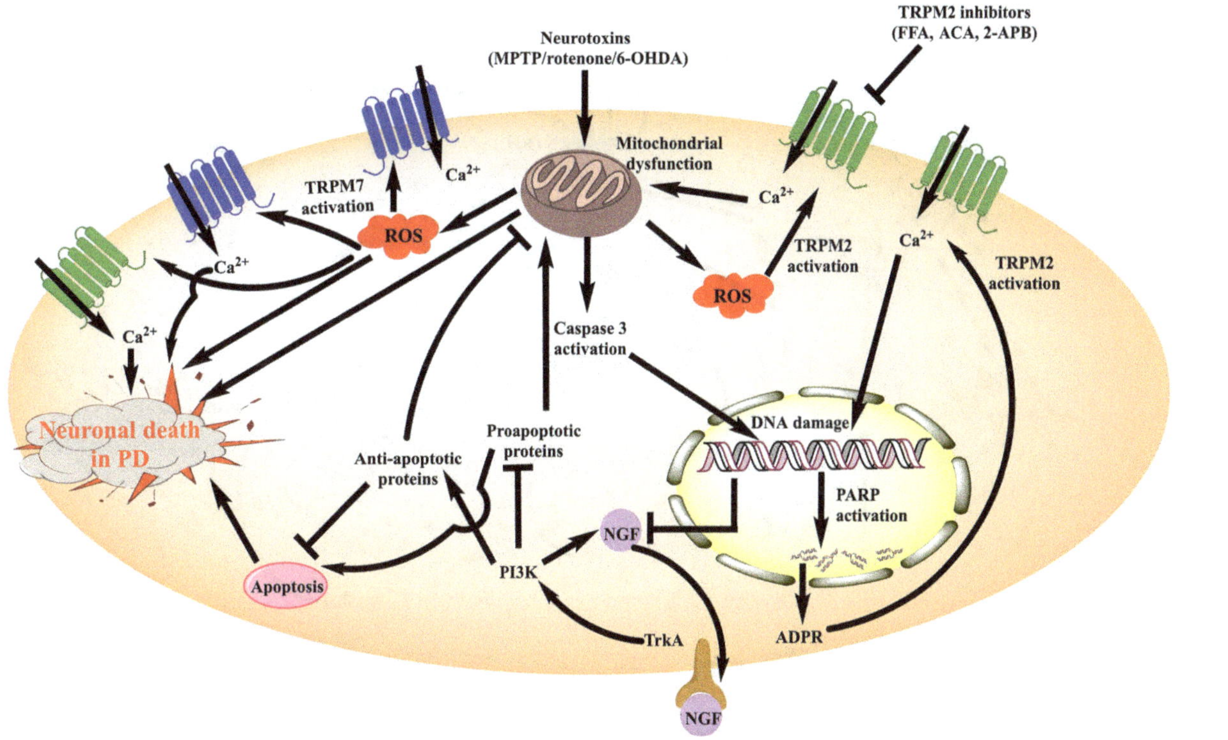

FIGURE 2 | Schematic diagram illustrating the role of TRPM channels in neuronal death associated with PD. Amongst the TRPM channels, TRPM2 and TRPM7 have been elucidated for their involvement in PD. Neurotoxins such as MPTP, 6-OHDA and rotenone inhibit the mitochondrial complexes producing mitochondrial dysfunction. It generates ROS which acts as an activator of both TRPM2 and TRPM7 leading to the increased Ca^{2+} influx within neurons. These events in totality increase the neuronal death in PD besides aggravating mitochondrial dysfunction. Moreover, cytochrome c (Cyt c) is released from the mitochondria in this process which promotes pro-apoptotic signaling and damages DNA. Damage to the DNA leads to poly ADP ribose polymerase (PARP) mediated ADPR formation which is also an activator of TRPM2 channel. Therefore, the cascade of events exhibits a positive feedback loop which aggravates neuronal death. Besides, there is a reduced expression of NGF and associated TrkA/PI3K signaling, which intensifies the pro-apoptotic response and plays its part in the TRPM2 and TRPM7 mediated neuronal death in PD. MPTP, 1-methyl-4-phenyl-1,2,3,6-tetrahydropyridine; 6-OHDA, 6-hydroxy dopamine; ROS, reactive oxygen species; FFA, Flufenamic acid; ACA, *N*-(*p*-amylcinnamoyl) anthranilic acid; 2-APB, 2-Aminoethoxydiphenyl borate; TRPM, Transient receptor potential melastatin 2; NGF, Nerve growth factor; PARP, poly ADP ribose polymerase; PI3K, phosphoinositide 3-kinase; ADPR, Adenosine di-phosphate ribose; TrkA, Tropomyosin receptor kinase A.

system and raised the possibility that these channels may contribute toward the pathogenesis of PD. Studies carried out using the MPP^+/MPTP model showed that the expression of TRPC1 was reduced in both the SNpc as well as PC12 neuronal cells in PD. Besides, $TRPC1^{-/-}$ mice also reported motor deficits and increased Terminal deoxynucleotidyl transferase dUTP nick end labeling (TUNEL)-positive cells in the basal ganglia suggesting the critical role of TRPC1 in regulating apoptotic signaling within the cell (He et al., 2016). Similar results were observed in other studies where TRPC1 overexpression protected from the effects of 6-OHDA, MPP^+ and α-synuclein toxicity in the neuronal cells (Bollimuntha et al., 2005; Sukumaran et al., 2018).

Several groups then looked at the downstream signaling associated with the neuroprotection offered by TRPC1 channels in PD models (Selvaraj et al., 2012). One of the possible mechanisms for this was the reduced endoplasmic reticulum (ER) stress which is otherwise increased in PD (Deng and Bai, 2012). It was shown that overexpression of TRPC1 channels in the SH-SY5Y cells treated with MPP^+ led to the restoration of phosphatidylinositol-3-kinase (PI3K)/mammalian target of rapamycin (Akt/mTOR) signaling and increased dopaminergic neuronal survival. Interestingly, similar findings were reported in the brains of the PD patients and $TRPC1^{-/-}$ mice which further showed an increased unfolded protein response (UPR) and reduced number of dopamine neurons in the brain (Selvaraj et al., 2012). On the other hand, TRPC1 deletion mediated ER stress was found to be associated with increased ROS, dysregulation of the glucose-regulated protein 78 (GRP78) and alteration in protein kinase RNA-like ER kinase (PERK) signaling pathways (Wang et al., 2018). In addition, potential crosstalk between the TRPC1-Stromal interaction molecule (STIM) and L-type calcium channels was also established using an electrophysiological study in the SNpc of the $TRPC1^{-/-}$ mice (Sun et al., 2017). As L-type calcium channel blockers like isradipine have already gone into clinical trials for PD, TRPC1 performing the same physiological function in dopaminergic neurons could be looked at as a molecular target in PD (Simuni et al., 2010; Sun et al., 2017). Consistent with these results are the findings of Sun et al. (2018a), where MPP^+ was found to reduce TRPC1 expression and store-operated calcium entry in the mesenchymal stem cell-derived dopaminergic neurons.

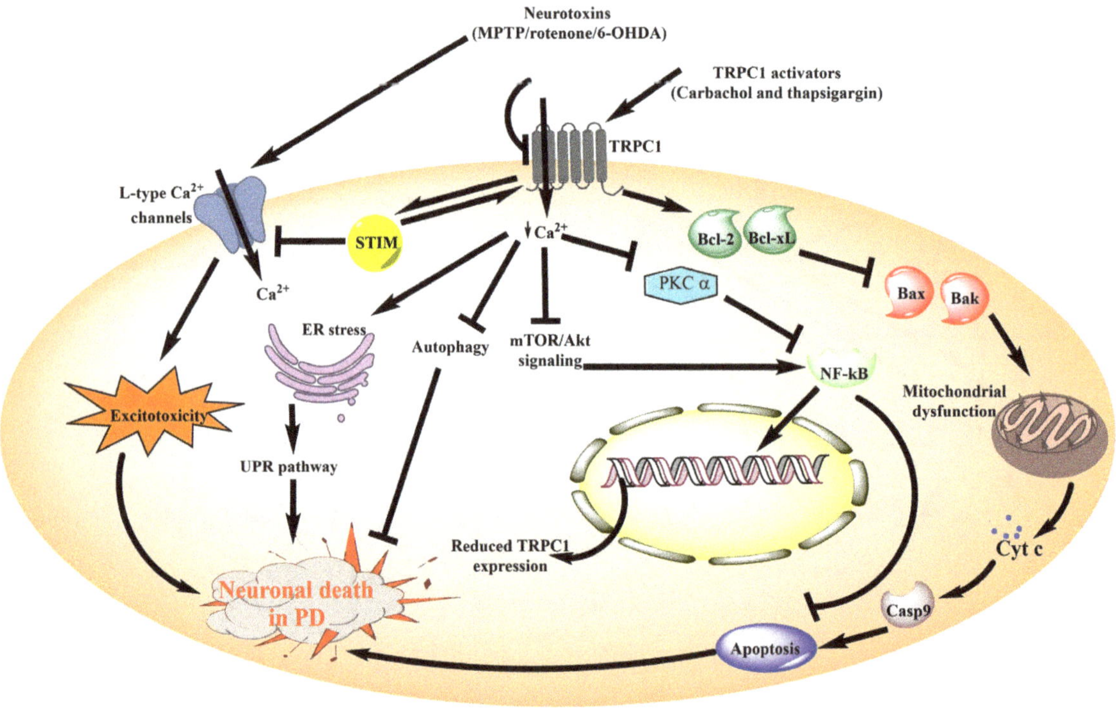

FIGURE 3 | Schematic diagram illustrating the role of TRPC1 channels in neuronal death associated with PD. TRPC1 channel is the most widely studied member of the TRPC subfamily for its involvement in PD. Ca^{2+} influx through TRPC1 channels is known to be neuroprotective in the PD models. Additionally, review of literature suggests that inhibition of Ca^{2+} influx from TRPC1 by the administration of neurotoxins causes aggravation of the PD pathology. It leads to inhibition of mTOR/Akt signaling as well as reduced levels of PKC α. These events reduce NF-κB expression which in turn increases the DNA damage and pro-apoptotic signaling to compromise neuronal survival. On the other hand, TRPC1 activation directly promotes anti-apoptotic signaling to reduce mitochondrial dysfunction and associated cell death in PD. In addition, diminished Ca^{2+} influx from the TRPC1 channels results in impaired autophagy and ER stress. Moreover, in association with STIM, TRPC1 channels inhibit the Ca^{2+} influx via L-type calcium channels which are one of the major contributors toward excitotoxicity mediated neuronal death in PD. MPTP, 1-methyl-4-phenyl-1,2,3,6-tetrahydropyridine; 6-OHDA, 6-hydroxy dopamine; TRPC1, Transient Receptor Potential Canonical 1; ER, endoplasmic reticulum; STIM, Stromal interaction molecule; UPR, unfolded protein response; mTOR, mammalian target of rapamycin; Akt, Protein kinase B; PKC, Protein kinase C; NF-κB, nuclear factor kappa-light-chain-enhancer of activated B cells; Cyt c, cytochrome c; Casp9, caspase 9; Bcl2, B-cell lymphoma 2; Bcl-xl, B-cell lymphoma-extra large; Bax, Bcl2-associated X protein; Bak, Bcl-2 homologous antagonist/killer.

Other pathways that were affected in PD due to reduced TRPC1 expression include attenuation of autophagy as well as impairment of nuclear factor kappa-light-chain-enhancer of activated B cells (NF-kB) and Tropomyosin receptor kinase A (TrkA) signaling (Yu et al., 2013; Sukumaran et al., 2018). In contrast to these findings, downregulation of STIM, a TRPC1 activator was shown to prevent oxidative stress and apoptosis mediated neuronal death in 6-OHDA treated PC-12 cells (Li et al., 2014; Sukumaran et al., 2017). However, despite this discrepancy, most of the other studies have suggested a beneficial role of TRPC1 channels in the pathophysiology of PD are shown in **Figure 3**.

Other TRPC channels such as TRPC3 are also expressed in the SNpc and striatal regions of the brain. These are important for the regulation of firing intensity and neuronal depolarization in these brain regions (Zhou et al., 2008; Xie and Zhou, 2014). Additionally, these channels are also required for synaptic transmission and motor coordination, making them an important target for investigation in the context of PD (Hartmann et al., 2008). Initial observation though suggested little to no change in the TRPC3 expression in PD, studies carried out much later have suggested otherwise (Selvaraj et al., 2009, 2012; Yu et al., 2013; Streifel et al., 2014). In the 6-OHDA model, data from RT-PCR studies showed reduced expression of TRPC3 in the SNpc (Yu et al., 2013). Similar results were reported by other groups which revealed that the inhibitory effects of neurotoxins, MPP^+ and 6-OHDA on TRPC3 was mediated through alteration in the purinergic calcium signaling (Lei et al., 2008; Streifel et al., 2014). However, drugs targeting TRPC3 have shown neuroprotective effects further challenging the role of molecular mechanisms related to TRPC3 in PD.

Besides the channels discussed in detail, most studies have invariably found no change in the expression of other TRPC channels including TRPC4/5/6 in different PD models as well as patients (Selvaraj et al., 2012; Lortet et al., 2013; Sukumaran et al., 2018). But, their ability to regulate the influx of calcium and other cations into the cell makes these channels an attractive candidate for studies in future.

TRPML Involvement in PD

TRPML channels are non-selective cation channels localized intracellularly on the endosomes and lysosomes. These are responsible for the intracellular calcium influx after activation by different cellular pathways (Grimm et al., 2012). Amongst the members of TRPML subfamily, mutations in TRPML1 have also been linked to the lysosomal storage disorder, mucolipidosis type IV (MLIV) which is also a form of neurodegeneration. It is known to produce motor and cognitive deficits, similar to those seen in PD patients (Dong et al., 2008). Moreover, the role of TRPML1 in the autophagy-related signaling has also been elucidated, making it an important channel for cell survival. Although there is no direct evidence as of now for its involvement, it has been hypothesized that TRPML1 activation could restore the impaired autophagy seen in PD patients (Anglade et al., 1997). Furthermore, mutations in GBA gene, which codes for lysosomal enzyme glucocerebrosidase is one of the potential risk factors for PD and has also been known to cause lysosomal dysfunction (DePaolo et al., 2009). Therefore, there are several studies currently underway to investigate the possible role of TRPML channels in PD (The Michael J. Fox Foundation for Parkinson's Research, 2019[1]; The Michael J. Fox Foundation for Parkinson's Research, 2020[2]). These studies are expected to provide deeper insights into the pathophysiology of PD and help in the identification of new molecules which could be useful for PD management.

[1]https://www.michaeljfox.org/grant/assessing-trpml1-agonists-gba-parkinsons-disease

[2]https://www.michaeljfox.org/grant/development-novel-trpml1-activator-parkinsons-disease

TRPA Involvement in PD

TRPA channel subfamily remains relatively unexplored in the context of PD. Though there is no study pertaining to its direct involvement, agents acting on these channels have provided important clues related to the development of side effects associated with current PD therapy. These have been discussed ahead in much more detail.

POTENTIAL PHARMACOLOGICAL INTERVENTIONS TARGETING TRP CHANNELS IN PD

A number of pharmacological agents have shown protective effects across different *in vitro* and *in vivo* studies. Detailed investigations pertaining to the beneficial effect of these agents has been discussed ahead and in **Table 2**.

TRPV1

A number of TRPV1 modulators have been studied by different groups in PD models. These include TRPV1 agonists (capsaicin and resiniferatoxin) as well as TRPV1 antagonists (capsazepine, AMG9810, oleoylethanolamide and iodo-resiniferatoxin). These agents exerted beneficial effects in the PD models. Capsaicin is an active phytochemical present in several *Capsicum* spp. which is highly selective toward TRPV1 channels (EC_{50} = 0.71 μM). It has been studied extensively for its disease-modifying effects

TABLE 2 | TRP channel modulators which accorded neuroprotection in the different PD models.

S No	TRP channel	Model	Pharmacological interventions	Major outcome	References
1	TRPM2	MPP^+	Flufenamic acid and *N*-(*p*-amylcinnamoyl) anthranilic acid	• Inhibition of ROS production and apoptosis • Increased neuronal cell viability by TRPM2 inhibition *in vitro*	Sun et al., 2018b
2	TRPM2	Rotenone	Flufenamic acid and 2-Aminoethoxydiphenyl borate	Inhibition of oxidative stress	Nazıroğlu et al., 2011
3	TRPV1	MPTP and 6-OHDA	Capsaicin	• Reduction in microglial activation, inflammation and oxidative stress • Improvement in neurobehavioral parameters and restoration of TH levels in the dopaminergic neurons	Chung et al., 2017; Zhao et al., 2017
4	TRPV1	Drosophila fly mutants expressing human α-synuclein	Capsaicin	• Reduction in oxidative stress and restoration of dopamine levels • Improvement in climbing ability	Siddique et al., 2012, 2018
5	TRPV1	6-OHDA	AMG9810	• Reduced neuronal death • Improved performance in the rotarod test	Razavinasab et al., 2013
6	TRPV1	6-OHDA	Capsazepine and Oleoylethanolamide	• Reduction in L-DOPA induced dyskinesias through crosstalk with endocannabinoid signaling	Morgese et al., 2007; González-Aparicio and Moratalla, 2014
7	TRPV1	AAV-A53T knock in mouse	Resiniferatoxin	• Improvement in motor function • No change in the dopamine levels	Sorrento Therapeutics Inc, 2020
8	TRPC1	MPP^+/MPTP	Carbachol and thapsigargin	• Accorded neuroprotection by increased AKT1 phosphorylation	Selvaraj et al., 2012
9	TRP3/6/7	MPP^+	SKF-96365	• Reduction of intracellular Ca^{2+} overload by reducing the overexpression of post synaptic scaffolding protein Homer1	Chen et al., 2013

in PD (Caterina et al., 1997; Musfiroh et al., 2013). It accorded neuroprotection in both the *in vitro* and *in vivo* rodent systems as well as in the drosophila model of PD. Capsaicin was further shown to improve rotarod performance and led to the restoration of dopaminergic signaling in the MPTP treated mice. Additionally, it also prevented glial cell activation and reduced oxidative stress in the astrocytes of MPTP induced PD mice. These effects were reversed after treatment with TRPV1 antagonists (capsazepine and iodo-resiniferatoxin) which confirmed that the beneficial effects were indeed attributed to the activation of TRPV1 channels (Chung et al., 2017). Similar observations were made in a study by Nam et al., which demonstrated that neuroprotective effects of capsaicin on TRPV1 were mediated through endogenous ciliary neurotrophic factor (CNTF) levels and CNTF-α receptors (Nam et al., 2015). It has been shown that the symptoms of PD first appear after 60–70% of the dopaminergic neuronal death has already taken place (Cheng et al., 2010). In a study, capsaicin was found to be capable of restoring the dopaminergic function even after the complete injury to the substantia nigra pars compacta (SNpc) and striatum (Kim et al., 2019). These results suggest the possibility for capsaicin to be effective in the later stages of PD when traditional medications fail to work. Besides, capsaicin also exerted a positive modulatory effect against oxidative insults and reversed the behavioral deficits induced by MPTP and 6-OHDA in the rodent models (Fong et al., 2016; Zhao et al., 2017). Capsaicin treated animals showed an increase in distance traveled in the open field and a significant reduction in the amphetamine-induced rotations after induction of PD. It was accompanied by a significant reduction in the malondialdehyde (MDA) levels and restoration of the superoxide dismutase (SOD) and catalase activity in the SNpc (Nam et al., 2015; Zhao et al., 2017).

The neuroprotective effects of capsaicin were further replicated in the drosophila fly mutants, which expressed a gene for human α-synuclein. These PD flies displayed a progressive form of neurodegeneration characterized by loss of dopamine function, oxidative stress and impaired performance in the climbing assay. Reversal of the pathological changes occurred in a dose-dependent manner which confirmed the therapeutic potential of capsaicin through TRPV1 activation for PD treatment (Siddique et al., 2012, 2018).

In contrast to these studies, other groups have shown that blockade of TRPV1 channels is also helpful in relieving some of the PD symptoms. A study involving the use of AMG9810, a selective TRPV1 blocker demonstrated a positive attenuation of the motor deficits after 6-OHDA administration which was evident from the rotarod test. Additionally, cresyl violet staining also showed that there was reduced neuronal death in the SNpc of the AMG9810 treated animals (Razavinasab et al., 2013). In line with the same, another TRPV1 blocker, capsazepine also exhibited neuroprotective effects in a number of PD models. Moreover, it was also found to reduce the occurrence of levodopa (L-DOPA) induced dyskinesia which is a prominent side effect seen with L-DOPA therapy in PD (Morgese et al., 2007). The most probable explanation for these effects came from a study where it was observed that TRPV1 blockade positively regulates the crosstalk between endocannabinoid receptors and TRPV1 downstream signaling which helps prevent L-DOPA induced dyskinesias (Lee et al., 2006; Giuffrida and Morgese, 2007; Morgese et al., 2007; Dos-Santos-Pereira et al., 2016). It is also supported by the findings in which oleoylethanolamide, another TRPV1 blocker showed protection in the 6-OHDA induced hemiparkinsonian model (González-Aparicio and Moratalla, 2014). Furthermore, blockade of TRPV1 has also been elucidated to play a crucial role in the modulation of pain pathways in PD (Li et al., 2020). TRPV1 expression was upregulated in the trigeminal subnucleus caudalis (Vc) which plays a role in central terminal sensitization of primary nociceptive neurons. In addition, its co-expression with 5-HT3A receptors in the rat dorsal root ganglion (DRG) and ability of TRPV1 blockers to inhibit the pain induced by 5-HT3A receptor agonists makes it a useful target for pain modulation in PD (Zeitz et al., 2002; Li et al., 2020).

Despite these promising results, the therapeutic window for the beneficial effects of TRPV1 modulators is very narrow and higher doses of TRPV1 blockers such as AMG9810 have been associated with learning and memory impairments in the preclinical studies (Razavinasab et al., 2013). Moreover, its interaction with endocannabinoids raised concern over the possible addictive potential and development of tolerance for these agents. However, when investigated, no such association was observed in studies involving TRPV1 blockers which makes them a viable option for studies in future (González-Aparicio and Moratalla, 2014).

In totality, these shreds of evidence suggested that targeting TRPV1 channels could be of therapeutic relevance for combating the motor and non-motor symptoms of PD. Therefore, to provide more proof to the speculation, Capsaicin is being investigated in patients for the elucidation of mechanisms related to swallowing and cough dysfunction in PD[3]. Another TRPV1 agonist, resiniferatoxin was shown to be effective in controlling the motor symptoms in the AAV-A53T knock-in PD mouse model (Sorrento Therapeutics Inc, 2020). According to the recent reports, it is soon expected to enter clinical trials which could open up new avenues of research for the management of PD.

Together, these studies capture a basic insight into the pharmacological modulation of TRPV channels which could be targeted in future for the treatment of PD. But, as the doubts over the clear molecular mechanisms, clinical efficacy and specificity persist, more detailed investigations are still necessary for the development of TRPV channel modulators as drug candidates in future.

TRPM2

Studies conducted in preclinical models as well as PD patients, showed an increase in TRPM2 expression, suggesting its possible involvement in PD (Sun et al., 2018b; An et al., 2019). It was also demonstrated that MPP^+ exposure leads to increased levels of TRPM2 accompanied by elevated oxidative stress and increased apoptosis in the SH-SY5Y neurons. It further resulted in reduced cell viability and caspase 3 activation in these neuronal cells (An et al., 2019; Ding et al., 2019). These effects were reversed by treatment with TRPM2 blockers, flufenamic acid (FFA) and *N*-(*p*-amylcinnamoyl) anthranilic acid (ACA). Moreover, similar results were obtained when knockdown of

[3]https://clinicaltrials.gov/ct2/show/NCT03321019

TRPM2 was carried out using a siRNA which resulted in reduced neuronal death and inhibition of apoptosis in the SH-SY5Y cells (Sun et al., 2018b). The detailed mechanism of this neuroprotection was delineated later in another study which attributed it to the working network of long non-coding RNA, p21 and microRNA, miR-625 present inside the neurons. It was also reported that long non-coding RNA, p21 is a positive modulator of TRPM2 expression and its knockdown could rescue from the toxicity induced by MPP^+ treatment (Ding et al., 2019).

Other authors have also confirmed the involvement of TRPM2 in PD with the help of different toxin-based models *in vitro* and *in vivo*. In a study by Yu et al. (2014) it was shown that TRPM2 expression was significantly increased in the SNpc of 6-OHDA treated rats. This increased expression was attenuated by treatment with nerve growth factor, which accorded neuroprotection through phosphatidylinositol 3-kinase (PI3K) signaling pathway (Yu et al., 2014). Furthermore, it was demonstrated that TRPM2 mediated increased ROS production and caspase 3 activity was suppressed by increased expression of transcription factor GATA3 binding protein (GATA3) (Zhou and Han, 2017). This suggests the involvement of multiple downstream pathways affected by TRPM2 associated neuronal death in PD. In line with these shreds of evidence, rotenone also led to increased TRPM2 activation by ROS dependent mechanisms (Freestone, 2009). These effects were reversed after treatment with TRPM2 blockers FFA and 2-aminoethoxydiphenyl borate (2-APB), which confirmed the potential of TRPM2 blockade in the treatment of PD (Nazıroğlu et al., 2011). Furthermore, electrophysiological findings have revealed that increased spontaneous firing of the substantia nigra pars reticulata (SNr) GABAergic neurons seen in PD is modulated by increased activation of the TRPM2 channels (Lee et al., 2013). Conclusively, the close association of TRPM2 and intracellular ionic homeostasis has been established and any change in it makes the individual more susceptible toward PD (Hermosura and Garruto, 2007). Though there is ample evidence available for its involvement, there is no report which has investigated the effect of pharmacological interventions targeting TRPM2 *in vivo*. This has largely hindered the development of more potent analogs which could be tried for their translational potential of TRPM2 in PD. Further, the neuroprotective potential of TRPM2 antagonists in neurodegenerative disorders like AD strengthens the claim of TRPM2 antagonists as neuroprotective agents (Thapak et al., 2020b).

TRPC1

Silencing of TRPC1 as well as its functional blockade was also associated with mitochondrial dysfunction and decrease in the TH levels after sub-chronic administration of MPTP to the C57BL/6 mice. These pathological changes were reversed after treatment with TRPC1 activators carbachol and thapsigargin or after TRPC1 overexpression which led to an increase in anti-apoptotic signaling (Selvaraj et al., 2009). Similar results were observed in other studies involving transgenic or toxin model-based systems (Bollimuntha et al., 2005; Sukumaran et al., 2018).

TRPC3/6/7

Studies have either reported reduced or no change in the expression of TRPC3/6/7 channels in PD (Selvaraj et al., 2009, 2012; Yu et al., 2013; Streifel et al., 2014). However, the neuroprotective effects of SKF-96365, a non-selective TRPC3/6/7 blocker in the MPP^+ model suggests a need to validate these findings (Chen et al., 2013). Therefore, challenging the reproducibility of these observations in other model systems could help resolve these concerns in the near future.

TRPA1

Expression of TRPA channels has not been directly correlated to the pathophysiology of PD. However, it was observed that apomorphine which is an approved medication for PD is a bimodal modulator of TRPA1 channels, the only known member of the TRPA subfamily (Schulze et al., 2013). Apomorphine is often used as an add-on therapy for the management of "off" episodes in PD but exhibits adverse effects like nausea and local reactions at the injection site (Carbone et al., 2019). Schulze et al. (2013) demonstrated with the help of cultured dorsal route ganglion (DRG) neurons and in the enterochromaffin model cell line QGP-1, that these adverse effects might be attributed to the activation of TRPA1 channels by apomorphine. Therefore, strategies targeting TRPA1 channels could be useful for the management of side-effects associated with apomorphine and other currently available medications for PD.

CHALLENGES IN THE DEVELOPMENT OF TRP CHANNEL MODULATORS AS DRUG CANDIDATES

TRP channels are involved in the regulation of a number of physiological processes in different organs of the body. Though alteration of their functions in some of the brain areas may be involved in the pathophysiology of PD, targeting these alterations in a selective and specific manner poses a greater challenge. This was evident during the studies of TRPV1 modulators in other conditions like pain where a number of clinical trials were terminated because of the off-target effects (Krarup et al., 2011; Rowbotham et al., 2011). Encouraging results obtained in rodent studies with these agents couldn't be replicated in patients due to a number of side effects like a diminished response to damaging heat, alteration in body temperature and reduced perception of taste were observed (Gavva et al., 2008). Therefore, management of safety and toxicity still remain the biggest hurdle for the translational success of TRP channel modulators. Another largely neglected area of research is the organellar distribution of TRP channels where they are coupled together to perform a plethora of unknown functions (Zhang et al., 2018). Besides, a report has also highlighted that the neuroprotection accorded by these agents is sex-specific which adds further complexity to the clinical development of these agents (Jia et al., 2011). Additionally, a number of agonists and antagonists of the same TRPs like TRPV1 and TRPM8 are together being investigated in the clinical trials which tell us that there is a lot more to the story than what we understand at present (Moran et al., 2011;

De Caro et al., 2019; Garami et al., 2020). This further raises the possibility of these modulators to be working through other unknown mechanisms that have not been investigated till date. To develop the understanding, several transgenic mice (TRP knock in and knock out) were made, but high embryonic or postnatal lethality has largely limited their use. This has further pushed back the progress of this field and necessitated the use of alternative approaches (Park et al., 2011; Woudenberg-Vrenken et al., 2011). Another pitfall in TRP research is the lack of selective agents as activators or inhibitors for any of the ion channel. As the structure and function of TRP channels are conserved across species, preclinical and animal data using selective agents could be highly useful for the further development of these agents (Hof et al., 2019). Therefore, increased knowledge of the TRP structure is also required and needs to be studied with the help of new approaches.

Despite these limitations, there are a number of clinically approved agents like probenecid and tranilast (TRPV2), glibenclamide (TRPM4), flufenamic acid and clotrimazole (TRPM2) and menthol (TRPM8) which have also been reported to modulate TRP channel activity. There are proof of concept studies which have found them to be effective in different CNS disorders (Thapak et al., 2020a; Zubov et al., 2020). Hence, it is possible that TRP channels may be indistinctly important for brain functions, and these molecules may pave the way for a completely new class of drugs for brain-related disorders including PD.

CONCLUSION

TRP channels perform a plethora of physiological functions in the CNS. The increased understanding of their role has led several researchers to investigate their likely contribution in the pathophysiology of neurodegenerative disorders, including PD. Moreover, their regulatory function in ionic homeostasis has made TRP channels an attractive pharmacological target where Ca^{2+} dyshomeostasis, oxidative stress and excitotoxicity mediated neuronal death are reported. The current review has presented a brief overview of the reports which have studied the pathophysiological involvement of TRP channels in PD. Additionally, beneficial effects of many of the pharmacological agents targeting TRP channels have also been highlighted, which suggests the possibility of a novel class of therapeutics for PD treatment in future. Amongst the agents known so far, ones targeting TRPV1, TRPM2 and TRPC1 have been most promising for PD treatment. Design of novel and selective analogs targeting these TRPs is expected to open up new avenues of research in future. Though these findings pertaining to the involvement of TRP channels in PD are encouraging, more studies highlighting the molecular mechanisms at length are required to ensure the translational success of these compounds in the clinical trials.

AUTHOR CONTRIBUTIONS

BV and SSS conceived the idea of the manuscript. BV wrote all the sections. SSS corrected the manuscript. Both authors approved the final proof for submission.

ACKNOWLEDGMENTS

We would like to acknowledge fellowship support provided by The Council of Scientific and Industrial Research to BV.

REFERENCES

Adhya, P., and Sharma, S. S. (2019). Redox TRPs in diabetes and diabetic complications: Mechanisms and pharmacological modulation. *Pharmacol. Res.* 146:104271. doi: 10.1016/j.phrs.2019.104271

Akyuva, Y., and Naziroglu, M. (2020). Resveratrol attenuates hypoxia-induced neuronal cell death, inflammation and mitochondrial oxidative stress by modulation of TRPM2 channel. *Sci. Rep.* 10:6449. doi: 10.1038/s41598-020-63577-5

An, X., Fu, Z., Mai, C., Wang, W., Wei, L., Li, D., et al. (2019). Increasing the TRPM2 Channel Expression in Human Neuroblastoma SH-SY5Y Cells Augments the Susceptibility to ROS-Induced Cell Death. *Cells* 8:28. doi: 10.3390/cells8010028

Anglade, P., Vyas, S., Javoy-Agid, F., Herrero, M. T., Michel, P. P., Marquez, J., et al. (1997). Apoptosis and autophagy in nigral neurons of patients with Parkinson's disease. *Histol Histopathol* 12, 25–31.

Bashiri, H., Hosseini-Chegeni, H., Alsadat Sharifi, K., Sahebgharani, M., and Salari, A. A. (2018). Activation of TRPV1 receptors affects memory function and hippocampal TRPV1 and CREB mRNA expression in a rat model of biliary cirrhosis. *Neurol. Res.* 40, 938–947. doi: 10.1080/01616412.2018.1504158

Beiske, A. G., Loge, J. H., Rønningen, A., and Svensson, E. (2009). Pain in Parkinson's disease: Prevalence and characteristics. *Pain* 141, 173–177. doi: 10.1016/j.pain.2008.12.004

Belrose, J. C., and Jackson, M. F. (2018). TRPM2: a candidate therapeutic target for treating neurological diseases. *Acta Pharmacol. Sin.* 39, 722–732. doi: 10.1038/aps.2018.31

Bodkin, J. V., Thakore, P., Aubdool, A. A., Liang, L., Fernandes, E. S., Nandi, M., et al. (2014). Investigating the potential role of TRPA1 in locomotion and cardiovascular control during hypertension. *Pharmacol. Res. Perspect.* 2:e00052. doi: 10.1002/prp2.52

Bollimuntha, S., Singh, B. B., Shavali, S., Sharma, S. K., and Ebadi, M. (2005). TRPC1-mediated inhibition of 1-methyl-4-phenylpyridinium ion neurotoxicity in human SH-SY5Y neuroblastoma cells. *J. Biol. Chem.* 280, 2132–2140. doi: 10.1074/jbc.M407384200

Carbone, F., Djamshidian, A., Seppi, K., and Poewe, W. (2019). Apomorphine for Parkinson's Disease: Efficacy and Safety of Current and New Formulations. *CNS Drugs* 33, 905–918. doi: 10.1007/s40263-019-00661-z

Caterina, M. J., Schumacher, M. A., Tominaga, M., Rosen, T. A., Levine, J. D., and Julius, D. (1997). The capsaicin receptor: a heat-activated ion channel in the pain pathway. *Nature* 389, 816–824. doi: 10.1038/39807

Chen, B., Ng, G., Gao, Y., Low, S. W., Sandanaraj, E., Ramasamy, B., et al. (2019). Non-Invasive Multimodality Imaging Directly Shows TRPM4 Inhibition Ameliorates Stroke Reperfusion Injury. *Transl. Stroke Res.* 10, 91–103. doi: 10.1007/s12975-018-0621-3

Chen, T., Zhu, J., Zhang, C., Huo, K., Fei, Z., and Jiang, X. F. (2013). Protective effects of SKF-96365, a non-specific inhibitor of SOCE, against MPP+-induced cytotoxicity in PC12 cells: potential role of Homer1. *PLoS One* 8:e55601. doi: 10.1371/journal.pone.0055601

Cheng, H. C., Ulane, C. M., and Burke, R. E. (2010). Clinical progression in Parkinson disease and the neurobiology of axons. *Ann. Neurol.* 67, 715–725. doi: 10.1002/ana.21995

Chung, Y. C., Baek, J. Y., Kim, S. R., Ko, H. W., Bok, E., Shin, W. H., et al. (2017). Capsaicin prevents degeneration of dopamine neurons by inhibiting glial activation and oxidative stress in the MPTP model of Parkinson's disease. *Exp. Mol. Med.* 49:e298. doi: 10.1038/emm.2016.159

Chung, Y. H., Kim, D., Moon, N. J., Oh, C. S., Lee, E., Shin, D. H., et al. (2007). Immunohistochemical study on the distribution of canonical transient receptor potential channels in rat basal ganglia. *Neurosci. Lett.* 422, 18–23. doi: 10.1016/j.neulet.2007.05.042

Cosens, D. J., and Manning, A. (1969). Abnormal electroretinogram from a Drosophila mutant. *Nature* 224, 285–287. doi: 10.1038/224285a0

Das, N. R., and Sharma, S. S. (2015). Peroxisome Proliferator Activated Receptor Gamma Coactivator 1 Alpha: An Emerging Target for Neuroprotection in Parkinson's Disease. *CNS Neurol. Disord. Drug Targets* 14, 1024–1030. doi: 10.2174/1871527314666150326000018

De Caro, C., Cristiano, C., Avagliano, C., Bertamino, A., Ostacolo, C., Campiglia, P., et al. (2019). Characterization of New TRPM8 Modulators in Pain Perception. *Int. J. Mol. Sci.* 20:5544. doi: 10.3390/ijms20225544

Deng, J., and Bai, J. (2012). The role of TRPC1 and Ca~(2+) in the endoplasmic reticulum stress of Parkinson's disease. *Chin. Bull. Life Sci.* 2012:15.

Denis, V., and Cyert, M. S. (2002). Internal Ca(2+) release in yeast is triggered by hypertonic shock and mediated by a TRP channel homologue. *J. Cell Biol.* 156, 29–34. doi: 10.1083/jcb.200111004

DePaolo, J., Goker-Alpan, O., Samaddar, T., Lopez, G., and Sidransky, E. (2009). The association between mutations in the lysosomal protein glucocerebrosidase and parkinsonism. *Mov. Disord.* 24, 1571–1578. doi: 10.1002/mds.22538

Ding, X. M., Zhao, L. J., Qiao, H. Y., Wu, S. L., and Wang, X. H. (2019). Long non-coding RNA-p21 regulates MPP(+)-induced neuronal injury by targeting miR-625 and derepressing TRPM2 in SH-SY5Y cells. *Chem. Biol. Interact* 307, 73–81. doi: 10.1016/j.cbi.2019.04.017

Dong, X. P., Cheng, X., Mills, E., Delling, M., Wang, F., Kurz, T., et al. (2008). The type IV mucolipidosis-associated protein TRPML1 is an endolysosomal iron release channel. *Nature* 455, 992–996. doi: 10.1038/nature07311

Dos-Santos-Pereira, M., Da-Silva, C. A., Guimarães, F. S., and Del-Bel, E. (2016). Co-administration of cannabidiol and capsazepine reduces L-DOPA-induced dyskinesia in mice: Possible mechanism of action. *Neurobiol. Dis.* 94, 179–195. doi: 10.1016/j.nbd.2016.06.013

Fonfria, E., Marshall, I. C., Boyfield, I., Skaper, S. D., Hughes, J. P., Owen, D. E., et al. (2005). Amyloid beta-peptide(1-42) and hydrogen peroxide-induced toxicity are mediated by TRPM2 in rat primary striatal cultures. *J. Neurochem.* 95, 715–723. doi: 10.1111/j.1471-4159.2005.03396.x

Fonfria, E., Murdock, P. R., Cusdin, F. S., Benham, C. D., Kelsell, R. E., and Mcnulty, S. (2006). Tissue distribution profiles of the human TRPM cation channel family. *J. Recept. Signal. Transduct. Res.* 26, 159–178. doi: 10.1080/10799890600637506

Fong, G. M., Johnstone, D., Antao, S., Stone, J., and Witting, P. (2016). Mechanism of Neuroprotection by Capsaicin in a Model of Parkinson's Disease. *Free Radical. Bio. Med.* 100:S54. doi: 10.1016/j.freeradbiomed.2016.10.141

Freestone, P. S. (2009). *Effects of rotenone and 6-OHDA on dopaminergic neurons of the Substantia nigra studied in vitro*, Doctor of Philosophy. Auckland: University of Auckland.

Garami, A., Shimansky, Y. P., Rumbus, Z., Vizin, R. C. L., Farkas, N., Hegyi, J., et al. (2020). Hyperthermia induced by transient receptor potential vanilloid-1 (TRPV1) antagonists in human clinical trials: Insights from mathematical modeling and meta-analysis. *Pharmacol. Ther.* 208:107474. doi: 10.1016/j.pharmthera.2020.107474

Gavva, N. R. (2009). Setbacks in the clinical development of TRPV1 antagonists: what next? *Open Drug Discover. J.* 1, 1–35. doi: 10.2174/1877381800901010001

Gavva, N. R., Treanor, J. J., Garami, A., Fang, L., Surapaneni, S., Akrami, A., et al. (2008). Pharmacological blockade of the vanilloid receptor TRPV1 elicits marked hyperthermia in humans. *Pain* 136, 202–210. doi: 10.1016/j.pain.2008.01.024

Giuffrida, A., and Morgese, M. G. (2007). Direct and indirect cannabinoid agonists reduce L-dopa-induced-dyskinesias via CB1-and TRPV1-mediated mechanisms. *Feder. Am. Soc. Exp. Biol.* 21, A787–A787.

González-Aparicio, R., and Moratalla, R. (2014). Oleoylethanolamide reduces L-DOPA-induced dyskinesia via TRPV1 receptor in a mouse model of Parkinson's disease. *Neurobiol. Dis.* 62, 416–425. doi: 10.1016/j.nbd.2013.10.008

Grimm, C., Hassan, S., Wahl-Schott, C., and Biel, M. (2012). Role of TRPML and two-pore channels in endolysosomal cation homeostasis. *J. Pharmacol. Exp. Ther.* 342, 236–244. doi: 10.1124/jpet.112.192880

Guatteo, E., Chung, K. K., Bowala, T. K., Bernardi, G., Mercuri, N. B., and Lipski, J. (2005). Temperature sensitivity of dopaminergic neurons of the substantia nigra pars compacta: involvement of transient receptor potential channels. *J. Neurophysiol.* 94, 3069–3080. doi: 10.1152/jn.00066.2005

Hardie, R. C. (2007). TRP channels and lipids: from Drosophila to mammalian physiology. *J. Physiol.* 578, 9–24. doi: 10.1113/jphysiol.2006.118372

Hartmann, J., Dragicevic, E., Adelsberger, H., Henning, H. A., Sumser, M., Abramowitz, J., et al. (2008). TRPC3 channels are required for synaptic transmission and motor coordination. *Neuron* 59, 392–398. doi: 10.1016/j.neuron.2008.06.009

He, K., Qi, F., Guo, C., Zhan, S., Xu, H., Liu, J., et al. (2016). Movement deficits and neuronal loss in basal ganglia in TRPC1 deficient mice. *Oncotarget* 7, 69337–69346. doi: 10.18632/oncotarget.12567

Hermosura, M. C., and Garruto, R. M. (2007). TRPM7 and TRPM2-Candidate susceptibility genes for Western Pacific ALS and PD? *Biochim. Biophys. Acta* 1772, 822–835. doi: 10.1016/j.bbadis.2007.02.008

Hermosura, M. C., Nayakanti, H., Dorovkov, M. V., Calderon, F. R., Ryazanov, A. G., Haymer, D. S., et al. (2005). A TRPM7 variant shows altered sensitivity to magnesium that may contribute to the pathogenesis of two Guamanian neurodegenerative disorders. *Proc. Natl. Acad. Sci. U S A.* 102, 11510–11515. doi: 10.1073/pnas.0505149102

Hof, T., Chaigne, S., Récalde, A., Sallé, L., Brette, F., and Guinamard, R. (2019). Transient receptor potential channels in cardiac health and disease. *Nat. Rev. Cardiol.* 16, 344–360. doi: 10.1038/s41569-018-0145-2

Jia, J., Verma, S., Nakayama, S., Quillinan, N., Grafe, M. R., Hurn, P. D., et al. (2011). Sex differences in neuroprotection provided by inhibition of TRPM2 channels following experimental stroke. *J. Cereb. Blood Flow Metab.* 31, 2160–2168. doi: 10.1038/jcbfm.2011.77

Kaneko, Y., and Szallasi, A. (2014). Transient receptor potential (TRP) channels: a clinical perspective. *Br. J. Pharmacol.* 171, 2474–2507. doi: 10.1111/bph.12414

Kim, K. I., Baek, J. Y., Jeong, J. Y., Nam, J. H., Park, E. S., Bok, E., et al. (2019). Delayed Treatment of Capsaicin Produces Partial Motor Recovery by Enhancing Dopamine Function in MPP(+)-lesioned Rats via Ciliary Neurotrophic Factor. *Exp. Neurobiol.* 28, 289–299. doi: 10.5607/en.2019.28.2.289

Krarup, A. L., Ny, L., Astrand, M., Bajor, A., Hvid-Jensen, F., Hansen, M. B., et al. (2011). Randomised clinical trial: the efficacy of a transient receptor potential vanilloid 1 antagonist AZD1386 in human oesophageal pain. *Aliment Pharmacol. Ther.* 33, 1113–1122. doi: 10.1111/j.1365-2036.2011.04629.x

Kumar, P., Kaundal, R. K., More, S., and Sharma, S. S. (2009). Beneficial effects of pioglitazone on cognitive impairment in MPTP model of Parkinson's disease. *Behav. Brain Res.* 197, 398–403. doi: 10.1016/j.bbr.2008.10.010

Kumar, S., Singh, U., Goswami, C., and Singru, P. S. (2017). Transient receptor potential vanilloid 5 (TRPV5), a highly Ca(2+)-selective TRP channel in the rat brain: relevance to neuroendocrine regulation. *J. Neuroendocrinol.* 29:28235149. doi: 10.1111/jne.12466

Kunert-Keil, C., Bisping, F., Krüger, J., and Brinkmeier, H. (2006). Tissue-specific expression of TRP channel genes in the mouse and its variation in three different mouse strains. *BMC Genomics* 7:159. doi: 10.1186/1471-2164-7-159

Lee, C. R., Machold, R. P., Witkovsky, P., and Rice, M. E. (2013). TRPM2 channels are required for NMDA-induced burst firing and contribute to H(2)O(2)-dependent modulation in substantia nigra pars reticulata GABAergic neurons. *J. Neurosci.* 33, 1157–1168. doi: 10.1523/jneurosci.2832-12.2013

Lee, J., Di Marzo, V., and Brotchie, J. M. (2006). A role for vanilloid receptor 1 (TRPV1) and endocannabinnoid signalling in the regulation of spontaneous and L-DOPA induced locomotion in normal and reserpine-treated rats. *Neuropharmacology* 51, 557–565. doi: 10.1016/j.neuropharm.2006.04.016

Lee, N., Chen, J., Sun, L., Wu, S., Gray, K. R., Rich, A., et al. (2003). Expression and characterization of human transient receptor potential melastatin 3 (hTRPM3). *J. Biol. Chem.* 278, 20890–20897. doi: 10.1074/jbc.M211232200

Lehen'kyi, V., Raphaël, M., and Prevarskaya, N. (2012). The role of the TRPV6 channel in cancer. *J. Physiol.* 590, 1369–1376. doi: 10.1113/jphysiol.2011.225862

Lei, Z., Junfeng, W., Ruiliang, G., and Xiaomin, W. (2008). TRPC3-mediated Inhibition of MPP~+ Neurotoxicity in MN9D Cells. *J. Cap. Med. Univ.* 2008:15.

Li, B., Xiao, L., Wang, Z. Y., and Zheng, P. S. (2014). Knockdown of STIM1 inhibits 6-hydroxydopamine-induced oxidative stress through attenuating calcium-dependent ER stress and mitochondrial dysfunction in undifferentiated PC12 cells. *Free Radic. Res.* 48, 758–768. doi: 10.3109/10715762.2014.905687

Li, H. (2017). TRP Channel Classification. *Adv. Exp. Med. Biol.* 976, 1–8. doi: 10.1007/978-94-024-1088-4_1

Li, J., Sun, Y., and Chen, J. (2019). Transcriptome sequencing in a 6-hydroxydopamine rat model of Parkinson's disease. *Genes Genet. Syst.* 94, 61–69. doi: 10.1266/ggs.18-00036

Li, M., Zhu, M., Xu, Q., Ding, F., Tian, Y., and Zhang, M. (2020). Sensation of TRPV1 via 5-hydroxytryptamine signaling modulates pain hypersensitivity in a 6-hydroxydopamine induced mice model of Parkinson's disease. *Biochem. Biophys. Res. Commun.* 521, 868–873. doi: 10.1016/j.bbrc.2019.10.204

Lortet, S., Lacombe, E., Boulanger, N., Rihet, P., Nguyen, C., Kerkerian-Le Goff, L., et al. (2013). Striatal molecular signature of subchronic subthalamic nucleus high frequency stimulation in parkinsonian rat. *PLoS One* 8:e60447. doi: 10.1371/journal.pone.0060447

Martorana, A., Giampà, C., Demarch, Z., Viscomi, M. T., Patassini, S., Sancesario, G., et al. (2006). Distribution of TRPC1 receptors in dendrites of rat substantia nigra: a confocal and electron microscopy study. *Eur. J. Neurosci.* 24, 732–738. doi: 10.1111/j.1460-9568.2006.04932.x

Moran, M. M., Mcalexander, M. A., Bíró, T., and Szallasi, A. (2011). Transient receptor potential channels as therapeutic targets. *Nat. Rev. Drug. Discov.* 10, 601–620. doi: 10.1038/nrd3456

Morgese, M. G., Cassano, T., Cuomo, V., and Giuffrida, A. (2007). Anti-dyskinetic effects of cannabinoids in a rat model of Parkinson's disease: role of CB(1) and TRPV1 receptors. *Exp. Neurol.* 208, 110–119. doi: 10.1016/j.expneurol.2007.07.021

Mrejeru, A., Wei, A., and Ramirez, J. M. (2011). Calcium-activated non-selective cation currents are involved in generation of tonic and bursting activity in dopamine neurons of the substantia nigra pars compacta. *J. Physiol.* 589, 2497–2514. doi: 10.1113/jphysiol.2011.206631

Musella, A., De Chiara, V., Rossi, S., Prosperetti, C., Bernardi, G., Maccarrone, M., et al. (2009). TRPV1 channels facilitate glutamate transmission in the striatum. *Mol. Cell Neurosci.* 40, 89–97. doi: 10.1016/j.mcn.2008.09.001

Musfiroh, I., Mutakin, M., Angelina, T., and Muchtaridi, M. (2013). Capsaicin level of various capsicum fruits. *Int. J. Pharm. Pharm. Sci.* 5, 248–251.

Nam, J. H., Park, E. S., Won, S. Y., Lee, Y. A., Kim, K. I., Jeong, J. Y., et al. (2015). TRPV1 on astrocytes rescues nigral dopamine neurons in Parkinson's disease via CNTF. *Brain* 138, 3610–3622. doi: 10.1093/brain/awv297

Nazıroğlu, M., Özgül, C., Çelik, Ö, Çiğ, B., and Sözbir, E. (2011). Aminoethoxydiphenyl borate and flufenamic acid inhibit Ca2+ influx through TRPM2 channels in rat dorsal root ganglion neurons activated by ADP-ribose and rotenone. *J. Membr. Biol.* 241, 69–75. doi: 10.1007/s00232-011-9363-9

Ordás, P., Hernández-Ortego, P., Vara, H., Fernández-Peña, C., Reimúndez, A., Morenilla-Palao, C., et al. (2019). Expression of the cold thermoreceptor TRPM8 in rodent brain thermoregulatory circuits. *J. Comp. Neurol.* 2019:30942489. doi: 10.1002/cne.24694

Ostapchenko, V. G., Chen, M., Guzman, M. S., Xie, Y. F., Lavine, N., Fan, J., et al. (2015). The Transient Receptor Potential Melastatin 2 (TRPM2) Channel Contributes to β-Amyloid Oligomer-Related Neurotoxicity and Memory Impairment. *J. Neurosci.* 35, 15157–15169. doi: 10.1523/jneurosci.4081-14.2015

Park, U., Vastani, N., Guan, Y., Raja, S. N., Koltzenburg, M., and Caterina, M. J. (2011). TRP vanilloid 2 knock-out mice are susceptible to perinatal lethality but display normal thermal and mechanical nociception. *J. Neurosci.* 31, 11425–11436. doi: 10.1523/jneurosci.1384-09.2011

Parkinson's News Today. (2020). *Parkinsons disease statistics.* Available online at: https://parkinsonsnewstoday.com/parkinsons-disease-statistics/ (accessed on July 13, 2020).

Razavinasab, M., Shamsizadeh, A., Shabani, M., Nazeri, M., Allahtavakoli, M., Asadi-Shekaari, M., et al. (2013). Pharmacological blockade of TRPV1 receptors modulates the effects of 6-OHDA on motor and cognitive functions in a rat model of Parkinson's disease. *Fundam Clin. Pharmacol.* 27, 632–640. doi: 10.1111/fcp.12015

Roberts, J. C., Davis, J. B., and Benham, C. D. (2004). [3H]Resiniferatoxin autoradiography in the CNS of wild-type and TRPV1 null mice defines TRPV1 (VR-1) protein distribution. *Brain Res.* 995, 176–183. doi: 10.1016/j.brainres.2003.10.001

Rowbotham, M. C., Nothaft, W., Duan, W. R., Wang, Y., Faltynek, C., Mcgaraughty, S., et al. (2011). Oral and cutaneous thermosensory profile of selective TRPV1 inhibition by ABT-102 in a randomized healthy volunteer trial. *Pain* 152, 1192–1200. doi: 10.1016/j.pain.2011.01.051

Samanta, A., Hughes, T. E. T., and Moiseenkova-Bell, V. Y. (2018). Transient Receptor Potential (TRP) Channels. *Subcell Biochem.* 87, 141–165. doi: 10.1007/978-981-10-7757-9_6

Schulze, A., Oehler, B., Urban, N., Schaefer, M., and Hill, K. (2013). Apomorphine is a bimodal modulator of TRPA1 channels. *Mol. Pharmacol.* 83, 542–551. doi: 10.1124/mol.112.081976

Selvaraj, S., Sun, Y., Watt, J. A., Wang, S., Lei, S., Birnbaumer, L., et al. (2012). Neurotoxin-induced ER stress in mouse dopaminergic neurons involves downregulation of TRPC1 and inhibition of AKT/mTOR signaling. *J. Clin. Invest.* 122, 1354–1367. doi: 10.1172/jci61332

Selvaraj, S., Watt, J. A., and Singh, B. B. (2009). TRPC1 inhibits apoptotic cell degeneration induced by dopaminergic neurotoxin MPTP/MPP(+). *Cell Calcium.* 46, 209–218. doi: 10.1016/j.ceca.2009.07.008

Shibasaki, K., Ishizaki, Y., and Mandadi, S. (2013). Astrocytes express functional TRPV2 ion channels. *Biochem. Biophys. Res. Commun.* 441, 327–332. doi: 10.1016/j.bbrc.2013.10.046

Shindo, Y., Yamanaka, R., Suzuki, K., Hotta, K., and Oka, K. (2015). Intracellular magnesium level determines cell viability in the MPP(+) model of Parkinson's disease. *Biochim. Biophys. Acta* 1853, 3182–3191. doi: 10.1016/j.bbamcr.2015.08.013

Siddique, Y. H., Naz, F., and Jyoti, S. (2018). Effect of capsaicin on the oxidative stress and dopamine content in the transgenic Drosophila model of Parkinson's disease. *Acta Biol. Hung* 69, 115–124. doi: 10.1556/018.69.2018.2.1

Siddique, Y., Ara, G., Jyoti, S., and Afzal, M. (2012). Effect of capsaicin on the climbing ability in Drosophila model of Parkinson's disease. *Am. J. Drug Discov. Dev.* 2, 50–54. doi: 10.3923/ajdd.2012.50.54

Simuni, T., Borushko, E., Avram, M. J., Miskevics, S., Martel, A., Zadikoff, C., et al. (2010). Tolerability of isradipine in early Parkinson's disease: a pilot dose escalation study. *Mov. Disord.* 25, 2863–2866. doi: 10.1002/mds.23308

Skogar, O., and Lokk, J. (2016). Pain management in patients with Parkinson's disease: challenges and solutions. *J. Multidiscip. Healthc.* 9, 469–479. doi: 10.2147/jmdh.s105857

Sorrento Therapeutics Inc. (2020). *Sorrento Therapeutics Announces Discovery of a Potential Non-Dopaminergic Approach to Controlling Parkinson's Motor Symptoms With Resiniferatoxin (RTX) Intrathecal Administration.* California: Sorrento Therapeutics, Inc. Available online at: https://investors.sorrentotherapeutics.com/node/10481/pdf (accessed on May 6, 2020).

Steinberg, X., Lespay-Rebolledo, C., and Brauchi, S. (2014). A structural view of ligand-dependent activation in thermoTRP channels. *Front. Physiol.* 5:171. doi: 10.3389/fphys.2014.00171

Streifel, K. M., Gonzales, A. L., De Miranda, B., Mouneimne, R., Earley, S., and Tjalkens, R. (2014). Dopaminergic neurotoxicants cause biphasic inhibition of purinergic calcium signaling in astrocytes. *PLoS One* 9:e110996. doi: 10.1371/journal.pone.0110996

Sukumaran, P., Sun, Y., Antonson, N., and Singh, B. B. (2018). Dopaminergic neurotoxins induce cell death by attenuating NF-κB-mediated regulation of TRPC1 expression and autophagy. *FASEB J.* 32, 1640–1652. doi: 10.1096/fj.201700662RR

Sukumaran, P., Sun, Y., Schaar, A., Selvaraj, S., and Singh, B. B. (2017). TRPC Channels and Parkinson's Disease. *Adv. Exp. Med. Biol.* 976, 85–94. doi: 10.1007/978-94-024-1088-4_8

Sun, Y., Selvaraj, S., Pandey, S., Humphrey, K. M., Foster, J. D., Wu, M., et al. (2018a). MPP(+) decreases store-operated calcium entry and TRPC1 expression in Mesenchymal Stem Cell derived dopaminergic neurons. *Sci. Rep.* 8:11715. doi: 10.1038/s41598-018-29528-x

Sun, Y., Sukumaran, P., Selvaraj, S., Cilz, N. I., Schaar, A., Lei, S., et al. (2018b). TRPM2 Promotes Neurotoxin MPP(+)/MPTP-Induced Cell Death. *Mol. Neurobiol.* 55, 409–420. doi: 10.1007/s12035-016-0338-9

Sun, Y., Zhang, H., Selvaraj, S., Sukumaran, P., Lei, S., Birnbaumer, L., et al. (2017). Inhibition of L-Type Ca(2+) Channels by TRPC1-STIM1 Complex Is Essential for the Protection of Dopaminergic Neurons. *J. Neurosci.* 37, 3364–3377. doi: 10.1523/jneurosci.3010-16.2017

Thapak, P., Bishnoi, M., and Sharma, S. S. (2020a). Amelioration of diabetes-induced cognitive impairment by Transient Receptor Potential Vanilloid 2 (TRPV2) channel inhibitor: Behavioral and mechanistic study. *Neurochem. Int.* 139:104783. doi: 10.1016/j.neuint.2020.104783

Thapak, P., Bishnoi, M., and Sharma, S. S. (2020b). Pharmacological inhibition of Transient Receptor Potential Melastatin 2 (TRPM2) Channels Attenuates Diabetes-induced Cognitive Deficits in Rats: A Mechanistic Study. *Curr. Neurovasc. Res.* 17, 249–258. doi: 10.2174/1567202617666200415142211

Thapak, P., Vaidya, B., Joshi, H. C., Singh, J. N., and Sharma, S. S. (2020c). Therapeutic potential of pharmacological agents targeting TRP channels in CNS disorders. *Pharmacol. Res.* 159:105026. doi: 10.1016/j.phrs.2020.105026

Tjaša, O., Kolmančič, K., Tratnjek, L., Živin, A., and Živin, M. (2016). "Immunohistochemical Staining of Trpv4 Channels in Rat Parkinson Disease Model," in *Proceedings of the MEi: CogSci Conference 2016*, (Bratislava: Comenius University).

Uppalapati, D., Das, N. R., Gangwal, R. P., Damre, M. V., Sangamwar, A. T., and Sharma, S. S. (2014). Neuroprotective Potential of Peroxisome Proliferator Activated Receptor- α Agonist in Cognitive Impairment in Parkinson's Disease: Behavioral, Biochemical, and PBPK Profile. *PPAR Res.* 2014:753587. doi: 10. 1155/2014/753587

Venkatachalam, K., and Montell, C. (2007). TRP channels. *Annu. Rev. Biochem.* 76, 387–417. doi: 10.1146/annurev.biochem.75.103004.142819

Voets, T., Talavera, K., Owsianik, G., and Nilius, B. (2005). Sensing with TRP channels. *Nat. Chem. Biol.* 1, 85–92. doi: 10.1038/nchembio0705-85

Wang, D., Yu, H., Xu, B., Xu, H., Zhang, Z., Ren, X., et al. (2018). TRPC1 Deletion Causes Striatal Neuronal Cell Apoptosis and Proteomic Alterations in Mice. *Front. Aging. Neurosci.* 10:72. doi: 10.3389/fnagi.2018.00072

Williams, N. M., Hubbard, L., Sandor, C., Webber, C., Hendry, H., Lawton, M., et al. (2020). Genome-Wide Association Study of Pain in Parkinson's Disease Implicates TRPM8 as a Risk Factor. *Mov. Disord.* 35, 705–707. doi: 10.1002/ mds.28001

Woudenberg-Vrenken, T. E., Sukinta, A., Van Der Kemp, A. W., Bindels, R. J., and Hoenderop, J. G. (2011). Transient receptor potential melastatin 6 knockout mice are lethal whereas heterozygous deletion results in mild hypomagnesemia. *Nephron. Physiol.* 117, 11–19. doi: 10.1159/000320580

Xie, Y. F., and Zhou, F. (2014). TRPC3 channel mediates excitation of striatal cholinergic interneurons. *Neurol. Sci.* 35, 1757–1761. doi: 10.1007/s10072-014-1827-0

Xu, H., Ramsey, I. S., Kotecha, S. A., Moran, M. M., Chong, J. A., Lawson, D., et al. (2002). TRPV3 is a calcium-permeable temperature-sensitive cation channel. *Nature* 418, 181–186. doi: 10.1038/nature00882

Yang, C. P., Zhang, Z. H., Zhang, L. H., and Rui, H. C. (2016). Neuroprotective Role of MicroRNA-22 in a 6-Hydroxydopamine-Induced Cell Model of Parkinson's Disease via Regulation of Its Target Gene TRPM7. *J. Mol. Neurosci.* 60, 445–452. doi: 10.1007/s12031-016-0828-2

Yu, Y.-P., Xie, A.-M., and Chi, X.-L. (2013). The effect of TrkA signaling pathway on the expressions of TRPC1, TRPC3 in 6-hydroxydopamine lesioned rat treated by electroacupuncture. *Glob. J. Card. Cereb. Dis.* 1:1. doi: 10.14725/ gjccd.v1n1a203

Yu, Y.-P., Xie, A.-M., and Yang, X.-H. (2014). TrkA Pathway (s) are Involves in the Regulation of TRPM2 and TRPM7 Expression in the Substantia Nigra of the Parkinson's Disease Rat Model Induced by 6-Hydroxydopamine. *Adv. Res.* 2, 782–796. doi: 10.9734/AIR/2014/10543

Zeitz, K. P., Guy, N., Malmberg, A. B., Dirajlal, S., Martin, W. J., Sun, L., et al. (2002). The 5-HT3 subtype of serotonin receptor contributes to nociceptive processing via a novel subset of myelinated and unmyelinated nociceptors. *J. Neurosci.* 22, 1010–1019. doi: 10.1523/jneurosci.22-03-01010. 2002

Zhang, X., Hu, M., Yang, Y., and Xu, H. (2018). Organellar TRP channels. *Nat. Struct. Mol. Biol.* 25, 1009–1018. doi: 10.1038/s41594-018-0148-z

Zhao, Z., Wang, J., Wang, L., Yao, X., Liu, Y., Li, Y., et al. (2017). Capsaicin Protects Against Oxidative Insults and Alleviates Behavioral Deficits in Rats with 6-OHDA-Induced Parkinson's Disease via Activation of TRPV1. *Neurochem. Res.* 42, 3431–3438. doi: 10.1007/s11064-017-2388-4

Zhen, X. C., and Chu, H. Y. (2020). Emerging novel approaches to drug research and diagnosis of Parkinson's disease. *Acta Pharmacol. Sin.* 41, 439–441. doi: 10.1038/s41401-020-0369-7

Zheng, J. (2013). Molecular mechanism of TRP channels. *Compr. Physiol.* 3, 221–242. doi: 10.1002/cphy.c120001

Zhou, F. W., Matta, S. G., and Zhou, F. M. (2008). Constitutively active TRPC3 channels regulate basal ganglia output neurons. *J. Neurosci.* 28, 473–482. doi: 10.1523/jneurosci.3978-07.2008

Zhou, Y., and Han, D. (2017). GATA3 modulates neuronal survival through regulating TRPM2 in Parkinson's disease. *Int. J. Clin. Exp. Med.* 10, 15178–15186.

Zubov, A., Muruzheva, Z., Tikhomirova, M., and Karpenko, M. (2020). Glibenclamide as a neuroprotective antidementia drug. *Arch. Physiol. Biochem.* 11, 1–4. doi: 10.1080/13813455.2020.1789170

2

Role of Oxidative Stress and Ca^{2+} Signaling in Psychiatric Disorders

Akito Nakao[1], Yoshihiro Matsunaga[1], Katsumi Hayashida[1] and Nobuaki Takahashi[2]**

[1] *Laboratory of Molecular Biology, Department of Synthetic Chemistry and Biological Chemistry, Graduate School of Engineering, Kyoto University, Kyoto, Japan,*

[2] *The Hakubi Center for Advanced Research, Kyoto University, Kyoto, Japan*

***Correspondence:**
Akito Nakao
nakao@sbchem.kyoto-u.ac.jp
Nobuaki Takahashi
takahashi@sbchem.kyoto-u.ac.jp

Psychiatric disorders are caused by complex and diverse factors, and numerous mechanisms have been proposed for the pathogenesis of these disorders. Accumulating evidence suggests that oxidative stress is one of the general factors involved in the pathogenesis/pathophysiology of major psychiatric disorders, including bipolar disorder, depression, anxiety disorder, and schizophrenia. Indeed, some clinical trials have shown improvement of the symptoms of these disorders by antioxidant supplementation. However, the molecular basis for the relationship between oxidative stress and the pathogenesis of psychiatric disorders remains largely unknown. In general, Ca^{2+} channels play central roles in neuronal functions, including neuronal excitability, neurotransmitter release, synaptic plasticity, and gene regulation, and genes that encode Ca^{2+} channels have been found to be associated with psychiatric disorders. Notably, a class of Ca^{2+}-permeable transient receptor potential (TRP) cation channels is activated by changes in cellular redox status, whereby these TRP channels can link oxidative stress to Ca^{2+} signals. Given the unique characteristic of redox-sensitive TRP channels, these channels could be a target for delineating the pathogenesis or pathophysiology of psychiatric disorders. In this review, we summarize the outcomes of clinical trials for antioxidant treatment in patients with psychiatric disorders and the current insights into the physiological/pathological significance of redox-sensitive TRP channels in the light of neural functions, including behavioral phenotypes, and discuss the potential role of TRP channels in the pathogenesis of psychiatric disorders. Investigation of redox-sensitive TRP channels may lead to the development of novel therapeutic strategies for the treatment of psychiatric disorders.

Keywords: oxidative stress, Ca^{2+} signaling, TRP channels, behavior, psychiatric disorders

INTRODUCTION

Psychiatric disorders, which are chronic, recurrent, and devastating disorders, are one of the main causes of disability worldwide, with the current understanding of psychiatric disorders remaining limited due to the complex and diverse nature of these disorders. Based on a 2017 survey, the number of patients with psychiatric disorders is extremely high worldwide (284 million cases of anxiety disorders; 264 million cases of depression; 46 million cases of bipolar disorder; 20 million cases of schizophrenia) (Ritchie and Roser, 2018); therefore, therapeutic strategies for the treatment of psychiatric disorders are urgently required.

Accumulating evidence suggests that oxidative stress is one of the general factors involved in the pathogenesis/pathophysiology of psychiatric disorders (Ng et al., 2008), with antioxidant levels seeming to correlate with the degree of severity of psychiatric disorders (Zhang et al., 2003; Machado-Vieira et al., 2007; Sarandol et al., 2007), and antioxidant treatment has been shown to improve psychiatric symptoms in some clinical trials (Dakhale et al., 2005; Sivrioglu et al., 2007; Ellegaard et al., 2019). Moreover, markers of oxidative stress, including lipid peroxidation products and oxidized DNA, have been shown to be elevated in the blood of patients with psychiatric disorders. While the molecular mechanisms by which oxidative stress induces psychiatric disorders are still largely unknown, the lines of evidence strongly suggest that oxidative stress is associated with the physiology/pathology of psychiatric disorders.

Ca^{2+} channels mediate a number of neuronal functions, including neuronal excitability, neurotransmitter release, synaptic plasticity, and gene regulation. Many lines of evidence from human studies have indicated a critical contribution of voltage-dependent Ca^{2+} channels (VDCC) to the pathogenesis/pathophysiology of psychiatric disorders (Sklar et al., 2002, 2011; Ferreira et al., 2008; Ripke et al., 2011, 2014). However, since VDCCs control multiple critical physiological functions in the central nervous system (CNS), targeting VDCCs could cause complicated and uncontrollable results. Thus, targeting the "cart" that modulates Ca^{2+} signaling upon oxidative stress rather than the "horse" that governs the CNS system may be a promising approach and could reduce unwanted side effects.

Among the Ca^{2+}-permeable cation channels, transient receptor potential (TRP) channels have attracted attention as unique sensors of a wide variety of stresses, including oxidative stress (Mori et al., 2016). Given that redox-sensitive TRP channels induce Ca^{2+} influx upon oxidative stress, these channels could be mediators that link oxidative stress to dysregulated Ca^{2+} signaling in the pathogenesis/pathophysiology of psychiatric disorders.

In the first part of this review, we introduce the literature that examines oxidative stress in psychiatric disorders. In the second part, we review the significance of Ca^{2+} signaling in psychiatric disorders and provide current insights into the roles of redox-sensitive TRP channels in the functioning of neurons and glia as well as the development of neuronal connectivity and the function of the higher brain.

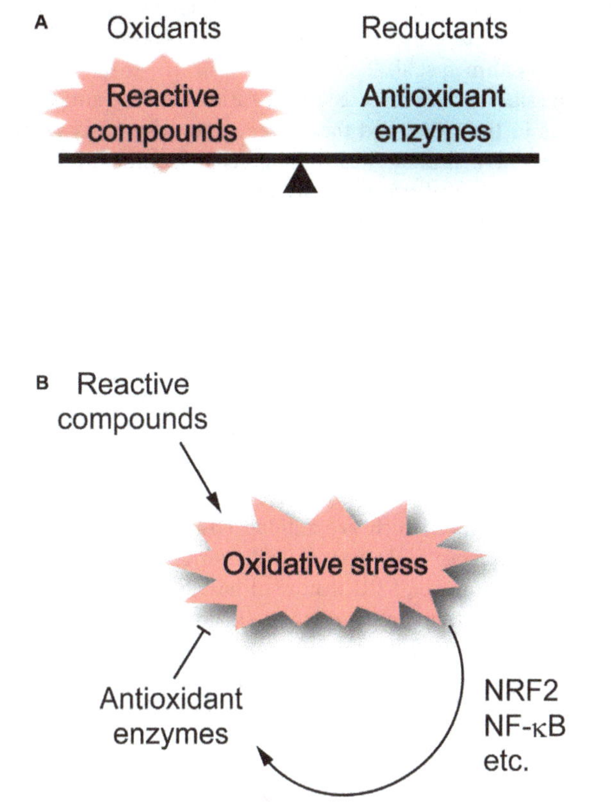

FIGURE 1 | Regulation of cellular redox homeostasis. **(A)** Cellular redox status is determined by the balance between the levels of intracellular reactive compounds and antioxidant enzymes. **(B)** Reactive compounds shift the cellular redox status to oxidative conditions, while antioxidant enzymes neutralize oxidative stress. The expression of antioxidant enzymes is induced upon oxidative stress via oxidant defense transcription factors, such as NRF2 and NF-κB.

OXIDATIVE STRESS IN PSYCHIATRIC DISORDERS

Cellular redox status is determined by the balance between the levels of intracellular antioxidants and redox reactive species, including reactive oxygen species (ROS) and other electrophilic molecules, which can cause oxidative damage to membrane lipids, proteins, and DNA (**Figure 1A**). While a decrease in antioxidant enzymes shifts the cellular redox status to oxidative conditions, intriguingly, the expression of antioxidant enzymes is induced upon oxidative stress via oxidant defense transcription factors, such as NRF2 and NF-κB; therefore, both enhanced and suppressed antioxidant expression can be associated with oxidative stress (**Figure 1B**).

It is highly controversial whether the antioxidant system is upregulated or downregulated in psychiatric disorders. In bipolar disorder, the activities of superoxide dismutases (SODs) and catalase (CAT) have been found to be decreased in the blood (Ranjekar et al., 2003), while the activity of glutathione peroxidases (GPXs) has been shown to be comparable between bipolar patients and healthy individuals (Kuloglu et al., 2002c; Ranjekar et al., 2003).

In contrast, several studies have demonstrated increased SOD activities in bipolar disorder (Abdalla et al., 1986; Kuloglu et al., 2002c). In major depression and anxiety disorders, such as obsessive-compulsive disorder, panic disorder, and social phobia, the activity of SODs alone or SODs and GPXs has been shown to be increased (Kuloglu et al., 2002a,b; Khanzode et al., 2003; Atmaca et al., 2004; Sarandol et al., 2007). In schizophrenia, higher activities of SODs (Abdalla et al., 1986; Kuloglu et al., 2002c) and GPXs have been reported in the blood of patients (Kuloglu et al., 2002c), while several other studies have reported that the activities of SODs, CAT, and GPXs are lower in schizophrenic patients than in healthy controls (Ranjekar et al., 2003; Ben Othmen et al., 2008).

Some studies have reported a correlation between antioxidant activities in the blood and the degree of severity of psychiatric disorders. In a finding which suggests that antioxidant level is an indicator of disease severity and that lithium, a primary treatment for bipolar disorder, directly or indirectly normalizes redox status, one study that compared healthy controls with either unmedicated or lithium-treated patients in manic episodes of bipolar disorder indicates that, while SOD activity was significantly higher in manic patients compared with controls, it was indistinguishable between the lithium-treated group and the control group (Machado-Vieira et al., 2007). In patients with major depressive disorder, a significant positive correlation was found between the severity of the disease and SOD activity (Sarandol et al., 2007). Interestingly, serotonin reuptake inhibitors (SSRIs), which are antidepressant drugs, have been shown to decrease SOD activity (Bilici et al., 2001; Khanzode et al., 2003); however, SSRI treatment has also been reported to increase SOD activity in patients with major depressive disorder (Herken et al., 2007). In schizophrenic patients, SOD activity is significantly increased in the serum compared to control subjects and is decreased after treatment with atypical antipsychotics, such as clozapine, risperidone, olanzapine, quetiapine, and ziprasidone, in schizophrenic patients (Dakhale et al., 2004). It has also been reported that treatment with risperidone, an atypical antipsychotic, significantly decreased the blood SOD levels in schizophrenic patients and that decreased SOD levels may correlate with an improvement in symptoms (Zhang et al., 2003).

In contrast to the controversy on the effects of antioxidant activity on psychiatric disorders, overall, markers of oxidative stress, such as lipid peroxidation and oxidized DNA, have been shown to be elevated in patients with psychiatric disorders. An increase in one lipid peroxidation product, malondialdehyde (MDA), was reported in both bipolar disorder and schizophrenia (Kuloglu et al., 2002c). The level of thiobarbituric acid-reactive substances, another marker of lipid peroxidation, has also been reported to be increased in schizophrenia (Herken et al., 2001; Akyol et al., 2002). In major depression, a number of factors that maintain or disturb redox homeostasis are altered: depletion of ω-3 fatty acids, which suppress lipid peroxidation (Peet et al., 1998), elevation of MDA (Bilici et al., 2001; Khanzode et al., 2003; Sarandol et al., 2007), and increases in 8-hydroxy-2′-deoxyguanosine, a marker of oxidized DNA damage (Forlenza and Miller, 2006). In anxiety disorders, elevated MDA levels have been reported in obsessive-compulsive disorder (Kuloglu et al., 2002a; Ersan et al., 2006), panic disorder (Kuloglu et al., 2002b), and social phobia (Atmaca et al., 2004). These results provide evidence that oxidative stress is induced in psychiatric disorders and suggest both that the antioxidant system is upregulated through oxidant defense mechanisms and that decreased antioxidant activities lead to enhanced oxidative stress in some types of psychiatric disorders (**Figure 1**).

The potential significance of oxidative stress in psychiatric disorders has been demonstrated by some clinical trials that reported an improvement in symptoms through antioxidant treatment (**Table 1**). In patients with bipolar disorder, a randomized, double-blind, multicenter, placebo-controlled study of individuals (n = 75) showed that 24-week treatment with *N*-acetyl cysteine (NAC) significantly improved depressive symptoms (Berk et al., 2008), while a three-arm, 16-week, double-blind, randomized, placebo-controlled NAC treatment trial (n = 181) with depressive symptoms in bipolar disorder provided overall negative results, with no significant differences between groups detected at the primary outcome but some positive secondary signals were detected (Berk et al., 2019), suggesting that longer-term supplementation of NAC is required for the amelioration. In patients with major depressive disorder, a double-blind, randomized, placebo-controlled, clinical trial was performed with NAC as an adjunctive treatment in 269 participants, and the results exhibited limited but significant effects of adjunctive NAC treatment in reducing depressive symptoms in patients with major depressive disorder (Berk et al., 2014). Notably, meta-analysis was carried out to aggregate the data on double-blind, randomized, placebo-controlled trials evaluating the effect of NAC treatment on depressive symptoms in a total of 574 participants, of whom 291 were randomized to receive NAC and 283 received a placebo, regardless of the main psychiatric conditions. The results demonstrated that treatment with NAC significantly improved depressive symptoms in patients with bipolar and major depressive disorders and in individuals with trichotillomania or heavy smoking (Fernandes et al., 2016). In patients with schizophrenia, a 12-week, double-blind, randomized, placebo-controlled, clinical trial has recently been performed to assess the effectiveness of NAC as an adjunctive treatment with conventional antipsychotic medications in 84 patients (Sepehrmanesh et al., 2018). This clinical trial demonstrated that NAC-treated patients showed significantly improved cognitive functions (Sepehrmanesh et al., 2018). In addition to NAC supplementation, co-treatment of antipsychotic drugs with both ω-3 fatty acids and vitamins E and C for 4 months improved psychotic symptoms in schizophrenic patients (Arvindakshan et al., 2003). There results suggest that oxidative stress is involved in the pathophysiology of psychiatric disorders and that antioxidant supplementation may have a suppressive effect on symptoms.

Ca^{2+} SIGNALING IN PSYCHIATRIC DISORDERS

In the CNS, Ca^{2+} signaling is pivotal for numerous cellular events, including neuronal excitability, neurotransmitter release, synaptic plasticity, and Ca^{2+}-induced gene regulation (Catterall, 2011; Sawamura et al., 2017). Due to the fundamental role of Ca^{2+} signaling in the CNS, Ca^{2+} channels are thought to be a prime target for the pathogenesis of psychiatric disorders. Indeed, genes encoding Ca^{2+} channels have been shown to be associated with psychiatric disorders (McQuillin et al., 2006; Ripke et al., 2014; Griesi-Oliveira et al., 2015).

Among the Ca^{2+} channels, *CACNA1C*-encoded $Ca_V1.2$, an L-type VDCC, is strongly associated with psychiatric disorders

TABLE 1 | Clinical trials for antioxidant treatment in patients with schizophrenia, bipolar disorder, and major depressive disorder.

Schizophrenia

Antioxidant	Trial design → Outcomes	Sample size	
NAC (Sepehrmanesh et al., 2018)	Adjunctive NAC 1,200 mg/day supplements 12 weeks double-blind treatment → Improvement in PANSS, MMSE, Digit Span Test, and SCWT scores	NAC: Placebo:	42 42
Vitamin C/E and ω-3 fatty acids (Sivrioglu et al., 2007)	Adjunctive vitamin C 1,000 mg/day, vitamin E 800 IU/day, EPA 360 mg/day, and DHA 240 mg/day supplements 4 months open-label treatment → Improvement in BPRS, BARS, SAS scores, and SANS total score	Vitamin C/E and ω-3 fatty acids:	17
Vitamin C (Dakhale et al., 2005)	Adjunctive vitamin C 500 mg/day supplements 8 weeks double-blind treatment → Improvement in BPRS score	Vitamin C: Placebo:	20 20
Vitamin C/E and ω-3 fatty acids (Arvindakshan et al., 2003)	Adjunctive vitamin C 1,000 mg/day, vitamin E 800 IU/day, EPA 360 mg/day, and DHA 240 mg/day supplements 4 months open-labeled treatment and 4 months follow up → 8 months; Improvement in BPRS-total, positive-PANSS, general psychopathology-PANSS, and PANSS-total scores	Vitamin C/E and ω-3 fatty acids:	33

Bipolar disorder

Antioxidant	Trial design → Outcomes	Sample size	
NAC (Berk et al., 2019)	Adjunctive NAC 2,000 mg/day and cocktail of 16 nutrient agents supplements 16 weeks double-blind treatment and 4 weeks follow up → 16 weeks; No significant change 20 weeks; Improvement in MADRS, BDRS, SOFAS, and LIFE-RIFT scores (Placebo v.s. NAC + nutrient agents)	NAC + nutrient agents: NAC: Placebo:	61 59 61
NAC (Ellegaard et al., 2019)	Adjunctive NAC 3,000 mg/day supplements 20 weeks double-blind treatment and 4 weeks follow up → 20 weeks; Improvement in YMRS score	NAC: Placebo:	40 40
NAC (Berk et al., 2008)	Adjunctive NAC 2000 mg/day supplements 24 weeks double-blind treatment and 4 weeks follow up → 24 weeks; Improvement in MADRS, BDRS, CGI-S-BP, Q-LES-Q, LIFE-RIFT, SLICE-LIFE, GAF, and SOFAS scores	NAC: Placebo:	38 37

Major depressive disorder

Antioxidant	Trial design → Outcomes	Sample size	
NAC (Berk et al., 2014)	Adjunctive NAC 2,000 mg/day supplements 12 weeks double-blind treatment and 4 weeks follow up → 16 weeks; Improvement in MADRS, CGI-S, SLICE-LIFE, and LIFE-RIFT scores	NAC: Placebo:	135 134

BARS, Barnes Akathisia Rating Scale; BDRS, Bipolar Depression Rating Scale; BPRS, Brief Psychiatric Rating Scale; CGI-S, Clinical Global Impressions-Severity of illness; CGI-S-BP, Clinical Global Impression Severity scale for Bipolar disorder; GAF, Global Assessment of Functioning Scale; LIFE-RIFT, Longitudinal Interval Follow-Up Evaluation-Range of Impaired Functioning Tool; MADRS, Montgomery-Åsberg Depression Rating Scale; MMSE, Mini-Mental State Examination; PANSS, Positive And Negative Syndrome Scale; Q-LES-Q, Quality of Life Enjoyment and Satisfaction Questionnaire; SANS, Scale for the Assessment of Negative Symptoms; SAS, Simpson-Angus Scale; SCWT, Stroop Color and Word test; SLICE-LIFE, Streamlined Longitudinal Interview Clinical Evaluation from the Longitudinal Interval Follow-up Evaluation; SOFAS, Social and Occupational Functioning Assessment Scale; YMRS, Young Mania Rating Scale.

(Sklar et al., 2002, 2011; Ferreira et al., 2008; Ripke et al., 2011, 2014). In humans, a risk-associated single nucleotide polymorphism (rs1006737) in *CACNA1C* predicts both increased hippocampal activity during emotional processing and higher prefrontal activity during executive cognition (Bigos et al., 2010). In rodents, conditional deletion of *Cacna1c* in the hippocampus and cortex results in severe impairment of hippocampus-dependent spatial memory based on the Morris water maze test (Moosmang et al., 2005; White et al., 2008). Acute pharmacological blockade of $Ca_V1.2$, but not chronic genetic inactivation, impairs the acquisition of fear learning (Langwieser et al., 2010), while anterior cingulate cortex-limited deletion of *Cacna1c* in mice impairs observational fear learning (Jeon et al., 2010). Constitutive *Cacna1c* heterozygous knockout (KO) mice, forebrain-specific conditional *Cacna1c* KO mice, and prefrontal cortex-specific *Cacna1c* knockdown mice show increased anxiety-like behavior in the elevated-plus maze test (Lee et al., 2012). The behavioral phenotypes in mice with genetic or pharmacological inhibition of $Ca_V1.2$ are summarized in the previous literature (Nakao et al., 2015).

Clinical studies with $Ca_V1.2$ blockers for psychiatric disorders have been summarized in a previous review paper (Kabir et al., 2017). While some clinical trials using $Ca_V1.2$ blockers have demonstrated improved symptoms of psychiatric disorders, the effect remains controversial (Kabir et al., 2017). Notably, since $Ca_V1.2$ controls multiple critical physiological functions in various organs and tissues, including the vascular system, the sinoatrial node, cardiomyocytes, pancreatic islets, adrenal medulla, and intestinal smooth muscle (Zamponi et al., 2015), the use of $Ca_V1.2$ blockers could cause highly complicated and uncontrollable results.

REDOX-SENSITIVE TRP CHANNELS

Among the Ca^{2+}-permeable channels, a class of TRP channels is activated by oxidative stress (so-called redox-sensitive TRP channels). Given the critical role of oxidative stress and aberrant Ca^{2+} signaling in psychiatry disorders, it is possible that redox-sensitive TRP channels serve as a cue for understanding the molecular pathogenesis of these disorders.

The *trp* was originally identified through the genetic studies of the *Drosophila* phototransduction mutant (Montell and Rubin, 1989). The term "TRP" is derived from "transient receptor potential" as the *trp* mutant photoreceptors fail to generate the Ca^{2+}-dependent sustained phase of receptor potential and therefore fail to induce subsequent Ca^{2+}-dependent adaptation to light in *Drosophila*. In mammals, 28 TRP homologs have been identified since the cloning of the *Drosophila trp* gene (Montell and Rubin, 1989). They are divided into six subfamilies: TRPC (canonical), TRPV (vanilloid), TRPM (melastatin), TRPP (polycystin), TRPML (mucolipin), and TRPA (ankyrin) groups, according to the amino acid homology (Clapham, 2003; Nilius et al., 2007). TRP channels are putative six-transmembrane polypeptide subunits and assemble as tetramers to form a variety of Ca^{2+}-permeable cation channels. Because of their distinct activation mechanisms and biophysical properties, TRP channels are highly suited to function in sensory receptor cells, either as molecular sensors for environmental or endogenous stimuli or as modulators of signal transduction cascades downstream of metabotropic receptors. Indeed, TRP channels play crucial roles in many types of senses, including touch, taste, and smell in mammals (Clapham, 2003; Voets et al., 2005; Moran et al., 2011). Thus, in marked contrast to VDCCs and fast ligand-gated Ca^{2+}-permeable channels that participate in specialized cellular functions, TRP channels play divergent roles in cell physiology and pathophysiology.

Among TRP channels, one particular group of TRP channels, including TRPM2, TRPC5, TRPV1–V4, and TRPA1 channels, function as exquisite sensors of redox status. The redox-sensitive TRP channels induce Ca^{2+} entry into the cells in response to cellular redox perturbation and can convert oxidative stress information into Ca^{2+} signals. Details of redox-sensitive TRP channels have been summarized in several review papers from our group (Takahashi and Mori, 2011; Takahashi et al., 2011a; Kozai et al., 2013; Sakaguchi and Mori, 2020).

TRPM2 channel, the first redox-sensitive TRP channel to be identified, is activated by H_2O_2 through the production of nicotinamide adenine dinucleotide and its metabolites, ADP-ribose and cyclic ADP-ribose (Hara et al., 2002; Perraud et al., 2005). A later study proposed that oxidation of the methionine located in the ADP-ribose binding region of TRPM2 sensitizes the channel activities (Kashio et al., 2012). H_2O_2-activated Ca^{2+} or cation influx through TRPM2 induces cell death (Hara et al., 2002) and insulin secretion in pancreatic β-cells (Togashi et al., 2006; Uchida et al., 2011). Furthermore, studies using *Trpm2* KO mice have shown that TRPM2 widely contributes to the innate immune system in monocytes, macrophages, neutrophils, and natural killer cells (Yamamoto et al., 2008; Knowles et al., 2011; Di et al., 2012; Hiroi et al., 2013; Rah et al., 2015).

In addition to the indirect redox-sensing mechanism via TRPM2, direct redox-sensing mechanisms involving cysteine (Cys) modification have emerged as mechanisms that underly the activation of various TRP channels (Yoshida et al., 2006; Takahashi and Mori, 2011; Takahashi et al., 2011b). TRPC5 channel, for example, is activated by nitric oxide (NO), reactive disulfides, and H_2O_2 via the oxidative modification of Cys residues (Cys553 and Cys558) located on the N-terminal side of the pore-forming region between S5 and S6 transmembrane helices in mouse TRPC5 (Yoshida et al., 2006). Interestingly, TRPC5 is also activated by the reducing agent dithiothreitol and extracellular-reduced thioredoxin (Xu et al., 2008). Both thermosensor channels (TRPV1, TRPV3, and TRPV4) and the closest relatives of TRPC5 (TRPC1 and TRPC4) have Cys residues corresponding to Cys553 and Cys558 on the TRPC5 protein and are activated by NO, reactive disulfides, and H_2O_2 (Yoshida et al., 2006). The mustard oil or wasabi sensor TRPA1 channel, which is predominantly expressed in sensory and vagal neurons, is also activated via modification of Cys residues located in the N-terminal ankyrin repeat domain (Hinman et al., 2006; Macpherson et al., 2007; Takahashi et al., 2008) and has the highest oxidation sensitivity among all TRP channel family members (Takahashi et al., 2011b).

Notably, all the redox-sensitive TRP channels are expressed to some extent in the CNS and affect neuronal and glial functions. Given this fact, together with the evidence that both Ca^{2+} signals and oxidative stress are critical mediators in psychiatric disorders, it is possible that redox-sensitive TRP channels could be a target for delineating the pathogenesis or pathophysiology of psychiatric disorders.

NEURONAL AND GLIAL FUNCTIONS OF REDOX-SENSITIVE TRP CHANNELS

In neuronal circuits, excitation-inhibition balance is considered a framework for understanding the mechanisms of psychiatric disorders (Sohal and Rubenstein, 2019). TRPM2 channel is abundantly expressed in the brain (Hara et al., 2002; Kraft et al., 2004; Fonfria et al., 2006) and H_2O_2-induced Ca^{2+} influx via TRPM2 in neurons was initially identified to induce cell death (Kaneko et al., 2006). Later studies have suggested several important roles for TRPM2 in the physiology of the CNS. TRPM2 activation by ADPR has been suggested as a regulator of VDCC and NMDAR via a rise in intracellular Ca^{2+} concentration ($[Ca^{2+}]_i$) in cultured hippocampal pyramidal neurons (Olah et al., 2009). In CA3-CA1 synapses, the loss of TRPM2 selectively impairs NMDAR-dependent long-term depression (LTD), while it does not affect long-term potentiation (LTP) (Xie et al., 2011). The impaired LTD in *Trpm2* KO mice is rescued by dopamine D2 receptor stimulation through the reduction of phosphorylated GSK-3β, suggesting that TRPM2 plays a key role in hippocampal synaptic plasticity via the GSK-3β signaling pathway. In guinea pig midbrain slices, TRPM2 has been shown to be required for NMDA-induced burst firing and to contribute to H_2O_2-dependent modulation of substantia nigra pars reticulata (SNr) GABAergic neurons (Lee et al., 2013). Given that an increase in burst firing in SNr GABAergic neurons is observed in Parkinson's disease and that oxidative stress is linked to Parkinson's disease, TRPM2 could be associated with the pathophysiology of Parkinson's disease.

Quantitative post-mortem investigations have convincingly demonstrated abnormalities in the glial cells of patients with psychiatric disorders (Cotter et al., 2001). In addition to neurons and immune cells, TRPM2 has been shown to be functionally expressed in glial cells, such as the microglia and astrocytes (Kraft et al., 2004; Kaneko et al., 2006; Bond and Greenfield, 2007). Oxidative stress induced by the inhibition of intracellular GSH biosynthesis with D,L-buthionine-*S*,*R*-sulfoximine (BSO) elicits Ca^{2+} influx potentially via TRPM2 in astrocytes isolated from humans (Lee et al., 2010). In rat cultured astrocytes, *tert*-butyl hydroperoxide-induced oxidative stress upregulates TRPM2 mRNA within 1 h – the transcripts were peaked at 4 h and were still apparent at 24 h post-stress (Bond and Greenfield, 2007), suggesting that glial TRPM2 expression is enhanced upon oxidative stress in disease conditions, including psychiatric disorders, and mediates the pathophysiology of disease.

TRPC5 is predominantly expressed in the brain, where it can form heterotetrameric complexes with TRPC1 and TRPC4 channel subunits. Recently, TRPC1, TRPC4, and TRPC5 have been demonstrated to assemble into heteromultimers in mouse brains, but not with other TRP family members, based on quantitative high-resolution mass spectrometry (Bröker-Lai et al., 2017). Brain slices prepared from *Trpc5* KO and *Trpc4* KO mice exhibit significant reductions in the synaptic responses that are mediated by the activation of $G_{q/11}$ protein-coupled receptors (e.g., group I metabotropic glutamate receptors and cholecystokinin [CCK] 2 receptors) in the amygdala (Riccio et al., 2009, 2014). As a consequence, deficiency of *Trpc5* or *Trpc4* induces anxiolytic behavior in mice (Riccio et al., 2009, 2014) (see "Redox-Sensitive TRP Channels in Higher Brain Functions" section). In hippocampal neurons from *Trpc1*/*Trpc4*/*Trpc5* triple KO mice, action potential-triggered excitatory postsynaptic currents (EPSCs) are significantly reduced, whereas the frequency, amplitude, and kinetics of quantal miniature EPSC signaling remains unchanged (Bröker-Lai et al., 2017). Consistent with this observation, evoked postsynaptic responses in hippocampal slice recordings and transient potentiation after tetanic stimulation have been reported to be decreased in triple KO mice (Bröker-Lai et al., 2017). In layer III pyramidal neurons in the entorhinal cortex, enhancement of neuronal excitability induced by CCK, one of the most abundant neuropeptides in the brain, is significantly inhibited by intracellular application of the antibody to TRPC5, suggesting the involvement of TRPC5 channels in neuropeptide-mediated neuronal excitability (Wang et al., 2011). TRPC5 has been also demonstrated to mediate muscarinic receptor-induced slowing after depolarization, which is observed in the pyramidal cells of the cerebral cortex (Yan et al., 2009). Interestingly, TRPC1, TRPC4, and TRPC5 channels are activated by leptin, a hormone that plays a key role in appetite, overeating, and obesity, via the Jak2-PI3 kinase-PLCγ1 pathway in hypothalamic proopiomelanocortin neurons (Qiu et al., 2010). Taken together, these lines of evidence suggest that TRPC1, TRPC4, and TRPC5 channels are involved in various physiological processes, including memory and appetite, by regulating neuronal functions.

TRPC1, TRPC4, and TRPC5 channels have also been shown to be expressed in astrocytes (Song et al., 2005; Malarkey et al., 2008). In the results suggesting that the TRPC1, TRPC4, and TRPC5 channels are functionally expressed in astrocytes and also modulate neuronal circuits, high-resolution imaging revealed that store-operated Ca^{2+} entry (SOCE) mediated by TRPC1 is linked not only functionally but also structurally to the ER Ca^{2+} stores in mouse astrocytes (Golovina, 2005). TRPC1-mediated Ca^{2+} entry in response to mechanical and pharmacological stimulation has been shown to contribute to glutamate release from rat astrocytes (Malarkey et al., 2008).

TRPV1 is broadly expressed in the brain regions, including the olfactory nuclei, cerebral cortex, dentate gyrus, thalamus, hypothalamus, periaqueductal gray, superior colliculus, locus coeruleus, and cerebellar cortex (Roberts et al., 2004). TRPV1 is involved in various forms of synaptic plasticity, which have been well-summarized in previous review papers (Kauer and Gibson, 2009; Ramírez-Barrantes et al., 2016; Sawamura et al., 2017). In the hippocampus, TRPV1 mediates LTD at excitatory synapses onto CA1 interneurons (Gibson et al., 2008). The excitatory synapses of the hippocampal CA1 interneurons are depressed by TRPV1 agonist capsaicin and the potent endogenous TRPV1 activator 12-(S)-HPETE (Gibson et al., 2008). TRPV1 activation by capsaicin or by endocannabinoid anandamide depressed somatic but not dendritic inhibitory inputs onto dentate granule cells, suggesting that TRPV1 modulates GABAergic synaptic transmission in a compartment-specific manner (Chávez et al., 2014). Interestingly, acute inescapable stress on an elevated platform suppressed LTP and facilitated LTD at the hippocampal CA3-CA1 synapse, but the TRPV1 agonist capsaicin effectively prevented these effects, suggesting that TRPV1 contributes to stress-induced impairment of spatial memory (Li et al., 2008) (see "Redox-Sensitive TRP Channels in Higher Brain Functions" section).

TRPA1, the channel that has the highest oxidation sensitivity among the TRP channels, is expressed in the brain (Stokes et al., 2006), including in the hippocampus (Lee et al., 2016), the dentate gyrus (Koch et al., 2011), the supraoptic nucleus (Yokoyama et al., 2011), the nucleus tractus solitarii (Sun et al., 2009), and the somatosensory cortex (Kheradpezhouh et al., 2017). TRPA1 is also expressed in astrocytes and regulates basal $[Ca^{2+}]_i$ (Shigetomi et al., 2012, 2013; Takizawa et al., 2018). TRPA1 inhibition, which decreases resting $[Ca^{2+}]_i$ in astrocytes, impairs interneuron inhibitory synapse efficacy by reducing GAT-3-mediated GABA transport, resulting in the elevation of extracellular GABA (Shigetomi et al., 2012). Furthermore, astrocyte TRPA1 channels are required for constitutive D-serine release into the extracellular space, which contributes to NMDA receptor-dependent LTP in CA3-CA1 synapses (Shigetomi et al., 2013). In rat astrocyte cell line C6 cells and primary cultured astrocytes, a TRPA1-mediated spontaneous rise of $[Ca^{2+}]_i$ modulated the spontaneous release of peptide hormones from astrocytes (Takizawa et al., 2018). Recently, our group reported that TRPA1 acts as an acute hypoxia sensor in brainstem astrocytes through O_2-dependent protein translocation and triggers ATP release from astrocytes, which potentiates respiratory center activity (Uchiyama et al., 2020). Interestingly, vascular endothelial cell-specific *Trpa1* KO exacerbates cerebral infarcts following permanent middle cerebral artery occlusion in mice (Pires and Earley, 2018), suggesting that TRPA1 in cerebral artery endothelial cells is activated by oxidative stress under ischemia and protects from cerebral ischemia through the secretion of vasodilators, including NO. Taken together, TRPA1 is expressed in diverse cell types within the brain, including glial and endothelial cells, and promotes the secretion of factors that modulate neuronal circuits and vascular tonus upon oxidative stress in disease conditions.

REDOX-SENSITIVE TRP CHANNELS IN THE ESTABLISHMENT OF NEURONAL CONNECTIVITY

Abnormalities in neurites are considered to be involved in the pathogenesis of psychiatric disorders because they can cause impaired neuronal connectivity (Penzes et al., 2011). TRPC1 positively regulates netrin-1-induced growth-cone turning in cultured *Xenopus* spinal neurons (Wang and Poo, 2005; Shim et al., 2009), while it is not involved in brain-derived neurotrophic factor (BDNF)-induced growth-cone turning in cultured rat cerebellar granule cells (Li et al., 2005). Both TRPC1 and TRPC3 channels are required for leptin-sensitive current and leptin-induced spine formation in cultured hippocampal neurons (Dhar et al., 2014). Interestingly, SOCE mediated by TRPC1 is required for the proliferation of adult hippocampal neural progenitor cells (Li et al., 2012). Activation of TRPC4 induces inhibition and arborization of neurite growth in cultured hippocampal neurons (Jeon et al., 2013). TRPC5 that interacts with the growth-cone-enriched protein stathmin 2 has been shown to be a negative regulator of neurite extension and growth-cone morphology (Greka et al., 2003). In semaphorin 3A-induced neuronal growth-cone collapse, calpain has been demonstrated to cleave and activate TRPC5 channels, suggesting that TRPC5 acts downstream of the semaphorin signaling that causes changes in neuronal growth-cone morphology (Kaczmarek et al., 2012). Neurotrophin-3-induced Ca^{2+} influx via TRPC5 inhibits neuronal dendritic growth through activation of Ca^{2+}/calmodulin kinase (CaMK) IIα (He et al., 2012). TRPC5 channels have also been shown to induce the activation of Ca^{2+}/calmodulin kinase kinase (CaMKK) and the γ-isoform of CaMKI (CaMKIγ), followed by the promotion of axon formation in cultured hippocampal neurons (Davare et al., 2009). In the cerebellar cortex, *Trpc5* deficiency causes the formation of long and highly branched granule neuron dendrites with impaired dendritic claw differentiation, resulting in gait and motor coordination deficits (Puram et al., 2011). Mechanistically, TRPC5 forms a complex specifically with CaMKIIβ and induces the CaMKIIβ-dependent phosphorylation of ubiquitin ligase Cdc20-APC at the centrosome, suggesting the significance of the TRPC5/CaMKIIβ/Cdc20-APC signaling axis in the regulation of dendritic morphology (Puram et al., 2011). Thus, the TRPC1, TRPC4, and TRPC5 channels are key regulators for proper establishment of neuronal connectivity.

In cultured cortical neurons, pharmacological perturbation of TRPM2 markedly increases the axonal growth, and the neurons isolated from *Trpm2* KO mice have significantly longer neurites and a greater number of spines than those isolated from control mice (Jang et al., 2014). In addition, the blockage of TRPM2 reverses lysophosphatidic acid induced suppression of neurite growth (Jang et al., 2014), suggesting that TRPM2 is a negative regulator of neurite outgrowth.

REDOX-SENSITIVE TRP CHANNELS IN HIGHER BRAIN FUNCTIONS

Genome scanning for 47 bipolar disorder families has shown that there is a susceptibility locus near the telomere on chromosome 21q (Straub et al., 1994). Fine mapping linkage analysis identified that *TRPM2* on chromosome 21q is associated with bipolar disorder (McQuillin et al., 2006). Two SNPs of *TRPM2* were found in the analysis: a base pair change in exon 11 of *TRPM2*, which causes an amino acid substitution (aspartic acid to glutamic acid: D543E), and a non-conservative change from

TABLE 2 | Behavioral phenotypes in mice with genetic or pharmacological inactivation of redox-sensitive TRP channels.

	Anxiety	Memory	Other behavioral phenotype
TRPM2 KO mice (Jang et al., 2015)	**Increased anxiety-like behavior** Decreased time spent in open arms in EP Increased latency to Light part in LD	N/D	Decreased interaction time in social interaction test
TRPM2 KO mice (Andoh et al., 2019)	Normal in LD and EP Normal in social interaction test	Normal in radial maze and Y-maze tests Decreased flexibility in Barnes maze test	Normal in rotarod, forced swim, tail suspension, and prepulse inhibition tests Increased resiliency to repeated social defeat stress
Middle-aged TRPM2 KO mice (Kakae et al., 2019) Middle-aged: 12–16 months old Aged: 20–24 months old	N/D	**Enhanced spatial working memory** Middle-aged TRPM2 KO mice show increased alternation behavior compared with middle-aged WT in Y-maze test. **Enhanced spatial reference memory** Middle-aged TRPM2 KO mice show increased exploratory preference compared with middle-aged WT in novel object recognition test. Aged TRPM2 KO mice show increased exploratory preference compared with aged WT in novel location recognition test.	N/D
Stressed TRPM2 KO mice (Ko et al., 2019) **Stressed**	**Decreased anxiety-like behavior** Stressed TRPM2 KO mice show more sucrose consumption compared with stressed WT in sucrose consumption test. Stressed TRPM2 KO mice show less escaped latency compared with stressed WT in learned helplessness test. Stressed TRPM2 KO mice show less latency to feed compared with stressed WT in novelty suppressed feeding test. Stressed TRPM2 KO mice show less immobility time compared with stressed WT in forced swim test.	N/D	N/D
Normal	**Decreased anxiety-like behavior** Non-stressed TRPM2 KO mice show less latency to feed compared with non-stressed WT in novelty suppressed feeding test. Non-stressed TRPM2 KO mice show less immobility time compared with non-stressed WT in forced swim test.	N/D	N/D
TRPC5 KO mice (Riccio et al., 2009)	**Decreased anxiety-like behavior** Increased entries in open arms in EP in center region in OF (first 5 min) Increased number of nose contacts in social interaction test	Normal in fear conditioning test	Decrease tendency in acoustic startle response Normal in novelty-suppressed feeding test Normal in locomotor activity in OF

(Continued)

TABLE 2 | Continued

	Anxiety	Memory	Other behavioral phenotype
TRPC4 KO mice (Riccio et al., 2014)	**Decreased anxiety-like behavior** Increased entry and time spent in open arms in EP in center region in OF	Normal in auditory and contextual fear conditioning tests	Normal in acoustic startle, tail suspension, and beam walking tests Normal in gait analysis Normal in total distance in OF (red light) Increased total distance in OF
TRPC1 KO mice (Lepannetier et al., 2018)	Normal in OF and EP	**Impaired fear memory** Decreased freezing response in contextual and trace fear conditioning tests **Impaired spatial working memory** Decreased alternance in Y-maze tests Decreased correct arm entry in spatial novelty preference test (modified Y-maze) Normal in Morris water maze and radial maze tests	Increased distance traveled in OF in total 2 days
TRPC1,4,5 KO mice (Bröker-Lai et al., 2017)	N/D	**Impaired spatial working memory** Increased number of errors in T-maze and radial maze tests Normal spatial reference memory in Morris water maze test	N/D
TRPC4/TRPC5 channel inhibitor (M084) (Yang et al., 2015)	**M084 decreased anxiety-like behavior** Increased number of entries in light part in the LD Increased number of entries and time spent in open arms in EP	N/D	Normal in locomotor activity (no difference among control, CUS, and CUS + M084) M084 rescues the immobility which is increased by CUS in forced swim test M084 rescues the latency to feed which is increased by CUS in novelty suppressed feeding test
TRPC4/TRPC5 channel inhibitor (HC-070) (Just et al., 2018)	**HC-070 decreased anxiety-like behavior** HC-070 rescues open arm entries decreased by CCK-4 in EP Decreased number of buried marble in marble burying test	Rescued the freezing time which is increased by CSD in auditory and contextual freezing tests (HC-070 inhibited formation of trauma.)	Decreased immobility time in tail suspension and forced swim tests Normal locomotor activity in OF
TRPV1 KO mice (Marsch et al., 2007)	**Decreased anxiety-like behavior** Increased total distance moved in light part in LD Increased time and entries in open arms in EP Normal in OF	**Impaired fear memory** Decreased freezing response in auditory and contextual fear conditioning tests	Normal in auditory response
TRPA1 KO mice (Lee et al., 2017)	**Decreased anxiety-like behavior** Increased time spent in open arms in EP	**Enhanced fear memory** Increased freezing in auditory fear conditioning test **Enhanced spatial reference memory** Increased cross numbers in probe trial in Morris water maze test Increased discrimination index in novel location recognition	Enhanced social recognition behavior

(Continued)

TABLE 2 | Continued

	Anxiety	Memory	Other behavioral phenotype
Aged TRPA1 KO mice (Borbély et al., 2019) Young: 3–4 months old. Old: 18 months old	**Decreased anxiety-like behavior** Young TRPA1 KO mice show increased number of entries in center region compared with young WT in OF.	**Enhanced reference memory** Old TRPA1 KO mice show higher discrimination index compared with old WT in novel object recognition test. **Enhanced spatial working memory** Young TRPA1 KO mice show less reference memory error compared with young WT in radial maze test. Old TRPA1 KO mice show less exploration time compared with WT in radial maze test.	Young TRPA1 KO mice show higher velocity compared with young WT in radial maze test.

CSD, chronic social defeat; CUS, chronic unpredictable stress; EP, elevated plus-maze test; LD, light-dark transition test; N/D, not determined; OF, open field test

arginine to cysteine (R755C). Notably, the D543E mutation induces loss of function of TRPM2 activities, and *Trpm2* KO mice exhibit bipolar disorder-related behaviors, such as mood disturbances and impairments in social cognition (Jang et al., 2015) (**Table 2**). Interestingly, disruption of *Trpm2* increases phosphorylation of GSK-3, which is implicated as one of the main targets of lithium (Xie et al., 2011; Jang et al., 2015). Although the significance of GSK-3 in the pathology of bipolar disorder is still debated (Alda, 2015), these observations suggest that dysregulation of GSK-3 could, at least in part, account for the bipolar disorder-related behaviors induced by hypoactive TRPM2 mutations. Furthermore, a SNP of *TRPM2* has recently been identified as a risk factor for bipolar disorder in a Japanese population (Mahmuda et al., 2020). These lines of evidence suggest a link between defects in TRPM2 activities and the pathology of bipolar disorder.

In addition to the connection between TRPM2 and bipolar disorder, accumulating evidence has indicated the impact of TRPM2 on major depressive disorder. In a mouse model of depression via chronic unpredictable stress, disruption of *Trpm2* produced antidepressant-like behaviors accompanied by reduced ROS, suppressed ROS-induced calpain activation, and enhanced phosphorylation of two Cdk5 targets, synapsin 1 and histone deacetylase 5, which are linked to synaptic function and gene expression, respectively (Ko et al., 2019). Notably, while middle-aged (12–16 months) and aged (20–24 months) wild-type (WT) mice exhibited memory dysfunction compared with young (2–3 months) WT mice, these characteristics were undetectable in *Trpm2* KO mice (Kakae et al., 2019) (**Table 2**), potentially owing to defects in the sensing of oxidative stress, whose levels are increased by aging (Tan et al., 2018). *Trpm2* deficiency also attenuates social avoidance induced by repeated social defeat stress in mice (Andoh et al., 2019). Under physiological conditions, a comprehensive behavioral test battery has shown that *Trpm2* KO mice exhibit no behavioral phenotypes in light/dark transition, rotarod, elevated plus maze, social interaction, prepulse inhibition, Y-maze, forced swim, cued and contextual fear conditioning, and tail suspension tests (Andoh et al., 2019), whereas *Trpm2* KO mice were also reported to exhibit bipolar disorder-related behaviors (Jang et al., 2015) (**Table 2**). Differences in the genetic backgrounds of mice or the animal facilities and equipment used in the behavioral analyses could explain the inconsistency of the results. Collectively, these findings suggest that disruption of *Trpm2* potentially induces behavioral phenotypes in pathological conditions that could be related to oxidative stress.

TRPC4 and TRPC5 are highly expressed in the cortex and amygdala, the regions thought to be crucial in regulating anxiety (Riccio et al., 2009, 2014). Importantly, previous works with transgenic mice suggest that TRPC4 and TRPC5 play important roles in amygdala function, and thus inhibition of TRPC4 and TRPC5 have anxiolytic effects (Riccio et al., 2009, 2014). This implicates the significance of both TRPC4 and TRPC5 in innate fear function, which represents a key response to environmental stress. *Trpc5* KO mice exhibited diminished innate fear levels in response to innately aversive stimuli (Riccio et al., 2009) (**Table 2**). *Trpc4* KO mice also showed suppressed $G_{\alpha\ q/11}$-dependent responses in the amygdala, which regulate fear-related behavioral processes, and decreased anxiety-like behaviors (Riccio et al., 2014) (see "Neuronal and Glial Functions of Redox-Sensitive TRP Channels" section) (**Table 2**). *Trpc4* knockdown in the lateral amygdala via lentivirus-mediated gene delivery of RNAi mirrored the behavioral phenotype of constitutive *Trpc4* KO mice. Given that the animal model for the analysis of innate fear responses is limited, *Trpc4* and *Trpc5* KO mice may be useful animal models for investigating the mechanisms underlying the regulation of innate fear responses. It is worth noting that there is a caveat regarding interpretation of the behavioral data because *Trpc5* KO mice have deficits in gait and motor coordination (Puram et al., 2011).

In contrast to *Trpc4* and *Trpc5* KO mice, deletion of the *Trpc1* gene impairs fear memory formation but not innate fear behavior (Lepannetier et al., 2018), suggesting that TRPC1 regulates fear-related behavioral processes through distinct mechanisms from the TRPC5- and TRPC4-mediated pathways. In hippocampal functions, deletion of *Trpc1* impaired functioning in the Y-maze task, and the triple deficiency of *Trpc1/Trpc4/Trpc5* induced reduced performance in the T-maze and radial maze tests, while both *Trpc1* single KO and *Trpc1/Trpc4/Trpc5* triple KO mice showed normal acquisition in the Morris water maze task (Bröker-Lai et al., 2017; Lepannetier et al., 2018), suggesting that TRPC1 and possibly both TRPC4 and TRPC5 regulate spatial working memory but not spatial reference memory.

Pharmacological analysis in rats revealed that the TRPV1 antagonist, capsazepine, attenuates anxiety-like behaviors in the elevated-plus maze test (Kasckow et al., 2004). Consistent with this observation, *Trpv1* KO mice exhibited less anxiety-related behaviors in the elevated-plus maze test and in the light/dark test compared to their WT littermates (Marsch et al., 2007) (**Table 2**). Furthermore, *Trpv1* KO mice showed less freezing in auditory and contextual fear conditioning tests, suggesting that TRPV1 regulates fear memory formation (Marsch et al., 2007). Under stressful conditions, *in vivo* activation of TRPV1 by intrahippocampal or intragastrical infusion of capsaicin prevented the impairing spatial memory retrieval caused by acute inescapable stress by placing mice on an elevated platform (Li et al., 2008), suggesting that activation of TRPV1 induces anti-stress effects.

Trpa1 KO mice displayed decreased anxiety-like behaviors in elevated-plus maze, better performance in the fear conditioning and novel location recognition tests, and enhanced social

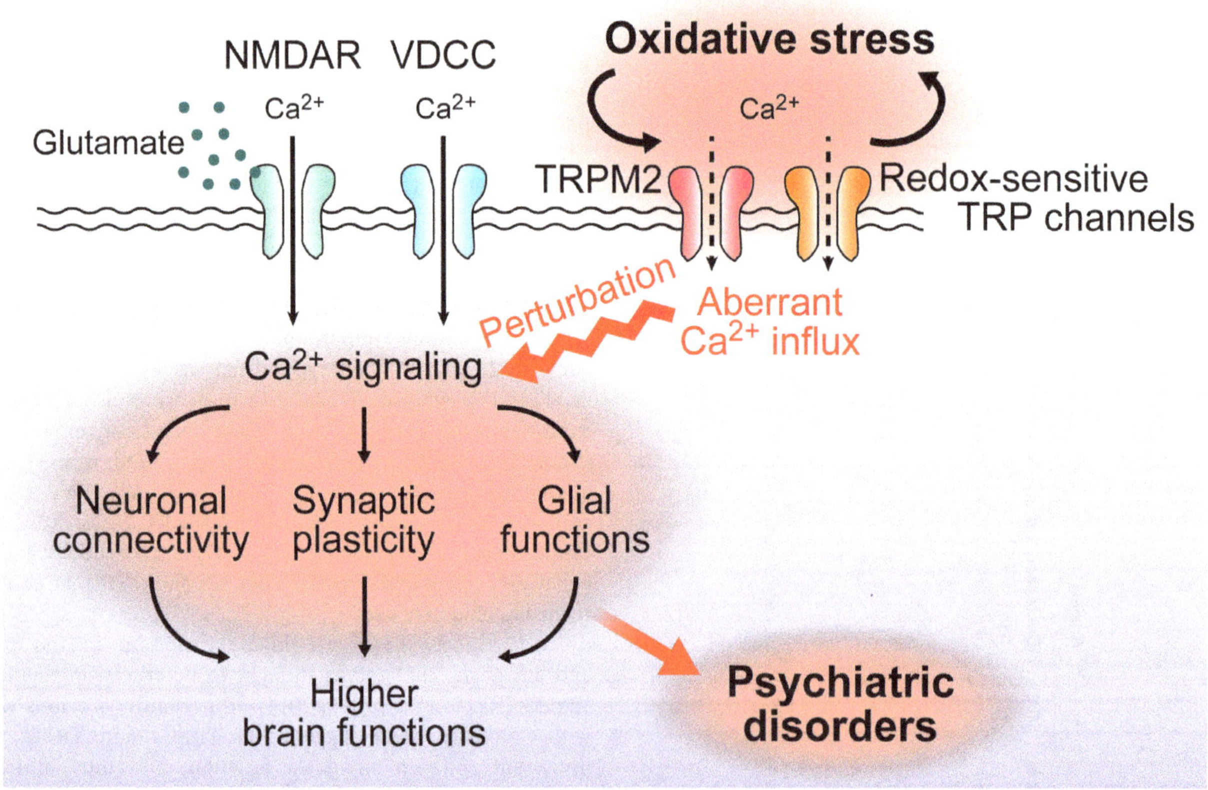

FIGURE 2 | A putative model for the impact of redox-sensitive TRP channels in the pathogenesis/pathophysiology of psychiatric disorders. VDCC- or NMDAR-mediated Ca^{2+} signaling plays fundamental roles in neural functions such as neuronal connectivity, synaptic plasticity, and glial functions, contributing to higher brain functions. Oxidative stress alters expression and activities of redox-sensitive TRP channels, which further enhances oxidative stress and induces a perturbation of the Ca^{2+} signaling mediated by VDCC or NMDAR. This could be associated with the pathogenesis/pathophysiology of psychiatric disorders. Notably, SNPs of *TRPM2* have been identified as a risk factor for bipolar disorder.

recognition behavior (Lee et al., 2017) (**Table 2**), possibly due, at least in part, to the evidence that TRPA1 negatively regulates hippocampal functions potentially through the suppression of neurite outgrowth (Lee et al., 2017). However, there is a caveat regarding the interpretation of the behavioral data because *Trpa1* KO mice are suggested to exhibit impaired motor function through axonal bundle fragmentation, downregulation of myelin basic protein, and decreased mature oligodendrocyte population in the brain (Lee et al., 2017); therefore, the observed behavioral phenotypes could be merely due to impaired motor functions rather than hippocampal functions. Interestingly, TRPA1 in astrocytes is implicated to partially contribute to cuprizone-induced demyelination, which is frequently used for the animal model of multiple sclerosis (Kriszta et al., 2020), raising the possibility that there is a connection between TRPA1 expression or function and psychiatric disorders. Notably, another behavioral analysis using aged (18-month-old) *Trpa1* KO mice supports the notion that TRPA1 negatively regulates hippocampal functions in an age-dependent manner (Borbély et al., 2019) (**Table 2**). Thus, these lines of evidence suggest that TRPA1 is a negative regulator of brain functions, raising the possibility that there is a connection between TRPA1 expression or function and psychiatric disorders; however, further studies are required to validate this hypothesis.

PERSPECTIVE

As described above, accumulating evidence has indicated that most redox-sensitive TRP channels have significant impacts on higher brain functions even though the role of oxidative stress as the activation trigger of the channels in this context is not fully understood. Comprehensive analysis of gene expression in normal brains and the brains of patients with psychiatric disorders would delineate the significance of redox-sensitive TRP channels in these disorders, where notably, TRPM2 expression is enhanced in hippocampal tissue samples from patients with major depressive disorder (Ko et al., 2019), and, furthermore, TRPA1 is upregulated in astrocytes of the hippocampus in the mouse model of Alzheimer's disease, in which oxidative stress is deeply involved (Lee et al., 2016). Given that oxidative stress is associated with psychiatric disorders and that the expression of redox-sensitive TRP channels is induced by oxidative stress partly via the activation of NRF2, an oxidant defense transcription factor (Takahashi et al., 2018), it is possible that upregulated redox-sensitive TRP channels are involved in the pathogenesis or pathophysiology of psychiatric disorders (**Figures 1, 2**).

The concept of excitation-inhibition balance in neuropsychiatric disorders has been considered as a framework for investigating their mechanisms (Sohal and Rubenstein, 2019). Given that TRPA1 has the highest oxidation sensitivity among the TRP channels (Takahashi et al., 2011b; Mori et al., 2016), it is likely that TRPA1 senses oxidative stress acutely and moderates the excitation-inhibition balance by regulating astrocyte resting $[Ca^{2+}]_i$, which affects inhibitory synapse efficacy through the reduction of GABA transport (Shigetomi et al., 2012). Recently, several studies have shown that treatment with novel TRPC4/TRPC5 channel inhibitors produce antidepressant and anxiolytic-like effects in mice, suggesting that TRPC4 and TRPC5 channels are novel molecular candidates for the treatment of psychiatric symptoms (Yang et al., 2015; Just et al., 2018) (**Table 2**). Thus, the investigation of redox-sensitive TRP channels in the pathogenesis/pathophysiology of psychiatric disorders may lead to the development of novel therapeutic strategies for the treatment of these disorders.

AUTHOR CONTRIBUTIONS

AN and NT generated the first draft of the manuscript. All authors contributed to the revisions.

REFERENCES

Abdalla, D. S., Monteiro, H. P., Oliveira, J. A., and Bechara, E. J. (1986). Activities of superoxide dismutase and glutathione peroxidase in schizophrenic and manic-depressive patients. *Clin. Chem.* 32, 805–807. doi: 10.1093/clinchem/32.5.805

Akyol, Ö, Herken, H., Uz, E., Fadıllıoğlu, E., Ünal, S., Sögüt, S., et al. (2002). The indices of endogenous oxidative and antioxidative processes in plasma from schizophrenic patients: the possible role of oxidant/antioxidant imbalance. *Prog. Neuropsychopharmacol. Biol. Psychiatry* 26, 995–1005. doi: 10.1016/S0278-5846(02)00220-8

Alda, M. (2015). Lithium in the treatment of bipolar disorder: pharmacology and pharmacogenetics. *Mol. Psychiatry* 20, 661–670. doi: 10.1038/mp.2015.4

Andoh, C., Nishitani, N., Hashimoto, E., Nagai, Y., Takao, K., Miyakawa, T., et al. (2019). TRPM2 confers susceptibility to social stress but is essential for behavioral flexibility. *Brain Res.* 1704, 68–77. doi: 10.1016/j.brainres.2018.09.031

Arvindakshan, M., Ghate, M., Ranjekar, P. K., Evans, D. R., and Mahadik, S. P. (2003). Supplementation with a combination of ω-3 fatty acids and antioxidants (vitamins E and C) improves the outcome of schizophrenia. *Schizophr. Res.* 62, 195–204. doi: 10.1016/S0920-9964(02)00284-0

Atmaca, M., Tezcan, E., Kuloglu, M., Ustundag, B., and Tunckol, H. (2004). Antioxidant enzyme and malondialdehyde valuesin social phobia before and after citalopram treatment. *Eur. Arch. Psychiatry Clin. Neurosci.* 254, 231–235. doi: 10.1007/s00406-004-0484-3

Ben Othmen, L., Mechri, A., Fendri, C., Bost, M., Chazot, G., Gaha, L., et al. (2008). Altered antioxidant defense system in clinically stable patients with schizophrenia and their unaffected siblings. *Prog. Neuropsychopharmacol. Biol. Psychiatry* 32, 155–159. doi: 10.1016/j.pnpbp.2007.08.003

Berk, M., Copolov, D. L., Dean, O., Lu, K., Jeavons, S., Schapkaitz, I., et al. (2008). N-acetyl cysteine for depressive symptoms in bipolar disorder—a double-blind randomized placebo-controlled trial. *Biol. Psychiatry* 64, 468–475. doi: 10.1016/j.biopsych.2008.04.022

Berk, M., Dean, O. M., Cotton, S. M., Jeavons, S., Tanious, M., Kohlmann, K., et al. (2014). The efficacy of adjunctive N-acetylcysteine in major depressive disorder: a double-blind, randomized, placebo-controlled trial. *J. Clin. Psychiatry* 75, 628–636. doi: 10.4088/JCP.13m08454

Berk, M., Turner, A., Malhi, G. S., Ng, C. H., Cotton, S. M., Dodd, S., et al. (2019). A randomised controlled trial of a mitochondrial therapeutic target for bipolar depression: mitochondrial agents, N-acetylcysteine, and placebo. *BMC Med.* 17:18. doi: 10.1186/s12916-019-1257-1

Bigos, K. L., Mattay, V. S., Callicott, J. H., Straub, R. E., Vakkalanka, R., Kolachana, B., et al. (2010). Genetic variation in CACNA1C affects brain circuitries related to mental illness. *Arch. Gen. Psychiatry* 67, 939–945. doi: 10.1001/archgenpsychiatry.2010.96

Bilici, M., Efe, H., Köroğlu, M. A., Uydu, H. A., Bekaroğlu, M., and Değer, O. (2001). Antioxidative enzyme activities and lipid peroxidation in major depression: alterations by antidepressant treatments. *J. Affect. Disord.* 64, 43–51. doi: 10.1016/S0165-0327(00)00199-3

Bond, C. E., and Greenfield, S. A. (2007). Multiple cascade effects of oxidative stress on astroglia. *Glia* 55, 1348–1361. doi: 10.1002/glia.20547

Borbély, É, Payrits, M., Hunyady, Á, Mezö, G., and Pintér, E. (2019). Important regulatory function of transient receptor potential ankyrin 1 receptors in age-related learning and memory alterations of mice. *GeroScience* 41, 643–654. doi: 10.1007/s11357-019-00083-1

Bröker-Lai, J., Kollewe, A., Schindeldecker, B., Pohle, J., Nguyen Chi, V., Mathar, I., et al. (2017). Heteromeric channels formed by TRPC1, TRPC4 and TRPC5 define hippocampal synaptic transmission and working memory. *EMBO J.* 36, 2770–2789. doi: 10.15252/embj.201696369

Catterall, W. A. (2011). Voltage-gated calcium channels. *Cold Spring Harb. Perspect. Biol.* 3:a003947. doi: 10.1101/cshperspect.a003947

Chávez, A. E., Hernández, V. M., Rodenas-Ruano, A., Chan, C. S., and Castillo, P. E. (2014). Compartment-specific modulation of GABAergic synaptic transmission by TRPV1 channels in the dentate gyrus. *J. Neurosci.* 34, 16621–16629. doi: 10.1523/JNEUROSCI.3635-14.2014

Clapham, D. E. (2003). TRP channels as cellular sensors. *Nature* 426, 517–524. doi: 10.1038/nature02196

Cotter, D. R., Pariante, C. M., and Everall, I. P. (2001). Glial cell abnormalities in major psychiatric disorders: the evidence and implications. *Brain Res. Bull.* 55, 585–595. doi: 10.1016/S0361-9230(01)00527-5

Dakhale, G., Khanzode, S., Khanzode, S., Saoji, A., Khobragade, L., and Turankar, A. (2004). Oxidative damage and schizophrenia: the potential benefit by atypical antipsychotics. *Neuropsychobiology* 49, 205–209. doi: 10.1159/000077368

Dakhale, G. N., Khanzode, S. D., Khanzode, S. S., and Saoji, A. (2005). Supplementation of vitamin C with atypical antipsychotics reduces oxidative stress and improves the outcome of schizophrenia. *Psychopharmacology* 182, 494–498. doi: 10.1007/s00213-005-0117-1

Davare, M. A., Fortin, D. A., Saneyoshi, T., Nygaard, S., Kaech, S., Banker, G., et al. (2009). Transient receptor potential canonical 5 channels activate Ca^{2+}/calmodulin kinase Iγ to promote axon formation in hippocampal neurons. *J. Neurosci.* 29, 9794–9808. doi: 10.1523/JNEUROSCI.1544-09.2009

Dhar, M., Wayman, G. A., Zhu, M., Lambert, T. J., Davare, M. A., and Appleyard, S. M. (2014). Leptin-induced spine formation requires TrpC channels and the CaM kinase cascade in the hippocampus. *J. Neurosci.* 34, 10022–10033. doi: 10.1523/JNEUROSCI.2868-13.2014

Di, A., Gao, X.-P., Qian, F., Kawamura, T., Han, J., Hecquet, C., et al. (2012). The redox-sensitive cation channel TRPM2 modulates phagocyte ROS production and inflammation. *Nat. Immunol.* 13, 29–34. doi: 10.1038/ni.2171

Ellegaard, P. K., Licht, R. W., Nielsen, R. E., Dean, O. M., Berk, M., Poulsen, H. E., et al. (2019). The efficacy of adjunctive N-acetylcysteine in acute bipolar depression: a randomized placebo-controlled study. *J. Affect. Disord.* 245, 1043–1051. doi: 10.1016/j.jad.2018.10.083

Ersan, S., Bakir, S., Erdal Ersan, E., and Dogan, O. (2006). Examination of free radical metabolism and antioxidant defence system elements in patients with obsessive-compulsive disorder. *Prog. Neuropsychopharmacol. Biol. Psychiatry* 30, 1039–1042. doi: 10.1016/j.pnpbp.2006.03.034

Fernandes, B. S., Dean, O. M., Dodd, S., Malhi, G. S., and Berk, M. (2016). N-acetylcysteine in depressive symptoms and functionality: a systematic review and meta-analysis. *J. Clin. Psychiatry* 77, 457–466. doi: 10.4088/JCP.15r09984

Ferreira, M. A. R., O'Donovan, M. C., Meng, Y. A., Jones, I. R., Ruderfer, D. M., Jones, L., et al. (2008). Collaborative genome-wide association analysis supports a role for ANK3 and CACNA1C in bipolar disorder. *Nat. Genet.* 40, 1056–1058. doi: 10.1038/ng.209

Fonfria, E., Murdock, P. R., Cusdin, F. S., Benham, C. D., Kelsell, R. E., and McNulty, S. (2006). Tissue distribution profiles of the human TRPM cation channel family. *J. Recept. Signal Transduct. Res.* 26, 159–178. doi: 10.1080/10799890600637506

Forlenza, M. J., and Miller, G. E. (2006). Increased serum levels of 8-Hydroxy-2′-deoxyguanosine in clinical depression. *Psychosom. Med.* 68, 1–7. doi: 10.1097/01.psy.0000195780.37277.2a

Gibson, H. E., Edwards, J. G., Page, R. S., Van Hook, M. J., and Kauer, J. A. (2008). TRPV1 channels mediate long-term depression at synapses on hippocampal interneurons. *Neuron* 57, 746–759. doi: 10.1016/j.neuron.2007.12.027

Golovina, V. A. (2005). Visualization of localized store-operated calcium entry in mouse astrocytes. Close proximity to the endoplasmic reticulum. *J. Physiol.* 564, 737–749. doi: 10.1113/jphysiol.2005.085035

Greka, A., Navarro, B., Oancea, E., Duggan, A., and Clapham, D. E. (2003). TRPC5 is a regulator of hippocampal neurite length and growth cone morphology. *Nat. Neurosci.* 6, 837–845. doi: 10.1038/nn1092

Griesi-Oliveira, K., Acab, A., Gupta, A. R., Sunaga, D. Y., Chailangkarn, T., Nicol, X., et al. (2015). Modeling non-syndromic autism and the impact of TRPC6 disruption in human neurons. *Mol. Psychiatry* 20, 1350–1365. doi: 10.1038/mp.2014.141

Hara, Y., Wakamori, M., Ishii, M., Maeno, E., Nishida, M., Yoshida, T., et al. (2002). LTRPC2 Ca^{2+}-permeable channel activated by changes in redox status confers susceptibility to cell death. *Mol. Cell* 9, 163–173. doi: 10.1016/S1097-2765(01)00438-5

He, Z., Jia, C., Feng, S., Zhou, K., Tai, Y., Bai, X., et al. (2012). TRPC5 channel is the mediator of neurotrophin-3 in regulating dendritic growth via CaMKIIα in rat hippocampal neurons. *J. Neurosci.* 32, 9383–9395. doi: 10.1523/JNEUROSCI.6363-11.2012

Herken, H., Gurel, A., Selek, S., Armutcu, F., Ozen, M. E., Bulut, M., et al. (2007). Adenosine deaminase, nitric oxide, superoxide dismutase, and xanthine oxidase in patients with major depression: impact of antidepressant treatment. *Arch. Med. Res.* 38, 247–252. doi: 10.1016/j.arcmed.2006.10.005

Herken, H., Uz, E., Özyurt, H., Söğüt, S., Virit, O., and Akyol, Ö (2001). Evidence that the activities of erythrocyte free radical scavenging enzymes and the products of lipid peroxidation are increased in different forms of schizophrenia. *Mol. Psychiatry* 6, 66–73. doi: 10.1038/sj.mp.4000789

Hinman, A., Chuang, H., Bautista, D. M., and Julius, D. (2006). TRP channel activation by reversible covalent modification. *Proc. Natl. Acad. Sci. U.S.A.* 103, 19564–19568. doi: 10.1073/pnas.0609598103

Hiroi, T., Wajima, T., Negoro, T., Ishii, M., Nakano, Y., Kiuchi, Y., et al. (2013). Neutrophil TRPM2 channels are implicated in the exacerbation of myocardial ischaemia/reperfusion injury. *Cardiovasc. Res.* 97, 271–281. doi: 10.1093/cvr/cvs332

Jang, Y., Lee, M. H., Lee, J., Jung, J., Lee, S. H., Yang, D.-J., et al. (2014). TRPM2 mediates the lysophosphatidic acid-induced neurite retraction in the developing brain. *Pflüg. Arch. Eur. J. Physiol.* 466, 1987–1998. doi: 10.1007/s00424-013-1436-4

Jang, Y., Lee, S. H., Lee, B., Jung, S., Khalid, A., Uchida, K., et al. (2015). TRPM2, a susceptibility gene for bipolar disorder, regulates glycogen synthase kinase-3 activity in the brain. *J. Neurosci.* 35, 11811–11823. doi: 10.1523/JNEUROSCI.5251-14.2015

Jeon, D., Kim, S., Chetana, M., Jo, D., Ruley, H. E., Lin, S.-Y., et al. (2010). Observational fear learning involves affective pain system and Cav1.2 Ca^{2+} channels in ACC. *Nat. Neurosci.* 13, 482–488. doi: 10.1038/nn.2504

Jeon, J.-P., Roh, S.-E., Wie, J., Kim, J., Kim, H., Lee, K.-P., et al. (2013). Activation of TRPC4β by Gαi subunit increases Ca^{2+} selectivity and controls neurite morphogenesis in cultured hippocampal neuron. *Cell Calcium* 54, 307–319. doi: 10.1016/j.ceca.2013.07.006

Just, S., Chenard, B. L., Ceci, A., Strassmaier, T., Chong, J. A., Blair, N. T., et al. (2018). Treatment with HC-070, a potent inhibitor of TRPC4 and TRPC5, leads to anxiolytic and antidepressant effects in mice. *PLoS One* 13:e0191225. doi: 10.1371/journal.pone.0191225

Kabir, Z. D., Martínez-Rivera, A., and Rajadhyaksha, A. M. (2017). From gene to behavior: L-type calcium channel mechanisms underlying neuropsychiatric symptoms. *Neurotherapeutics* 14, 588–613. doi: 10.1007/s13311-017-0532-0

Kaczmarek, J. S., Riccio, A., and Clapham, D. E. (2012). Calpain cleaves and activates the TRPC5 channel to participate in semaphorin 3A-induced neuronal growth cone collapse. *Proc. Natl. Acad. Sci. U.S.A.* 109, 7888–7892. doi: 10.1073/pnas.1205869109

Kakae, M., Miyanohara, J., Morishima, M., Nagayasu, K., Mori, Y., Shirakawa, H., et al. (2019). Pathophysiological role of TRPM2 in age-related cognitive impairment in mice. *Neuroscience* 408, 204–213. doi: 10.1016/j.neuroscience.2019.04.012

Kaneko, S., Kawakami, S., Hara, Y., Wakamori, M., Itoh, E., Minami, T., et al. (2006). A Critical Role of TRPM2 in neuronal cell death by hydrogen peroxide. *J. Pharmacol. Sci.* 101, 66–76. doi: 10.1254/jphs.FP0060128

Kasckow, J. W., Mulchahey, J. J., and Geracioti, T. D. Jr. (2004). Effects of the vanilloid agonist olvanil and antagonist capsazepine on rat behaviors. *Prog.*

Neuropsychopharmacol. Biol. Psychiatry 28, 291–295. doi: 10.1016/j.pnpbp.2003.10.007

Kashio, M., Sokabe, T., Shintaku, K., Uematsu, T., Fukuta, N., Kobayashi, N., et al. (2012). Redox signal-mediated sensitization of transient receptor potential melastatin 2 (TRPM2) to temperature affects macrophage functions. *Proc. Natl. Acad. Sci. U.S.A.* 109, 6745–6750. doi: 10.1073/pnas.1114193109

Kauer, J. A., and Gibson, H. E. (2009). Hot flash: TRPV channels in the brain. *Trends Neurosci.* 32, 215–224. doi: 10.1016/j.tins.2008.12.006

Khanzode, S. D., Dakhale, G. N., Khanzode, S. S., Saoji, A., and Palasodkar, R. (2003). Oxidative damage and major depression: the potential antioxidant action of selective serotonin re-uptake inhibitors. *Redox Rep.* 8, 365–370. doi: 10.1179/135100003225003393

Kheradpezhouh, E., Choy, J. M. C., Daria, V. R., and Arabzadeh, E. (2017). TRPA1 expression and its functional activation in rodent cortex. *Open Biol.* 7:160314. doi: 10.1098/rsob.160314

Knowles, H., Heizer, J. W., Li, Y., Chapman, K., Ogden, C. A., Andreasen, K., et al. (2011). Transient Receptor Potential Melastatin 2 (TRPM2) ion channel is required for innate immunity against Listeria monocytogenes. *Proc. Natl. Acad. Sci. U.S.A.* 108, 11578–11583. doi: 10.1073/pnas.1010678108

Ko, S. Y., Wang, S. E., Lee, H. K., Jo, S., Han, J., Lee, S. H., et al. (2019). Transient receptor potential melastatin 2 governs stress-induced depressive-like behaviors. *Proc. Natl. Acad. Sci. U.S.A.* 116, 1770–1775. doi: 10.1073/pnas.1814335116

Koch, M., Kreutz, S., Böttger, C., Grabiec, U., Ghadban, C., Korf, H.-W., et al. (2011). The cannabinoid WIN 55,212-2-mediated protection of dentate gyrus granule cells is driven by CB1 receptors and modulated by TRPA1 and Cav2.2 channels. *Hippocampus* 21, 554–564. doi: 10.1002/hipo.20772

Kozai, D., Ogawa, N., and Mori, Y. (2013). Redox regulation of transient receptor potential channels. *Antioxid. Redox Signal.* 21, 971–986. doi: 10.1089/ars.2013.5616

Kraft, R., Grimm, C., Grosse, K., Hoffmann, A., Sauerbruch, S., Kettenmann, H., et al. (2004). Hydrogen peroxide and ADP-ribose induce TRPM2-mediated calcium influx and cation currents in microglia. *Am. J. Physiol. Cell Physiol.* 286, C129–C137. doi: 10.1152/ajpcell.00331.2003

Kriszta, G., Nemes, B., Sándor, Z., Ács, P., Komoly, S., Berente, Z., et al. (2020). Investigation of cuprizone-induced demyelination in mGFAP-driven conditional transient receptor potential ankyrin 1 (TRPA1) receptor knockout mice. *Cells* 9:81. doi: 10.3390/cells9010081

Kuloglu, M., Atmaca, M., Tezcan, E., Gecici, Ö, Tunckol, H., and Ustundag, B. (2002a). Antioxidant enzyme activities and malondialdehyde levels in patients with obsessive-compulsive disorder. *Neuropsychobiology* 46, 27–32. doi: 10.1159/000063573

Kuloglu, M., Atmaca, M., Tezcan, E., Ustundag, B., and Bulut, S. (2002b). Antioxidant enzyme and malondialdehyde levels in patients with panic disorder. *Neuropsychobiology* 46, 186–189. doi: 10.1159/000067810

Kuloglu, M., Ustundag, B., Atmaca, M., Canatan, H., Tezcan, A. E., and Cinkilinc, N. (2002c). Lipid peroxidation and antioxidant enzyme levels in patients with schizophrenia and bipolar disorder. *Cell Biochem. Funct.* 20, 171–175. doi: 10.1002/cbf.940

Langwieser, N., Christel, C. J., Kleppisch, T., Hofmann, F., Wotjak, C. T., and Moosmang, S. (2010). Homeostatic switch in hebbian plasticity and fear learning after sustained loss of Cav1.2 calcium channels. *J. Neurosci.* 30, 8367–8375. doi: 10.1523/JNEUROSCI.4164-08.2010

Lee, A. S., Ra, S., Rajadhyaksha, A. M., Britt, J. K., De Jesus-Cortes, H., Gonzales, K. L., et al. (2012). Forebrain elimination of cacna1c mediates anxiety-like behavior in mice. *Mol. Psychiatry* 17, 1054–1055. doi: 10.1038/mp.2012.71

Lee, C. R., Machold, R. P., Witkovsky, P., and Rice, M. E. (2013). TRPM2 channels are required for NMDA-induced burst firing and contribute to H2O2-dependent modulation in substantia nigra pars reticulata GABAergic neurons. *J. Neurosci.* 33, 1157–1168. doi: 10.1523/JNEUROSCI.2832-12.2013

Lee, K.-I., Lee, H.-T., Lin, H.-C., Tsay, H.-J., Tsai, F.-C., Shyue, S.-K., et al. (2016). Role of transient receptor potential ankyrin 1 channels in Alzheimer's disease. *J. Neuroinflammation* 13:92. doi: 10.1186/s12974-016-0557-z

Lee, K.-I., Lin, H.-C., Lee, H.-T., Tsai, F.-C., and Lee, T.-S. (2017). Loss of transient receptor potential ankyrin 1 channel deregulates emotion, learning and memory, cognition, and social behavior in mice. *Mol. Neurobiol.* 54, 3606–3617. doi: 10.1007/s12035-016-9908-0

Lee, M., Cho, T., Jantaratnotai, N., Wang, Y. T., McGeer, E., and McGeer, P. L. (2010). Depletion of GSH in glial cells induces neurotoxicity: relevance to aging and degenerative neurological diseases. *FASEB J.* 24, 2533–2545. doi: 10.1096/fj.09-149997

Lepannetier, S., Gualdani, R., Tempesta, S., Schakman, O., Seghers, F., Kreis, A., et al. (2018). Activation of TRPC1 channel by metabotropic glutamate receptor mGluR5 modulates synaptic plasticity and spatial working memory. *Front. Cell. Neurosci.* 12:318. doi: 10.3389/fncel.2018.00318

Li, H.-B., Mao, R.-R., Zhang, J.-C., Yang, Y., Cao, J., and Xu, L. (2008). Antistress effect of TRPV1 channel on synaptic plasticity and spatial memory. *Biol. Psychiatry* 64, 286–292. doi: 10.1016/j.biopsych.2008.02.020

Li, M., Chen, C., Zhou, Z., Xu, S., and Yu, Z. (2012). A TRPC1-mediated increase in store-operated Ca^{2+} entry is required for the proliferation of adult hippocampal neural progenitor cells. *Cell Calcium* 51, 486–496. doi: 10.1016/j.ceca.2012.04.014

Li, Y., Jia, Y.-C., Cui, K., Li, N., Zheng, Z.-Y., Wang, Y., et al. (2005). Essential role of TRPC channels in the guidance of nerve growth cones by brain-derived neurotrophic factor. *Nature* 434, 894–898. doi: 10.1038/nature03477

Machado-Vieira, R., Andreazza, A. C., Viale, C. I., Zanatto, V., Cereser, V., Vargas, R., et al. (2007). Oxidative stress parameters in unmedicated and treated bipolar subjects during initial manic episode: a possible role for lithium antioxidant effects. *Neurosci. Lett.* 421, 33–36. doi: 10.1016/j.neulet.2007.05.016

Macpherson, L. J., Dubin, A. E., Evans, M. J., Marr, F., Schultz, P. G., Cravatt, B. F., et al. (2007). Noxious compounds activate TRPA1 ion channels through covalent modification of cysteines. *Nature* 445, 541–545. doi: 10.1038/nature05544

Mahmuda, N. A., Yokoyama, S., Munesue, T., Hayashi, K., Yagi, K., Tsuji, C., et al. (2020). One single nucleotide polymorphism of the TRPM2 channel gene identified as a risk factor in bipolar disorder associates with autism spectrum disorder in a japanese population. *Diseases* 8:4. doi: 10.3390/diseases8010004

Malarkey, E. B., Ni, Y., and Parpura, V. (2008). Ca^{2+} entry through TRPC1 channels contributes to intracellular Ca^{2+} dynamics and consequent glutamate release from rat astrocytes. *Glia* 56, 821–835. doi: 10.1002/glia.20656

Marsch, R., Foeller, E., Rammes, G., Bunck, M., Kössl, M., Holsboer, F., et al. (2007). Reduced anxiety, conditioned fear, and hippocampal long-term potentiation in transient receptor potential vanilloid type 1 receptor-deficient mice. *J. Neurosci.* 27, 832–839. doi: 10.1523/JNEUROSCI.3303-06.2007

McQuillin, A., Bass, N. J., Kalsi, G., Lawrence, J., Puri, V., Choudhury, K., et al. (2006). Fine mapping of a susceptibility locus for bipolar and genetically related unipolar affective disorders, to a region containing the C21ORF29 and TRPM2 genes on chromosome 21q22.3. *Mol. Psychiatry* 11, 134–142. doi: 10.1038/sj.mp.4001759

Montell, C., and Rubin, G. M. (1989). Molecular characterization of the drosophila trp locus: a putative integral membrane protein required for phototransduction. *Neuron* 2, 1313–1323. doi: 10.1016/0896-6273(89)90069-X

Moosmang, S., Haider, N., Klugbauer, N., Adelsberger, H., Langwieser, N., Müller, J., et al. (2005). Role of hippocampal Cav1.2 Ca^{2+} channels in NMDA receptor-independent synaptic plasticity and spatial memory. *J. Neurosci.* 25, 9883–9892. doi: 10.1523/JNEUROSCI.1531-05.2005

Moran, M. M., McAlexander, M. A., Bíró, T., and Szallasi, A. (2011). Transient receptor potential channels as therapeutic targets. *Nat. Rev. Drug Discov.* 10, 601–620. doi: 10.1038/nrd3456

Mori, Y., Takahashi, N., Polat, O. K., Kurokawa, T., Takeda, N., and Inoue, M. (2016). Redox-sensitive transient receptor potential channels in oxygen sensing and adaptation. *Pflüg. Arch. Eur. J. Physiol.* 468, 85–97. doi: 10.1007/s00424-015-1716-2

Nakao, A., Miki, T., Shoji, H., Nishi, M., Takeshima, H., Miyakawa, T., et al. (2015). Comprehensive behavioral analysis of voltage-gated calcium channel beta-anchoring and -regulatory protein knockout mice. *Front. Behav. Neurosci.* 9:141. doi: 10.3389/fnbeh.2015.00141

Ng, F., Berk, M., Dean, O., and Bush, A. I. (2008). Oxidative stress in psychiatric disorders: evidence base and therapeutic implications. *Int. J. Neuropsychopharmacol.* 11, 851–876. doi: 10.1017/S1461145707008401

Nilius, B., Owsianik, G., Voets, T., and Peters, J. A. (2007). Transient receptor potential cation channels in disease. *Physiol. Rev.* 87, 165–217. doi: 10.1152/physrev.00021.2006

Olah, M. E., Jackson, M. F., Li, H., Perez, Y., Sun, H.-S., Kiyonaka, S., et al. (2009). Ca^{2+}-dependent induction of TRPM2 currents in hippocampal neurons. *J. Physiol.* 587, 965–979. doi: 10.1113/jphysiol.2008.162289

Peet, M., Murphy, B., Shay, J., and Horrobin, D. (1998). Depletion of Omega-3 fatty acid levels in red blood cell membranes of depressive patients. *Biol. Psychiatry* 43, 315–319. doi: 10.1016/S0006-3223(97)00206-0

Penzes, P., Cahill, M. E., Jones, K. A., VanLeeuwen, J.-E., and Woolfrey, K. M. (2011). Dendritic spine pathology in neuropsychiatric disorders. *Nat. Neurosci.* 14, 285–293. doi: 10.1038/nn.2741

Perraud, A.-L., Takanishi, C. L., Shen, B., Kang, S., Smith, M. K., Schmitz, C., et al. (2005). Accumulation of free ADP-ribose from mitochondria mediates oxidative stress-induced gating of TRPM2 cation channels. *J. Biol. Chem.* 280, 6138–6148. doi: 10.1074/jbc.M411446200

Pires, P. W., and Earley, S. (2018). Neuroprotective effects of TRPA1 channels in the cerebral endothelium following ischemic stroke. *eLife* 7:e35316. doi: 10.7554/eLife.35316

Puram, S. V., Riccio, A., Koirala, S., Ikeuchi, Y., Kim, A. H., Corfas, G., et al. (2011). A TRPC5-regulated calcium signaling pathway controls dendrite patterning in the mammalian brain. *Genes Dev.* 25, 2659–2673. doi: 10.1101/gad.174060.111

Qiu, J., Fang, Y., Rønnekleiv, O. K., and Kelly, M. J. (2010). Leptin excites proopiomelanocortin neurons via activation of TRPC channels. *J. Neurosci.* 30, 1560–1565. doi: 10.1523/JNEUROSCI.4816-09.2010

Rah, S.-Y., Kwak, J.-Y., Chung, Y.-J., and Kim, U.-H. (2015). ADP-ribose/TRPM2-mediated Ca^{2+} signaling is essential for cytolytic degranulation and antitumor activity of natural killer cells. *Sci. Rep.* 5:9482. doi: 10.1038/srep09482

Ramírez-Barrantes, R., Cordova, C., Poblete, H., Muñoz, P., Marchant, I., Wianny, F., et al. (2016). Perspectives of TRPV1 function on the neurogenesis and neural plasticity. *Neural Plast.* 2016:e1568145. doi: 10.1155/2016/1568145

Ranjekar, P. K., Hinge, A., Hegde, M. V., Ghate, M., Kale, A., Sitasawad, S., et al. (2003). Decreased antioxidant enzymes and membrane essential polyunsaturated fatty acids in schizophrenic and bipolar mood disorder patients. *Psychiatry Res.* 121, 109–122. doi: 10.1016/S0165-1781(03)00220-8

Riccio, A., Li, Y., Moon, J., Kim, K.-S., Smith, K. S., Rudolph, U., et al. (2009). Essential role for TRPC5 in amygdala function and fear-related behavior. *Cell* 137, 761–772. doi: 10.1016/j.cell.2009.03.039

Riccio, A., Li, Y., Tsvetkov, E., Gapon, S., Yao, G. L., Smith, K. S., et al. (2014). Decreased anxiety-like behavior and Gαq/11-dependent responses in the amygdala of mice lacking TRPC4 channels. *J. Neurosci.* 34, 3653–3667. doi: 10.1523/JNEUROSCI.2274-13.2014

Ripke, S., Neale, B. M., Corvin, A., Walters, J. T. R., Farh, K.-H., Holmans, P. A., et al. (2014). Biological insights from 108 schizophrenia-associated genetic loci. *Nature* 511, 421–427. doi: 10.1038/nature13595

Ripke, S., Sanders, A. R., Kendler, K. S., Levinson, D. F., Sklar, P., Holmans, P. A., et al. (2011). Genome-wide association study identifies five new schizophrenia loci. *Nat. Genet.* 43, 969–976. doi: 10.1038/ng.940

Ritchie, H., and Roser, M. (2018). *Mental Health. Our World Data.* Available online at: https://ourworldindata.org/mental-health (accessed April 24, 2020).

Roberts, J. C., Davis, J. B., and Benham, C. D. (2004). [^{3}H]Resiniferatoxin autoradiography in the CNS of wild-type and TRPV1 null mice defines TRPV1 (VR-1) protein distribution. *Brain Res.* 995, 176–183. doi: 10.1016/j.brainres.2003.10.001

Sakaguchi, R., and Mori, Y. (2020). Transient receptor potential (TRP) channels: biosensors for redox environmental stimuli and cellular status. *Free Radic. Biol. Med.* 146, 36–44. doi: 10.1016/j.freeradbiomed.2019.10.415

Sarandol, A., Sarandol, E., Eker, S. S., Erdinc, S., Vatansever, E., and Kirli, S. (2007). Major depressive disorder is accompanied with oxidative stress: short-term antidepressant treatment does not alter oxidative–antioxidative systems. *Hum. Psychopharmacol. Clin. Exp.* 22, 67–73. doi: 10.1002/hup.829

Sawamura, S., Shirakawa, H., Nakagawa, T., Mori, Y., and Kaneko, S. (2017). "TRP channels in the brain: what are they there for?," in *Neurobiology of TRP Channels Frontiers in Neuroscience*, ed. T. L. R. Emir (Boca Raton, FL: CRC Press/Taylor & Francis).

Sepehrmanesh, Z., Heidary, M., Akasheh, N., Akbari, H., and Heidary, M. (2018). Therapeutic effect of adjunctive N-acetyl cysteine (NAC) on symptoms of chronic schizophrenia: a double-blind, randomized clinical trial. *Prog. Neuropsychopharmacol. Biol. Psychiatry* 82, 289–296. doi: 10.1016/j.pnpbp.2017.11.001

Shigetomi, E., Jackson-Weaver, O., Huckstepp, R. T., O'Dell, T. J., and Khakh, B. S. (2013). TRPA1 channels are regulators of astrocyte basal calcium levels and long-term potentiation via constitutive d-serine release. *J. Neurosci.* 33, 10143–10153. doi: 10.1523/JNEUROSCI.5779-12.2013

Shigetomi, E., Tong, X., Kwan, K. Y., Corey, D. P., and Khakh, B. S. (2012). TRPA1 channels regulate astrocyte resting calcium and inhibitory synapse efficacy through GAT-3. *Nat. Neurosci.* 15, 70–80. doi: 10.1038/nn.3000

Shim, S., Yuan, J. P., Kim, J. Y., Zeng, W., Huang, G., Milshteyn, A., et al. (2009). Peptidyl-Prolyl isomerase FKBP52 controls chemotropic guidance of neuronal growth cones via regulation of TRPC1 channel opening. *Neuron* 64, 471–483. doi: 10.1016/j.neuron.2009.09.025

Sivrioglu, E. Y., Kirli, S., Sipahioglu, D., Gursoy, B., and Sarandöl, E. (2007). The impact of ω-3 fatty acids, vitamins E and C supplementation on treatment outcome and side effects in schizophrenia patients treated with haloperidol: an open-label pilot study. *Prog. Neuropsychopharmacol. Biol. Psychiatry* 31, 1493–1499. doi: 10.1016/j.pnpbp.2007.07.004

Sklar, P., Gabriel, S. B., McInnis, M. G., Bennett, P., Lim, Y.-M., Tsan, G., et al. (2002). Family-based association study of 76 candidate genes in bipolar disorder: BDNF is a potential risk locus. *Mol. Psychiatry* 7, 579–593. doi: 10.1038/sj.mp.4001058

Sklar, P., Ripke, S., Scott, L. J., Andreassen, O. A., Cichon, S., Craddock, N., et al. (2011). Large-scale genome-wide association analysis of bipolar disorder identifies a new susceptibility locus near ODZ4. *Nat. Genet.* 43, 977–983. doi: 10.1038/ng.943

Sohal, V. S., and Rubenstein, J. L. R. (2019). Excitation-inhibition balance as a framework for investigating mechanisms in neuropsychiatric disorders. *Mol. Psychiatry* 24, 1248–1257. doi: 10.1038/s41380-019-0426-0

Song, X., Zhao, Y., Narcisse, L., Duffy, H., Kress, Y., Lee, S., et al. (2005). Canonical transient receptor potential channel 4 (TRPC4) co-localizes with the scaffolding protein ZO-1 in human fetal astrocytes in culture. *Glia* 49, 418–429. doi: 10.1002/glia.20128

Stokes, A., Wakano, C., Koblan-Huberson, M., Adra, C. N., Fleig, A., and Turner, H. (2006). TRPA1 is a substrate for de-ubiquitination by the tumor suppressor CYLD. *Cell. Signal.* 18, 1584–1594. doi: 10.1016/j.cellsig.2005.12.009

Straub, R. E., Lehner, T., Luo, Y., Loth, J. E., Shao, W., Sharpe, L., et al. (1994). A possible vulnerability locus for bipolar affective disorder on chromosome 21q22.3. *Nat. Genet.* 8, 291–296. doi: 10.1038/ng1194-291

Sun, B., Bang, S.-I., and Jin, Y.-H. (2009). Transient receptor potential A1 increase glutamate release on brain stem neurons. *NeuroReport* 20, 1002–1006. doi: 10.1097/WNR.0b013e32832d2219

Takahashi, N., Chen, H.-Y., Harris, I. S., Stover, D. G., Selfors, L. M., Bronson, R. T., et al. (2018). Cancer cells co-opt the neuronal redox-sensing channel TRPA1 to promote oxidative-stress tolerance. *Cancer Cell* 33, 985.e7–1003.e7. doi: 10.1016/j.ccell.2018.05.001

Takahashi, N., Kozai, D., Kobayashi, R., Ebert, M., and Mori, Y. (2011a). Roles of TRPM2 in oxidative stress. *Cell Calcium* 50, 279–287. doi: 10.1016/j.ceca.2011.04.006

Takahashi, N., Kuwaki, T., Kiyonaka, S., Numata, T., Kozai, D., Mizuno, Y., et al. (2011b). TRPA1 underlies a sensing mechanism for O_2. *Nat. Chem. Biol.* 7, 701–711. doi: 10.1038/nchembio.640

Takahashi, N., Mizuno, Y., Kozai, D., Yamamoto, S., Kiyonaka, S., Shibata, T., et al. (2008). Molecular characterization of TRPA1 channel activation by cysteine-reactive inflammatory mediators. *Channels* 2, 287–298. doi: 10.4161/chan.2.4.6745

Takahashi, N., and Mori, Y. (2011). TRP channels as sensors and signal integrators of redox status changes. *Front. Pharmacol.* 2:58. doi: 10.3389/fphar.2011.00058

Takizawa, M., Harada, K., Nakamura, K., and Tsuboi, T. (2018). Transient receptor potential ankyrin 1 channels are involved in spontaneous peptide hormone release from astrocytes. *Biochem. Biophys. Res. Commun.* 501, 988–995. doi: 10.1016/j.bbrc.2018.05.097

Tan, B. L., Norhaizan, M. E., Liew, W.-P.-P., and Sulaiman Rahman, H. (2018). Antioxidant and oxidative stress: a mutual interplay in age-related diseases. *Front. Pharmacol.* 9:1162. doi: 10.3389/fphar.2018.01162

Togashi, K., Hara, Y., Tominaga, T., Higashi, T., Konishi, Y., Mori, Y., et al. (2006). TRPM2 activation by cyclic ADP-ribose at body temperature is involved in insulin secretion. *EMBO J.* 25, 1804–1815. doi: 10.1038/sj.emboj.7601083

Uchida, K., Dezaki, K., Damdindorj, B., Inada, H., Shiuchi, T., Mori, Y., et al. (2011). Lack of TRPM2 impaired insulin secretion and glucose metabolisms in mice. *Diabetes Metab. Res. Rev.* 60, 119–126. doi: 10.2337/db10-0276

Uchiyama, M., Nakao, A., Kurita, Y., Fukushi, I., Takeda, K., Numata, T., et al. (2020). O_2-dependent protein internalization underlies astrocytic sensing of acute hypoxia by restricting multimodal TRPA1 channel responses. *Curr. Biol.* 30, 3378.e7–3396.e7. doi: 10.1016/j.cub.2020.06.047

Voets, T., Talavera, K., Owsianik, G., and Nilius, B. (2005). Sensing with TRP channels. *Nat. Chem. Biol.* 1, 85–92. doi: 10.1038/nchembio0705-85

Wang, G. X., and Poo, M. (2005). Requirement of TRPC channels in netrin-1-induced chemotropic turning of nerve growth cones. *Nature* 434, 898–904. doi: 10.1038/nature03478

Wang, S., Zhang, A.-P., Kurada, L., Matsui, T., and Lei, S. (2011). Cholecystokinin facilitates neuronal excitability in the entorhinal cortex via activation of TRPC-like channels. *J. Neurophysiol.* 106, 1515–1524. doi: 10.1152/jn.00025.2011

White, J. A., McKinney, B. C., John, M. C., Powers, P. A., Kamp, T. J., and Murphy, G. G. (2008). Conditional forebrain deletion of the L-type calcium channel CaV1.2 disrupts remote spatial memories in mice. *Learn. Mem.* 15, 1–5. doi: 10.1101/lm.773208

Xie, Y.-F., Belrose, J. C., Lei, G., Tymianski, M., Mori, Y., MacDonald, J. F., et al. (2011). Dependence of NMDA/GSK-3β Mediated Metaplasticity on TRPM2 Channels at Hippocampal CA3-CA1 Synapses. *Mol. Brain* 4:44. doi: 10.1186/1756-6606-4-44

Xu, S.-Z., Sukumar, P., Zeng, F., Li, J., Jairaman, A., English, A., et al. (2008). TRPC channel activation by extracellular thioredoxin. *Nature* 451, 69–72. doi: 10.1038/nature06414

Yamamoto, S., Shimizu, S., Kiyonaka, S., Takahashi, N., Wajima, T., Hara, Y., et al. (2008). TRPM2-mediated Ca^{2+} influx induces chemokine production in monocytes that aggravates inflammatory neutrophil infiltration. *Nat. Med.* 14, 738–747. doi: 10.1038/nm1758

Yan, H.-D., Villalobos, C., and Andrade, R. (2009). TRPC channels mediate a muscarinic receptor-induced afterdepolarization in cerebral cortex. *J. Neurosci.* 29, 10038–10046. doi: 10.1523/JNEUROSCI.1042-09.2009

Yang, L.-P., Jiang, F.-J., Wu, G.-S., Deng, K., Wen, M., Zhou, X., et al. (2015). Acute Treatment with a Novel TRPC4/C5 channel inhibitor produces antidepressant and anxiolytic-like effects in mice. *PLoS One* 10:e0136255. doi: 10.1371/journal.pone.0136255

Yokoyama, T., Ohbuchi, T., Saito, T., Sudo, Y., Fujihara, H., Minami, K., et al. (2011). Allyl isothiocyanates and cinnamaldehyde potentiate miniature excitatory postsynaptic inputs in the supraoptic nucleus in rats. *Eur. J. Pharmacol.* 655, 31–37. doi: 10.1016/j.ejphar.2011.01.011

Yoshida, T., Inoue, R., Morii, T., Takahashi, N., Yamamoto, S., Hara, Y., et al. (2006). Nitric oxide activates TRP channels by cysteine S-nitrosylation. *Nat. Chem. Biol.* 2, 596–607. doi: 10.1038/nchembio821

Zamponi, G. W., Striessnig, J., Koschak, A., and Dolphin, A. C. (2015). The physiology, pathology, and pharmacology of voltage-gated calcium channels and their future therapeutic potential. *Pharmacol. Rev.* 67, 821–870. doi: 10.1124/pr.114.009654

Zhang, X. Y., Zhou, D. F., Cao, L. Y., Zhang, P. Y., Wu, G. Y., and Shen, Y. C. (2003). The effect of risperidone treatment on superoxide dismutase in schizophrenia. *J. Clin. Psychopharmacol.* 23, 128–131.

3

Contribution of NAADP to Glutamate-Evoked Changes in Ca^{2+} Homeostasis in Mouse Hippocampal Neurons

Julia Hermann[1], Melanie Bender[1], Dagmar Schumacher[1,2], Marcel S. Woo[3], Artem Shaposhnykov[3], Sina C. Rosenkranz[3], Vladimir Kuryshev[1,2], Chris Meier[4], Andreas H. Guse[5], Manuel A. Friese[3], Marc Freichel[1,2] and Volodymyr Tsvilovskyy[1,2]**

[1] Institute of Pharmacology, Heidelberg University, Heidelberg, Germany, [2] DZHK (German Centre for Cardiovascular Research), Partner Site Heidelberg/Mannheim, Heidelberg, Germany, [3] Institut für Neuroimmunologie und Multiple Sklerose, Universitätsklinikum Hamburg-Eppendorf, Hamburg, Germany, [4] Organic Chemistry, Department of Chemistry, University of Hamburg, Hamburg, Germany, [5] The Calcium Signaling Group, Department of Biochemistry and Molecular Cell Biology, University Medical Center Hamburg-Eppendorf, Hamburg, Germany

***Correspondence:**
Marc Freichel
marc.freichel@pharma.uni-heidelberg.de
Volodymyr Tsvilovskyy
volodymyr.tsvilovskyy@pharma.uni-heidelberg.de

Nicotinic acid adenine dinucleotide phosphate (NAADP) is a second messenger that evokes calcium release from intracellular organelles by the engagement of calcium release channels, including members of the Transient Receptor Potential (TRP) family, such as TRPML1, the (structurally) related Two Pore Channel type 1 (TPC1) and TPC2 channels as well as Ryanodine Receptors type 1 (RYR1; Guse, 2012). NAADP evokes calcium release from acidic calcium stores of many cell types (Guse, 2012), and NAADP-sensitive Ca^{2+} stores have been described in hippocampal neurons of the rat (Bak et al., 1999; McGuinness et al., 2007). Glutamate triggers Ca^{2+}-mediated neuronal excitotoxicity in inflammation-induced neurodegenerative pathologies such as Multiple Sclerosis (MS; Friese et al., 2014), and when applied extracellularly to neurons glutamate can elevate NAADP levels in these cells. Accordingly, glutamate-evoked Ca^{2+} signals from intracellular organelles were inhibited by preventing organelle acidification (Pandey et al., 2009). Analysis of reported RNA sequencing experiments of cultured hippocampal neurons revealed the abundance of Mcoln1 (encoding TRPML1), Tpcn1, and Tpcn2 (encoding TPC1 and TPC2, respectively) as potential NAADP target channels in these cells. Transcripts encoding Ryr1 were not found in contrast to Ryr2 and Ryr3. To study the contribution of NAADP signaling to glutamate-evoked calcium transients in murine hippocampal neurons we used the NAADP antagonists Ned-19 (Naylor et al., 2009) and BZ194 (Dammermann et al., 2009). Our results show that both NAADP antagonists significantly reduce glutamate-evoked calcium transients. In addition to extracellular glutamate application, we studied synchronized calcium oscillations in the cells of the neuronal cultures evoked by addition of the $GABA_A$ receptor antagonist bicuculline. Pretreatment with Ned-19 (50 μM) or BZ194 (100 μM) led to an increase in the frequency of bicuculline-induced calcium oscillations at the cost of calcium transient amplitudes. Interestingly, Ned-19 triggered a rise in intracellular calcium concentrations 25 min after bicuculline stimulation, leading to the question whether NAADP acts as a neuroprotective messenger in hippocampal neurons. Taken together, our results are in agreement with the concept that NAADP signaling significantly contributes to glutamate evoked Ca^{2+} rise in hippocampal neurons and to the amplitude and frequency of synchronized Ca^{2+} oscillations triggered by spontaneous glutamate release events.

Keywords: hippocampal neurons, glutamate, NAADP, Ca^{2+} homeostasis, neuronal excitotoxicity

INTRODUCTION

In neurons, changes of free intracellular calcium ion concentration [$(Ca^{2+})_i$] regulate many physiological functions such as neuronal plasticity, gene transcription and synaptic transmission (Ureshino et al., 2019). Defects in Ca^{2+} homeostasis are a reasonable cause for cell death and, eventually, neurodegeneration (Wojda et al., 2008; Szydlowska and Tymianski, 2010). Under these conditions, the homeostatic system, which assures low $[Ca^{2+}]_i$ in the range of 100 nM (in resting conditions), is defective (Nedergaard and Verkhratsky, 2010; Zundorf and Reiser, 2011). The tight equilibrium in $[Ca^{2+}]_i$ is usually maintained by a large number of ion channels and transporters in the plasma membrane as well as in the intracellular compartments of the cell.

Exaggerated rise in $[Ca^{2+}]_i$, which can be triggered by glutamate accumulation, e.g., after hypoxia, leads to apoptosis and necrotic cell death. Glutamate-evoked changes in intracellular Ca^{2+} homeostasis involve the activation of ionotropic NMDA, AMPA, and kainate (KA) receptors, as well as the mechanisms downstream of the activation of metabotropic glutamate receptors (mGluRs; Reiner and Levitz, 2018). The underlying processes of Ca^{2+}-overload mediated toxicity may include over-activation of several types of enzymes, e.g., proteases of the calpain family, phosphatase calcineurin, nitric oxide synthases, endonucleases (leading to DNA fragmentation), and phospholipid scramblase leading to phosphatidyl-choline PS exposure in the outer leaflet of the plasma membrane (Orrenius et al., 2003; Hardingham and Bading, 2010). In acute (e.g., following cerebral ischemia) or chronic neurodegenerative diseases, such as Alzheimer's disease (AD), Parkinson's disease (PD), and Multiple sclerosis (MS), glutamate elevations evoke an impairment of mitochondrial function, survival-promoting gene expression and the maintenance of structural integrity of neurons that all act in concert during the development of neurodegeneration (Bading, 2017). Impaired Ca^{2+} homeostasis in familial forms of AD is thought to occur from a dysfunction of presenilins, which act as Ca^{2+} release channel in the ER, a subsequent Ca^{2+} accumulation in the ER, and downregulation of neuronal store-operated Ca^{2+} entry (Popugaeva et al., 2017). Furthermore, Aß42/40 proteins fragments, which arise by proteolysis from the amyloid precursor protein (APP) and aggregate to neurotoxic oligomers, can form Ca^{2+}-permeable pores in the plasma membrane and modulate activity of voltage dependent calcium channels and NMDA receptors. Elevated ER Ca^{2+} content leads to enhanced Ca^{2+} release via D-*myo*-inositol 1, 4, 5-trisphosphate receptors (IP_3R), and ryanodine receptors (RYR) as well as Ca^{2+} accumulation in the cytosol (Popugaeva et al., 2017). In PD the impaired Ca^{2+} homeostasis leading to increased vulnerability in dopaminergic neurons of the substantia nigra is characterized by an activity-related oscillatory intracellular Ca^{2+} load potentially caused by the altered activity of multiple Ca^{2+} conducting channels including store-operated channels, ionotropic glutamate receptors, and voltage gated Ca_V1 channels (Duda et al., 2016). Notably, the application of dihydropyridines as negative allosteric modulators of Ca_V1 Ca^{2+} channels is associated with a decreased risk and progression of PD (Surmeier et al., 2017).

Glutamate-evoked neurotoxicity is also a key process in the pathogenesis of MS, and glutamate levels are elevated in the CSF and brains of MS patients. A growing body of evidence has suggested that the inflammatory insults in MS determine neurodegeneration by alterations of ion exchange mechanisms and here in particular Ca^{2+} handling (Friese et al., 2014). Dysregulation of cellular Ca^{2+} homeostasis evoked by glutamate was previously considered to be a result of Ca^{2+} entry via ionotropic glutamate receptors; however, our recent studies have identified that the neuronally expressed Na^+- and Ca^{2+}-permeable acid sensing ion channel-1 (ASIC1) and Ca^{2+}-activated transient receptor potential melastatin 4 (TRPM4) crucially contribute to maladaptive cation handling under inflammatory conditions (Friese et al., 2007; Schattling et al., 2012). Specifically, our studies showed that neuronal Ca^{2+} overload with excessive activation of Ca^{2+}-dependent processes may be one component of neuronal injury. However, the constituents of channels in both the plasmalemmal and intracellular organelles contributing to cytosolic Ca^{2+} rise, as well as the mechanisms by which intracellular Ca^{2+} homeostasis is orchestrated, e.g., by providing a sufficient buffering capacity during neuroinflammation, remain to be poorly understood.

The cellular Ca^{2+} homeostasis can be modulated not only by Ca^{2+} channels in the plasma membrane, but also by Ca^{2+} release from intracellular Ca^{2+} stores. Organelles that function as Ca^{2+} stores with a major impact on cytosolic Ca^{2+} homeostasis include (i) the mitochondrion, (ii) the endoplasmic reticulum, and (iii) the lysosomes that can buffer and release Ca^{2+}. Over the last years, numerous studies have revealed that glutamate stimulation in neurons evokes, in addition to IP_3, the synthesis of Nicotinic acid adenine dinucleotide phosphate (NAADP) and Ca^{2+} release from acidic stores. NAADP-sensitive Ca^{2+} stores have been described in brain microsomes (Bak et al., 1999) and in lysosome-related organelles in hippocampal neurons of the rat (Bak et al., 1999; McGuinness et al., 2007). Extracellular glutamate application is able to elevate cellular NAADP levels in hippocampal neurons, and glutamate-evoked Ca^{2+} signals from intracellular organelles were inhibited by antagonizing acidification of lysosomes (Pandey et al., 2009). A recent study has also shown that Ca^{2+} entry via voltage gated Ca^{2+} channels triggers Ca^{2+} release from the lysosome via an NAADP-sensitive channel and, subsequently, fusion of the lysosome with the plasma membrane (Padamsey et al., 2017). In addition, metabotropic glutamate receptor 1 (mGluR1) has been reported to couple to NAADP signaling eliciting Ca^{2+} release from acidic stores via TPC channels during synaptic plasticity (Foster et al., 2018). In non-neuronal cells the NAADP-evoked Ca^{2+} release depends on ryanodine receptors, such as on Ryanodine Receptors type 1 (RYR1) in *T* cells (Diercks et al., 2018), and on TRPML1 channels in fibroblasts (Zhang et al., 2011).

In this study we aimed to investigate the contribution of NAADP signaling to glutamate evoked calcium transients in murine hippocampal neurons following extracellular glutamate application using NAADP antagonists. A second set of experiments was performed under conditions of facilitated spontaneous glutamate release events by pharmacological inhibition of $GABA_A$ receptors that, while being active, exhibit an inhibitory influence on neurotransmitter exocytosis. The results of our experiments reveal that the NAADP antagonists Ned-19 (Naylor et al., 2009) and BZ194 (Dammermann et al., 2009), respectively, significantly reduced glutamate evoked calcium transients in neurons upon extracellularly applied glutamate and that these NAADP antagonists increase the frequencies of bicuculline-evoked calcium oscillations at the cost of lower calcium transient amplitudes supporting the concept that NAADP signaling significantly contributes to glutamate evoked Ca^{2+} rise in hippocampal neurons.

MATERIALS AND METHODS

Isolation of Hippocampal Neurons From Mouse Embryos

Pregnant females (E16.5) from timed mating were euthanized by CO_2 inhalation. Embryos were isolated after ovarian section. After removal of the placenta and the uterus the embryos were placed in a Petri dish with 25 ml ice cold Hanks' Balanced Salt Solution (ThermoFisher). Hippocampi were dissected from the embryo's head under a stereo microscope (8× magnification, Stemi SV4, Carl Zeiss) and digested with trypsin/EDTA (Sigma-Aldrich) and warmed to 37°C. For each independent cell preparation hippocampi from at least 4 Embryos were pooled. Cells were dissociated by repeated trituration steps using a Pasteur pipette and filtered using a cell strainer (40 μm, Corning). Thereafter, cells were centrifuged (1.700*g*, 2 min), and resuspended in Neurobasal medium (Neurobasal medium, ThermoFisher: 21103049, supplemented with 1% Penicillin-Streptomycin, 45 μM ß-Mercaptoethanol, 1× B27 Supplement, and 0.5 mM GlutaMAX-I). Cells were then plated on Poly-D-lysine coated coverslips (382.000 cells per coverslip, diameter 18 mm) and cultured in 12 well plates at 37°C and 5% CO_2 in Neurobasal medium supplemented with 1% Penicillin-Streptomycin, 45 μM ß-Mercaptoethanol, 1 × B27 Supplement, and 0.5 mM GlutaMAX-I. At day 3 after plating, cells were treated with Ara-C (500 nM) to prevent proliferation of glial cells. Medium was changed at day 6 or 7 and microfluorimetric calcium imaging experiments were performed at day 13 to 15 *in vitro* (d.i.v.).

All animal procedures were approved and performed according to the regulations of the Regierungspräsidium Karlsruhe and the University Heidelberg (*T* 25/16) and conformed to the guidelines from the directive 2010/63/EU of the European Parliament on the protection of animals used for scientific purposes.

Fluorimetric $[Ca^{2+}]_i$ Measurements

Cultured hippocampal neuronal cells were loaded with a fluorescent Ca^{2+} indicator Fura-2 by incubation in Physiological Salt Solution (PSS) supplemented with 2 μM Fura-2 AM (Thermo Fisher Scientific, Darmstadt, Germany) and 0.1% Pluronic F-127 (Sigma-Aldrich Chemie GmbH, Steinheim, Germany) for 30 min at room temperature and prior to imaging were washed with PSS. The PSS had the following composition (in mM): NaCl 140, KCl 5, $CaCl_2$ 2, $MgCl_2$ 1, HEPES 20, and Glucose 10. For the preparation of high potassium solution (60 mM), NaCl was equimolarly replaced by KCl. The imaging set-up was built on a base of a fluorescence microscope Axio Observer A1 equipped with a Fluar 20×/0.75 objective (both Zeiss, Germany). Excitation at 340 nm and 380 nm (exposure time 100 ms) was achieved using a polychrome V monochromator (Till Photonics, Germany) and the emitted light with a cut off filter >500 nm was collected by a CMOS camera (ORCA-flash 4.0, Hamamatsu Photonics, Japan). The acquisition frequency was 1 Hz. The monochromator and the CMOS camera were controlled by the ZEN 2.0 Pro (Zeiss, Germany) acquisition software. Regions of interest (ROIs) were placed at cell somata and the fluorescence signals were background corrected. The time course of $[Ca^{2+}]_i$ changes was presented as F340/F380 ratio. All experiments were performed at room temperature.

Glutamate and Bafilomycin A1 were purchased from Sigma-Aldrich, Ned-19 was purchased from Santa Cruz Biotechnology. BZ194 was synthesized as described (Dammermann et al., 2009). After 5 min of baseline recording glutamate or bicuculline were applied and changes in $[Ca^{2+}]_i$ were monitored for 15 (glutamate) or 25 min (bicuculline) treatment. Thereafter, high-potassium solution (60 mM) was applied to identify excitable cells.

The change of basal $[Ca^{2+}]_i$ (**Figures 5J,N,R**) was calculated from the F 340/380 ratios at the time point 30 min subtracted by the F340/380 values at the time point 5 min.

Gene Expression Analysis

Gene expression analysis was performed using the data of high throughput mRNA sequencing. Raw gene counts were taken from the gene expression omnibus (GEO) database under the accession numbers GSE104802 (Mao et al., 2018) and GSE142064 (unpublished[1]).For the unstimulated control samples of each dataset transcripts per kilobase million (TPM) were calculated and normalized to the mean mRNA expression

[1]https://www.ncbi.nlm.nih.gov/geo/query/acc.cgi?acc=GSE142064

value of the depicted genes from each dataset. Data processing and visualization were performed within the R environment (Version 1.2.5001).

Statistical Analysis

Analysis of $[Ca^{2+}]_i$ peak amplitudes and area under the curve (AUC) was performed using Origin PRO software (Origin Lab 2015). Oscillation peaks observed under bicuculline treatment were classified as "low" or "high" if their absolute ratio amplitude was <0.15 or ≥ 0.15, respectively. The Fura-2 measurements from each independent cell preparation (made out of at least 4 embryos) were performed at least three times. 50–100 hippocampal neurons were measured simultaneously during each independent measurement. For calculation of a mean preparation trace, all the cells recorded with a particular protocol from a particular independent cell preparation were pooled. For the determination of significant differences of mean values obtained from two groups, a two-sample Student's *t*-test was used ($p < 0.05$ for significance). *N* indicates the number of independent cell preparations and n indicates the number of measured cells unless otherwise stated.

RESULTS

Current Concepts About Glutamate-Evoked and NAADP-Mediated Calcium Homeostasis in Neurons and Potential NAADP Target Channels

In addition to ionotropic NMDA, AMPA, and KA receptors, glutamate activates mGluRs to elicit downstream signaling events in the cell (Reiner and Levitz, 2018). It was shown that stimulation of hippocampal neurons with glutamate triggers NAADP synthesis probably via activation of mGluR1 receptors and mediates calcium release from lysosomal stores via two-pore-channels (Bak et al., 1999; McGuinness et al., 2007; Pandey et al., 2009; Foster et al., 2018). The prerequisite for this process is the loading of acidic stores with calcium ions which depends on the activity of the V-ATPase (**Figure 1**) and acidification that then allows Ca^{2+} uptake via H^+/Ca^{2+} exchange. Recently, experimental evidence was reported that calcium entry into neurons mediated by voltage gated calcium channels can trigger calcium release from acidic stores via NAADP sensitive channels. In addition to Two Pore Channel type 1 (TPC1) and TPC2 channels (Rahman et al., 2014; Grimm et al., 2017), TRPML1 (Zhang et al., 2011), and ryanodine receptors such as RYR1 have been reported as a NAADP target channels in other cell types (Guse, 2012; Diercks et al., 2018). The current concepts of NAADP-mediated calcium release and potential NAADP target channels that also may operate in hippocampal neurons are summarized in **Figure 1A** based on two independent RNAseq expression analyses in primary cultured neurons from mouse hippocampus GSE104802 (Mao et al., 2018) and GSE142064 (unpublished). Our analysis of these studies revealed that transcripts of Mcoln1 (encoding TRPML1 channels) are abundantly expressed in murine hippocampal neuron cultures whereas Mcoln2 and Mcoln3 transcripts are virtually not detectable. Within the TPC channel family, Tpcn1 transcripts (encoding TPC1) were detected (**Figure 1B**) and Tpcn2 transcripts (encoding TPC2) were also present, however, to a lower extent. Amongst the ryanodine receptors, transcripts encoding Ryr2 and Ryr3 were readily detected, whereas expression of Ryr1 seems to be negligible in hippocampal neurons in both studies.

In the current study we aim to analyze the contribution of NAADP-mediated calcium release from acidic stores in primary hippocampal neurons. Representative images of cultured hippocampal neurons 14 days after isolation, which were analyzed in our study, are shown in **Figure 1C** and demonstrate a dense and complex network of synaptic connections between the neurons. Cell bodies are 13–20 μm in size, from which numerous axonal structures originate similarly as has been described in previous publications (Mao and Wang, 2001). We have studied a possible involvement of NAADP-mediated Ca^{2+}-release in $[Ca^{2+}]_i$ elevation events registered after extracellular application of glutamate or during endogenous glutamate release events triggered by inhibition of $GABA_A$ receptors. To this end, we tested different concentration of glutamate (1, 3, and 10 μM) and measured the time course of intracellular calcium rise using Fura-2-based microfluorimetry. The rise of $[Ca^{2+}]_i$ triggered by 1 μM glutamate was transient and completely returned to the baseline ~5 min after the beginning of stimulation (**Supplementary Figure 1A**), whereas the responses elicited by application of 3 μM glutamate had a higher amplitude and a much longer decay phase with a half-decay time from about ~8 min (**Supplementary Figure 1B**). Following application of 10 μM glutamate the calcium plateau did not revert within a time frame of 15 min (not shown). Thus, protocols using the application of 3 μM glutamate were used in the following to test its modulation by interference with NAADP antagonists.

Glutamate Evoked $[Ca^{2+}]_i$ Rise in Hippocampal Neurons Is Reduced by NAADP Antagonists

After Fura-2 loading, hippocampal neurons were pre-incubated with Ned-19 (50 μM) for 5 min before starting the recording. 5 min after beginning of the recording, the cells were stimulated with glutamate (3 μM) for 15 min. Finally, to exclude possible recording of $[Ca^{2+}]_i$ in glial cells, we stimulated the cells with high-potassium solution (60 mM) as a positive control for excitable cells. Representative recordings are shown in **Figure 2B** and demonstrate an instantaneous $[Ca^{2+}]_i$ rise followed by a continuous and more variable decay phase. In average, the fluorescence ratio declined during 15 min after glutamate application to ~30% of initial amplitude (**Figure 2D**, black traces).

The treatment with Ned-19 resulted in a significant reduction of the amplitude of glutamate-evoked $[Ca^{2+}]_i$ rise (**Figures 2C–E**). The F340/F380 ratio was reduced by ~27%. We also observed a ~54% reduction of the AUC of the fluorescence ratio for the time period of 15 min after glutamate application (**Figure 2F**). After application of high

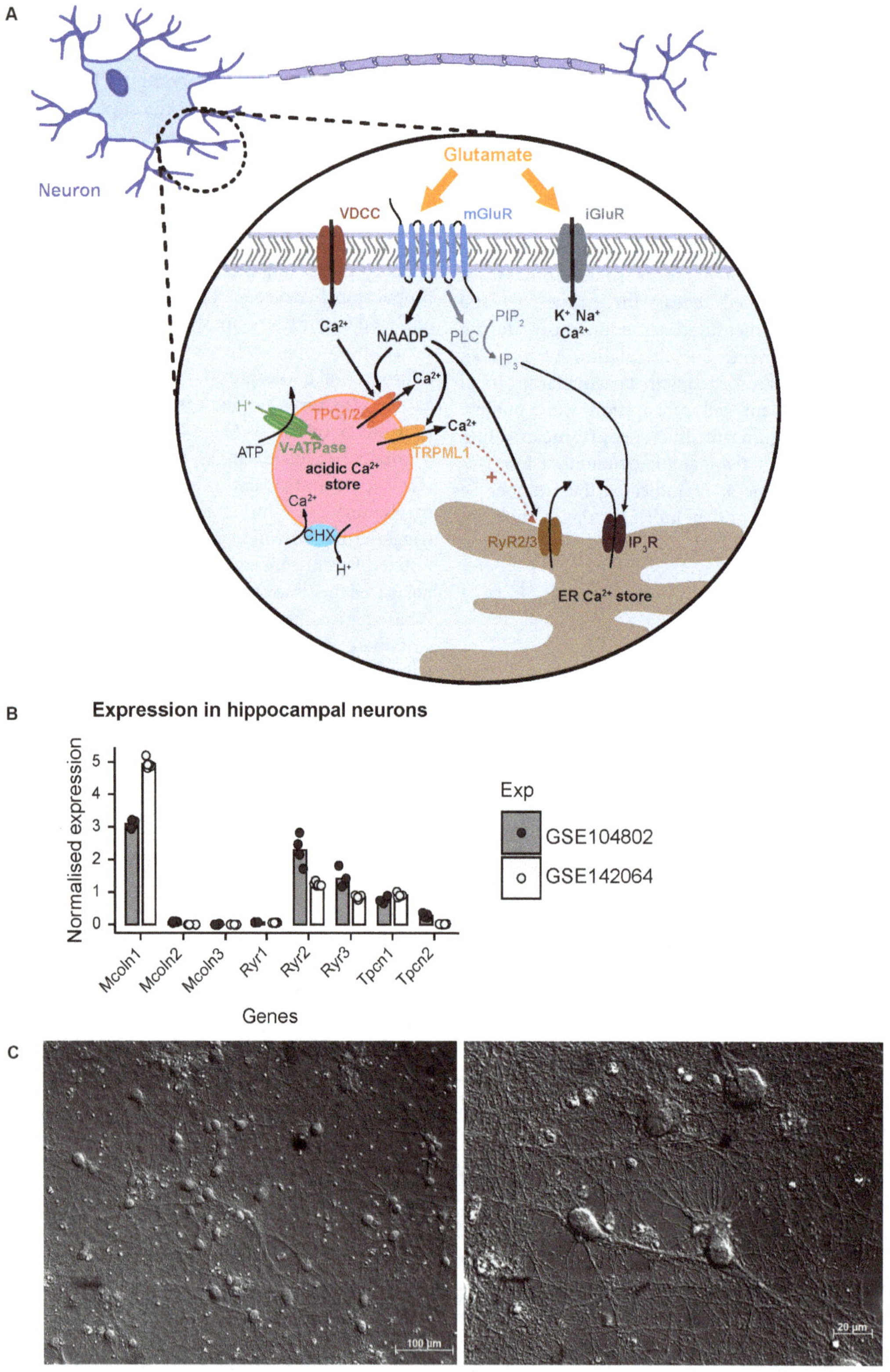

FIGURE 1 | A model based on current literature summarizing regulators of NAADP-mediated Ca^{2+} homeostasis following extracellular glutamate action in hippocampal neurons of mice. **(A)** Glutamate activates ionotropic NMDA, AMPA, and KA receptors (iGluR) resulting in Ca^{2+} influx across the plasma membrane. The activation of metabotropic glutamate receptors (mGluR) induces the synthesis of inositol trisphosphate (IP_3) which mediates Ca^{2+} release from the endoplasmic reticulum (ER). In the CNS and particularly in hippocampal neurons glutamate induces the synthesis of nicotinic acid adenine dinucleotide phosphate (NAADP) and

(Continued)

FIGURE 1 | Continued

subsequent Ca^{2+} release (Bak et al., 1999; McGuinness et al., 2007; Pandey et al., 2009). NAADP can be produced following activation of mGuR1 receptors and is known to mediate Ca^{2+} release into the cytosol via activation of two-pore channels 1/2 (TPC1/2) residing in the membrane of endo-lysosomal Ca^{2+} stores in many cell types including neurons (Bayraktar et al., 1990; Patel, 2015; Grimm et al., 2017; Foster et al., 2018) resulting in Ca^{2+} flux into the cytoplasm. Recently, it was also shown that Ca^{2+} entry via voltage gated Ca^{2+} channels triggers Ca^{2+} release from the lysosome via an NAADP-sensitive channel and, subsequently, fusion of the lysosome with the plasma membrane (Padamsey et al., 2017). In some cells the NAADP-evoked Ca^{2+} release depends on ryanodine receptors (RyR) such as the RyR1 in T cells (Diercks et al., 2018), and also TRPML1 channels were proposed as NAADP target channels (Zhang et al., 2011; Li et al., 2013). **(B)** Normalized mRNA expression of depicted genes in unstimulated primary hippocampal neuronal cultures. Transcripts per kilobase million (TPM) were calculated from GSE104802 (Mao et al., 2018; $n = 4$) and GSE142064 ($n = 5$) and were normalized to the mean expression from each dataset. **(C)** Representative images of primary hippocampal neurons of a C57BL/6N mice after 14 days *in vitro* as used in this study; photomicrography was performed using a transmitted light microscope with differential interference contrast (upper figure: objective EC Plan-Neofluar 20×/0.50 M27; lower figure: Plan Apochromat 63×/1.4 Oil DIC M27). Scale bars 100 μM, 20 μM.

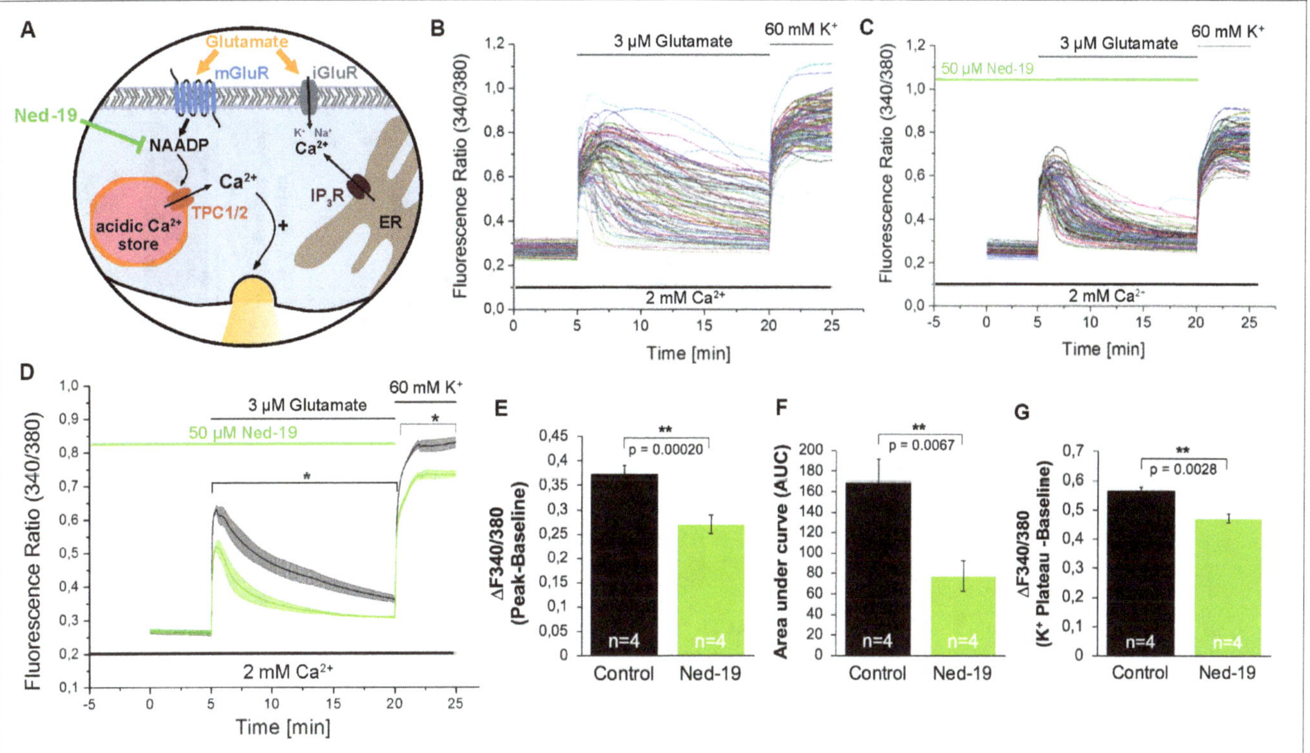

FIGURE 2 | The NAADP antagonist Ned-19 reduces the glutamate-induced Ca^{2+} increase in hippocampal neurons. **(A)** Ned-19 acts as a NAADP antagonist (Naylor et al., 2009). **(B,C)** Representative traces of the glutamate-induced changes in the F340/380 fluorescence intensity values in hippocampal neurons without **(B)** and with **(C)** pretreatment with Ned-19 (50 μM). **(D)** Average traces are given as the arithmetic mean ± SEM of the F340/380 fluorescence intensity values without (black, $n = 1057$ cells) and with (green, $n = 659$ cells) Ned-19 (50 μM) pre-incubation. Data from four independent C57Bl/6N preparations ($N = 4$) are shown. During all experiments, the cells were remained in physiological solution containing 2 mM Ca^{2+}. For measurements with Ned19, the cells were pre-incubated for 5 min. After 5 min of baseline recording, the cells were stimulated with glutamate (3 μM) for 15 min. For the last 5 min, the cells were stimulated with high potassium solution (60 mM K^{+}). The amplitude of the glutamate-induced calcium increase **(E)** as well as the AUC **(F)** and the amplitude of the high-potassium induced calcium transients **(G)** were analyzed. **: $p < 0{,}01$; *: $p < 0{,}05$.

potassium solution all cells in both conditions reacted with fast $[Ca^{2+}]_i$ rise reaching a plateau phase about 2 min after the stimulation. However, the F340/F380 fluorescence ratio amplitude of this high potassium-induced responses was reduced by ~16% in cells pretreated with the NAADP antagonist Ned-19 (**Figure 2G**).

In addition to Ned-19, we used BZ194 as an independent NAADP antagonist. BZ194 was shown to effectively reduce NAADP-dependent calcium transients at a concentration of 500 μM (Nebel et al., 2013) and (**Figure 3A**). As it is evident from the representative traces (**Figures 3B,C**) and the average traces (**Figure 3D**), it is obvious that BZ194 pretreatment at the concentration at 500 μM does not prevent immediate $[Ca^{2+}]_i$ rise although the peak ratio levels were reduced significantly by ~38% (**Figure 3E**), and the AUC of the $[Ca^{2+}]_i$ transients as a measure for the total calcium elevation over the period of stimulation is largely reduced by ~82% (**Figure 3F**). Similarly, like in case of Ned-19 (50 μM) pretreatment the amplitude of high potassium-evoked $[Ca^{2+}]_i$ transients was also reduced. The observed reduction was ~12% (**Figure 3G**). As the NAADP antagonist BZ194 was shown to affect calcium release in a dose-dependent manner in *T* lymphocytes and cardiomyocytes

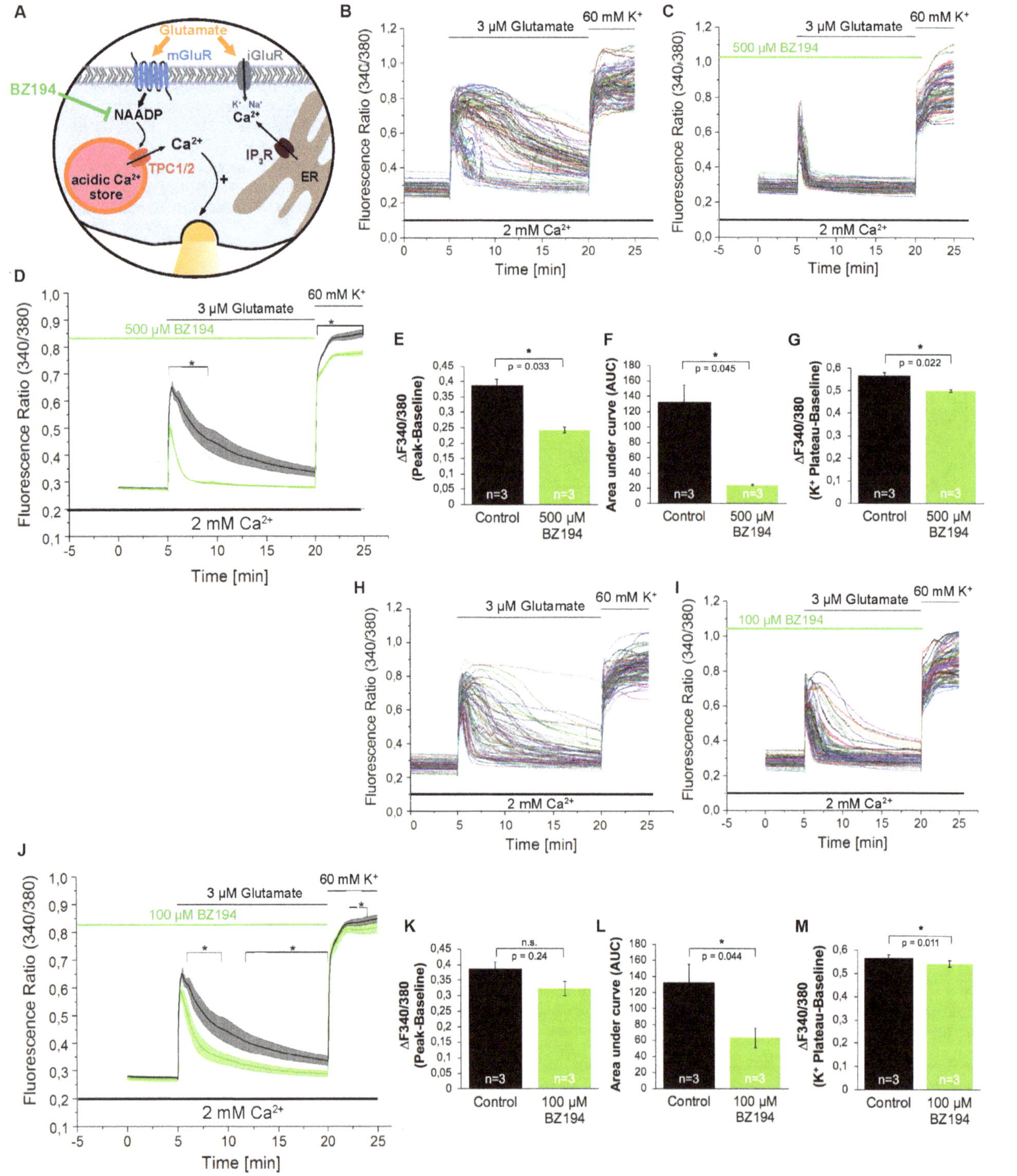

FIGURE 3 | The effect of the NAADP antagonist BZ194 on the time course of the glutamate-induced Ca^{2+} increase in hippocampal neurons. **(A)** BZ194 acts as a NAADP antagonist (Dammermann et al., 2009). **(B,C,H,I)** Representative traces of the glutamate-induced changes in the F340/380 fluorescence intensity values of hippocampal neurons without **(B,H)** and with 500 µM **(C)** or 100 µM **(I)** pre-incubation with BZ194. **(D,J)** Average traces are given as the arithmetic mean ± SEM of the averaged F340/380 fluorescence intensity values without (black, n = 719 cells in **D** and **J**) and with (green) 500 µM (**D**, n = 650 cells) or 100 µM (**J**, n = 611 cells) BZ194 pre-incubation. Data from independent C57Bl/6N preparations (n = 4) are shown. During all experiments, the cells were remained in physiological solution containing 2 mM Ca^{2+}. For measurements with BZ194, the cells were pre-incubated for 5 min. After 5 min recording, the cells were stimulated with glutamate (3 µM) for 15 min. For the last 5 min, the cells were stimulated with high potassium solution (60 mM K^+). Finally, the amplitude of the glutamate-induced calcium increase **(E,K)** as well as the AUC **(F,L)** and the amplitude of the high-potassium induced calcium transients **(G,M)** were analyzed. **: $p < 0{,}01$; *: $p < 0{,}05$.

(Dammermann et al., 2009; Nebel et al., 2013) we performed similar experiments with BZ194 pretreatment in hippocampal neurons using a lower concentration (100 μM, **Figures 3H–M**). Under these conditions the inhibition of glutamate evoked $[Ca^{2+}]_i$ rise was less pronounced as compared to BZ194 applied at the concentration of 500 μM. The AUC of the $[Ca^{2+}]_i$ transient was reduced by ~52% (**Figure 3L**) and the amplitude of glutamate evoked $[Ca^{2+}]_i$ rise was partially reduced in average, but was not significantly different from the non-treated cells (**Figure 3K**). High potassium-evoked calcium rise was still significantly reduced at some time points but the reduction was only ~5% in average (**Figure 3M**).

The acidification of endo-lysosomes depends on the activity of the Vacuolar-type H^+-ATPase (V-ATPase; **Figure 4A**), and by its inhibition using Bafilomycin A1 (Bowman et al., 1988) the calcium accumulation in the acidic stores can be prevented indirectly by inhibition of lysosomal acidification in many cell types (Yoshimori et al., 1991; Shen et al., 2012). Pre-incubation with Bafilomycin A1 (100 nM) for 60 min only slightly reduced the amplitude of glutamate evoked $[Ca^{2+}]_i$ transients by ~16% (**Figures 4B–E**) and the AUC of these responses was not significantly reduced under the conditions tested (**Figure 4F**). Nevertheless the fluorescence ratio amplitude of the high potassium solution-evoked responses was significantly reduced by ~23% (**Figure 4G**).

Calcium Transients Triggered by Bicuculline-Evoked Glutamate Release Events Are Modulated by NAADP Antagonists

In the next set of experiments, we aimed to investigate whether NAADP not only affects the calcium transients evoked by extracellular application of glutamate, but also by glutamate release events that occur endogenously in cells of our neuronal cultures. To facilitate such glutamate release events the cells were treated with bicuculline, a $GABA_A$ receptor antagonist, to prevent the inhibitory influence of these chloride channels on exocytosis of neurotransmitters (Hardingham et al., 2002). To this end, bicuculline (300 μM) was applied 5 min after recording of the resting $[Ca^{2+}]_i$. Representative traces of individual cells as well as the average traces are shown in **Figures 5A–F**. The bicuculline (300 μM) evoked changes in $[Ca^{2+}]_i$ appear as repetitive Ca^{2+} oscillations, were evoked within the first minute after bicuculline application and appeared synchronized between all tested cells of the culture dish. To assess whether NAADP antagonists affect the properties of these synchronized calcium transients, we quantified the oscillation frequency (**Figures 5G,K,O**), the AUC (**Figures 5I,M,Q**) as well as the amplitude of the corresponding calcium transients. To this end we compared calcium transients with high and low amplitudes (see method section for details) in bicuculline-evoked calcium transients with and without NAADP antagonist pretreatment (**Figures 5H,L,P**). In these experiments, cells were pretreated with Ned-19 in a concentration of 50 μM (**Figures 5A,B**), or 30 μM (**Figures 5C,D**) for 5 min. BZ194 (100 μM, **Figures 5E,F**) was pre-incubated for 60 min. The quantitative analysis of the time course of bicuculline-evoked calcium transients showed that pre-incubation with Ned-19 (50 μM) and BZ194 (100 μM), respectively, significantly altered the properties of bicuculline-evoked calcium transients, whereas Ned-19 at the concentration of 30 μM had no significant effect. In fact, the oscillation frequency was significantly increased by both NAADP antagonists (**Figures 5G,O**). Ned-19 (50 μM) pretreatment led to a significant increase in the number of calcium transients with a lower amplitude at the cost of transients with a higher amplitude although the reduction of the proportion of higher amplitudes itself was not statistically significant (**Figure 5H**). In average, there was a tendency toward an increase of the AUC upon Ned-19 (50 μM) pretreatment (**Figure 5I**). We noticed that the $[Ca^{2+}]_i$ continuously increased in most experiments particularly at the end of the observation time between 25 and 30 min after bicuculline application when cells were pretreated with Ned-19 (50 μM; **Figures 5A,B**, right panels). Therefore, we quantified the average change in $[Ca^{2+}]_i$ at the end of the bicuculline treatment compared to the calcium levels before bicuculline applications in cells without (black) and with Ned-19 (50 μM, green) pretreatment (**Figure 5J**). We found that Ned-19 treatment caused a significant calcium accumulation over this observation time period under bicuculline action and this increase in resting $[Ca^{2+}]_i$ was also observed to some degree when Ned-19 pretreatment was performed at the concentration of 30 μM, however, a similar effect was not observed with BZ194 (100 μM) pretreatment.

DISCUSSION

Over the last two decades, the concept of generation of NAADP in neurons following stimulation with glutamate has been first developed in brain microsomes (Bak et al., 1999) and then in lysosome-related organelles in hippocampal neurons (McGuinness et al., 2007). The generation of NAADP upon extracellular glutamate application has been directly measured (Pandey et al., 2009), however, the contribution of lysosomal stores due to glutamate evoked Ca^{2+} release relied on the depletion of lysosomal calcium stores by the dipeptide glycyl-l-phenylalanine 2-naphthylamide (GPN) that prevents organellar acidification. Yet, a recent study has demonstrated that GPN-evoked increase in $[Ca^{2+}]_i$ is not due to selective targeting of GPN on lysosomes, but increases cytosolic pH and subsequently Ca^{2+} release from the ER (Atakpa et al., 2019). However, our results using NAADP antagonists show that NAADP signaling contributes to glutamate-evoked $[Ca^{2+}]_i$ rise after extracellular glutamate application in hippocampal neurons. We also find that the nature of calcium transients, which occur in synchronous manner in all neurons throughout culture of hippocampal neurons after endogenous glutamate release, also depends on NAADP signaling as revealed by the use of the NAADP antagonists.

To analyze the contribution of NAADP-evoked signaling events during glutamate evoked $[Ca^{2+}]_i$ rise, in the present

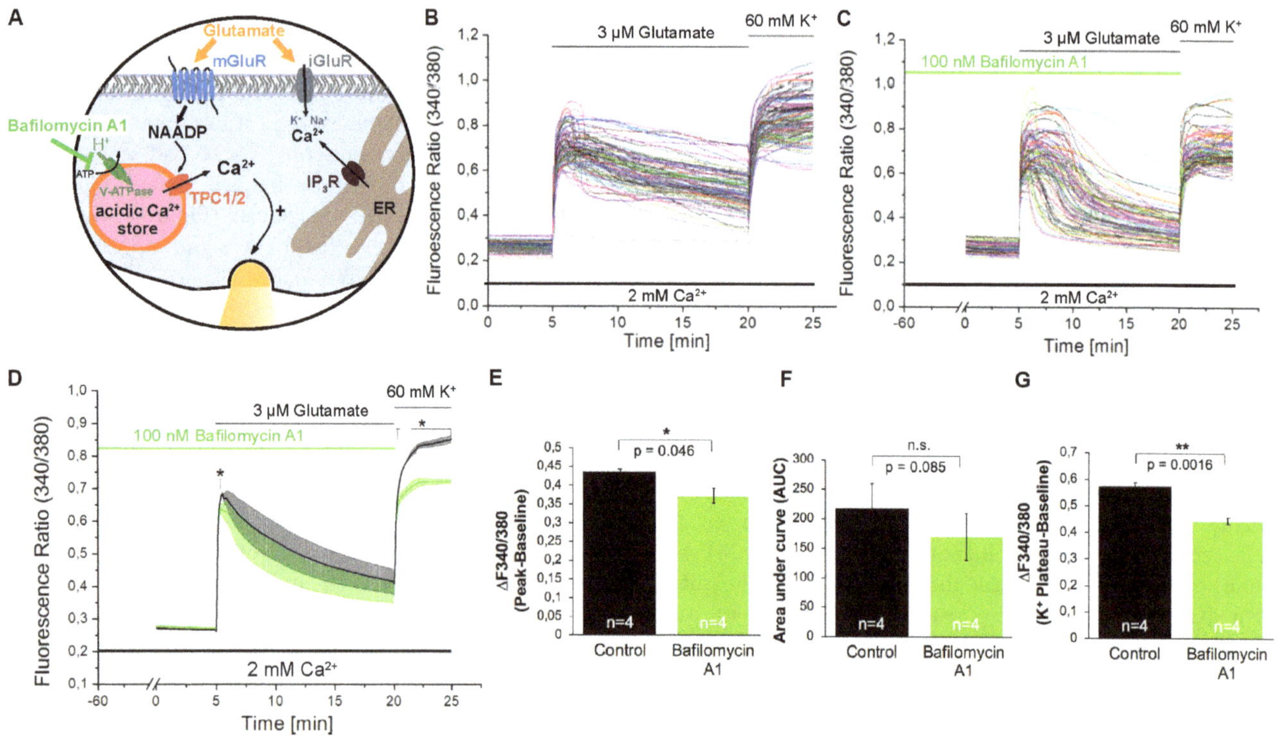

FIGURE 4 | The V-ATPase blocker Bafilomycin A1 does not affect glutamate-induced Ca^{2+} increase in hippocampal neurons. **(A)** Model depicting the action of Bafilomycin A1 as inhibitor of H^+ transport into acidic organelles. **(B,C)** Representative traces of the glutamate-induced changes in the F340/380 fluorescence intensity values in hippocampal neurons without **(B)** and with **(C)** pretreatment with Bafilomycin A1 (100 nM). **(D)** Average traces are given as the arithmetic mean ± SEM of the averaged F340/380 fluorescence intensity values without (black, n = 745 cells) and with (green, n = 849 cells) Bafilomycin A1 (100 nM) pre-incubation. Data from independent C57Bl/6N preparations (N = 4) are shown. During all experiments, the cells were remained in physiological solution containing 2 mM Ca^{2+}. For measurements with Bafilomycin A1, the cells were pre-incubated for 60 min. After 5 min of baseline recording, the cells were stimulated with glutamate (3 μM) for 15 min. For the last 5 min, the cells were stimulated with high potassium solution (60 mM K^+). The amplitude of the glutamate-induced calcium increase **(E)** as well as the AUC **(F)** and the amplitude of the high-potassium induced calcium transients **(G)** were analyzed. **: $p < 0{,}01$; *: $p < 0{,}05$.

study, we used two independent NAADP antagonists, Ned-19 (Naylor et al., 2009), and BZ194 (Dammermann et al., 2009). Pre-incubation with Ned-19 (50 μM) reduced peak amplitudes of glutamate evoked $[Ca^{2+}]_i$ rise by ~27%, after pretreatment with BZ194 (500 μM) peak amplitudes of glutamate-evoked calcium transients decreased by ~38%. In previous research, Ned-19 was used at this concentration in other cell types to antagonize NAADP action (Esposito et al., 2011), and BZ194 at this concentration was found to significantly reduce the Isoproterenol-evoked $[Ca^{2+}]_i$ rise from acidic stores in cardiomyocytes (Nebel et al., 2013). Pre-incubation with Bafilomycin A1, a V-ATPase blocker, which erases calcium accumulation in acidic stores indirectly by preventing their acidification (Bowman et al., 1988; Yoshimori et al., 1991), resulted only in a ~16% reduction of the amplitude of glutamate-evoked Ca^{2+} release. In a previous study, the Bafilomycin A1 effect on glutamate evoked $[Ca^{2+}]_i$ rise amplitude was more pronounced reaching ~50% reduction of the Ca^{2+} transient amplitude, however, in the aforementioned study, Bafilomycin A1 was used in a much higher concentration (1 μM vs. 100 nM in this study) and glutamate was applied at a concentration of 10 μM to stimulate the cells (Pandey et al., 2009). Another reason behind this discrepancy might also be that this study analyzed calcium transients in the absence of extracellular calcium levels, which was not pursued in our study, as the removal of extracellular calcium ions repeatedly triggered spontaneous calcium transients in mouse hippocampal neurons (data not shown). In addition, the fact that glutamate evokes Ca^{2+} entry also via ionotropic glutamate receptors in the presence of extracellular Ca^{2+}, as well as via voltage-gated calcium channels (Bading et al., 1993; Hardingham et al., 2001), can also contribute to the differences in the effectivity of Bafilomycin A1 between the two studies. Nevertheless, our study, using two independent NAADP antagonists and Bafilomycin A1, provide evidence about the contribution of NAADP-mediated calcium release and acidic stores to the amplitude of glutamate-evoked global calcium rise in hippocampal neurons of the mouse. Additional evidence comes from the analysis of the AUC of the glutamate-evoked $[Ca^{2+}]_i$ rise as Ned-19 (50 μM) pretreatment reduced AUC by ~54%, and pretreatment with BZ194 reduced AUC by ~82% and ~52% when used at concentrations of 500 μM and 100 μM, respectively. Bafilomycin A1 did not affect this parameter, which can be attributed to the differences in the kinetics, and/or in the ability to evoke alkalization of acidic calcium stores by

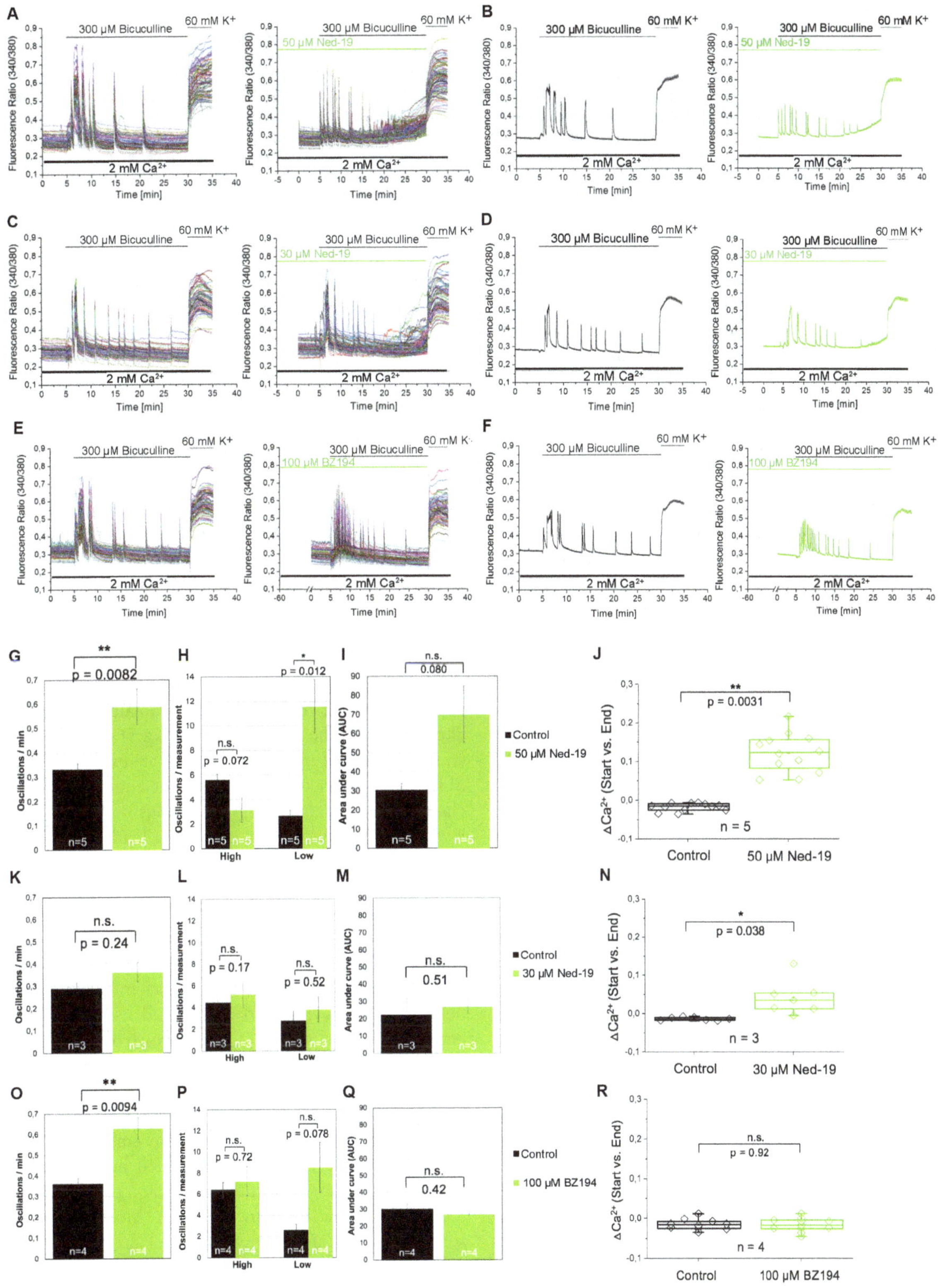

FIGURE 5 | The effect of the NAADP antagonists Ned19 and BZ194 on Ca^{2+} transients triggered by glutamate release events following inhibition of $GABA_A$ receptors in hippocampal neurons. **(A,C,E)** Representative traces of the bicuculline-induced changes in the F340/380 fluorescence intensity values in hippocampal neurons without (left) and with (right) preincubation with Ned-19 (50 µM; **A** or 30 µM; **C**) or BZ194 (100 µM; **E**). **(B,D,F)** Average traces are given as the arithmetic mean ± SEM without (black) and with (green) the corresponding NAADP antagonists (50 µM Ned-19, *n* = 89 cells, **B**; 30 µM Ned-19, *n* = 86 cells, **D**;

(Continued)

FIGURE 5 | Continued
and 100 μM BZ194, $n = 79$ cells, **F**). During all experiments, the cells were remained in physiological solution containing 2 mM Ca^{2+}. For measurements with Ned19, the cells were pre-incubated for 5 min; for measurements with BZ194, the cells were pre-incubated for 60 min. After 5 min recording, the cells were stimulated with bicuculline (300 μM) for 25 min. For the last 5 min, the cells were stimulated with high potassium solution (60 mM K^+). For each antagonist, several independent preparations (50 μM Ned19: $N = 5$: upper line; 30 μM Ned19: $N = 3$: middle line; and 100 μM BZ194: $N = 4$: lower line) were pooled. The oscillation frequency **(G,K,O)**, the number of high and low peaks **(H,L,P)** as well as the AUC **(I,M,Q)** were determined for each preparation without (black) and with (green) pre-incubation of the respective NAADP antagonist. **(J,N,R)** The change of the intracellular Ca^{2+} levels before and 25 min after bicuculline application (ΔCa^{2+}) was determined for each measurement without (black) und with (green) pre-incubation of the respective NAADP antagonist. For each p-value: $n = 5$ (50 μM Ned19); $n = 3$ (30 μM Ned19), and $n = 4$ (100 μM BZ194). **: $p < 0,01$; *: $p < 0,05$.

Bafilomycin A1 in the mouse and rat's hippocampal neurons. There could be some differences in effectivity of Bafilomycin A1 depending on cell type and time window (Klionsky et al., 2008).

Stimulation of the neuronal cultures with a high potassium solution led to an instantaneous increase that in contrast to glutamate stimulation was characterized by a continuous plateau. This response is similar to previously reported findings (Verkhratsky and Petersen, 2010). Interestingly, the high potassium-evoked $[Ca^{2+}]_i$ rise, which is supposed to be mediated by voltage gated calcium channels, was significantly reduced by both NAADP antagonists, Ned-19 and BZ194, as well as by pretreatment with the V-ATPase inhibitor Bafilomycin A1. A possible explanation for this result is that calcium entry via voltage-gated calcium channels can lead to a subsequent activation of Ca^{2+} release from NAADP-sensitive lysosomal calcium stores (Padamsey et al., 2017). An alternative explanation can be that endo-lysosomal calcium release supports the trafficking of *N*-type calcium channels into the plasma membrane (Hui et al., 2015). In agreement with the results reported by Padamsey et al. (2017) and Hui et al. (2015), the functional inactivation of endo-lysosomal calcium stores, which we performed in the present study using NAADP antagonists and Bafilomycin A1, would disrupt mutually facilitating interaction between lysosomal Ca^{2+} release and voltage-dependent calcium entry resulting in the reduced depolarization-induced calcium entry (see **Figures 3D,J, 4D**). However, it remains to be determined in further research whether the Ca^{2+} release from the acidic stores precedes the activation of voltage-gated channels or vice versa.

In order to corroborate the relevance of NAADP signaling found after extracellular application of glutamate in micromolar concentrations we aimed to study conditions that are more similar to those occurring *in vivo* where glutamate is released locally by exocytotic release, e.g., in the synaptic cleft or even extrasynaptically. To this end, we performed experiments in which we applied the $GABA_A$ receptor antagonist bicuculline. This experimental strategy has been commonly used to remove the inhibitory influence of the $GABA_A$-mediated chloride currents on the exocytosis in glutamatergic neurons. Bicuculline-evoked calcium signals were characterized by $[Ca^{2+}]_i$ oscillations synchronized through all neuronal cells in the cell culture dish. Both Ned-19 (50 μM) and BZ194 (100 μM) pretreatments resulted in a significant increase in the frequency of bicuculline-evoked $[Ca^{2+}]_i$ oscillations, accompanied by a significant increase in the occurrence of calcium transients with a lower amplitude. While further research is needed to identify physiological and pathophysiological consequences of such changes in the nature of these glutamate-evoked $[Ca^{2+}]_i$ oscillations, it is already known that a precise regulation of Ca^{2+} release from acidic stores via two-pore channels is essential for regulation of synaptic plasticity, since deletion of TPC channels leads to a reversal from long-term potentiation to long-term depression in mice (Foster et al., 2018).

Potential NAADP Target Channels in Hippocampal Neurons

To get an idea which channels might be present in our cell system to mediate glutamate-evoked calcium release we analyzed the expression of candidate NAADP target channels in two independent RNA seq experiments that were performed in murine hippocampal neurons, i.e., GSE104802 (Mao et al., 2018) and GSE142064 (unpublished). The analysis suggests that both TPC channel subtypes, TPC1 and TPC2, were expressed in murine hippocampal neurons and might operate as NAADP target channels upon glutamate stimulation similarly like TRPML1. The causal contribution of any of these channels could be revealed by studying glutamate evoked Ca^{2+} transients in hippocampal neurons that are deficient for the corresponding channels or by patch clamp recordings performed in the endo-lysosomes of these cells as was done before in other cell types (Chen et al., 2017). Alternatively, agonists and antagonists that specifically target individual channel subtypes, as recently reported for members of these channel families (Plesch et al., 2018; Gerndt et al., 2020), might be useful tools to pinpoint the contribution of distinct channel entities in this process. TRPML1 protein expression in cultured mouse embryonic hippocampal neurons was previously demonstrated using Western blotting analysis (Zhang et al., 2017). RYR1, which operates as an NAADP target channel early during *T* cell activation (Wolf et al., 2015; Diercks et al., 2018), seems to be not expressed in cultured murine hippocampal neurons. In contrast to RYR2 and RYR3, we did not find RYR1 expression in mouse embryonic hippocampal neurons. Similar results were reported in the study analyzing developmental changes in the expression of the three ryanodine receptor mRNAs in the mouse brain (Mori et al., 2000). These authors report that in the hippocampal CA1 region RYR1 mRNA appeared only at P1 and reached its peak level at P7. Also in the adult mouse hippocampal CA region, RYR1 had the lowest expression level compared to RYR2 and RYR3. A contribution of RYR2 and/or RYR3 for intracellular Ca^{2+} rise downstream of NAADP generation has not been reported so far, although these receptors appear to be regulated by cyclic ADP-ribose (Fritz et al., 2005; Dabertrand et al., 2007). However, RYR2 and RYR3 should be studied in the future with similar approaches as discussed for TPC and TRPML1 channels above.

Taken together, the results of this study provide evidence that NAADP-sensitive calcium stores contribute to the alteration in cellular calcium homeostasis in neurons evoked by glutamate. Whether calcium release from these acidic stores aggravates excitotoxicity in disease models with inflammatory neuronal degeneration such as Multiple Sclerosis needs to be elaborated in further research by the inhibition of endo-lysosomal channels with specific antagonists or their genetic deletion.

ETHICS STATEMENT

The animal study was reviewed and approved by Regierungspräsidium Karlsruhe and the University Heidelberg.

AUTHOR CONTRIBUTIONS

MF and VT: Conceptualization. JH and MW: Data curation. JH, VT, MW, VK, and MF: Formal analysis. MAF and MF: Funding acquisition. JH, VT, and MF: Investigation. JH, MB, DS, MW, AS, SR, and VT: Methodology. VT, MAF, and MF: Project administration. CM and AG: Resources. VT, MAF, and MF: Supervision. JH, MW, and MF: Visualization. JH, VT, and MF: Writing - original draft. Writing - review and editing, all authors.

ACKNOWLEDGMENTS

We are thankful to Xenia Tolksdorf, Christin Richter, Manuela Ritzal, and Hans-Peter Gensheimer for expert technical assistance, to Angela Wirth for her critical revision of the manuscript.

REFERENCES

Atakpa, P., van Marrewijk, L. M., Apta-Smith, M., Chakraborty, S., and Taylor, C. W. (2019). GPN does not release lysosomal Ca(2+) but evokes Ca(2+) release from the ER by increasing the cytosolic pH independently of cathepsin C. *J. Cell Sci.* 132:223883.

Bading, H. (2017). Therapeutic targeting of the pathological triad of extrasynaptic NMDA receptor signaling in neurodegenerations. *J. Exp. Med.* 214, 569–578. doi: 10.1084/jem.20161673

Bading, H., Ginty, D. D., and Greenberg, M. E. (1993). Regulation of gene expression in hippocampal neurons by distinct calcium signaling pathways. *Science* 260, 181–186. doi: 10.1126/science.8097060

Bak, J., White, P., Timar, G., Missiaen, L., Genazzani, A. A., and Galione, A. (1999). Nicotinic acid adenine dinucleotide phosphate triggers Ca2+ release from brain microsomes. *Curr. Biol.* 9, 751–754. doi: 10.1016/s0960-9822(99)80335-2

Bayraktar, M., Gedik, O., Akalin, S., Usman, A., Adalar, N., and Telatar, F. (1990). The effect of radioactive iodine treatment on thyroid C cells. *Clin. Endocrinol.* 33, 625–630. doi: 10.1111/j.1365-2265.1990.tb03901.x

Bowman, E. J., Siebers, A., and Altendorf, K. (1988). Bafilomycins: a class of inhibitors of membrane ATPases from microorganisms, animal cells, and plant cells. *Proc. Natl. Acad. Sci. U.S.A.* 85, 7972–7976. doi: 10.1073/pnas.85.21.7972

Chen, C. C., Cang, C., Fenske, S., Butz, E., Chao, Y. K., Biel, M., et al. (2017). Patch-clamp technique to characterize ion channels in enlarged individual endolysosomes. *Nat. Protoc.* 12, 1639–1658. doi: 10.1038/nprot.2017.036

Dabertrand, F., Fritz, N., Mironneau, J., Macrez, N., and Morel, J. L. (2007). Role of RYR3 splice variants in calcium signaling in mouse nonpregnant and pregnant myometrium. *Am. J. Physiol. Cell Physiol.* 293, C848–C854.

Dammermann, W., Zhang, B., Nebel, M., Cordiglieri, C., Odoardi, F., Kirchberger, T., et al. (2009). NAADP-mediated Ca2+ signaling via type 1 ryanodine receptor in T cells revealed by a synthetic NAADP antagonist. *Proc. Natl. Acad. Sci. U.S.A.* 106, 10678–10683. doi: 10.1073/pnas.0809997106

Diercks, B. P., Werner, R., Weidemuller, P., Czarniak, F., Hernandez, L., Lehmann, C., et al. (2018). ORAI1, STIM1/2, and RYR1 shape subsecond Ca(2+) microdomains upon T cell activation. *Sci. Signal.* 11:eaat0358. doi: 10.1126/scisignal.aat0358

Duda, J., Potschke, C., and Liss, B. (2016). Converging roles of ion channels, calcium, metabolic stress, and activity pattern of Substantia nigra dopaminergic neurons in health and Parkinson's disease. *J. Neurochem.* 139(Suppl. 1), 156–178. doi: 10.1111/jnc.13572

Esposito, B., Gambara, G., Lewis, A. M., Palombi, F., D'Alessio, A., Taylor, L. X., et al. (2011). NAADP links histamine H1 receptors to secretion of von Willebrand factor in human endothelial cells. *Blood* 117, 4968–4977. doi: 10.1182/blood-2010-02-266338

Foster, W. J., Taylor, H. B. C., Padamsey, Z., Jeans, A. F., Galione, A., and Emptage, N. J. (2018). Hippocampal mGluR1-dependent long-term potentiation requires NAADP-mediated acidic store Ca(2+) signaling. *Sci. Signal.* 11:558.

Friese, M. A., Craner, M. J., Etzensperger, R., Vergo, S., Wemmie, J. A., Welsh, M. J., et al. (2007). Acid-sensing ion channel-1 contributes to axonal degeneration in autoimmune inflammation of the central nervous system. *Nat. Med.* 13, 1483–1489. doi: 10.1038/nm1668

Friese, M. A., Schattling, B., and Fugger, L. (2014). Mechanisms of neurodegeneration and axonal dysfunction in multiple sclerosis. *Nat. Rev. Neurol.* 10, 225–238. doi: 10.1038/nrneurol.2014.37

Fritz, N., Macrez, N., Mironneau, J., Jeyakumar, L. H., Fleischer, S., and Morel, J. L. (2005). Ryanodine receptor subtype 2 encodes Ca2+ oscillations activated by acetylcholine via the M2 muscarinic receptor/cADP-ribose signalling pathway in duodenum myocytes. *J. Cell Sci.* 118(Pt 10), 2261–2270. doi: 10.1242/jcs.02344

Gerndt, S., Chen, C. C., Chao, Y. K., Yuan, Y., Burgstaller, S., Scotto Rosato, A., et al. (2020). Agonist-mediated switching of ion selectivity in TPC2 differentially promotes lysosomal function. *eLife* 9:e54712.

Grimm, C., Butz, E., Chen, C. C., Wahl-Schott, C., and Biel, M. (2017). From mucolipidosis type IV to Ebola: TRPML and two-pore channels at the crossroads of endo-lysosomal trafficking and disease. *Cell Calcium* 67, 148–155. doi: 10.1016/j.ceca.2017.04.003

Guse, A. H. (2012). Linking NAADP to ion channel activity: a unifying hypothesis. *Sci. Signal.* 5:e18.

Hardingham, G. E., Arnold, F. J., and Bading, H. (2001). Nuclear calcium signaling controls CREB-mediated gene expression triggered by synaptic activity. *Nat. Neurosci.* 4, 261–267. doi: 10.1038/85109

Hardingham, G. E., and Bading, H. (2010). Synaptic versus extrasynaptic NMDA receptor signalling: implications for neurodegenerative disorders. *Nat. Rev. Neurosci.* 11, 682–696. doi: 10.1038/nrn2911

Hardingham, G. E., Fukunaga, Y., and Bading, H. (2002). Extrasynaptic NMDARs oppose synaptic NMDARs by triggering CREB shut-off and cell death pathways. *Nat. Neurosci.* 5, 405–414. doi: 10.1038/nn835

Hui, L., Geiger, N. H., Bloor-Young, D., Churchill, G. C., Geiger, J. D., and Chen, X. (2015). Release of calcium from endolysosomes increases calcium influx through N-type calcium channels: evidence for acidic store-operated calcium entry in neurons. *Cell Calcium* 58, 617–627. doi: 10.1016/j.ceca.2015.10.001

Klionsky, D. J., Elazar, Z., Seglen, P. O., and Rubinsztein, D. C. (2008). Does bafilomycin A1 block the fusion of autophagosomes with lysosomes? *Autophagy* 4, 849–850. doi: 10.4161/auto.6845

Li, P. L., Zhang, Y., Abais, J. M., Ritter, J. K., and Zhang, F. (2013). Cyclic ADP-Ribose and NAADP in vascular regulation and diseases. *Messenger* 2, 63–85. doi: 10.1166/msr.2013.1022

Mao, L., and Wang, J. Q. (2001). Upregulation of preprodynorphin and preproenkephalin mRNA expression by selective activation of group I metabotropic glutamate receptors in characterized primary cultures of rat striatal neurons. *Brain Res. Mol. Brain Res.* 86, 125–137. doi: 10.1016/s0169-328x(00)00276-x

Mao, W., Salzberg, A. C., Uchigashima, M., Hasegawa, Y., Hock, H., Watanabe, M., et al. (2018). Activity-induced regulation of synaptic strength through the chromatin reader L3mbtl1. *Cell Rep.* 23, 3209–3222. doi: 10.1016/j.celrep.2018.05.028

McGuinness, L., Bardo, S. J., and Emptage, N. J. (2007). The lysosome or lysosome-related organelle may serve as a Ca2+ store in the boutons of hippocampal pyramidal cells. *Neuropharmacology* 52, 126–135. doi: 10.1016/j.neuropharm.2006.07.029

Mori, F., Fukaya, M., Abe, H., Wakabayashi, K., and Watanabe, M. (2000). Developmental changes in expression of the three ryanodine receptor mRNAs in the mouse brain. *Neurosci. Lett.* 285, 57–60. doi: 10.1016/s0304-3940(00)01046-6

Naylor, E., Arredouani, A., Vasudevan, S. R., Lewis, A. M., Parkesh, R., Mizote, A., et al. (2009). Identification of a chemical probe for NAADP by virtual screening. *Nat. Chem. Biol.* 5, 220–226. doi: 10.1038/nchembio.150

Nebel, M., Schwoerer, A. P., Warszta, D., Siebrands, C. C., Limbrock, A. C., Swarbrick, J. M., et al. (2013). Nicotinic acid adenine dinucleotide phosphate (NAADP)-mediated calcium signaling and arrhythmias in the heart evoked by beta-adrenergic stimulation. *J. Biol. Chem.* 288, 16017–16030. doi: 10.1074/jbc.m112.441246

Nedergaard, M., and Verkhratsky, A. (2010). Calcium dyshomeostasis and pathological calcium signalling in neurological diseases. *Cell Calcium* 47, 101–102. doi: 10.1016/j.ceca.2009.12.011

Orrenius, S., Zhivotovsky, B., and Nicotera, P. (2003). Regulation of cell death: the calcium-apoptosis link. *Nat. Rev. Mol. Cell Biol.* 4, 552–565. doi: 10.1038/nrm1150

Padamsey, Z., McGuinness, L., Bardo, S. J., Reinhart, M., Tong, R., Hedegaard, A., et al. (2017). Activity-dependent exocytosis of lysosomes regulates the structural plasticity of dendritic spines. *Neuron* 93, 132–146. doi: 10.1016/j.neuron.2016.11.013

Pandey, V., Chuang, C. C., Lewis, A. M., Aley, P. K., Brailoiu, E., Dun, N. J., et al. (2009). Recruitment of NAADP-sensitive acidic Ca2+ stores by glutamate. *Biochem. J.* 422, 503–512. doi: 10.1042/bj20090194

Patel, S. (2015). Function and dysfunction of two-pore channels. *Sci. Signal.* 8:re7. doi: 10.1126/scisignal.aab3314

Plesch, E., Chen, C. C., Butz, E., Scotto Rosato, A., Krogsaeter, E. K., Yinan, H., et al. (2018). Selective agonist of TRPML2 reveals direct role in chemokine release from innate immune cells. *eLife* 7: e39720.

Popugaeva, E., Pchitskaya, E., and Bezprozvanny, I. (2017). Dysregulation of neuronal calcium homeostasis in Alzheimer's disease - a therapeutic opportunity? *Biochem. Biophys. Res. Commun.* 483, 998–1004. doi: 10.1016/j.bbrc.2016.09.053

Rahman, T., Cai, X., Brailoiu, G. C., Abood, M. E., Brailoiu, E., and Patel, S. (2014). Two-pore channels provide insight into the evolution of voltage-gated Ca2+ and Na+ channels. *Sci. Signal.* 7:ra109. doi: 10.1126/scisignal.2005450

Reiner, A., and Levitz, J. (2018). Glutamatergic signaling in the central nervous system: ionotropic and metabotropic receptors in concert. *Neuron* 98, 1080–1098. doi: 10.1016/j.neuron.2018.05.018

Schattling, B., Steinbach, K., Thies, E., Kruse, M., Menigoz, A., Ufer, F., et al. (2012). TRPM4 cation channel mediates axonal and neuronal degeneration in experimental autoimmune encephalomyelitis and multiple sclerosis. *Nat. Med.* 18, 1805–1811. doi: 10.1038/nm.3015

Shen, D., Wang, X., Li, X., Zhang, X., Yao, Z., Dibble, S., et al. (2012). Lipid storage disorders block lysosomal trafficking by inhibiting a TRP channel and lysosomal calcium release. *Nat. Commun.* 3:731.

Surmeier, D. J., Halliday, G. M., and Simuni, T. (2017). Calcium, mitochondrial dysfunction and slowing the progression of Parkinson's disease. *Exp. Neurol.* 298(Pt B), 202–209. doi: 10.1016/j.expneurol.2017.08.001

Szydlowska, K., and Tymianski, M. (2010). Calcium, ischemia and excitotoxicity. *Cell Calcium* 47, 122–129. doi: 10.1016/j.ceca.2010.01.003

Ureshino, R. P., Erustes, A. G., Bassani, T. B., Wachilewski, P., Guarache, G. C., Nascimento, A. C., et al. (2019). The interplay between Ca(2+) signaling pathways and neurodegeneration. *Int. J. Mol. Sci.* 20:6004. doi: 10.3390/ijms20236004

Verkhratsky, A., and Petersen, O. (2010). "Principles of the Ca2+ homeostatic/signalling system," in *Calcium Measurement Methods*, eds A. Verkhratsky and O. Petersen (Totowa: NJ: Humana Press), 1–11. doi: 10.1007/978-1-60761-476-0_1

Wojda, U., Salinska, E., and Kuznicki, J. (2008). Calcium ions in neuronal degeneration. *IUBMB Life* 60, 575–590. doi: 10.1002/iub.91

Wolf, I. M., Diercks, B. P., Gattkowski, E., Czarniak, F., Kempski, J., Werner, R., et al. (2015). Frontrunners of T cell activation: Initial, localized Ca2+ signals mediated by NAADP and the type 1 ryanodine receptor. *Sci. Signal.* 8:ra102. doi: 10.1126/scisignal.aab0863

Yoshimori, T., Yamamoto, A., Moriyama, Y., Futai, M., and Tashiro, Y. (1991). Bafilomycin A1, a specific inhibitor of vacuolar-type H(+)-ATPase, inhibits acidification and protein degradation in lysosomes of cultured cells. *J. Biol. Chem.* 266, 17707–17712.

Zhang, F., Xu, M., Han, W. Q., and Li, P. L. (2011). Reconstitution of lysosomal NAADP-TRP-ML1 signaling pathway and its function in TRP-ML1(-/-) cells. *Am. J. Physiol. Cell Physiol.* 301, C421–C430.

Zhang, L., Fang, Y., Cheng, X., Lian, Y., Xu, H., Zeng, Z., et al. (2017). TRPML1 participates in the progression of Alzheimer's disease by regulating the PPARgamma/AMPK/Mtor signalling pathway. *Cell Physiol. Biochem.* 43, 2446–2456. doi: 10.1159/000484449

Zundorf, G., and Reiser, G. (2011). Calcium dysregulation and homeostasis of neural calcium in the molecular mechanisms of neurodegenerative diseases provide multiple targets for neuroprotection. *Antioxid. Redox. Signal.* 14, 1275–1288. doi: 10.1089/ars.2010.3359

4

TRPM3 in Brain (Patho)Physiology

Katharina Held[1,2*†] *and Balázs István Tóth*[3*†]

[1] *Laboratory of Endometrium, Endometriosis and Reproductive Medicine, Department of Development and Regeneration, KU Leuven, Leuven, Belgium,* [2] *Laboratory of Ion Channel Research, Department of Cellular and Molecular Medicine and VIB-KU Leuven Center for Brain and Disease Research, KU Leuven, Leuven, Belgium,* [3] *Laboratory of Cellular and Molecular Physiology, Department of Physiology, Faculty of Medicine, University of Debrecen, Debrecen, Hungary*

Correspondence:
Katharina Held
kathi.held@kuleuven.vib.be
Balázs István Tóth
toth.istvan@med.unideb.hu

† *These authors have contributed equally to this work*

Already for centuries, humankind is driven to understand the physiological and pathological mechanisms that occur in our brains. Today, we know that ion channels play an essential role in the regulation of neural processes and control many functions of the central nervous system. Ion channels present a diverse group of membrane-spanning proteins that allow ions to penetrate the insulating cell membrane upon opening of their channel pores. This regulated ion permeation results in different electrical and chemical signals that are necessary to maintain physiological excitatory and inhibitory processes in the brain. Therefore, it is no surprise that disturbances in the functions of cerebral ion channels can result in a plethora of neurological disorders, which present a tremendous health care burden for our current society. The identification of ion channel-related brain disorders also fuel the research into the roles of ion channel proteins in various brain states. In the last decade, mounting evidence has been collected that indicates a pivotal role for transient receptor potential (TRP) ion channels in the development and various physiological functions of the central nervous system. For instance, TRP channels modulate neurite growth, synaptic plasticity and integration, and are required for neuronal survival. Moreover, TRP channels are involved in numerous neurological disorders. TRPM3 belongs to the melastatin subfamily of TRP channels and represents a non-selective cation channel that can be activated by several different stimuli, including the neurosteroid pregnenolone sulfate, osmotic pressures and heat. The channel is best known as a peripheral nociceptive ion channel that participates in heat sensation. However, recent research identifies TRPM3 as an emerging new player in the brain. In this review, we summarize the available data regarding the roles of TRPM3 in the brain, and correlate these data with the neuropathological processes in which this ion channel may be involved.

Keywords: ion channels, channelopathies, transient receptor potential melastatin 3 channel, pregnenolone sulfate, brain, neurological disorders, gating pore current

INTRODUCTION

The brain forms the control center of our body and is responsible for processing tremendous amounts of data to monitor and regulate our bodily functions at day and night. Such a precise control needs to be fast and accurate and requires highly sophisticated information processing. Our body accomplishes this task via neuronal cells, which form a complex connectome within the nervous system (Purves, 2004). Within the nervous system, information is delivered and processed in form of electrical signals and synaptic events. Electrical signals occur, propagate and get transduced by neurons due to a diverse set of ion channels present in the membranes of the nerve cells (Hille, 2001). Ion channel proteins allow the permeation of ions over the otherwise ion-impermeable cell membrane, which results in a potential difference between the extracellular space and the intracellular side of the cell known as the membrane potential. Practically, changes in membrane potential serve as the information bearing electrical signals and are strictly controlled by ion channels (Hille, 2001; Purves, 2004). Therefore, genetic or acquired alterations in function of ion channels can result in severe disturbances of the electrical signaling in our nervous system causing several neurological or psychiatric diseases. For this reason, ion channels are primary targets for pharmacological interventions to treat such diseases (Kullmann, 2002; Kumar et al., 2016).

Among the hundreds of ion channels expressed in the human brain, Transient Receptor Potential (TRP) channels form a diverse group of poly-modally activated cation channels and they are generally considered as molecular sensors of external and internal stimuli (Clapham, 2003; Voets et al., 2005; Nilius, 2012). In total, 28 different TRP channels exist in mammals, which are divided into seven subfamilies according to their sequence homology. Functionally active TRP channels are composed of four individual subunits (Clapham et al., 2005) as recently evidenced by high resolution structural models (Liao et al., 2013; Yin et al., 2018; Cao, 2020; Huang et al., 2020) (**Figure 1**). Once activated, TRP channels allow the influx of cations into the intracellular space resulting in the depolarization of the plasma membrane and possible subsequent modulation of voltage-gated ion channels (Clapham et al., 2005; Gees et al., 2010; Wu et al., 2010; Nilius and Szallasi, 2014). Importantly, most TRP channels possess a substantial permeability for calcium, which is a vital signaling molecule throughout several cellular and molecular processes and therefore, plays a leading role in brain homeostasis and excitability (McBurney and Neering, 1987; Zündorf and Reiser, 2011). It is generally believed that TRP channels can play a substantial role in fine-tuning the membrane potential and neuronal excitability (Sawamura et al., 2017).

Abbreviations: 2-APB, 2-aminoethoxydiphenyl borate; CA1, Cornu Ammonis 1; DEE, developmental and epileptic encephalopathies; DHEA, dehydroepiandrosterone; DRG, dorsal root ganglia; GABA, γ-aminobutyric acid; Gβγ, G beta-gamma complex; GIRK, G-protein-coupled inward rectifier potassium channel; ICFR, *r*egion *i*ndispensable for *c*hannel *f*unctions in TRPM3; *I-V* plot, current-voltage plot; KS, Kabuki syndrome; K_V, voltage-gated potassium channel; MCA/MR, multiple congenital anomaly/mental retardation syndrome; MITF, microphthalmia/melanogenesis-associated transcription factor; N.at-K_V3.2, flatworm voltage-gated potassium channel 3; Na_V, voltage-gated sodium channel; NFATc1, nuclear factor of activated T cells type c1; NMDA, N-methyl-D-aspartate; Pax6, paired-box 6 transcription factor; PD, pore domain; PtdIns(4,5)P_2, phosphatidylinositol 4,5-bisphosphate; PtdIns(3,4,5)P_3, phosphatidylinositol 3,4,5-trisphosphate; PregS, pregnenolone sulfate; RANKL, receptor activator of nuclear factor kappa-B ligand; S1-6, transmembrane segments 1-6; STS, steroid sulfatase; TRPM, transient receptor potential channel melastatin; TRPC, transient receptor potential channel canonical; TRPV, transient receptor potential channel vanilloid; VM/PQ mutation, human TRPM3 DEE point mutations with amino acid substitutions valine to methionine (VM) and proline to glutamine (PQ); VSD, voltage-sensing domain; WT, wild type.

Some members of the TRP channel family are functionally expressed in various brain regions and their involvement in diverse physiological and pathological processes of the brain has already been described (Moran et al., 2004; Nilius, 2012; Reboreda, 2012; Sawamura et al., 2017). Among them, the TRP canonical (TRPC) channel subfamily presents probably the most-studied TRP channel subfamily in the brain (Sawamura et al., 2017). TRPCs were reported in various brain regions (Riccio et al., 2002; Huang et al., 2011), where they were implicated in excitatory post-synaptic conduction (Kim et al., 2003), neuronal cell death and survival (Jia et al., 2007; Narayanan et al., 2008), and dendritic growth and spine formation (Amaral and Pozzo-Miller, 2007; Tai et al., 2008), among other things. Another well-studied TRP channel in the brain is TRP **v**anilloid 1 (TRPV1), which is of importance in descending modulatory pain pathways and seems to play an extended role in other brain functions, by enhancing glutamatergic neurotransmission (Martins et al., 2014).

The TRP **m**elastatin (TRPM) channel subfamily represents an especially heterogeneous group within the TRP superfamily and includes eight members in total (TRPM1-8). Most of them are non-selective calcium-permeable cation channels. As an exception, TRPM4 and TRPM5 are calcium-impermeable channels activated by intracellular calcium. As such, all TRPM family members can evoke calcium increases in cells, either by conducting calcium ions through their pores or by regulating the membrane potential, thereby activating/modulating calcium channels or transporters (Clapham et al., 2005; Wu et al., 2010; Huang et al., 2020). Moreover, three members (TRPM2, TRPM6 and TRPM7) are so-called "chanzymes," bearing an enzyme (kinase or hydrolase) domain in addition to their ion channel pore (Nilius and Owsianik, 2011; Huang et al., 2020). Furthermore, several TRPM channels are also thermosensitive, covering a wide range of physiological temperatures (TRPM2, TRPM3, TRPM4, TRPM5 and TRPM8) (Talavera et al., 2005; Dhaka et al., 2007; Vriens et al., 2011; Tan and McNaughton, 2018; Vandewauw et al., 2018). The diverse properties of the TRPM family explain their involvement in a multitude of biological processes. They are regulating sensory processes, including vision (TRPM1) (Morgans et al., 2009), taste (TRPM5) (Pérez et al., 2002; Talavera et al., 2005), temperature sensation and nociception (TRPM2, TRPM3, TRPM8) (Dhaka et al., 2007; Voets et al., 2007; Vriens et al., 2011; Held et al., 2015b; Tan and McNaughton, 2018; Vandewauw et al., 2018). Moreover, they play important roles in ion homeostasis (Mg^{2+} uptake and reabsorption by TRPM6 and TRPM7) (Schlingmann et al., 2007), and modulate secretory processes (TRPM2, TRPM3, TRPM4, TRPM5) in various cells all over the body (Cheng et al., 2007; Wagner et al., 2008; Brixel et al., 2010; Mathar et al., 2010; Uchida et al., 2011; Held et al., 2015a; Philippaert et al., 2017).

TRPM2 represents the best characterized member in the brain, where it exhibits an ubiquitous expression pattern (Allen Mouse Brain Atlas, 2004; Fonfria et al., 2006; Lein et al., 2007). It is intensively studied with regards to its role in the response to oxidative stress, which occurs during aging and neurodegenerative diseases (Sita et al., 2018). Recently, TRPM2 was also described as a hypothalamic heat sensor involved

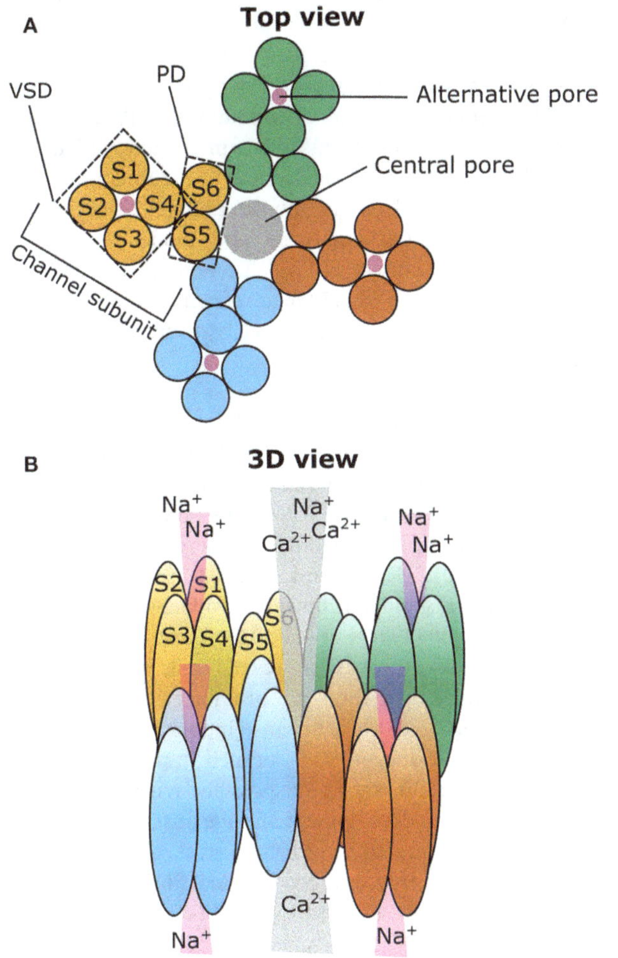

FIGURE 1 | Cartoon illustrating the putative localization of the central and alternative ion pore in TRPM3. **(A)** Top view on a representation of the four TRPM3 channel subunits (individually colored) that come together to form a functional ion channel. The voltage-sensing domain (VSD) and the pore domain (PD) are indicated in one of the subunits as well as the path of the central pore (gray circle) and the putative path(s) for the alternative ion pore(s) (four magenta circles). **(B)** Same as in **(A)** but in a three-dimensional representation looking from the diagonal top on TRPM3. S1–6: Transmembrane segment 1–6.

in central thermoregulation (Song et al., 2016). Furthermore, TRPM7 is widely expressed in the brain, and was shown to be involved in cell growth (Turlova et al., 2016) and cell death after ischemic and hypoxic brain injuries (Aarts et al., 2003; Sun et al., 2009; Chen et al., 2015; Sun, 2017). TRPM4 was also reported to be involved in cognitive functions, as well as in (patho)physiological processes, such as hippocampal plasticity (Menigoz et al., 2016; Bovet-Carmona et al., 2018) or development of trauma induced brain edema (Gerzanich et al., 2019; Woo et al., 2020).

TRPM3, a less studied member of the melastatin subfamily (Grimm et al., 2003; Lee et al., 2003), recently came into the focus of attention due to its involvement in human brain pathologies. In fact, TRPM3 is best characterized in the peripheral nervous system, where it functions as a noxious heat sensor in somatosensory neurons (Vriens et al., 2011; Vriens and Voets, 2018). Although several groups had indicated an abundant expression of TRPM3 in the brain in the past (Oberwinkler and Philipp, 2014), only few studies investigated its roles in the central nervous system, showing its functional presence in cerebellar Purkinje cells (Zamudio-Bulcock et al., 2011) and oligodendrocytes (Hoffmann et al., 2010). The more surprising were two recent publications that reported *de novo* mutations in TRPM3 as the cause of developmental and epileptic encephalopathies (DEEs) in a total of nine patients (Dyment et al., 2019; de Sainte Agathe et al., 2020). These findings motivated further functional studies on these mutant channels (Van Hoeymissen et al., 2020; Zhao et al., 2020).

In this review, we summarize our current knowledge and knowledge gaps related to TRPM3, focusing on channel properties that are relevant to understand its role in brain function and pathology.

ION CHANNEL PROPERTIES AND FUNCTIONS OF TRPM3—LESSONS FROM THE PERIPHERAL NERVOUS SYSTEM AND NON-NEURAL TISSUES

General Properties of TRPM3 Splice Variants

TRPM3 was identified <20 years ago as a functional ion channel-forming TRP protein (Grimm et al., 2003; Lee et al., 2003). In 2007, it was even labeled as an enigmatic channel (Oberwinkler, 2007), based on the fact that the *Trpm3* gene appears to encode the highest number of channel isoforms reported within the TRP family (Oberwinkler and Philipp, 2014; Shiels, 2020). The different isoforms arise from alternative splicing at the N terminal part of the channel and from alternative splicing of exons spread all over the gene. The mouse isoforms are classified into TRPM3α and TRPM3β groups depending on the start exon. TRPM3α isoforms start with exon 1 and do not express exon 2, while TRPM3β isoforms start with exon 2 (Oberwinkler et al., 2005; Oberwinkler, 2007; Oberwinkler and Philipp, 2014). Recently, the novel splice variants, TRPM3γ2 and TRPM3γ3 were identified, which start with exon2 and have a truncation in exon 28 (Uchida et al., 2019). As in mouse, several splice variants exist in humans, labeled as TRPM3a-f following their relative abundance (Lee et al., 2003). Even more transcript variants and predicted protein sequences are deposited in the public NCBI reference sequence (RefSeq) database (Shiels, 2020). The splicing pattern seems to be well-conserved between species (Oberwinkler and Phillipp, 2007; Oberwinkler and Philipp, 2014). However, most of the reported isoforms are not yet functionally characterized and their roles are largely unknown. Whether they form functional cation channels seems to depend on a specific *r*egion *i*ndispensable for *c*hannel *f*unctions (ICFR), which was identified to be essential for the channel formation. Isoforms lacking ICFR, like TRPM3α7, do not form functional ion channels, probably due to a disturbed tetrameric channel complex formation and a decreased plasma membrane expression. Therefore, when co-expressed with the functional TRPM3α2, TRPM3α7 acts as a dominant negative regulator of the channel activity (Frühwald et al., 2012). Although TRPM3α7 transcripts were detected and estimated to form about 15% of the total TRPM3 transcripts in the brain (Frühwald et al., 2012), its impact on brain-specific function is yet to be discovered.

Upon cloning, both human and mouse TRPM3 were identified as Ca^{2+} entry channels (Grimm et al., 2003; Lee et al., 2003), but their permeability and functional features can vary tremendously between different isoforms. At this point, only a few of the TRPM3 isoforms have been functionally characterized in detail, with the most comprehensive analyses comparing the isoforms TRPM3α1 and TRPM3α2 (Oberwinkler et al., 2005; Held et al., 2020), which differ only in the presence (TRPM3α1) or absence (TRPM3α2) of a 12 amino acid-long sequence insertion into the pore-forming loop. This seemingly minor difference results in a massive change in their biophysical characteristics, which dramatically affects their permeability. Homotetrameric ion channels formed by TRPM3α2 subunits are permeable for Ca^{2+}, Mg^{2+}, and even for Zn^{2+} and other divalent cations. In contrast, TRPM3α1 displays strongly reduced permeability for divalent cations and high selectivity toward monovalent cations (Oberwinkler et al., 2005; Wagner et al., 2010). Similar to other TRP channels, both isoforms are strongly inhibited by intracellular Mg^{2+} and show reduced ionic currents in the presence of extracellular divalent cations. The permeability of TRPM3α2, but not TRPM3α1, is also markedly reduced by extracellular monovalent cations (Oberwinkler et al., 2005). In addition to differences in selectivity, there are also marked differences in the pharmacological properties of the short and long pore loop variants. For instance, the long pore loop variant TRPM3α1 is insensitive to pregnenolone sulfate (PregS), a well-characterized agonist of the short pore loop variants TRPM3α2-6, and the isoforms show different sensitivities to several other agonists and antagonists, as well (Held et al., 2020), as detailed later in this review. The recently described isoforms TRPM3γ2 and TRPM3γ3 (Uchida et al., 2019) exhibit biophysical and pharmacological characteristics that appear very similar to those of TRPM3α2, although they show a generally decreased channel activity.

The high diversity amongst TRPM3 isoforms raises the physiologically highly relevant question to what extent do they contribute to the formation of the native TRPM3 channels in the various tissues. Although the answer is uncertain, the data discussed below suggest that most native TRPM3 channels exhibit biophysical and pharmacological properties that are similar to those of TRPM3α2. Indeed, publicly available transcriptome data from mouse tissues demonstrate that the short pore loop isoforms generally dominate, although to varying degrees in different tissues (Held et al., 2020). The transcripts of the recently described γ isoforms are also highly expressed in dorsal root ganglia (DRGs), but their expression in the brain is not known. Moreover, these γ isoforms were suggested not to interact with TRPM3α2 and not to alter pharmacological properties of TRPM3α2 when co-expressed in a recombinant system (Uchida et al., 2019).

The most abundant and characterized human isoform TRPM3a also shares the short pore loop with TRPM3α2 (Oberwinkler and Phillipp, 2007) and both their pharmacological properties and functional features are very similar (Badheka et al., 2015, 2017; Held et al., 2015a). Native human TRPM3 expressed in the sensory ganglia also seems to be functionally similar to the mouse TRPM3α2 channel (Vangeel et al., 2020). Cumulatively, these data indicate that the mouse channel, especially the TRPM3α2 variant, is a highly relevant model to study the function of (native) human TRPM3. Therefore, in the following parts we use the term TRPM3 when referring to the TRPM3α2 variant or to native channels, and specify distinct other variants when relevant.

It is important to mention that, besides the various isoforms, the *Trpm3* gene also codes a microRNA, miR-204, in intron 9 in both humans and mice. It is often co-expressed with the TRPM3 ion channel and should be considered in certain situations when investigating TRPM3 functions, especially when analyzing gene-deleted animal models (Oberwinkler and Philipp, 2014; Shiels, 2020). TRPM3 and miR-204 are co-expressed in pancreatic beta cells and affect insulin production and secretion (Wagner et al., 2008; Thiel et al., 2013; Xu et al., 2013). They are also highly co-expressed in several cells of the eye and seem to be regulated by the same promoter and transcription factors, including paired-box 6 transcription factor (Pax6) and microphthalmia/melanogenesis-associated transcription factor (MITF). These results suggest a possible synergism between their function in eye development and the onset of some ocular diseases (Karali et al., 2007; Adijanto et al., 2012; Xie et al., 2014; Shiels, 2020). Interestingly, TRPM1, the closest relative of TRPM3, also hosts a microRNA, miR-211, which belongs to the same microRNA family as miR-204 and also plays a significant role in the eye (Shiels, 2020). Moreover, in clear cell renal cell carcinoma, TRPM3 and miR-204 were found to play an antagonistic role in the control of oncogenic autophagy (Hall et al., 2014).

(Patho)physiological Roles of TRPM3 in the Periphery

TRPM3 was originally described as a constitutively active Ca^{2+} entry channel in the plasma membrane, which can contribute to store-operated Ca^{2+} entry in certain conditions (Lee et al., 2003), although later studies suggested that store depletion is not significant in regulating TRPM3 activity (Grimm et al., 2003, 2005; Oberwinkler and Phillipp, 2007). The activity of recombinant TRPM3 expressed in HEK293 cells can be stimulated by hypotonic solutions (Grimm et al., 2003; Held et al., 2020), although it remains unclear whether TRPM3 is directly activated by hypotonicity-related membrane stretching or the hypoosmotic environment activates the channel indirectly (Oberwinkler and Phillipp, 2007). TRPM3 was reported to mediate the effects of hypotonic stress in different context: decreased serum osmolarity stimulated the constriction of ductus arteriosus via activation of TRPM3 (Aoki et al., 2014) and hypotonic stress-induced upregulation of the receptor activator of nuclear factor kappa-B ligand (RANKL) and the nuclear factor of activated T cells type c1 (NFATc1) was mediated by both TRPM3 and TRPV4 in periodontal ligament cells and osteoblasts (Son et al., 2015, 2018). These results suggest that TRPM3 can contribute to the mechanical stress-induced bone remodeling. Oppositely, inhibition of TRPM3 by hypertonic solutions may contribute to hypertonicity-induced gene expression in ciliated renal epithelial cells. However, conclusions of this study may be regarded with some caution, as the expression of TRPM3 was confirmed with antibodies and at RNA level, but TRPM3-mediated currents were not reported. Furthermore, the pharmacological effect of the TRPM3 agonist PregS on the hypertonic (500 mosM NaCl) solution-induced gene expression was only very partial, although it could be reversed by the TRPM3 antagonist isosakuranetin (Siroky et al., 2017). Another study, using pharmacological tools, suggested the presence of TRPP2-TRPM3 heteromeric channels in renal primary cilia (Kleene et al., 2019). In contrast to the most widespread variant, the long pore loop isoform TRPM3α1 is not sensitive to hypotonic clues (Held et al., 2020).

TRPM3 is also expressed in vascular smooth muscle cells, where its activation evoked smooth muscle contraction resulting in vasoconstriction, and inhibited IL-6 secretion (Naylor et al., 2010). However, activation of TRPM3 in the perivascular nerves resulted in vasodilation via release of vasoactive substances from perivascular nerve endings (Alonso-Carbajo et al., 2019). Stimulation of TRPM3 also inhibited secretory activity in fibroblast-like synoviocytes from rheumatoid arthritis patients, as TRPM3 agonist inhibited hyaloronan release (Ciurtin et al., 2010). The pharmacological activation of TRPM3 channels expressed in pancreatic beta cells induced insulin secretion (Wagner et al., 2008; Colsoul et al., 2011; Becker et al., 2020). Upon its activation, TRPM3 stimulated the opening of voltage-gated Ca^{2+} channels and initiated complex signaling pathways, upregulating the expression of different transcription factors (Mayer et al., 2011; Müller et al., 2011; Thiel et al., 2013; Becker et al., 2020). The opening of TRPM3 also serves as a regulated Zn^{2+} entry pathway in beta cells (Wagner et al., 2010), where zinc plays a relevant role in the biosynthesis and storage of insulin (Dunn, 2005). Interestingly, extracellular zinc entering via TRPM3 or voltage-gated Ca^{2+} channels can inhibit gene expression initiated by Ca^{2+} entry via the same channels. Therefore, the zinc release accompanying insulin release is hypothesized to act as a negative feedback on exocytosis (Loviscach et al., 2020). Zinc plays an important role in the central nervous system as well, by regulating excitability of ion channels and it can be released together with glutamate (Frederickson et al., 2005; Sensi et al., 2009), but until today, the role of TRPM3 in zinc-related signaling in the brain remains elusive.

TRPM3 is intensely studied in the somatosensory neurons of DRGs and trigeminal ganglia. In 2011, it was introduced as a new member of the thermosensitive TRP channels activated by warming. Elevation of temperature from room temperature to 33°C potentiates agonist induced TRPM3 activation, but its sensitivity toward warming is more dominant in the noxious heat range (>42°C) (Vriens et al., 2011, 2014b; Voets, 2012; Held et al., 2015b). Interestingly, heat sensitivity is completely lost in the long pore loop variant TRPM3α1 (Held et al., 2020). Compared to the well-characterized heat sensor TRPV1, the current–temperature relationship curve of TRPM3 is shifted slightly toward higher temperatures and its temperature-dependent increase in open probability is less steep (Vriens et al., 2011, 2014b; Voets, 2012; Held et al., 2015b). In good accordance with its thermosensitivity and expression by small-sized somatosensory neurons, TRPM3 plays a role in noxious heat sensation together with TRPV1 and TRPA1 (Vriens et al., 2011; Vandewauw et al., 2018; Vriens and Voets, 2018, 2019). TRPM3 activation results in neuropeptide release from the sensory terminals (Held et al., 2015a) and the channel is sensitized by inflammatory conditions, which may contribute to inflammatory hyperalgesia (Vriens et al., 2011; Mulier et al., 2020). In contrast to TRPV1, TRPM3 does not to appear to play a role in central thermoregulation and neither agonists nor antagonists induce noticeable changes in core body temperature (Vriens et al., 2011; Straub et al., 2013a). It selectively mediates pain, and is not involved in itch evoked by pruritic mediators such as histamine or serotonin (Kelemen et al., 2021), which are known to signal via TRPV1 (Shim et al., 2007) and TRPA1 (Morita et al., 2015), respectively.

In addition to somatosensory afferents, TRPM3 is also functional in the vagal afferents of the nodose ganglion (Staaf et al., 2010; Fenwick et al., 2014; Wu et al., 2014; Ragozzino et al., 2020). These channels contribute to basal and temperature-driven spontaneous glutamate release from the central terminals in the nucleus tractus solitarii, while not affecting the synchronous or asynchronous glutamate release (Ragozzino et al., 2020).

Regulation of the Channel Activity and Pharmacology of TRPM3

Intrinsic Regulation by Signaling Molecules

Until today, only a few intracellular signaling molecules were reported to interact with TRPM3. Like other TRP channels, TRPM3 activity is reduced by intracellular Mg^{2+} (Oberwinkler et al., 2005) and Ca^{2+} (Przibilla et al., 2018), and potentiated by phosphatidylinositol 4,5-bisphosphate [PtdIns(4,5)P_2] and other phosphoinositides, among which PtdIns(3,4,5)P_3 was found to be the most effective (Badheka and Rohacs, 2015; Badheka et al., 2015; Tóth et al., 2015, 2016; Uchida et al., 2016). Multiple Ca^{2+}-calmodulin binding sites on the N-terminus were identified, which may interact with PtdIns(4,5)P_2, and S100A protein (Holakovska et al., 2012; Holendova et al., 2012; Przibilla et al., 2018). In good accordance, signaling pathways decreasing endogenous PtdIns(4,5)P_2, like phospholipase C activation evoked by M1 or M3 muscarinic acetylcholine receptors, inhibited both recombinant and native TRPM3 (Badheka et al., 2015; Tóth et al., 2015). $G_{\beta\gamma}$ subunits of trimeric G-proteins were also shown to be negatively coupled to TRPM3 activity, which underlies inhibition of TRPM3 upon stimulation of several G-protein-coupled receptors, including G_q-coupled M1 muscarinic acetylcholine, B2 bradykinin receptors and G_i-coupled M2 muscarinic acetylcholine, D2 dopamine, $GABA_B$, neuropeptide Y, μ-opioid receptors and G_s-coupled EP-2 prostaglandin, and

A2B adenosine receptors or receptors of somatostatin (Badheka et al., 2017; Dembla et al., 2017; Quallo et al., 2017; Alkhatib et al., 2019). A 10-amino-acid-long domain in TRPM3 was identified that interacted with $G_{\beta\gamma}$ proteins. This domain is encoded in an alternatively spliced exon, and is absent in the TRPM3α4 and TRPM3α5 variants, rendering them insensitive to μ-opioid receptor activation or overexpressed $G\beta_1\gamma_2$ subunits. X-ray crystallographic analysis of the corresponding peptide bound to $G\beta_1\gamma_2$ revealed that this domain of TRPM3 interacts exclusively with the $G\beta_1$ (and not $G\gamma_2$) subunit, and amino acids on both the TRPM3 peptide and the $G\beta_1$-proteins that mediate the interaction were identified. Interestingly, the interacting residues in $G\beta_1$ only partially overlap with those involved in the inhibitory interaction with G-protein-coupled inward rectifier K^+ (GIRK) channels (Behrendt et al., 2020). These results suggest that pharmacological targeting of TRPM3 may have a great potential to influence several signaling pathways relevant in various brain functions and in peripheral pain sensation.

TRPM3 Is a Steroid Regulated Channel

The first chemical activator of TRPM3 to be identified was D-erythro sphingosine, which was known from earlier studies to inhibit other ion channels. Two structural analogs, dihydro-D-erythro-sphingosine and N,N-dimethyl-D-erythro-sphingosine, although less effectively, also activated TRPM3, while neither ceramide and 1-sphingosine-phosphate (other significant signaling lipids of the sphingolipid pathway), nor arachidonic acid, anandamide, linoleic acid, linolenic acid, and diacylglycerol analogs affected the channel (Grimm et al., 2005). However, the TRPM3 specificity of D-erythro sphingosine was questioned later (Wagner et al., 2008). The L-type Ca^{2+} channel blocker nifedipine also activated TRPM3 in a reversible way (Wagner et al., 2008), but the long pore loop variant TRPM3α1 was found to be insensitive for nifedipine (Held et al., 2020).

The best characterized and most widely used endogenous TRPM3 agonist is the steroid compound PregS. It activates the channel by shifting its current-voltage activation curve toward more negative membrane potentials and also potentiates temperature-induced activation (Wagner et al., 2008; Vriens et al., 2011; Held et al., 2018). These mechanisms of action are typical features of the agonist-evoked activation of thermosensitive TRP channels in general (Voets et al., 2004). Although PregS activated TRPM3 only in supraphysiological concentrations in most of the experiments carried out at room temperature, a marked activation was evoked by only 100 nM PregS at 37°C, which is in the range of the physiological plasma concentrations (Vriens et al., 2011). Therefore, PregS can be considered as an endogenous activator of TRPM3, even in physiological circumstances. Due to the presence of the negatively charged sulfate group, pregS is a quite lipophobic substance and it behaves as a membrane-impermeable ligand that activates the channel only if applied to the extracellular side (Wagner et al., 2008). This finding suggests that the steroid-binding pocket of TRPM3 is located on the extracellular surface. The steroid (PregS) sensitivity is conserved in the short pore loop (TRPM3α2-α6) variants but completely lost in the long pore loop (TRPM3α1) variant, arguing for the importance of the pore region in the steroid activation of the channel (Held et al., 2020). Analysis of the structure-activity relationship of the steroid ligands revealed that the natural PregS is more effective than its enantiomer and the position and orientation of the sulfate group is also very important to preserve TRPM3 activation (Majeed et al., 2010; Drews et al., 2014). A few other, structurally similar steroid compounds [pregnenolone, dehydroepiandrosterone (DHEA) and DHEA-sulfate] also evoked a moderate activation of TRPM3 (Wagner et al., 2008).

Other steroids were also tested for activity toward the channel. In contrast to PregS, dihydrotestosterone, 17β-estradiol, and progesterone and its metabolites inhibited TRPM3 activation. The inhibitory effect of progesterone was independent of the used TRPM3 activator, whereas dihydrotestosterone behaved as competitive antagonist of PregS (Majeed et al., 2012).

Opening of a Non-canonical Pore and Its Significance

We found that activation by PregS is strongly potentiated by the co-application of the antifungal clotrimazole or its structural analogs TRAM34, senicapoc, and tamoxifen. Importantly, clotrimazole did not only potentiate the outwardly rectifying PregS evoked currents flowing through the well-established central pore of the channel, but also evoked monovalent-selective inwardly rectifying currents at negative membrane potentials (Vriens et al., 2014a). The biophysical characteristics of these currents resemble the so-called omega currents or gating pore currents described earlier in mutated voltage-gated Na^+ and K^+ channels (Sokolov et al., 2005, 2007; Tombola et al., 2005, 2007). The existence of an alternative ion permeation pathway conducting "omega-like" currents in TRPM3 is supported by several lines of evidence. Among others, the voltage sensitivity and permeability of this alternative ion permeation pathway strikingly differs from the main pore, and, in contrast to the main pore, it is resistant to Ca^{2+}-induced desensitization, as well as to classical pore blockers like La^{3+}. Importantly, mutations in the pore domain disrupting the channel's permeability did not affect the alternative pore current, but several mutations generated in the voltage-sensing domain affected the gating pore current, underlining the fundamental role of the voltage sensor domain in forming the non-canonical pore (**Figure 1**). Furthermore, introducing an arginine residue (Trp982Arg) into the S4 segment of the voltage sensor domain prevented PregS and clotrimazole from activating the alternative pore current without inhibiting the main pore-related conductance (Vriens et al., 2014a; Held et al., 2018). Indeed, arginine residues are essential components of the S4 segment of voltage-gated ion channels, and eliminating these positively charged residues results in the appearance of the gating pore current in the above mentioned mutated K^+ and Na^+ channels (Sokolov et al., 2005; Tombola et al., 2005; Held et al., 2016). Based on our best knowledge, until today, the opening of non-canonical pores was revealed only in three naturally occurring wild type ion channels: a flatworm K_v3 channel (N.at-$K_v3.2$), the H_v proton channel, which even does not possess a classical pore domain (Ramsey et al., 2006, 2010; Sasaki et al., 2006; Okamura et al., 2015), and the mammalian TRPM3 (Vriens et al., 2014a). Alignment of the S4 segment of these channels to other voltage-gated ion channels reveals that some of the arginine residues are substituted by uncharged or negatively charged amino acid residues, thereby further highlighting that the loss of positively charged residues from the S4 plays a crucial role in the appearance of an alternative ion permeation pathway [For a comparative review about non-canonical pores in ion channels, we refer to our recent work (Held et al., 2016)]. Recently, we also identified CIM0216 as the currently available most potent and highly effective exogenous activator of TRPM3. Application of CIM0216 alone (i.e., without any other agonist) results in the simultaneous opening of both the classical and the non-canonical pore of the channel (Held et al., 2015a). However, until now, no endogenous ligand was identified that opens this alternative permeation pathway through TRPM3. Interestingly, clotrimazole applied on its own activated the PregS-insensitive long pore loop variant TRPM3α1, which resulted in a linear *I-V* relationship, including large inward currents at negative membrane potentials. The clotrimazole-evoked currents were found to be largely resistant to the classical pore blocker La^{3+} and to Ca^{2+} desensitization, suggesting a potential contribution of the non-canonical pore (Held et al., 2020).

Although, the physiological circumstances that may open the non-canonical pore of TRPM3 remain elusive, it may have important pathological significance. Compared to the exclusive activation of the main pore conductance, the additional opening of the non-canonical pore in TRPM3 increases the discharge rate of somatosensory neurons and exacerbates TRPM3-mediated nociception (Vriens et al., 2014a; Held et al., 2015a). Mutations in the voltage-sensing domain of Na_V and Ca_V channels that result in the appearance of ion conducting non-canonical pores are known to cause muscle (periodic paralysis) and heart diseases (Mixed Arrhythmias and Dilated Cardiomyopathy). Some mutations in the voltage sensor of $K_V7.2$ and $K_V7.3$ subunits also result in the development of non-canonical pore currents. These currents can contribute to the hyperexcitability of neurons and are associated with benign familial neonatal seizures. Recently, two mutations in TRPM3 were found in patients with developmental and epileptic encephalopathies (DEE) (Dyment et al., 2019; de Sainte Agathe et al., 2020). Notably, the mutations were characterized as gain of function mutations (Van Hoeymissen et al., 2020; Zhao et al., 2020), and in one of them the natural ligand PregS activated the gating pore currents (Van Hoeymissen et al., 2020).

Antagonists of TRPM3

Only few blockers of TRPM3 have been described. As nifedipine was recognized as an agonist of the channel, other dihydropyridines were also tested and found to inhibit TRPM3 (Drews et al., 2014). 2-aminoethoxydiphenyl borate (2-APB), an inhibitor of the IP_3 receptor, interacts with several TRP channels. It activates the warm sensitive TRPV1-3, and inhibits several other members of the family, including TRPM3 (Xu et al., 2005). The non-steroidal anti-inflammatory fenamates also inhibited multiple TRP channels, but only mefenamic acid was found to be selective for TRPM3 (Klose et al., 2011). The phospholipase C inhibitor compound U73122 is also suggested to inhibit TRPM3 activation (Leitner et al., 2016).

TRPM3 is inhibited by ononetin, a deoxybenzoin from the plant Ononis spinosa (spiny restharrow), which belongs to the *Fabaceae*. The channel is also blocked by the citrus fruit flavanones hesperetin, naringenin, eriodictyol, liquiritigenin, and isosakuranetin, among which isosakuranetin is the most potent blocker reported until today (Straub et al., 2013a,b). Isosakuranetin and related compounds were also shown to inhibit acute thermal nociception (Straub et al., 2013a) and neuropathic pain (Jia et al., 2017). Another non-steroidal anti-inflammatory drug, diclofenac was also characterized as a TRPM3 blocker, inhibiting agonist-induced currents (Suzuki et al., 2016). The anticonvulsant primidone and the tetracyclic antidepressant maprotiline are also effective blockers of TRPM3. Primidone was found to block the main pore currents evoked by heat, Nifedipine, and PregS, as well as the alternative pore current induced by PregS and clotrimazole. Primidone also attenuated TRPM3-mediated acute thermal pain and heat hyperalgesia. Importantly the IC_{50} value of primidone is in the range of its therapeutic plasma concentrations (Krügel et al., 2017). Recently, we demonstrated that volatile anesthetics can also inhibit TRPM3 in slightly higher concentrations than reached in the plasma during general anesthesia (Kelemen et al., 2020). Although antidepressants, anticonvulsants and volatile anesthetics probably target ion channels in the central nervous system, the putative role of TRPM3 in their therapeutic effect remains to be elucidated.

Interestingly, primidone and volatile anesthetics inhibited both the classical and the non-canonical pore mediated currents, which suggests that these inhibitors do not act as classical pore-blockers but rather inhibit a more general conformational change in the proteins (Krügel et al., 2017; Kelemen et al., 2020).

ROLE OF TRPM3 IN THE BRAIN

Expression of TRPM3 in Various Brain Regions

The brain represents, next to the kidney, one of the tissues with the highest indicated TRPM3 expression. High levels of TRPM3 mRNA were found in several studies of whole brain tissues from rodent and human (Fantozzi et al., 2003; Grimm et al., 2003; Lee et al., 2003; Oberwinkler et al., 2005; Fonfria et al., 2006; Inoue et al., 2006; Wagner et al., 2008; Gilliam and Wensel, 2011; Jang et al., 2012). More detailed expression analysis showed a high abundance of TRPM3 in the choroid plexus, the cerebellum, the forebrain and the hippocampus (dentate gyrus), among others (Lee et al., 2003; Oberwinkler et al., 2005; Kunert-Keil et al., 2006; Hasselblatt et al., 2009; Hoffmann et al., 2010; Zamudio-Bulcock et al., 2011; Oberwinkler and Philipp, 2014) (**Table 1**). Likewise, TRPM3 also displays a diverse distribution pattern over several different cell types within the brain. TRPM3 expression was found in neuronal cells, epithelial cells as well as in oligodendrocytes (Hasselblatt et al., 2009; Hoffmann et al., 2010; Zamudio-Bulcock et al., 2011), but on a functional level it was only confirmed in cerebellar Purkinje neurons (Zamudio-Bulcock et al., 2011) and in oligodendrocytes isolated from whole brain tissue (Hoffmann et al., 2010) (**Table 1**). Actually, to date

TABLE 1 | Overview of reported brain regions expressing TRPM3.

Brain region	Cell type	Tested expression level
Whole brain	Not specified (n.s.)	mRNA Protein
	Oligodendrocytes	mRNA Protein Functional
Basal ganglia	n.s.	mRNA
Substantia nigra	n.s.	mRNA
Brain stem	Neuronal cells	Protein
	Oligodendrocytes	Protein
Cerebrum	n.s.	mRNA
Corpus callosum	Oligodendrocytes	Protein
Choroid plexus	n.s.	mRNA
	Epithelial cells	mRNA
Cerebellum	n.s.	mRNA
		Protein
	Purkinje cell	Protein
		Functional
Cortex	Neuronal cells	protein
Fimbria hippocampi	Oligodendrocytes	protein
Forebrain	n.s.	mRNA
Hippocampus	n.s.	mRNA
Dentate gyrus	n.s.	mRNA
Hypothalamus	n.s.	mRNA
Locus coeruleus	n.s.	mRNA
Tenia tecta	n.s.	mRNA
-	Oli-neu/OLN-93 cells	Protein Functional

Brain regions, cell types and the levels of the reported expression for TRPM3 are summarized; n.s., not specified.

no structured analysis of the TRPM3 expression was carried out in the different brain areas and the variety of used detection techniques makes it almost impossible to compare the TRPM3 expression between different brain regions (Oberwinkler and Philipp, 2014).

It is interesting to note that several different splice variants of TRPM3 were described to be expressed in the mouse brain, with a total of seven alpha (Oberwinkler et al., 2005; Frühwald et al., 2012) and 17 beta variants (Frühwald et al., 2012; Oberwinkler and Philipp, 2014). Although it was reported that certain splice variant mRNA levels are tissue- and development-dependent in the brain (Hoffmann et al., 2010; Held et al., 2020), it remains unknown whether these different splice variants are functionally expressed in the reported tissues and whether they may be involved in mechanisms regulating TRPM3 activity in a cell-specific manner.

Function of TRPM3 in the Brain

Since TRPM3 is a non-selective, calcium-permeable cation channel, TRPM3 activity will result in a depolarization of the neuronal membrane. So far, the only studies that showed functional TRPM3 in brain cells were performed in primary oligodendrocytes isolated from the whole brain (Hoffmann et al., 2010) and in cerebellar Purkinje neurons in brain slices (Zamudio-Bulcock et al., 2011). Furthermore, a functional role of TRPM3 in the choroid plexus was suggested (Millar and Brown, 2006; Millar et al., 2007). These studies provided molecular evidence of TRPM3 activity, using allegedly TRPM3-specific pharmacology or a dominant-negative TRPM3 protein block. Despite this molecular evidence, no further efforts have been made to investigate potential effects of TRPM3 activation on a behavioral or (patho)physiological level in these or other studies. Given the expression of TRPM3 in the brain areas mentioned above, certain assumptions can be made concerning the potential physiological roles of TRPM3 in the brain. For instance, the high mRNA expression and functional activity of TRPM3 in cerebellar Purkinje neurons suggests a role of TRPM3 in the coordination of movement (Beckstead, 1996; Purves, 2004). Furthermore, the high expression of TRPM3 in the choroid plexus (Oberwinkler et al., 2005; Millar and Brown, 2006; Millar et al., 2007), may indicate a potential role of TRPM3 in the ion homoeostasis that is necessary for the production of the cerebrospinal fluid (Damkier et al., 2013). Moreover, high levels of TRPM3 in the hippocampus (Oberwinkler et al., 2005; Kunert-Keil et al., 2006; Hoffmann et al., 2010) hint at a potential role in memory formation and consolidation (Andersen, 2007). Fittingly, some endogenous TRPM3 (ant)agonists are known to influence synaptic signaling and memory functions. For instance, the endogenous TRPM3 activator PregS was reported to increase long-term potentiation at hippocampal CA1 synapses (Sabeti et al., 2007), which may lead to memory-improving effects (Dastgheib et al., 2015). Although these actions of PregS were often attributed to effects on NMDA and $GABA_A$ receptors (Paul and Purdy, 1992; Mayo et al., 1993; Akk et al., 2001; Horak, 2004), it is equally plausible that effects of PregS were partially mediated via TRPM3 channel activation (Wagner et al., 2008). Similarly, estradiol, a reported TRPM3 antagonist, was shown to enhance memory consolidation mediated via the dorsal hippocampus (Tuscher et al., 2019). In addition, three recent studies reported in parallel on the modulation of TRPM3 by $G_{\beta\gamma}$-proteins via a signaling cascade with GPCRs, such as $GABA_B$-, μ-opioid- and NPY receptors (Badheka et al., 2017; Dembla et al., 2017; Quallo et al., 2017). Of note, all of these receptors can be found abundantly in the brain (Hill and Bowery, 1981; Delfs et al., 1994; Reichmann and Holzer, 2016), and the inhibitory effects of endogenous, brain-relevant GPCR ligands such as somatostatin (Martel et al., 2012) and morphine (Beltrán-Campos et al., 2015) on TRPM3 currents were illustrated in these studies (Badheka et al., 2017; Dembla et al., 2017; Quallo et al., 2017). However, all of these studies were performed in heterologous expression systems or peripheral sensory neurons and no brain tissue was used to confirm similar actions. Nevertheless, it can be hypothesized that these mechanisms are not exclusive to peripheral nerves, and that receptor-mediated modulation of TRPM3 may also occur in brain tissue. Undoubtedly, the identification of several brain-relevant receptors and ligands that are either directly or indirectly modulating TRPM3 strengthens the evidence that TRPM3 might present an important player in various brain functions. However, such assumptions still have to be confirmed in experiments specifically designed to investigate the here hypothesized or other functions.

TRPM3 in Brain Disorders

The first link between TRPM3 and brain pathologies was reported in 2009, when Kuniba et al. (2009) performed molecular karyotyping in 17 patients and mutation screening in 41 patients with Kabuki syndrome (KS), a multiple congenital anomaly/mental retardation syndrome (MCA/MR). They identified a chromosomal region that also contains the *TRPM3* gene as a potentially contributing factor in the manifestation of KS. A few years later, Pagnamenta et al. reported a rare *TRPM3* exon deletion in a family with autism and proposed this deletion to contribute to the autism phenotype that was observed in these patients (Pagnamenta et al., 2011). Additionally, TRPM3 overexpression was observed in benign and malignant choroid plexus tumors (Hasselblatt et al., 2009; Japp et al., 2015, 2016). Very recently, TRPM3 was suggested to be involved in mood and anxiety disorders, as an interesting potential player in post-partum mood disorders (Thippeswamy and Davies, 2020). This suggestion was based on the facts that the PregS level-regulating steroid sulfatase (STS) enzyme deficiency is positively linked to mental health conditions and depression in human patients (Cavenagh et al., 2019) and PregS levels were reportedly increased in STS-deficient patients (Sánchez-Guijo et al., 2016). Fittingly, it was also shown that TRPM3 expression was altered in a mouse model of bipolar disorder due to serotonin depletion (Maddaloni et al., 2018), thereby supporting the idea that TRPM3 may regulate mood conditions. However, no hard evidence was provided yet for the mechanistic involvement of TRPM3 in the development and/or manifestation of the above-studied diseases. Considering that several other genes were found to be altered in these patients, conclusions concerning the role of TRPM3 in the investigated pathologies should be regarded with caution.

Interestingly, more evidence for a role of TRPM3 in brain pathologies was provided by a Ca^{2+} influx assay-based drug screening study that identified the clinically approved and commonly used anticonvulsant drug primidone and the anti-depressant maprotiline as potent and relatively selective TRPM3 inhibitors (Krügel et al., 2017). Both drugs were able to completely block the channel activity with IC_{50} values of $\sim$0.6 μM for primidone and $\sim$1.3 μM for maprotiline. However, despite this promising pharmacological profile of maprotiline, reported plasma concentrations during patient treatment are not reaching the concentration ranges necessary to inhibit TRPM3. In contrast, the plasma concentrations of primidone that are obtained in patients treated for epilepsy are in the range of concentrations needed to induce a full block of the PregS-induced TRPM3 currents in a HEK cell culture model (Krügel et al., 2017). Given that there is no consensus on the mechanism for the anticonvulsant action of primidone, TRPM3 represents a potential novel target of this anti-epileptic drug. It can be speculated that a downregulation of the TRPM3 activity might stabilize neuronal membrane potential and/or decrease presynaptic calcium release, thereby rendering the cells less susceptible to damaging overexcitation.

Finally, a recent case study reported two *de novo* mutations in the *TRPM3* gene to be the cause of DEE in a total of eight patients between the age of 4 and 38 (Dyment et al., 2019). All eight patients in this study were heterozygous for a *TRPM3* mutation and the majority of them were male (six out of eight). From all eight patients, seven carried an identical point mutation in the linker region between transmembrane segments 4 and 5. This mutation resulted in the substitution of a valine with a methionine (VM mutation) (**Figure 2A**). The remaining patient carried a proline to glutamine substitution (PQ mutation) at the boundary of the TRPM3 pore-forming loop (Dyment et al., 2019) (**Figure 2A**). More supporting evidence of these findings was given last year by de Sainte Agathe et al. (2020) who reported about another female DEE patient carrying the VM TRPM3 mutation. Interestingly, this patient did not have epilepsy at the moment of assessment, although it could not be excluded that this might occur in a later stage of life, as was observed in one patient described in Dyment et al. (2019) Although both studies did not further investigate the molecular mechanisms surrounding the disease phenotype, two other research teams performed thorough biophysical characterizations of the two reported TRPM3 disease mutations in *in vitro* cell systems (Van Hoeymissen et al., 2020; Zhao et al., 2020). Both studies concluded that the mutations are causing a gain-of-function in TRPM3, which results in an increased basal channel activity with elevated calcium concentrations at rest, a leftward shift of the concentration-response curve for the endogenous agonist PregS and an increased sensitivity to heat stimuli (**Figures 2B–D**). Of note, it was shown that the VM mutation additionally results in the opening of the earlier described alternative ion permeation pathway (Vriens et al., 2014a; Held et al., 2015a, 2016) in TRPM3 upon sole application of PregS (Van Hoeymissen et al., 2020). This causes a dramatic increase of the inward currents at physiological resting membrane potentials (**Figure 2E**). Despite these detailed biophysical characterizations, it remains uncertain how a gain-of-function in the TRPM3 protein causes the observed DEE disease phenotype. Considering the essential role of calcium as a signaling molecule in several neuronal pre- and post-synaptic mechanisms, such as vesicle release, cell depolarization, receptor (de)phosphorylation and internalization as well as in the expressional regulation of proteins (Beattie et al., 2000; Brini et al., 2014), it is not unlikely that the recently studied TRPM3 DEE mutants may have detrimental effects in disease-carrying patients. High calcium levels in the pre- or post-synaptic site of excitatory synapses, which can be caused by an elevated basal channel activity (**Figure 2B**) or an increased neurosteroid-induced activity (PregS) (**Figures 2C,E**), might lead to an elevated firing frequency of excitatory post-synaptic neurons. This may subsequently result in hyper-excitable neuronal cells and explain the observed epileptic phenotype (Badawy et al., 2009). Moreover, the patients show initial developmental deficits prior to the epileptic phenotype (Dyment et al., 2019; de Sainte Agathe et al., 2020). It is hard to predict the exact mechanisms that lead to such developmental abnormalities, but it can be speculated that high calcium levels in mutant TRPM3-expressing

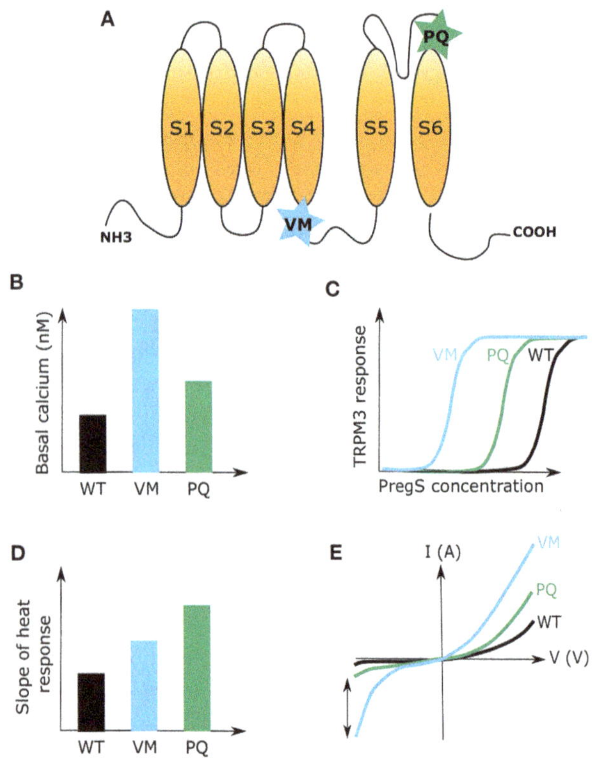

FIGURE 2 | Summary of the two reported developmental and epileptogenic encephalopathy (DEE) disease mutations in TRPM3. **(A)** Cartoon of a TRPM3 channel subunit indicating the positions of the valine to methionine (VM) and proline to glutamine (PQ) substitution mutations. **(B)** Representative graph indicating differences in basal calcium levels between HEK cells that express the TRPM3 wild type channel or the mutant channels VM or PQ. **(C)** Representative graph showing the leftward shift of the concentration-response curve of pregnenolone sulfate (PregS) for the two TRPM3 mutations (VM and PQ) causing developmental and epileptic encephalopathies (DEE). **(D)** Illustration of the heat sensitivity increase for the two DEE mutations compared to wild type (WT) TRPM3. **(E)** Typical examples of current-voltage (I-V) plots for wild type TRPM3 and the DEE mutants VM and PQ during activation with PregS. Note the increase in inward currents for both channel mutants. The two-sided arrow is indicating the high increase in inward currents for the VM mutant, which was attributed to the opening of the alternative ion pore in TRPM3.

brain cells may cause neuronal cell death (Toescu, 1998) or that mutated TRPM3 is abundantly expressed in certain inhibitory neurons, which could lead to abnormal synaptic plasticity (Baroncelli et al., 2011). It is definitely intriguing that the sensitivity of TRPM3 to hormonal clues is increased in the TRPM3 DEE mutant channels (**Figures 2C,E**) (Van Hoeymissen et al., 2020; Zhao et al., 2020), as hormones are known to be centrally involved in developmental regulations (McEwen, 1988, 1992). However, at this point, our knowledge regarding the functional roles of TRPM3 in the brain is very confined, and any kind of mechanistic speculation is rather premature. To illuminate the disease-causing processes in the brain, it first seems necessary to understand, which exact brain areas are affected in the disease-carrying patients, and subsequently confirm and

TABLE 2 | Overview of reported diseases that were linked with *TRPM3* alterations.

Disease	TRPM3 related changes	References
Autism	Deletion of exons 1-9 of *TRPM3*	Pagnamenta et al., 2011
Choroid plexus tumors	Up-regulation of *TRPM3* expression	Hasselblatt et al., 2009; Japp et al., 2015, 2016
Developmental and epileptic encephalopathies (DEE)	*De novo* substitutions in TRPM3 (V837M and P937Q)	Dyment et al., 2019; de Sainte Agathe et al., 2020
Kabuki syndrome	Deletion of chromosomal region that encodes *TRPM3* (9q21.11-q21.12)	Kuniba et al., 2009

For each disease the reported gene or protein alterations of TRPM3 are presented together with the according case studies.

determine specific TRPM3 functions in the various cell types of these brain regions. Clearly, a genetic animal disease-model would be of high scientific value to address such questions, and to shed light on the disease-causing mechanisms of TRPM3 mutations in the brain.

DISCUSSION

Several lines of evidence suggest TRPM3 as an emerging interesting novel player in brain physiology and pathology. First, TRPM3 was shown to be abundantly expressed and functionally active in different brain regions (Oberwinkler and Philipp, 2014). Furthermore, TRPM3 can be modulated by several endogenous brain ligands and receptors (Held et al., 2015b; Badheka et al., 2017; Csanády, 2017; Dembla et al., 2017; Quallo et al., 2017). In addition, TRPM3 was also shown to be targeted by a commonly used anti-convulsion drug, primidone (Krügel et al., 2017), a compound of which the exact molecular actions are up until today still illusive. However, a brain-specific interaction of these drugs and receptors with TRPM3, and the resulting consequences for brain functions still have to be demonstrated. Finally, various genetic alterations in the *TRPM3* gene were linked to several neurological disorders in human patients (Kuniba et al., 2009; Pagnamenta et al., 2011; Japp et al., 2016; Dyment et al., 2019; de Sainte Agathe et al., 2020) (**Table 2**). It is interesting to note that almost all of the neuropathologies that were linked to the *TRPM3* gene resulted in a state of intellectual disability in the affected patients. This may suggest a vital role of TRPM3 in neuronal development and could indicate that TRPM3 is of particular importance in defined brain regions. However, so far there are no studies that investigated genetic *Trpm3* alterations in a systematic way, by linking molecular TRPM3 functions directly to the *in vivo* phenotypes that are caused by these alterations. Clearly, there is an urgent need for more detailed functional studies of TRPM3 in the brain.

As TRPM3 represents a non-selective, cation permeable ion channel with a high permeability for calcium, it is very likely that TRPM3 has an impact on neuronal functions and development by affecting electrical and chemical signals in brain regions where it is expressed. Therefore, thorough morphological, molecular and electrophysiological assessments of different brain areas, circuits, and cells that were shown to express TRPM3 RNA or protein, are warranted in the future in healthy and diseased brains. Additionally, behavioral screening experiments to specifically address selected brain functions linked to the investigated areas, in combination with (brain region-specific) pharmacological targeting or genetic alterations in animal models would be of immense value for our future quest to explore the role(s) of TRPM3 in the brain. Considering the broad hormonal regulation profile of TRPM3 (as discussed in section TRPM3 Is a Steroid Regulated Channel), it would be of further scientific value to apply behavioral tests to animals of different gender and different developmental stages. Such experiments will not only provide insights into the physiological roles of TRPM3 in the brain but could also illuminate the mechanisms of disease in selected TRPM3 animal disease models.

Obviously, more research is required to investigate TRPM3 expression, regulation and function in different brain regions and cell types, and to validate its role in brain (patho)physiology. Nevertheless, given our current knowledge about the molecular and biophysical properties of TRPM3 and its recent genetic links to brain pathologies, it is tempting to imagine TRPM3 as an attractive potential new target for future drug interventions in neurological diseases such as epilepsy or autism spectrum disorders.

AUTHOR CONTRIBUTIONS

KH and BIT drafted, corrected, and wrote this article. BIT was responsible for the funding acquisition. All listed authors qualify for authorship and all authors qualifying for authorship are listed above.

ACKNOWLEDGMENTS

We thank all members of the Laboratory of Endometrium, Endometriosis and Reproductive Medicine (LEERM) and of the Laboratory of Ion Channel Research (LICR) from the KU Leuven, as well as the Laboratory of Cellular and Molecular Physiology (LCMP) in the Department of Physiology at the University of Debrecen for their helpful comments and discussions. We especially thank Prof. Thomas Voets (LICR) for his indispensable support and valuable advice in writing the manuscript.

REFERENCES

Aarts, M., Iihara, K., Wei, W.-L., Xiong, Z.-G., Arundine, M., Cerwinski, W., et al. (2003). A key role for TRPM7 channels in anoxic neuronal death. *Cell* 115, 863–877. doi: 10.1016/S0092-8674(03)01017-1

Adijanto, J., Castorino, J. J., Wang, Z.-X., Maminishkis, A., Grunwald, G. B., and Philp, N. J. (2012). Microphthalmia-associated transcription factor (MITF) promotes differentiation of human retinal pigment epithelium (RPE) by regulating microRNAs-204/211 expression. *J. Biol. Chem.* 287, 20491–20503. doi: 10.1074/jbc.M112.354761

Akk, G., Bracamontes, J., and Steinbach, J. H. (2001). Pregnenolone sulfate block of GABA $_A$ receptors: mechanism and involvement of a residue in the M2 region of the α subunit. *J. Physiol.* 532, 673–684. doi: 10.1111/j.1469-7793.2001.0673e.x

Alkhatib, O., da Costa, R., Gentry, C., Quallo, T., Bevan, S., and Andersson, D. A. (2019). Promiscuous G-protein-coupled receptor inhibition of transient receptor potential melastatin 3 ion channels by Gβγ subunits. *J. Neurosci. Off. J. Soc. Neurosci.* 39, 7840–7852. doi: 10.1523/JNEUROSCI.0882-19.2019

Allen Mouse Brain Atlas (2004). Available online at: mouse.brain-map.org (accessed January 21, 2021).

Alonso-Carbajo, L., Alpizar, Y. A., Startek, J. B., López-López, J. R., Pérez-García, M. T., and Talavera, K. (2019). Activation of the cation channel TRPM3 in perivascular nerves induces vasodilation of resistance arteries. *J. Mol. Cell. Cardiol.* 129, 219–230. doi: 10.1016/j.yjmcc.2019.03.003

Amaral, M. D., and Pozzo-Miller, L. (2007). TRPC3 channels are necessary for brain-derived neurotrophic factor to activate a nonselective cationic current and to induce dendritic spine formation. *J. Neurosci.* 27, 5179–5189. doi: 10.1523/JNEUROSCI.5499-06.2007

Andersen, P. (ed.). (2007). *The Hippocampus Book*. Oxford; New York, NY: Oxford University Press.

Aoki, R., Yokoyama, U., Ichikawa, Y., Taguri, M., Kumagaya, S., Ishiwata, R., et al. (2014). Decreased serum osmolality promotes ductus arteriosus constriction. *Cardiovasc. Res.* 104, 326–336. doi: 10.1093/cvr/cvu199

Badawy, R. A. B., Harvey, A. S., and Macdonell, R. A. L. (2009). Cortical hyperexcitability and epileptogenesis: understanding the mechanisms of epilepsy - part 2. *J. Clin. Neurosci.* 16, 485–500. doi: 10.1016/j.jocn.2008.10.001

Badheka, D., Borbiro, I., and Rohacs, T. (2015). Transient receptor potential melastatin 3 is a phosphoinositide-dependent ion channel. *J. Gen. Physiol.* 146, 65–77. doi: 10.1085/jgp.201411336

Badheka, D., and Rohacs, T. (2015). TRPM3 joins the ranks of PI(4,5)P2 sensitive ion channels. *Channels* 9, 233–234. doi: 10.1080/19336950.2015.1089072

Badheka, D., Yudin, Y., Borbiro, I., Hartle, C. M., Yazici, A., Mirshahi, T., et al. (2017). Inhibition of transient receptor potential melastatin 3 ion channels by G-protein βγ subunits. *eLife* 6:e26147. doi: 10.7554/eLife.26147.018

Baroncelli, L., Braschi, C., Spolidoro, M., Begenisic, T., Maffei, L., and Sale, A. (2011). Brain plasticity and disease: a matter of inhibition. *Neural Plast.* 2011, 1–11. doi: 10.1155/2011/286073

Beattie, E. C., Carroll, R. C., Yu, X., Morishita, W., Yasuda, H., von Zastrow, M., et al. (2000). Regulation of AMPA receptor endocytosis by a signaling mechanism shared with LTD. *Nat. Neurosci.* 3, 1291–1300. doi: 10.1038/81823

Becker, A., Mannebach, S., Mathar, I., Weissgerber, P., Freichel, M., Loodin, A. P., et al. (2020). Control of insulin release by transient receptor potential melastatin 3 (TRPM3) ion channels. *Cell. Physiol. Biochem. Int. J. Exp. Cell. Physiol. Biochem. Pharmacol.* 54, 1115–1131. doi: 10.33594/000000304

Beckstead, R. M. (ed). (1996). "The cerebellum and movement precision," in *A Survey of Medical Neuroscience*, (New York, NY: Springer), 226–237. doi: 10.1007/978-1-4419-8570-5_19

Behrendt, M., Gruss, F., Enzeroth, R., Dembla, S., Zhao, S., Crassous, P.-A., et al. (2020). The structural basis for an on-off switch controlling Gβγ-mediated inhibition of TRPM3 channels. *Proc. Natl. Acad. Sci. U.S.A.* 117, 29090–29100. doi: 10.1073/pnas.2001177117

Beltrán-Campos, V., Silva-Vera, M., García-Campos, M. L., and Díaz-Cintra, S. (2015). Effects of morphine on brain plasticity. *Neurol. Engl. Ed.* 30, 176–180. doi: 10.1016/j.nrleng.2014.08.001

Bovet-Carmona, M., Menigoz, A., Pinto, S., Tambuyzer, T., Krautwald, K., Voets, T., et al. (2018). Disentangling the role of TRPM4 in hippocampus-dependent plasticity and learning: an electrophysiological, behavioral and FMRI approach. *Brain Struct. Funct.* 223, 3557–3576. doi: 10.1007/s00429-018-1706-1

Brini, M., Calì, T., Ottolini, D., and Carafoli, E. (2014). Neuronal calcium signaling: function and dysfunction. *Cell. Mol. Life Sci.* 71, 2787–2814. doi: 10.1007/s00018-013-1550-7

Brixel, L. R., Monteilh-Zoller, M. K., Ingenbrandt, C. S., Fleig, A., Penner, R., Enklaar, T., et al. (2010). TRPM5 regulates glucose-stimulated insulin secretion. *Pflugers Arch.* 460, 69–76. doi: 10.1007/s00424-010-0835-z

Cao, E. (2020). Structural mechanisms of transient receptor potential ion channels. *J. Gen. Physiol.* 152:e201811998. doi: 10.1085/jgp.201811998

Cavenagh, A., Chatterjee, S., and Davies, W. (2019). Behavioural and psychiatric phenotypes in female carriers of genetic mutations associated with X-linked ichthyosis. *PLoS ONE* 14:e0212330. doi: 10.1371/journal.pone.0212330

Chen, W., Xu, B., Xiao, A., Liu, L., Fang, X., Liu, R., et al. (2015). TRPM7 inhibitor carvacrol protects brain from neonatal hypoxic-ischemic injury. *Mol. Brain* 8:11. doi: 10.1186/s13041-015-0102-5

Cheng, H., Beck, A., Launay, P., Gross, S. A., Stokes, A. J., Kinet, J.-P., et al. (2007). TRPM4 controls insulin secretion in pancreatic beta-cells. *Cell Calcium* 41, 51–61. doi: 10.1016/j.ceca.2006.04.032

Ciurtin, C., Majeed, Y., Naylor, J., Sukumar, P., English, A. A., Emery, P., et al. (2010). TRPM3 channel stimulated by pregnenolone sulphate in synovial fibroblasts and negatively coupled to hyaluronan. *BMC Musculoskelet. Disord.* 11:111. doi: 10.1186/1471-2474-11-111

Clapham, D. E. (2003). TRP channels as cellular sensors. *Nature* 426, 517–524. doi: 10.1038/nature02196

Clapham, D. E., Julius, D., Montell, C., and Schultz, G. (2005). International union of pharmacology. XLIX. Nomenclature and structure-function relationships of transient receptor potential channels. *Pharmacol. Rev.* 57, 427–450. doi: 10.1124/pr.57.4.6

Colsoul, B., Vennekens, R., and Nilius, B. (2011). Transient receptor potential cation channels in pancreatic β cells. *Rev. Physiol. Biochem. Pharmacol.* 161, 87–110. doi: 10.1007/112_2011_2

Csanády, L. (2017). A new target for G protein signaling. *eLife* 6:e31106. doi: 10.7554/eLife.31106

Damkier, H. H., Brown, P. D., and Praetorius, J. (2013). Cerebrospinal fluid secretion by the choroid plexus. *Physiol. Rev.* 93, 1847–1892. doi: 10.1152/physrev.00004.2013

Dastgheib, M., Dehpour, A. R., Heidari, M., and Moezi, L. (2015). The effects of intra-dorsal hippocampus infusion of pregnenolone sulfate on memory function and hippocampal BDNF mRNA expression of biliary cirrhosis-induced memory impairment in rats. *Neuroscience* 306, 1–9. doi: 10.1016/j.neuroscience.2015.08.018

de Sainte Agathe, J.-M., Van-Gils, J., Lasseaux, E., Arveiler, B., Lacombe, D., Pfirrmann, C., et al. (2020). Confirmation and expansion of the phenotype associated with the recurrent p.Val837Met variant in TRPM3. *Eur. J. Med. Genet.* 63:103942. doi: 10.1016/j.ejmg.2020.103942

Delfs, J. M., Kong, H., Mestek, A., Chen, Y., Yu, L., Reisine, T., et al. (1994). Expression of Mu opioid receptor mRNA in rat brain: an *in situ* hybridization study at the single cell level. *J. Comp. Neurol.* 345, 46–68. doi: 10.1002/cne.903450104

Dembla, S., Behrendt, M., Mohr, F., Goecke, C., Sondermann, J., Schneider, F. M., et al. (2017). Anti-nociceptive action of peripheral mu-opioid receptors by G-beta-gamma protein-mediated inhibition of TRPM3 channels. *eLife* 6:e26280. doi: 10.7554/eLife.26280.035

Dhaka, A., Murray, A. N., Mathur, J., Earley, T. J., Petrus, M. J., and Patapoutian, A. (2007). TRPM8 is required for cold sensation in mice. *Neuron* 54, 371–378. doi: 10.1016/j.neuron.2007.02.024

Drews, A., Mohr, F., Rizun, O., Wagner, T. F. J., Dembla, S., Rudolph, S., et al. (2014). Structural requirements of steroidal agonists of transient receptor potential melastatin 3 (TRPM3) cation channels. *Br. J. Pharmacol.* 171, 1019–1032. doi: 10.1111/bph.12521

Dunn, M. F. (2005). Zinc-ligand interactions modulate assembly and stability of the insulin hexamer – a review. *Biometals Int. J. Role Met. Ions Biol. Biochem. Med.* 18, 295–303. doi: 10.1007/s10534-005-3685-y

Dyment, D. A., Terhal, P. A., Rustad, C. F., Tveten, K., Griffith, C., Jayakar, P., et al. (2019). *De novo* substitutions of TRPM3 cause intellectual disability and epilepsy. *Eur. J. Hum. Genet.* 27, 1611–1618. doi: 10.1038/s41431-019-0462-x

Fantozzi, I., Zhang, S., Platoshyn, O., Remillard, C. V., Cowling, R. T., and Yuan, J. X.-J. (2003). Hypoxia increases AP-1 binding activity by enhancing capacitative Ca $^{2+}$ entry in human pulmonary artery endothelial cells. *Am. J. Physiol. Lung Cell. Mol. Physiol.* 285, L1233–L1245. doi: 10.1152/ajplung.00445.2002

Fenwick, A. J., Wu, S.-W., and Peters, J. H. (2014). Isolation of TRPV1 independent mechanisms of spontaneous and asynchronous glutamate release at primary afferent to NTS synapses. *Front. Neurosci.* 8:6. doi: 10.3389/fnins.2014.00006

Fonfria, E., Murdock, P. R., Cusdin, F. S., Benham, C. D., Kelsell, R. E., and Mcnulty, S. (2006). Tissue distribution profiles of the human TRPM cation channel family. *J. Recept. Signal Transduct.* 26, 159–178. doi: 10.1080/10799890600637506

Frederickson, C. J., Koh, J.-Y., and Bush, A. I. (2005). The neurobiology of zinc in health and disease. *Nat. Rev. Neurosci.* 6, 449–462. doi: 10.1038/nrn1671

Frühwald, J., Camacho Londoño, J., Dembla, S., Mannebach, S., Lis, A., Drews, A., et al. (2012). Alternative splicing of a protein domain indispensable for function of transient receptor potential melastatin 3 (TRPM3) ion channels. *J. Biol. Chem.* 287, 36663–36672. doi: 10.1074/jbc.M112.396663

Gees, M., Colsoul, B., and Nilius, B. (2010). The role of transient receptor potential cation channels in Ca2+ signaling. *Cold Spring Harb. Perspect. Biol.* 2, a003962–a003962. doi: 10.1101/cshperspect.a003962

Gerzanich, V., Stokum, J. A., Ivanova, S., Woo, S. K., Tsymbalyuk, O., Sharma, A., et al. (2019). Sulfonylurea receptor 1, transient receptor potential cation channel subfamily M member 4, and KIR6.2: role in hemorrhagic progression of contusion. *J. Neurotrauma* 36, 1060–1079. doi: 10.1089/neu.2018.5986

Gilliam, J. C., and Wensel, T. G. (2011). TRP channel gene expression in the mouse retina. *Vision Res.* 51, 2440–2452. doi: 10.1016/j.visres.2011.10.009

Grimm, C., Kraft, R., Sauerbruch, S., Schultz, G., and Harteneck, C. (2003). Molecular and functional characterization of the melastatin-related cation channel TRPM3. *J. Biol. Chem.* 278, 21493–21501. doi: 10.1074/jbc.M300945200

Grimm, C., Kraft, R., Schultz, G., and Harteneck, C. (2005). Activation of the melastatin-related cation channel TRPM3 by D-erythro-sphingosine [corrected]. *Mol. Pharmacol.* 67, 798–805. doi: 10.1124/mol.104.006734

Hall, D. P., Cost, N. G., Hegde, S., Kellner, E., Mikhaylova, O., Stratton, Y., et al. (2014). TRPM3 and miR-204 establish a regulatory circuit that controls oncogenic autophagy in clear cell renal cell carcinoma. *Cancer Cell* 26, 738–753. doi: 10.1016/j.ccell.2014.09.015

Hasselblatt, M., Mertsch, S., Koos, B., Riesmeier, B., Stegemann, H., Jeibmann, A., et al. (2009). TWIST-1 is overexpressed in neoplastic choroid plexus epithelial cells and promotes proliferation and invasion. *Cancer Res.* 69, 2219–2223. doi: 10.1158/0008-5472.CAN-08-3176

Held, K., Aloi, V. D., Freitas, A. C. N., Janssens, A., Segal, A., Przibilla, J., et al. (2020). Pharmacological properties of TRPM3 isoforms are determined by the length of the pore loop. *Br. J. Pharmacol.* doi: 10.1111/bph.15223. [Epub ahead of print].

Held, K., Gruss, F., Aloi, V. D., Janssens, A., Ulens, C., Voets, T., et al. (2018). Mutations in the voltage-sensing domain affect the alternative ion permeation pathway in the TRPM3 channel. *J. Physiol.* 596, 2413–2432. doi: 10.1113/JP274124

Held, K., Kichko, T., De Clercq, K., Klaassen, H., Van Bree, R., Vanherck, J.-C., et al. (2015a). Activation of TRPM3 by a potent synthetic ligand reveals a role in peptide release. *Proc. Natl. Acad. Sci. U.S.A.* 112, E1363–E1372. doi: 10.1073/pnas.1419845112

Held, K., Voets, T., and Vriens, J. (2015b). TRPM3 in temperature sensing and beyond. *Temperature* 2, 201–213. doi: 10.4161/23328940.2014.988524

Held, K., Voets, T., and Vriens, J. (2016). "Signature and pathophysiology of non-canonical pores in voltage-dependent cation channels," in *Reviews of Physiology, Biochemistry and Pharmacology Vol. 170 Reviews of Physiology, Biochemistry and Pharmacology*, eds B. Nilius, P. de Tombe, T. Gudermann, R. Jahn, R. Lill, and O. H. Petersen (Cham: Springer International Publishing), 67–99. doi: 10.1007/112_2015_5003

Hill, D. R., and Bowery, N. G. (1981). 3H-baclofen and 3H-GABA bind to bicuculline-insensitive GABAB sites in rat brain. *Nature* 290, 149–152. doi: 10.1038/290149a0

Hille, B. (2001). *Ion Channels of Excitable Membranes, 3rd Edn.* Sunderland, Mass: Sinauer.

Hoffmann, A., Grimm, C., Kraft, R., Goldbaum, O., Wrede, A., Nolte, C., et al. (2010). TRPM3 is expressed in sphingosine-responsive myelinating oligodendrocytes: TRPM3 in oligodendrocytes. *J. Neurochem.* 114, 654–665. doi: 10.1111/j.1471-4159.2010.06644.x

Holakovska, B., Grycova, L., Jirku, M., Sulc, M., Bumba, L., and Teisinger, J. (2012). Calmodulin and S100A1 protein interact with N terminus of TRPM3 channel. *J. Biol. Chem.* 287, 16645–16655. doi: 10.1074/jbc.M112.350686

Holendova, B., Grycova, L., Jirku, M., and Teisinger, J. (2012). PtdIns(4,5)P2 interacts with CaM binding domains on TRPM3 N-terminus. *Channels Austin Tex* 6, 479–482. doi: 10.4161/chan.22177

Horak, M. (2004). Molecular mechanism of pregnenolone sulfate action at NR1/NR2B receptors. *J. Neurosci.* 24, 10318–10325. doi: 10.1523/JNEUROSCI.2099-04.2004

Huang, J., Du, W., Yao, H., and Wang, Y. (2011). "TRPC channels in neuronal survival," in *TRP Channels*, ed M. X. Zhu (Boca Raton, FL: CRC Press/Taylor and Francis). Available online at: http://www.ncbi.nlm.nih.gov/books/NBK92826/ (accessed October 6, 2020).

Huang, Y., Fliegert, R., Guse, A. H., Lü, W., and Du, J. (2020). A structural overview of the ion channels of the TRPM family. *Cell Calcium* 85:102111. doi: 10.1016/j.ceca.2019.102111

Inoue, R., Jensen, L. J., Shi, J., Morita, H., Nishida, M., Honda, A., et al. (2006). Transient receptor potential channels in cardiovascular function and disease. *Circ. Res.* 99, 119–131. doi: 10.1161/01.RES.0000233356.10630.8a

Jang, Y., Lee, Y., Kim, S. M., Yang, Y. D., Jung, J., and Oh, U. (2012). Quantitative analysis of TRP channel genes in mouse organs. *Arch. Pharm. Res.* 35, 1823–1830. doi: 10.1007/s12272-012-1016-8

Japp, A. S., Gessi, M., Messing-Jünger, M., Denkhaus, D., zur Mühlen, A., Wolff, J. E., et al. (2015). High-resolution genomic analysis does not qualify atypical plexus papilloma as a separate entity among choroid plexus tumors. *J. Neuropathol. Exp. Neurol.* 74, 110–120. doi: 10.1097/NEN.0000000000000154

Japp, A. S., Klein-Hitpass, L., Denkhaus, D., and Pietsch, T. (2016). OTX2 defines a subgroup of atypical teratoid rhabdoid tumors with close relationship to choroid plexus tumors. *J. Neuropathol. Exp. Neurol.* 76, 32–38. doi: 10.1093/jnen/nlw101

Jia, S., Zhang, Y., and Yu, J. (2017). Antinociceptive effects of isosakuranetin in a rat model of peripheral neuropathy. *Pharmacology* 100, 201–207. doi: 10.1159/000478986

Jia, Y., Zhou, J., Tai, Y., and Wang, Y. (2007). TRPC channels promote cerebellar granule neuron survival. *Nat. Neurosci.* 10, 559–567. doi: 10.1038/nn1870

Karali, M., Peluso, I., Marigo, V., and Banfi, S. (2007). Identification and characterization of microRNAs expressed in the mouse eye. *Invest. Ophthalmol. Vis. Sci.* 48, 509–515. doi: 10.1167/iovs.06-0866

Kelemen, B., Lisztes, E., Vladár, A., Hanyicska, M., Almássy, J., Oláh, A., et al. (2020). Volatile anaesthetics inhibit the thermosensitive nociceptor ion channel transient receptor potential melastatin 3 (TRPM3). *Biochem. Pharmacol.* 174:113826. doi: 10.1016/j.bcp.2020.113826

Kelemen, B., Pinto, S., Kim, N., Lisztes, E., Hanyicska, M., Vladár, A., et al. (2021). The TRPM3 ion channel mediates nociception but not itch evoked by endogenous pruritogenic mediators. *Biochem. Pharmacol.* 183:114310. doi: 10.1016/j.bcp.2020.114310

Kim, S. J., Kim, Y. S., Yuan, J. P., Petralia, R. S., Worley, P. F., and Linden, D. J. (2003). Activation of the TRPC1 cation channel by metabotropic glutamate receptor mGluR1. *Nature* 426, 285–291. doi: 10.1038/nature02162

Kleene, S. J., Siroky, B. J., Landero-Figueroa, J. A., Dixon, B. P., Pachciarz, N. W., Lu, L., et al. (2019). The TRPP2-dependent channel of renal primary cilia also requires TRPM3. *PLoS ONE* 14:e0214053. doi: 10.1371/journal.pone.0214053

Klose, C., Straub, I., Riehle, M., Ranta, F., Krautwurst, D., Ullrich, S., et al. (2011). Fenamates as TRP channel blockers: mefenamic acid selectively blocks TRPM3. *Br. J. Pharmacol.* 162, 1757–1769. doi: 10.1111/j.1476-5381.2010.01186.x

Krügel, U., Straub, I., Beckmann, H., and Schaefer, M. (2017). Primidone inhibits TRPM3 and attenuates thermal nociception *in vivo*. *Pain* 158, 856–867. doi: 10.1097/j.pain.0000000000000846

Kullmann, D. M. (2002). The neuronal channelopathies. *Brain* 125, 1177–1195. doi: 10.1093/brain/awf130

Kumar, P., Kumar, D., Jha, S. K., Jha, N. K., and Ambasta, R. K. (2016). "Ion channels in neurological disorders," in *Advances in Protein Chemistry and Structural Biology*, ed R. Donev (London; Oxford; San Diego, CA; Cambridge: Elsevier), 97–136. doi: 10.1016/bs.apcsb.2015.10.006

Kunert-Keil, C., Bisping, F., Krüger, J., and Brinkmeier, H. (2006). Tissue-specific expression of TRP channel genes in the mouse and its variation in three different mouse strains. *BMC Genomics* 7:159. doi: 10.1186/1471-2164-7-159

Kuniba, H., Yoshiura, K., Kondoh, T., Ohashi, H., Kurosawa, K., Tonoki, H., et al. (2009). Molecular karyotyping in 17 patients and mutation screening in 41 patients with Kabuki syndrome. *J. Hum. Genet.* 54, 304–309. doi: 10.1038/jhg.2009.30

Lee, N., Chen, J., Sun, L., Wu, S., Gray, K. R., Rich, A., et al. (2003). Expression and Characterization of human transient receptor potential melastatin 3 (hTRPM3). *J. Biol. Chem.* 278, 20890–20897. doi: 10.1074/jbc.M211232200

Lein, E. S., Hawrylycz, M. J., Ao, N., Ayres, M., Bensinger, A., Bernard, A., et al. (2007). Genome-wide atlas of gene expression in the adult mouse brain. *Nature* 445, 168–176. doi: 10.1038/nature05453

Leitner, M. G., Michel, N., Behrendt, M., Dierich, M., Dembla, S., Wilke, B. U., et al. (2016). Direct modulation of TRPM4 and TRPM3 channels by the phospholipase C inhibitor U73122. *Br. J. Pharmacol.* 173, 2555–2569. doi: 10.1111/bph.13538

Liao, M., Cao, E., Julius, D., and Cheng, Y. (2013). Structure of the TRPV1 ion channel determined by electron cryo-microscopy. *Nature* 504, 107–112. doi: 10.1038/nature12822

Loviscach, L., Backes, T. M., Langfermann, D. S., Ulrich, M., and Thiel, G. (2020). Zn2+ ions inhibit gene transcription following stimulation of the Ca2+ channels Cav1.2 and TRPM3. *Met. Integr. Biometal Sci.* 12, 1735–1747. doi: 10.1039/D0MT00180E

Maddaloni, G., Migliarini, S., Napolitano, F., Giorgi, A., Nazzi, S., Biasci, D., et al. (2018). Serotonin depletion causes valproate-responsive manic-like condition and increased hippocampal neuroplasticity that are reversed by stress. *Sci. Rep.* 8:11847. doi: 10.1038/s41598-018-30291-2

Majeed, Y., Agarwal, A. K., Naylor, J., Seymour, V. A. L., Jiang, S., Muraki, K., et al. (2010). Cis-isomerism and other chemical requirements of steroidal agonists and partial agonists acting at TRPM3 channels. *Br. J. Pharmacol.* 161, 430–441. doi: 10.1111/j.1476-5381.2010.00892.x

Majeed, Y., Tumova, S., Green, B. L., Seymour, V. A. L., Woods, D. M., Agarwal, A. K., et al. (2012). Pregnenolone sulphate-independent inhibition of TRPM3 channels by progesterone. *Cell Calcium* 51, 1–11. doi: 10.1016/j.ceca.2011.09.005

Martel, G., Dutar, P., Epelbaum, J., and Viollet, C. (2012). Somatostatinergic systems: an update on brain functions in normal and pathological aging. *Front. Endocrinol.* 3:154. doi: 10.3389/fendo.2012.00154

Martins, D., Tavares, I., and Morgado, C. (2014). "Hotheaded": the role of TRPV1 in brain functions. *Neuropharmacology* 85, 151–157. doi: 10.1016/j.neuropharm.2014.05.034

Mathar, I., Vennekens, R., Meissner, M., Kees, F., Van der Mieren, G., Camacho Londoño, J. E., et al. (2010). Increased catecholamine secretion contributes to hypertension in TRPM4-deficient mice. *J. Clin. Invest.* 120, 3267–3279. doi: 10.1172/JCI41348

Mayer, S. I., Müller, I., Mannebach, S., Endo, T., and Thiel, G. (2011). Signal Transduction of Pregnenolone sulfate in insulinoma cells activation of EGR-1 expression involving TRPM3, voltage-gated calcium channels, erk, and ternary complex factors. *J. Biol. Chem.* 286, 10084–10096. doi: 10.1074/jbc.M110.202697

Mayo, W., Dellu, F., Robel, P., Cherkaoui, J., Le Moal, M., Baulieu, E.-E., et al. (1993). Infusion of neurosteroids into the nucleus basalis magnocellularis affects cognitive processes in the rat. *Brain Res.* 607, 324–328. doi: 10.1016/0006-8993(93)91524-V

McBurney, R. N., and Neering, I. R. (1987). Neuronal calcium homeostasis. *Trends Neurosci.* 10, 164–169. doi: 10.1016/0166-2236(87)90042-7

McEwen, B. S. (1988). Steroid hormones and the brain: linking "nature" and "nurture" *Neurochem. Res.* 13, 663–669. doi: 10.1007/BF00973285

McEwen, B. S. (1992). Steroid hormones: effect on brain development and function. *Horm. Res.* 37, 1–10. doi: 10.1159/000182393

Menigoz, A., Ahmed, T., Sabanov, V., Philippaert, K., Pinto, S., Kerselaers, S., et al. (2016). TRPM4-dependent post-synaptic depolarization is essential for the induction of NMDA receptor-dependent LTP in CA1 hippocampal neurons. *Pflugers Arch.* 468, 593–607. doi: 10.1007/s00424-015-1764-7

Millar, I., and Brown, P. (2006). Characterisation of a non-selective cation channel in mouse choroid plexus epithelial cells. *Proc. Physiol Soc.* 2:PC16.

Millar, I. D., Bruce, J. I., and Brown, P. D. (2007). Ion channel diversity, channel expression and function in the choroid plexuses. *Cerebrospinal Fluid Res.* 4:8. doi: 10.1186/1743-8454-4-8

Moran, M. M., Xu, H., and Clapham, D. E. (2004). TRP ion channels in the nervous system. *Curr. Opin. Neurobiol.* 14, 362–369. doi: 10.1016/j.conb.2004.05.003

Morgans, C. W., Zhang, J., Jeffrey, B. G., Nelson, S. M., Burke, N. S., Duvoisin, R. M., et al. (2009). TRPM1 is required for the depolarizing light response in retinal ON-bipolar cells. *Proc. Natl. Acad. Sci. U.S.A.* 106, 19174–19178. doi: 10.1073/pnas.0908711106

Morita, T., McClain, S. P., Batia, L. M., Pellegrino, M., Wilson, S. R., Kienzler, M. A., et al. (2015). HTR7 mediates serotonergic acute and chronic itch. *Neuron* 87, 124–138. doi: 10.1016/j.neuron.2015.05.044

Mulier, M., Van Ranst, N., Corthout, N., Munck, S., Vanden Berghe, P., Vriens, J., et al. (2020). Upregulation of TRPM3 in nociceptors innervating inflamed tissue. *eLife* 9:e61103. doi: 10.7554/eLife.61103.sa2

Müller, I., Rössler, O. G., and Thiel, G. (2011). Pregnenolone sulfate activates basic region leucine zipper transcription factors in insulinoma cells: role of voltage-gated Ca2+ channels and transient receptor potential melastatin 3 channels. *Mol. Pharmacol.* 80, 1179–1189. doi: 10.1124/mol.111.074781

Narayanan, K. L., Irmady, K., Subramaniam, S., Unsicker, K., and von Bohlen und Halbach, O. (2008). Evidence that TRPC1 is involved in hippocampal glutamate-induced cell death. *Neurosci. Lett.* 446, 117–122. doi: 10.1016/j.neulet.2008.09.034

Naylor, J., Li, J., Milligan, C. J., Zeng, F., Sukumar, P., Hou, B., et al. (2010). Pregnenolone sulphate- and cholesterol-regulated TRPM3 channels coupled to vascular smooth muscle secretion and contraction. *Circ. Res.* 106, 1507–1515. doi: 10.1161/CIRCRESAHA.110.219329

Nilius, B. (2012). Transient receptor potential (TRP) channels in the brain: the good and the ugly. *Eur. Rev.* 20, 343–355. doi: 10.1017/S1062798711000597

Nilius, B., and Owsianik, G. (2011). The transient receptor potential family of ion channels. *Genome Biol.* 12:218. doi: 10.1186/gb-2011-12-3-218

Nilius, B., and Szallasi, A. (2014). Transient receptor potential channels as drug targets: from the science of basic research to the art of medicine. *Pharmacol. Rev.* 66, 676–814. doi: 10.1124/pr.113.008268

Oberwinkler, J. (2007). TRPM3, a biophysical enigma? *Biochem. Soc. Trans.* 35, 89–90. doi: 10.1042/BST0350089

Oberwinkler, J., Lis, A., Giehl, K. M., Flockerzi, V., and Philipp, S. E. (2005). Alternative splicing switches the divalent cation selectivity of TRPM3 channels. *J. Biol. Chem.* 280, 22540–22548. doi: 10.1074/jbc.M503092200

Oberwinkler, J., and Philipp, S. E. (2014). "TRPM3," in mammalian transient receptor potential (TRP) cation channels handbook of experimental pharmacology. eds B. Nilius, and V. Flockerzi (Berlin, Heidelberg: Springer), 427–459. doi: 10.1007/978-3-642-54215-2_17

Oberwinkler, J., and Phillipp, S. E. (2007). TRPM3. *Handb. Exp. Pharmacol.* 179, 253–267. doi: 10.1007/978-3-540-34891-7_15

Okamura, Y., Fujiwara, Y., and Sakata, S. (2015). Gating mechanisms of voltage-gated proton channels. *Annu. Rev. Biochem.* 84, 685–709. doi: 10.1146/annurev-biochem-060614-034307

Pagnamenta, A. T., Holt, R., Yusuf, M., Pinto, D., Wing, K., Betancur, C., et al. (2011). A family with autism and rare copy number variants disrupting the duchenne/becker muscular dystrophy gene DMD and TRPM3. *J. Neurodev. Disord.* 3, 124–131. doi: 10.1007/s11689-011-9076-5

Paul, S. M., and Purdy, R. H. (1992). Neuroactive steroids. *FASEB J.* 6, 2311–2322. doi: 10.1096/fasebj.6.6.1347506

Pérez, C. A., Huang, L., Rong, M., Kozak, J. A., Preuss, A. K., Zhang, H., et al. (2002). A transient receptor potential channel expressed in taste receptor cells. *Nat. Neurosci.* 5, 1169–1176. doi: 10.1038/nn952

Philippaert, K., Pironet, A., Mesuere, M., Sones, W., Vermeiren, L., Kerselaers, S., et al. (2017). Steviol glycosides enhance pancreatic beta-cell function and taste sensation by potentiation of TRPM5 channel activity. *Nat. Commun.* 8:14733. doi: 10.1038/ncomms14733

Przibilla, J., Dembla, S., Rizun, O., Lis, A., Jung, M., Oberwinkler, J., et al. (2018). Ca2+-dependent regulation and binding of calmodulin to multiple sites of transient receptor potential melastatin 3 (TRPM3) ion channels. *Cell Calcium* 73, 40–52. doi: 10.1016/j.ceca.2018.03.005

Purves, D. (ed.). (2004). *Neuroscience, 3rd Edn.* Sunderland, MA: Sinauer Associates, Publishers.

Quallo, T., Alkhatib, O., Gentry, C., Andersson, D. A., and Bevan, S. (2017). G protein βγ subunits inhibit TRPM3 ion channels in sensory neurons. *eLife* 6:e26138. doi: 10.7554/eLife.26138.013

Ragozzino, F. J., Arnold, R. A., Fenwick, A. J., Riley, T. P., Lindberg, J. E. M., Peterson, B., et al. (2020). TRPM3 expression and control of glutamate release from primary vagal afferent neurons. *J. Neurophysiol.* 125, 199–210. doi: 10.1152/jn.00229.2020

Ramsey, I. S., Mokrab, Y., Carvacho, I., Sands, Z. A., Sansom, M. S. P., and Clapham, D. E. (2010). An aqueous H+ permeation pathway in the voltage-gated proton channel Hv1. *Nat. Struct. Mol. Biol.* 17, 869–875. doi: 10.1038/nsmb.1826

Ramsey, I. S., Moran, M. M., Chong, J. A., and Clapham, D. E. (2006). A voltage-gated proton-selective channel lacking the pore domain. *Nature* 440, 1213–1216. doi: 10.1038/nature04700

Reboreda, A. (2012). "TRP channels in the brain," in *TRP Channels in Drug Discovery Methods in Pharmacology and Toxicology*, eds A. Szallasi, and T. Bíró (Totowa, NJ: Humana Press), 115–140. doi: 10.1007/978-1-62703-095-3_7

Reichmann, F., and Holzer, P. (2016). Neuropeptide Y: a stressful review. *Neuropeptides* 55, 99–109. doi: 10.1016/j.npep.2015.09.008

Riccio, A., Medhurst, A. D., Mattei, C., Kelsell, R. E., Calver, A. R., Randall, A. D., et al. (2002). mRNA distribution analysis of human TRPC family in CNS and peripheral tissues. *Mol. Brain Res.* 109, 95–104. doi: 10.1016/S0169-328X(02)00527-2

Sabeti, J., Nelson, T. E., Purdy, R. H., and Gruol, D. L. (2007). Steroid pregnenolone sulfate enhances NMDA-receptor-independent long-term potentiation at hippocampal CA1 synapses: role for L-type calcium channels and sigma-receptors. *Hippocampus* 17, 349–369. doi: 10.1002/hipo.20273

Sánchez-Guijo, A., Neunzig, J., Gerber, A., Oji, V., Hartmann, M. F., Schuppe, H.-C., et al. (2016). Role of steroid sulfatase in steroid homeostasis and characterization of the sulfated steroid pathway: evidence from steroid sulfatase deficiency. *Mol. Cell. Endocrinol.* 437, 142–153. doi: 10.1016/j.mce.2016.08.019

Sasaki, M., Takagi, M., and Okamura, Y. (2006). A voltage sensor-domain protein is a voltage-gated proton channel. *Science* 312, 589–592. doi: 10.1126/science.1122352

Sawamura, S., Shirakawa, H., Nakagawa, T., Mori, Y., and Kaneko, S. (2017). "TRP channels in the brain," in *Neurobiology of TRP Channels*, eds T. L. R. Emir (Boca Raton: CRC Press), 295–322. doi: 10.4324/9781315152837-16

Schlingmann, K. P., Waldegger, S., Konrad, M., Chubanov, V., and Gudermann, T. (2007). TRPM6 and TRPM7—gatekeepers of human magnesium metabolism. *Biochim. Biophys. Acta BBA Mol. Basis Dis.* 1772, 813–821. doi: 10.1016/j.bbadis.2007.03.009

Sensi, S. L., Paoletti, P., Bush, A. I., and Sekler, I. (2009). Zinc in the physiology and pathology of the CNS. *Nat. Rev. Neurosci.* 10, 780–791. doi: 10.1038/nrn2734

Shiels, A. (2020). TRPM3_miR-204: a complex locus for eye development and disease. *Hum. Genomics* 14:7. doi: 10.1186/s40246-020-00258-4

Shim, W.-S., Tak, M.-H., Lee, M.-H., Kim, M., Kim, M., Koo, J.-Y., et al. (2007). TRPV1 mediates histamine-induced itching via the activation of phospholipase A2 and 12-lipoxygenase. *J. Neurosci. Off. J. Soc. Neurosci.* 27, 2331–2337. doi: 10.1523/JNEUROSCI.4643-06.2007

Siroky, B. J., Kleene, N. K., Kleene, S. J., Varnell, C. D., Comer, R. G., Liu, J., et al. (2017). Primary cilia regulate the osmotic stress response of renal epithelial cells through TRPM3. *Am. J. Physiol. Renal Physiol.* 312, F791–F805. doi: 10.1152/ajprenal.00465.2015

Sita, G., Hrelia, P., Graziosi, A., Ravegnini, G., and Morroni, F. (2018). TRPM2 in the brain: role in health and disease. *Cells* 7:82. doi: 10.3390/cells7070082

Sokolov, S., Scheuer, T., and Catterall, W. A. (2005). Ion permeation through a voltage- sensitive gating pore in brain sodium channels having voltage sensor mutations. *Neuron* 47, 183–189. doi: 10.1016/j.neuron.2005.06.012

Sokolov, S., Scheuer, T., and Catterall, W. A. (2007). Gating pore current in an inherited ion channelopathy. *Nature* 446, 76–78. doi: 10.1038/nature05598

Son, A., Kang, N., Kang, J. Y., Kim, K. W., Yang, Y.-M., and Shin, D. M. (2018). TRPM3/TRPV4 regulates Ca2+-mediated RANKL/NFATc1 expression in osteoblasts. *J. Mol. Endocrinol.* 61, 207–218. doi: 10.1530/JME-18-0051

Son, G. Y., Yang, Y. M., Park, W. S., Chang, I., and Shin, D. M. (2015). Hypotonic stress induces RANKL via transient receptor potential melastatin 3 (TRPM3) and vaniloid 4 (TRPV4) in human PDL cells. *J. Dent. Res.* 94, 473–481. doi: 10.1177/0022034514567196

Song, K., Wang, H., Kamm, G. B., Pohle, J., Reis, F., de, C., et al. (2016). The TRPM2 channel is a hypothalamic heat sensor that limits fever and can drive hypothermia. *Science* 353, 1393–1398. doi: 10.1126/science.aaf7537

Staaf, S., Franck, M. C. M., Marmigère, F., Mattsson, J. P., and Ernfors, P. (2010). Dynamic expression of the TRPM subgroup of ion channels in developing mouse sensory neurons. *Gene Expr. Patterns GEP* 10, 65–74. doi: 10.1016/j.gep.2009.10.003

Straub, I., Krügel, U., Mohr, F., Teichert, J., Rizun, O., Konrad, M., et al. (2013a). Flavanones that selectively inhibit TRPM3 attenuate thermal nociception *in vivo*. *Mol. Pharmacol.* 84, 736–750. doi: 10.1124/mol.113.086843

Straub, I., Mohr, F., Stab, J., Konrad, M., Philipp, S. E., Oberwinkler, J., et al. (2013b). Citrus fruit and fabacea secondary metabolites potently and selectively block TRPM3. *Br. J. Pharmacol.* 168, 1835–1850. doi: 10.1111/bph.12076

Sun, H.-S. (2017). Role of TRPM7 in cerebral ischaemia and hypoxia: TRPM7 in cerebral ischaemia. *J. Physiol.* 595, 3077–3083. doi: 10.1113/JP273709

Sun, H.-S., Jackson, M. F., Martin, L. J., Jansen, K., Teves, L., Cui, H., et al. (2009). Suppression of hippocampal TRPM7 protein prevents delayed neuronal death in brain ischemia. *Nat. Neurosci.* 12, 1300–1307. doi: 10.1038/nn.2395

Suzuki, H., Sasaki, E., Nakagawa, A., Muraki, Y., Hatano, N., and Muraki, K. (2016). Diclofenac, a nonsteroidal anti-inflammatory drug, is an antagonist of human TRPM3 isoforms. *Pharmacol. Res. Perspect.* 4:e00232. doi: 10.1002/prp2.232

Tai, Y., Feng, S., Ge, R., Du, W., Zhang, X., He, Z., et al. (2008). TRPC6 channels promote dendritic growth via the CaMKIV-CREB pathway. *J. Cell Sci.* 121, 2301–2307. doi: 10.1242/jcs.026906

Talavera, K., Yasumatsu, K., Voets, T., Droogmans, G., Shigemura, N., Ninomiya, Y., et al. (2005). Heat activation of TRPM5 underlies thermal sensitivity of sweet taste. *Nature* 438, 1022–1025. doi: 10.1038/nature04248

Tan, C.-H., and McNaughton, P. A. (2018). TRPM2 and warmth sensation. *Pflugers Arch.* 470, 787–798. doi: 10.1007/s00424-018-2139-7

Thiel, G., Müller, I., and Rössler, O. G. (2013). Signal transduction via TRPM3 channels in pancreatic β-cells. *J. Mol. Endocrinol.* 50, R75–83. doi: 10.1530/JME-12-0237

Thippeswamy, H., and Davies, W. (2020). A new molecular risk pathway for postpartum mood disorders: clues from steroid sulfatase-deficient individuals. *Arch. Womens Ment. Health.* doi: 10.1007/s00737-020-01093-1. [Epub ahead of print].

Toescu, E. C. (1998). Apoptosis and cell death in neuronal cells: where does Ca2+ fit in? *Cell Calcium* 24, 387–403. doi: 10.1016/S0143-4160(98)90062-8

Tombola, F., Pathak, M. M., Gorostiza, P., and Isacoff, E. Y. (2007). The twisted ion-permeation pathway of a resting voltage-sensing domain. *Nature* 445, 546–549. doi: 10.1038/nature05396

Tombola, F., Pathak, M. M., and Isacoff, E. Y. (2005). Voltage-sensing arginines in a potassium channel permeate and occlude cation-selective pores. *Neuron* 45, 379–388. doi: 10.1016/j.neuron.2004.12.047

Tóth, B. I., Konrad, M., Ghosh, D., Mohr, F., Halaszovich, C. R., Leitner, M. G., et al. (2015). Regulation of the transient receptor potential channel TRPM3 by phosphoinositides. *J. Gen. Physiol.* 146, 51–63. doi: 10.1085/jgp.201411339

Tóth, B. I., Oberwinkler, J., and Voets, T. (2016). Phosphoinositide regulation of TRPM channels - TRPM3 joins the club! *Channels Austin Tex.* 10, 83–85. doi: 10.1080/19336950.2015.1113719

Turlova, E., Bae, C. Y. J., Deurloo, M., Chen, W., Barszczyk, A., Horgen, F. D., et al. (2016). TRPM7 regulates axonal outgrowth and maturation of primary hippocampal neurons. *Mol. Neurobiol.* 53, 595–610. doi: 10.1007/s12035-014-9032-y

Tuscher, J. J., Taxier, L. R., Schalk, J. C., Haertel, J. M., and Frick, K. M. (2019). Chemogenetic suppression of medial prefrontal-dorsal hippocampal interactions prevents estrogenic enhancement of memory consolidation in female mice. *Eneuro* 6:ENEURO.0451-18.2019. doi: 10.1523/ENEURO.0451-18.2019

Uchida, K., Demirkhanyan, L., Asuthkar, S., Cohen, A., Tominaga, M., and Zakharian, E. (2016). Stimulation-dependent gating of TRPM3 channel in planar lipid bilayers. *FASEB J. Off. Publ. Fed. Am. Soc. Exp. Biol.* 30, 1306–1316. doi: 10.1096/fj.15-281576

Uchida, K., Dezaki, K., Damdindorj, B., Inada, H., Shiuchi, T., Mori, Y., et al. (2011). Lack of TRPM2 impaired insulin secretion and glucose metabolisms in mice. *Diabetes* 60, 119–126. doi: 10.2337/db10-0276

Uchida, K., Fukuta, N., Yamazaki, J., and Tominaga, M. (2019). Identification and classification of a new TRPM3 variant (γ subtype). *J. Physiol. Sci. JPS* 69, 623–634. doi: 10.1007/s12576-019-00677-6

Van Hoeymissen, E., Held, K., Nogueira Freitas, A. C., Janssens, A., Voets, T., and Vriens, J. (2020). Gain of channel function and modified gating properties in TRPM3 mutants causing intellectual disability and epilepsy. *eLife* 9:e57190. doi: 10.7554/eLife.57190

Vandewauw, I., De Clercq, K., Mulier, M., Held, K., Pinto, S., Van Ranst, N., et al. (2018). A TRP channel trio mediates acute noxious heat sensing. *Nature* 555, 662–666. doi: 10.1038/nature26137

Vangeel, L., Benoit, M., Miron, Y., Miller, P. E., De Clercq, K., Chaltin, P., et al. (2020). Functional expression and pharmacological modulation of TRPM3 in human sensory neurons. *Br. J. Pharmacol.* 177, 2683–2695. doi: 10.1111/bph.14994

Voets, T. (2012). Quantifying and modeling the temperature-dependent gating of TRP channels. *Rev. Physiol. Biochem. Pharmacol.* 162, 91–119. doi: 10.1007/112_2011_5

Voets, T., Droogmans, G., Wissenbach, U., Janssens, A., Flockerzi, V., and Nilius, B. (2004). The principle of temperature-dependent gating in cold- and heat-sensitive TRP channels. *Nature* 430, 748–754. doi: 10.1038/nature02732

Voets, T., Owsianik, G., Janssens, A., Talavera, K., and Nilius, B. (2007). TRPM8 voltage sensor mutants reveal a mechanism for integrating thermal and chemical stimuli. *Nat. Chem. Biol.* 3, 174–182. doi: 10.1038/nchembio862

Voets, T., Talavera, K., Owsianik, G., and Nilius, B. (2005). Sensing with TRP channels. *Nat. Chem. Biol.* 1, 85–92. doi: 10.1038/nchembio0705-85

Vriens, J., Held, K., Janssens, A., Tóth, B. I., Kerselaers, S., Nilius, B., et al. (2014a). Opening of an alternative ion permeation pathway in a nociceptor TRP channel. *Nat. Chem. Biol.* 10, 188–195. doi: 10.1038/nchembio.1428

Vriens, J., Nilius, B., and Voets, T. (2014b). Peripheral thermosensation in mammals. *Nat. Rev. Neurosci.* 15, 573–589. doi: 10.1038/nrn3784

Vriens, J., Owsianik, G., Hofmann, T., Philipp, S. E., Stab, J., Chen, X., et al. (2011). TRPM3 is a nociceptor channel involved in the detection of noxious heat. *Neuron* 70, 482–494. doi: 10.1016/j.neuron.2011.02.051

Vriens, J., and Voets, T. (2018). Sensing the heat with TRPM3. *Pflüg. Arch. Eur. J. Physiol.* 470, 799–807. doi: 10.1007/s00424-017-2100-1

Vriens, J., and Voets, T. (2019). Heat sensing involves a TRiPlet of ion channels. *Br. J. Pharmacol.* 176, 3893–3898. doi: 10.1111/bph.14812

Wagner, T. F. J., Drews, A., Loch, S., Mohr, F., Philipp, S. E., Lambert, S., et al. (2010). TRPM3 channels provide a regulated influx pathway for zinc in pancreatic beta cells. *Pflugers Arch.* 460, 755–765. doi: 10.1007/s00424-010-0838-9

Wagner, T. F. J., Loch, S., Lambert, S., Straub, I., Mannebach, S., Mathar, I., et al. (2008). Transient receptor potential M3 channels are ionotropic steroid receptors in pancreatic β cells. *Nat. Cell Biol.* 10, 1421–1430. doi: 10.1038/ncb1801

Woo, S. K., Tsymbalyuk, N., Tsymbalyuk, O., Ivanova, S., Gerzanich, V., and Simard, J. M. (2020). SUR1-TRPM4 channels, not KATP, mediate brain swelling following cerebral ischemia. *Neurosci. Lett.* 718:134729. doi: 10.1016/j.neulet.2019.134729

Wu, L.-J., Sweet, T.-B., and Clapham, D. E. (2010). International union of basic and clinical pharmacology. LXXVI. Current progress in the mammalian TRP ion channel family. *Pharmacol. Rev.* 62, 381–404. doi: 10.1124/pr.110.002725

Wu, S., Fenwick, A. J., and Peters, J. H. (2014). Channeling satiation: a primer on the role of TRP channels in the control of glutamate release from vagal afferent neurons. *Physiol. Behav.* 136, 179–184. doi: 10.1016/j.physbeh.2014.09.003

Xie, Q., Ung, D., Khafizov, K., Fiser, A., and Cvekl, A. (2014). Gene regulation by PAX6: structural-functional correlations of missense mutants and transcriptional control of Trpm3/miR-204. *Mol. Vis.* 20, 270–282.

Xu, G., Chen, J., Jing, G., and Shalev, A. (2013). Thioredoxin-interacting protein regulates insulin transcription through microRNA-204. *Nat. Med.* 19, 1141–1146. doi: 10.1038/nm.3287

Xu, S.-Z., Zeng, F., Boulay, G., Grimm, C., Harteneck, C., and Beech, D. J. (2005). Block of TRPC5 channels by 2-aminoethoxydiphenyl borate: a differential, extracellular and voltage-dependent effect. *Br. J. Pharmacol.* 145, 405–414. doi: 10.1038/sj.bjp.0706197

Yin, Y., Wu, M., Zubcevic, L., Borschel, W. F., Lander, G. C., and Lee, S.-Y. (2018). Structure of the cold- and menthol-sensing ion channel TRPM8. *Science* 359, 237–241. doi: 10.1126/science.aan4325

Zamudio-Bulcock, P. A., Everett, J., Harteneck, C., and Valenzuela, C. F. (2011). Activation of steroid-sensitive TRPM3 channels potentiates glutamatergic transmission at cerebellar Purkinje neurons from developing rats: TRPM3 channels modulate glutamate release. *J. Neurochem.* 119, 474–485. doi: 10.1111/j.1471-4159.2011.07441.x

Zhao, S., Yudin, Y., and Rohacs, T. (2020). Disease-associated mutations in the human TRPM3 render the channel overactive via two distinct mechanisms. *eLife* 9:e55634. doi: 10.7554/eLife.55634.sa2

Zündorf, G., and Reiser, G. (2011). Calcium dysregulation and homeostasis of neural calcium in the molecular mechanisms of neurodegenerative diseases provide multiple targets for neuroprotection. *Antioxid. Redox Signal.* 14, 1275–1288. doi: 10.1089/ars.2010.3359

5

The Role of TRP Channels and PMCA in Brain Disorders: Intracellular Calcium and pH Homeostasis

Sung-Min Hwang [1†]***, Ji Yeon Lee*** [2†]***, Chul-Kyu Park*** [1*] ***and Yong Ho Kim*** [1*]

[1] *Gachon Pain Center, Department of Physiology, Gachon University College of Medicine, Incheon, South Korea,*

[2] *Gil Medical Center, Department of Anesthesiology and Pain Medicine, Gachon University, Incheon, South Korea*

***Correspondence:**
Yong Ho Kim
euro16@gachon.ac.kr
Chul-Kyu Park
pck0708@gachon.ac.kr

† *These authors have contributed equally to this work*

Brain disorders include neurodegenerative diseases (NDs) with different conditions that primarily affect the neurons and glia in the brain. However, the risk factors and pathophysiological mechanisms of NDs have not been fully elucidated. Homeostasis of intracellular Ca^{2+} concentration and intracellular pH (pH_i) is crucial for cell function. The regulatory processes of these ionic mechanisms may be absent or excessive in pathological conditions, leading to a loss of cell death in distinct regions of ND patients. Herein, we review the potential involvement of transient receptor potential (TRP) channels in NDs, where disrupted Ca^{2+} homeostasis leads to cell death. The capability of TRP channels to restore or excite the cell through Ca^{2+} regulation depending on the level of plasma membrane Ca^{2+} ATPase (PMCA) activity is discussed in detail. As PMCA simultaneously affects intracellular Ca^{2+} regulation as well as pH_i, TRP channels and PMCA thus play vital roles in modulating ionic homeostasis in various cell types or specific regions of the brain where the TRP channels and PMCA are expressed. For this reason, the dysfunction of TRP channels and/or PMCA under pathological conditions disrupts neuronal homeostasis due to abnormal Ca^{2+} and pH levels in the brain, resulting in various NDs. This review addresses the function of TRP channels and PMCA in controlling intracellular Ca^{2+} and pH, which may provide novel targets for treating NDs.

Keywords: TRP channels, brain pathology, neurodegenerative diseases, calcium, pH, homeostasis, neuron

INTRODUCTION

Calcium (Ca^{2+}) is a second messenger involved in numerous signal transduction pathways, including cell proliferation, cell growth, neuronal excitability, metabolism, apoptosis, and differentiation (Berridge et al., 2000; Gleichmann and Mattson, 2011; Maklad et al., 2019). Intracellular Ca^{2+} has a complex role in brain signaling and regulates brain physiology to maintain neuronal integrity (Marambaud et al., 2009; Bezprozvanny, 2010; Kawamoto et al., 2012). Ca^{2+} influx across the plasma membrane is important for fundamental brain functions which are mainly mediated by glutamate receptor channels, voltage-gated Ca^{2+} channels, sodium-calcium exchanger, and transient receptor potential (TRP) channels (Bezprozvanny, 2010; Cross et al., 2010; Gees et al., 2010; Cuomo et al., 2015; Kumar et al., 2016). Thus, Ca^{2+} signaling affects a variety of neuronal functions in diverse physiological roles, and Ca^{2+} must be tightly regulated to avoid uncontrolled responses that can lead to pathological conditions (Kumar et al., 2016). However, sustained increase in Ca^{2+} influx induces endoplasmic reticulum stress, mitochondrial dysfunction, and various proteases, resulting in neuronal cell death

(Bezprozvanny, 2010; Kawamoto et al., 2012). Indeed, impaired cell function caused by reactive nitrogen (oxygen) species and abnormal pH homeostasis also underpins the pathophysiology of neurodegenerative diseases (NDs) (Piacentini et al., 2008; Bezprozvanny, 2010; Gleichmann and Mattson, 2011; Zundorf and Reiser, 2011; Harguindey et al., 2017, 2019; Popugaeva et al., 2017). In particular, the maintenance of Ca^{2+} and pH levels is involved in a variety of NDs, including Alzheimer's disease (AD), Parkinson's disease (PD), Huntington's disease (HD), amyotrophic lateral sclerosis (ALS), and age-related disorders (Harguindey et al., 2007; Kumar et al., 2009; Smaili et al., 2009; Ruffin et al., 2014; Hong et al., 2020; Thapak et al., 2020). Extensive literature indicates that an excessive increase in cytosolic Ca^{2+} and H^+ constitutes both direct and indirect ND-induced processes (Marambaud et al., 2009; Smaili et al., 2009; Bezprozvanny, 2010; Ruffin et al., 2014; Zhao et al., 2016; Harguindey et al., 2017).

TRP channels constitute a large family of membrane Ca^{2+} channels involved in a wide range of processes including thermoregulation, osmosis, pH, stretch, and chemical signaling (Kaneko and Szallasi, 2014). Functionally, activation of TRP channels influences Ca^{2+} signaling by allowing Ca^{2+} to enter the cell (cell depolarization), which may activate voltage-gated Ca^{2+} channels (Nilius and Owsianik, 2011; Vennekens et al., 2012). TRP channels in neuronal cells regulate voltage-gated Ca^{2+}, K^+, and Na^+ channels, whereas TRP channel regulation in glial cells results in reduced Ca^{2+} entry via ORAI by membrane depolarization, or increased Ca^{2+} influx through the hyperpolarization of the membrane (Gees et al., 2010). In the central nervous system, TRP channels are widely expressed throughout the brain and play an essential role in regulating Ca^{2+} homeostasis associated with various cellular functions, including synaptic plasticity, synaptogenesis, and synaptic transmission in a specific region of the brain (Venkatachalam and Montell, 2007; Kaneko and Szallasi, 2014; Jardin et al., 2017; Chi et al., 2018; Hong et al., 2020). In addition, TRP subtype channels are expressed simultaneously or separately in neurons and glia, fulfilling critical roles in cell homeostasis, development, neurogenesis, and synaptic plasticity (Vennekens et al., 2012). Several members of the TRP subtype are highly expressed in neurons and glia (Moran et al., 2004; Butenko et al., 2012; Ho et al., 2014; Ronco et al., 2014; Verkhratsky et al., 2014; Liu et al., 2017; Rakers et al., 2017) (**Table 1**). Thus, diverse TRP channels expressed in the brain are involved in the progression of NDs such as Parkinson's and Alzheimer's. In particular, increased intracellular Ca^{2+} via TRP channels contributes to various pathophysiological events (Venkatachalam and Montell, 2007; Kaneko and Szallasi, 2014; Moran, 2018; Hong et al., 2020) as well as brain disorders such as AD, PD, stroke, epilepsy, and migraine (**Table 1**)(Morelli et al., 2013; Kaneko and Szallasi, 2014; Kumar et al., 2016; Moran, 2018; Hong et al., 2020; Liu et al., 2020).

The normal regulation of intracellular Ca^{2+} levels involves mechanisms that control the specific uptake and extrusion mechanisms across the cell membrane (Kawamoto et al., 2012; Strehler and Thayer, 2018). Ca^{2+} influx is mediated by several voltage- and ligand-gated channels as well as transporters. Conversely, Ca^{2+} extrusion is dependent on Ca^{2+} pumps and Na^+/Ca^{2+} exchangers (Strehler and Thayer, 2018). Among these, plasma membrane Ca^{2+} ATPases (PMCAs) actively extrude Ca^{2+} ions out of cells (Boczek et al., 2019). Thus, these pumps are important gatekeepers for maintaining intracellular Ca^{2+} homeostasis in cells (Stafford et al., 2017; Boczek et al., 2019). However, PMCA dysfunction causes altered Ca^{2+} homeostasis and leads to a persistent increase in cytosolic Ca^{2+}, which can be neurotoxic and can accelerate the development of NDs and cognitive impairments as the person ages (Strehler and Thayer, 2018; Boczek et al., 2019). In particular, it is possible that the regulation of Ca^{2+} concentration might be more sensitive in which the cells are expressed both TRP and PMCA in the particular brain region (**Figure 1**). Thereby, abnormal expression of either TRP or PMCA subtype may be more likely to cause ND than other parts of the brain (**Figure 2**) (Minke, 2006; Stafford et al., 2017). In addition, PMCA activity is associated with intracellular acidification (Hwang et al., 2011) which is associated with neurological conditions observed among AD patients and other ND patients (Kato et al., 1998; Hamakawa et al., 2004; Mandal et al., 2012; Ruffin et al., 2014; Tyrtyshnaia et al., 2016).

It is crucial to investigate whether increased Ca^{2+} and (or) acidification are risk factors that affects ND-induced processes (Chesler, 2003; Hwang et al., 2011; Ruffin et al., 2014; Cuomo et al., 2015; Stafford et al., 2017; Boczek et al., 2019). Here, we review the involvement of TRP channels and PMCA in the pathophysiology of NDs.

BRAIN DISORDERS

Neurodegenerative Diseases

NDs such as AD, PD, HD, and ALS are age-related conditions characterized by uncontrolled neuronal death in the brain (Hong et al., 2020; Slanzi et al., 2020; Thapak et al., 2020). To date, several studies have reported that NDs are associated with protein aggregation, oxidative stress, inflammation, and abnormal Ca^{2+} homeostasis (Sprenkle et al., 2017). The impairment of Ca^{2+} homeostasis is known to result in increased susceptibility to NDs (Kumar et al., 2009; Smaili et al., 2009; Bezprozvanny, 2010; Gleichmann and Mattson, 2011; Kawamoto et al., 2012; Bagur and Hajnoczky, 2017). In particular, this impairment is associated with changes in Ca^{2+} buffering capacity, deregulation of Ca^{2+} channel activity, and alteration in other calcium regulatory proteins that occur in some types of neurons and glial cells in certain brain regions (Zundorf and Reiser, 2011; Nikoletopoulou and Tavernarakis, 2012). There is also increased Ca^{2+} influx mediated by abnormal TRP channel activation (Sawamura et al., 2017). Similarly, Ca^{2+} extrusion through PMCA has been shown to decrease in aged neurons (Jiang et al., 2012). For this reason, these NDs are associated with Ca^{2+} channels in neurons and glial cells (astrocytes, microglia, and oligodendrocytes), which are important for neuronal survival, myelin formation, neuronal support, and regulation of local neuron activity (neurons-glial signaling) (Zhang and Liao, 2015; Cornillot et al., 2019; Enders et al., 2020).

TABLE 1 | A summary of the transient receptor potential (TRP) subtypes found in distribution of central nervous system (CNS) cell types.

TRP channels		Expression in brain	Expression in glia	Disorders	References
TRPC subfamily	TRPC1	- Cerebellum, hippocampus, forebrain - Dopaminergic neuron (Human/mouse)	Astrocyte, microglia,	NDs, ADs, PD, HD,	Riccio et al., 2002; Bollimuntha et al., 2005, 2006; Selvaraj et al., 2009, 2012; Hong et al., 2015
	TRPC3	- Cerebellum, hippocampus, forebrain - Dopaminergic neuron (Human)	Astrocyte,	NDs, ADs, PDs	Rosker et al., 2004; Wu et al., 2004; Yamamoto et al., 2007; Mizoguchi et al., 2014
	TRPC4	Cerebellum, hippocampus, forebrain	Astrocyte,	Epilepsy	Wang et al., 2007; Wu et al., 2008; Von Spiczak et al., 2010; Tai et al., 2011
	TRPC5	- Cerebellum, forebrain - Hippocampus (mouse)	Astrocyte,	NDs, PDs, Epilepsy	Shin et al., 2010; Tai et al., 2011; Kaczmarek et al., 2012
	TRPC6	Cerebellum, hippocampus, forebrain, striatum	Astrocyte, microglia	NDs, ADs	Lessard et al., 2005; Wang et al., 2015; Liu et al., 2017; Lu et al., 2017
TRPM subfamily	TRPM2	- Hippocampus, forebrain - Cerebellum (human), cortex (rat)	Astrocyte, microglia	NDs, ADs, PDs	Fonfria et al., 2005; Kaneko et al., 2006; Hermosura et al., 2008; Ostapchenko et al., 2015
	TRPM7	- Cerebellum, forebrain, - Hippocampus (human) - cortex (mouse)	Astrocyte, microglia	NDs, ADs, PDs, Epilepsy	Aarts and Tymianski, 2005; Hermosura et al., 2005; Chen X. et al., 2010; Coombes et al., 2011; Oakes et al., 2019
TRPV subfamily	TRPV1	- Basal ganglia, hindbrain Cerebellum - Hippocampus (rat/mouse),	Astrocyte, microglia	NDs, AD, HD, epilepsy	Lastres-Becker et al., 2003; Kim et al., 2005; Gibson et al., 2008; Li et al., 2008; Lee et al., 2011; Balleza-Tapia et al., 2018
	TRPV4	Cerebellum, hippocampus,	Astrocyte, microglia	NDs, AD,	Auer-Grumbach et al., 2010; Chen D. H. et al., 2010; Landoure et al., 2010; Klein et al., 2011; Wang et al., 2019
TRPA subfamily	TRPA1	Cerebellum, hippocampus,	Astrocyte, oligodendrocyte	AD	Shigetomi et al., 2011; Lee et al., 2016; Saghy et al., 2016; Bolcskei et al., 2018

PMCA, plasma membrane Ca^{2+} ATPase; AD, Alzheimer's disease; PD, Parkinson's disease; ND, neurodegenerative disease.

Pathophysiological Role of TRP Channels

TRP channels are non-selective, Ca^{2+}-permeable channels that regulate diverse cellular functions in neurons (Nilius, 2007; Venkatachalam and Montell, 2007; Sawamura et al., 2017). Based on functional characterization of TRP channels by a wide range of stimuli (Zheng, 2013), aberrant activity of TRP channels likely initiates and/or propagates ND processes, especially cell death, via increased intracellular Ca^{2+} in various brain regions (Moran, 2018; Hong et al., 2020; Huang et al., 2020). Here, we focus on the function of TRP channels associated with Ca^{2+} signaling in neurons and glial cells (**Figure 1A**) (Nilius, 2007; Bollimuntha et al., 2011; Zheng, 2013; Zhang and Liao, 2015; Jardin et al., 2017; Sawamura et al., 2017; Hasan and Zhang, 2018; Samanta et al., 2018; Cornillot et al., 2019; Enders et al., 2020; Wang et al., 2020). Based on sequence homology, the TRP family currently comprises 28 mammalian channels and is subdivided into six subfamilies: TRP canonical (TRPC), TRP vanilloid (TRPV), TRP ankyrin (TRPA), TRP melastatin (TRPM), TRP polycystin (TRPP), and TRP mucolipin (TRPML) (Nilius, 2007; Selvaraj et al., 2010; Nishida et al., 2015; Sawamura et al., 2017). Most TRP channels are non-selective channels with consistent Ca^{2+} permeability (Samanta et al., 2018) and each TRP subtype responds to various temperatures, ligands, as well as specific agonists and activators (**Figure 1B**) (Luo et al., 2020). TRP channels are tetramers formed by monomers that share a common structure comprising six transmembrane domains and containing cation-selective pores (Hellmich and Gaudet, 2014). Numerous studies have reported that these TRP channels are related to neuronal cell death that is associated with abnormal Ca^{2+} homeostasis (Gees et al., 2010; Sawamura et al., 2017).

TRPC (Classic or Canonical)

TRPC was the first TRP group identified in mammals (Selvaraj et al., 2010). The TRPC subfamily contains members: TRPC1-7

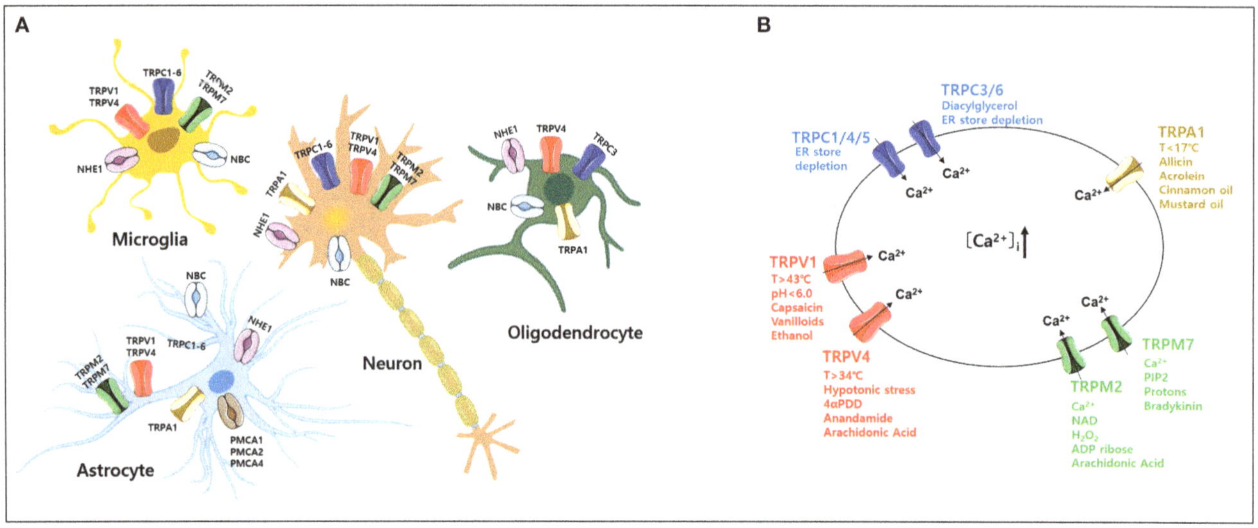

FIGURE 1 | Expression of various transient receptor potential (TRP) subtypes and calcium (Ca^{2+}) influx by their agonists in the mammalian central nervous system (CNS). **(A)** Expression profile of various TRP channels, NHE1, and NBC, in mammalian CNS cell types. **(B)** Ca^{2+} influx through activation of TRP subtypes by various agonists or activators in the mammalian CNS. TRP, transient receptor potential; PMCA, plasma membrane Ca^{2+} ATPase; NBC, Na^+/HCO_3^- cotransporters; NHE, Na^+/H^+ exchangers.

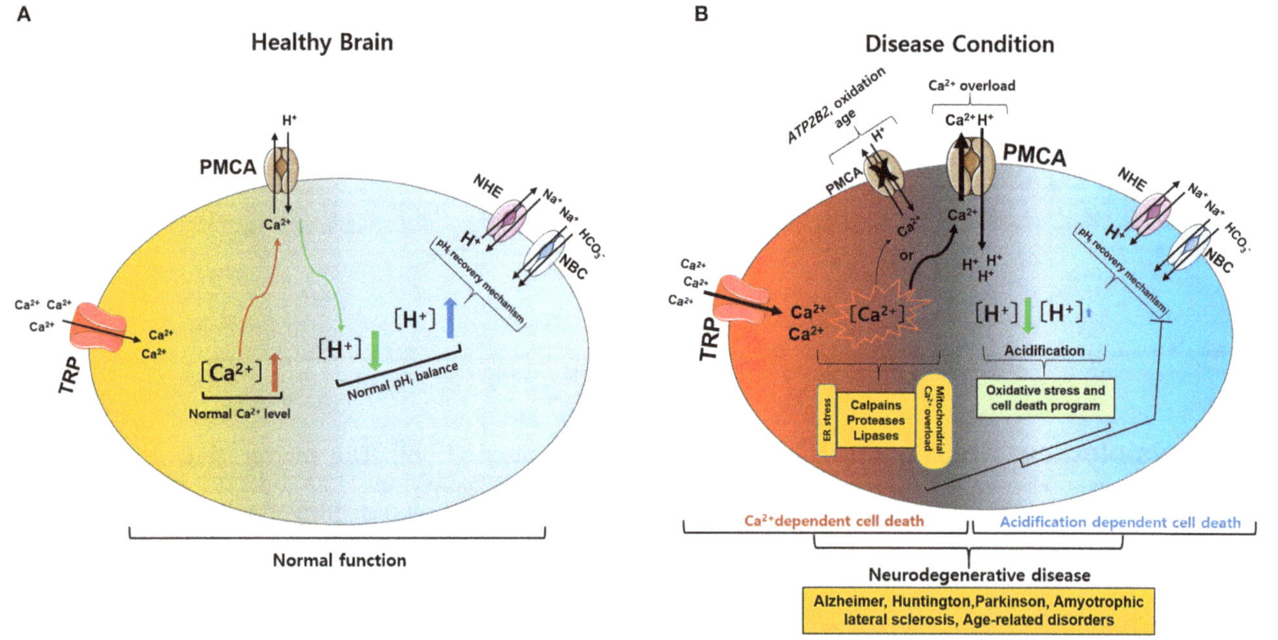

FIGURE 2 | Intracellular calcium (Ca^{2+}) and pH (pH_i) signaling by activation of TRP and PMCA in healthy and diseased condition of the brain. **(A)** Normal physiological function of intracellular Ca^{2+} and pH_i homeostasis. The activation of TRP channels leads to Ca^{2+} influx into the cytosol. Increased Ca^{2+} levels are regulated by PMCA. The activation of PMCA can cause acidification. Acidification conditions are mediated by pH_i recovery functions regulated by NBC and NHE. **(B)** Neurodegenerative diseases caused by pathophysiological functions of intracellular Ca^{2+} and pH_i homeostasis. (1) The activation of TRP channels leads to excess Ca^{2+} influx and overload Ca^{2+} is maintained due to *ATP2B2*, oxidation, and age-related downregulation of PMCA: Ca^{2+}-dependent cell death. (2) PMCA overexpression due to cytoplasmic Ca^{2+} overload cause persistent acidification from inhibition of the pH_i recovery mechanism by oxidative stress or cell death program: acidification dependent cell death. Ultimately, abnormal intracellular Ca^{2+} and pH_i levels impair neuronal function, resulting in neurodegenerative diseases. TRP, transient receptor potential; PMCA, plasma membrane Ca^{2+} ATPase; NBC, Na^+/HCO_3^- cotransporters; NHE, Na^+/H^+ exchangers.

(Wang et al., 2020). With the exception of TRPC2, all TRPC channels are widely expressed in the brain from the embryonic period to adulthood (Douglas et al., 2003). TRPC channels can form functional channels by heteromeric interactions, functioning as non-selective Ca^{2+} entry channels with distinct activation modes (Villereal, 2006). Thus, TRPC channels play an important role in regulating basic neuronal processes. TRPC1 is highly expressed and involved in the early development and proliferation of neurons (Yamamoto et al., 2005; Hentschke et al., 2006) as well as synaptic transmission (Broker-Lai et al., 2017; Wang et al., 2020). TRPC1 and TRPC4 have been reported to regulate neuronal cell death in response to seizures in the hippocampus and septum (Broker-Lai et al., 2017). The TRPC1/4/5 channel has been expressed in the somatosensory cortex, hippocampus, and motor cortex of adult rats (Riccio et al., 2002; Moran et al., 2004; Fowler et al., 2007). In particular, the dense expression of TRPC3 regulates hippocampal neuronal excitability and memory function (Neuner et al., 2015). The abnormal increase in sustained cytosolic Ca^{2+} by TRPC5 activation causes neuronal damage through the calpain-caspase-dependent pathway and the CaM kinase as seen in HD (Hong et al., 2015). Spinocerebellar ataxia type 14 (SCA14) is an autosomal dominant ND caused by a mutation in protein kinase Cγ (Wong et al., 2018). This mutation of SCA14 has been demonstrated to cause phosphorylation failure in TRPC3 channels, resulting in persistent Ca^{2+} entry that may contribute to neurodegeneration (Adachi et al., 2008). On the other hand, TRPC3 or TRPC6 promotes neurotrophin action on brain-derived neurotrophic factor (BDNF) by improving neuronal survival through Ca^{2+} influx (Huang et al., 2011). All TRPC channels are expressed in astrocytes and TRPC1 and TRPC3 play a critical role in astrocyte store-operated Ca^{2+} entry, which is induced by endoplasmic reticulum depletion (Verkhratsky et al., 2014). TRPC1 and TRPC6 are also expressed in rat microglia (Zhang and Liao, 2015). Thus, some TRPC channels exhibit different functions in normal physiological or pathological events, depending on Ca^{2+} signaling in the brain (Huang et al., 2011; Li et al., 2012; Neuner et al., 2015).

TRPM (Melastatin)

Of all TRP channels, the TRPM subfamily has the largest and most diverse expression levels and has been strongly implicated in NDs (Samanta et al., 2018). The TRPM channel consists of eight members (TRPM1-8) and shares common structural characteristics with other TRP channels (Huang et al., 2020). However, they have a variety of C-terminal sections with active enzyme domains and a unique N-terminal without ankyrin repeats involved in channel assembly and trafficking (Huang et al., 2020). A distinctive feature of TRPM channels is the regulation of Ca^{2+} and magnesium (Mg^{2+}) homeostasis, and TRPM (2–7) are mainly expressed in the CNS. In addition, TRPM2 is activated by a wide range of factors including NAD^{+}-related metabolites, adenosine diphosphate-ribose, oxidative stress, and depletion of glutathione (GSH) (Sita et al., 2018). Increased levels of reactive oxygen species (ROS) due to GSH depletion causes TRPM2-dependent Ca^{2+} influx to induce neuronal cell death, suggesting that several neurological disorders, including AD, PD, and bipolar disorder (Akyuva and Naziroglu, 2020). In addition, an increase in intracellular Ca^{2+} and Aβ induced by TRPM2 activity induces neuronal cell death in the rat striatum (Belrose and Jackson, 2018). Mg^{2+} is the second most abundant cation and essential cofactor in various enzymatic reactions (Ryazanova et al., 2010). TRPM2 is expressed by both microglia and astrocytes, which regulate gliosis and immune cell function (Wang et al., 2016; Huang et al., 2017). TRPM7 is permeable to Mg^{2+} and maintains Mg^{2+} homeostasis (Ryazanova et al., 2010). In mouse cortical neurons, inhibition of TRPM7 expression protects against neuronal cell damage (Asrar and Aarts, 2013; Huang et al., 2020). TRPM7 is also found in astrocytes and microglia to control migration, proliferation, and invasion (Siddiqui et al., 2014; Zeng et al., 2015).

TRPV (Vanilloid)

TRPV channels form homo- or heterotetrameric complexes and are non-selective cation channels (Startek et al., 2019). The TRPV subfamily consists of six members (TRPV1-6) that are located mostly on the plasma membrane (Zhai et al., 2020). Recent studies on pathological TRPV1 expression in the brain have been performed (Mickle et al., 2015). TRPV1 activation induces caspase-3 dependent programmed cell death through Ca^{2+}-mediated signaling, resulting in cell death of cortical neurons (Ho et al., 2012; Song et al., 2013) and also triggers cell death through L-type Ca^{2+} channels and Ca^{2+} influx in rat cortical neurons (Shirakawa et al., 2008). The activation of cannabinoid 1 (CB1) receptors stimulates TRPV1 activity, leading to increased intracellular Ca^{2+} and cell death of mesencephalic dopaminergic neurons (Kim et al., 2005, 2008). TRPV1 activation induces apoptotic cell death in rat cortical neurons, leading to chronic epilepsy distinguished by abnormal brain activity (Fu et al., 2009). TRPV1 activation in microglia plays a positive role in promoting microglial phagocytosis in damaged cells while disrupting mitochondria and increasing ROS production (Kim et al., 2006; Hassan et al., 2014). TRPV1 has been shown to affect the migration of astrocytes (Ho et al., 2014). Abnormal function of TRPV4 leads to neuronal dysfunction and axonal degeneration due to increased Ca^{2+} via Ca^{2+}/calmodulin-dependent protein kinase II (CaMKII) (Woolums et al., 2020). TRPV4 plays a role in regulating the osmotic pressure in the brain and is highly expressed throughout glial cells associated with ND (Liedtke and Friedman, 2003; Rakers et al., 2017). Thus, these channels play an important role in Ca^{2+} homeostasis and are therapeutic targets for various disorders.

TRPA (Ankyrin)

TRPA1 was first identified as an ankyrin-like transmembrane protein and the solitary member of the mammalian TRPA subfamily (Yang and Li, 2016). TRPA1 is a non-selective cation channel formed by homo- or heterotetramer subunits with a cytosolic N-terminal domain (16 ankyrin repeat sequence) and C-terminal Ca^{2+}-binding domains (Nilius et al., 2011; Fernandes et al., 2012). The TRPA1 channel responds to a variety of ligands, such as temperature, osmotic changes, and endogenous compounds (Nishida et al., 2015). To date, the reported role of TRPA1 in neurons is the mediation of pain, cold, inflammation, and itch sensation (Fernandes et al., 2012). Recent reports indicate that TRPA1 hyperactivation causes Aβ oligomer-mediated rapid Ca^{2+} signaling (Bosson et al., 2017; Hong et al., 2020). Additionally, ablation of TRPA1 in APP/PS1 transgenic mice attenuated the progression of AD, improved learning and memory conditions, and reduced Aβ plaques and cytokines (Lee et al., 2016). Similarly, TRPA1 channels promote Ca^{2+} hyperactivity of astrocytes and then contribute to synaptic dysfunction due to the oligomeric forms of Aβ peptide (Lee et al., 2016; Bosson et al., 2017; Logashina et al., 2019; Alavi et al., 2020). In addition, TRPA1 mediates Ca^{2+} signaling in astrocytes, resulting in dysregulation of synaptic activity in AD (Bosson et al., 2017).

Other Channels

TRPML and TRPP have limited similarity to other TRP family members (Samanta et al., 2018; Huang et al., 2020). TRPML channels (TRPML1-3) are Ca^{2+} permeable cation channels that each contain six transmembrane segments with helices (S1–S6) and a pore site comprised of S5, S6, and two pore helices (PH1 and PH2) (Schmiege et al., 2018; Tedeschi et al., 2019). TRPML channels are mostly located in intracellular compartments instead of the plasma membrane (Clement et al., 2020). TRPP channels share high protein sequence similarity with TRPML channels and are located in the primary cilia consisting of TRPP1 (also known as PKD1) and TRPP2 (PKD2) (Samanta et al., 2018). To date, evidence indicates that various TRP channels are expressed in the CNS and play important roles in the development of several NDs (Sawamura et al., 2017; Samanta et al., 2018). In particular, TRP channels and Ca^{2+} homeostasis (Bezprozvanny, 2010) are likely to underpin Ca^{2+}-dependent neuronal death in NDs (Sawamura et al., 2017; Hong et al., 2020).

PATHOPHYSIOLOGICAL ROLE OF PLASMA MEMBRANE CALCIUM ATPases

Of the various proteins involved in Ca^{2+} signaling, PMCA is the most sensitive Ca^{2+} detector that regulates Ca^{2+} homeostasis (Boczek et al., 2019). PMCA exists in four known isoforms (Boczek et al., 2019). In both mice and humans, PMCAs 1–4 exhibit anatomically distinct expression patterns, such that isoforms 1 and 4 are ubiquitously expressed in all tissue types, whereas PMCA2 and PMCA3 are tissue-specific and exclusive in neurons of the brain (Kip et al., 2006). In addition, PMCA1, 2, and 4 were detected in rat cortical astrocytes (Fresu et al., 1999) (**Table 2**). The general structure of PMCA consists of 10 transmembrane domains (TM) with the N- and C-terminal ends on the cytosolic side (Stafford et al., 2017). The physiological functions of PMCA include the regulation and maintenance of optimal Ca^{2+} homeostasis (Bagur and Hajnoczky, 2017). PMCA is an ATP-driven Ca^{2+} pump that maintains low resting intracellular Ca^{2+} concentration ($[Ca^{2+}]i$) to prevent cytotoxic Ca^{2+}overload-mediated cell death through activation of ion channels such as TRP (Zundorf and Reiser, 2011). In addition, PMCA is involved in Ca^{2+}-induced intracellular acidification by countertransport of H^+ ions (Vale-Gonzalez et al., 2006; Majdi et al., 2016). Thus, PMCA plays a vital role in controlling cell survival and cell death (Stafford et al., 2017). PMCA expression changes significantly during brain development

TABLE 2 | A summary of the transient receptor potential (TRP) subtypes found in distribution of central nervous system (CNS) cell types.

PMCA subfamily	Expression in brain	Expression in glia	Disorders	References
PMCA1	- Ubiquitous in brain (human and rat). - Cerebellum, cerebral cortex, brain stem (Human)	Rat cortical astrocytes	AD, PD	Stauffer et al., 1995; Fresu et al., 1999; Brini et al., 2013
PMCA2	- Cerebellar purkinje neurons (human/mouse) - cerebellum, cerebral cortex, brain stem (Human)	Rat cortical astrocytes	AD, PD, cerebellar ataxias, sensory neuron diseases	Stauffer et al., 1995; Fresu et al., 1999; Kurnellas et al., 2007; Empson et al., 2010; Hajieva et al., 2018; Strehler and Thayer, 2018
PMCA3	- Cerebellum, cerebral cortex (Human) - Cerebellum and hippocampus (Rat)	Limited	Cerebellar ataxias, sensory neuron diseases	Stauffer et al., 1995; Zanni et al., 2012; Strehler and Thayer, 2018
PMCA4	- Ubiquitous in brain (human/rat) - Cerebellum, cerebral cortex, brain stem (Human)	Rat cortical astrocytes	AD, PD	Stauffer et al., 1995; Fresu et al., 1999; Brini et al., 2013; Zaidi et al., 2018

PMCA, plasma membrane Ca^{2+} ATPase; AD, Alzheimer's disease; PD, Parkinson's disease.

(Boczek et al., 2019). One of the characteristics of brain aging is a Ca^{2+} homeostasis disorder, which can result in detrimental consequences on neuronal function (Boczek et al., 2019). Overall, PMCAs have been attributed a housekeeping role in maintaining intracellular Ca^{2+} levels through precise regulation of Ca^{2+} homeostasis (Strehler et al., 2007). However, the altered composition of PMCA is associated with a less efficient Ca^{2+} extrusion system, increasing the risk of neurodegenerative processes (Strehler and Thayer, 2018). *ATP2B2* is a deafness-associated gene that encodes PMCA2 (Smits et al., 2019). A recent study reported a link between PMCA2 and autism spectrum disorder (ASD) (Yang et al., 2013). ASD is a group of neurodevelopmental disorders that results in deficits in social interaction (Chaste and Leboyer, 2012; Fatemi et al., 2012). Intracellular Ca^{2+} levels are crucial for regulating neuronal survival, differentiation, and migration (Bezprozvanny, 2010). Perturbations in these processes underlie the pathogenesis of autism spectrum disorders (Gilbert and Man, 2017). *ATP2B3* mutations are associated with X-linked cerebellar ataxia and Ca^{2+} extrusion disorders in patients with cerebellar ataxia and developmental delay (Zanni et al., 2012; Mazzitelli and Adamo, 2014; Cali et al., 2015). Several neurotoxic agents, such as oxidation and age, downregulate PMCA function and increase susceptibility to NDs (Zaidi, 2010). In particular, the internalization of PMCA2 initiated by protease function in rat hippocampal pyramidal cells after glutamate exposure or kainate-induced seizures, in which loss of PMCA function occurs, may contribute to Ca^{2+} dysregulation and lead to neuronal cell death (Pottorf et al., 2006; Stafford et al., 2017). A decrease in PMCA activity and increased Ca^{2+} may cause cell death depending on the degree of cytosolic accumulation of tau and Aβ in AD (Boczek et al., 2019). In addition, PMCA expression is decreased in the cortex of postmortem brains of patients with AD (Berrocal et al., 2019; Boczek et al., 2019).

pH REGULATION BY PMCA IN NEURODEGENERATIVE DISEASES

As mentioned above, PMCAs have a Ca^{2+} extrusion function on the membrane and another important function, namely H^+ uptake (Stafford et al., 2017). Since PMCA is responsible for control of Ca^{2+} extrusion and H^+ uptake rates, it provides an important link between Ca^{2+} signaling and intracellular pH (pH_i) in neurons (Hwang et al., 2011). Mechanisms that maintain strict pH homeostasis in the brain control neuronal excitability, synaptic transmission, neurotransmitter uptake, nociception, and inflammation (Chesler, 2003; Dhaka et al., 2009; Casey et al., 2010; Hwang et al., 2011). Changes in pH caused via pH-sensitive or pH-regulated ion channels are detrimental to brain function and can cause multiple degenerative diseases (Ruffin et al., 2014). Neuronal excitability is particularly sensitive to changes in intracellular and extracellular pH mediated by various ion channels (Parker and Boron, 2013). The activation of TRPV1 has been reported to induce a rise in Ca^{2+} and cause intracellular acidification via the activation of PMCA in the rat trigeminal ganglion (Hwang et al., 2011). Under normal conditions, acidification conditions are promptly returned to and maintained at normal pH levels through a physiological pH_i recovery mechanism involving the regulation of Na^+/H^+ exchangers (NHE) and Na^+-HCO_3^- cotransporter (NBCs) in the brain (Chesler, 2003; Sinning and Hubner, 2013; Ruffin et al., 2014; Bose et al., 2015). NHE1 is abundantly expressed in all neuronal cells and astrocytes, regulating cell volume homeostasis and pH_i (Song et al., 2020). NBC1 is also widely expressed in astrocytes throughout the brain (Annunziato et al., 2013) (**Figure 1A**). However, functional inhibition of pH_i recovery mechanism in pathological conditions leads to excessive intracellular acidification (Majdi et al., 2016). Therefore, although the exact underlying mechanism that causes intracellular acidification in brain neurons is unknown. However, it appears that persistent intracellular acidification condition promotes irreversible neuronal damage and induces amyloid aggregation in the brains of patients with AD (Xiong et al., 2008; Ruffin et al., 2014).

CONCLUSION

Intracellular Ca^{2+} and pH regulation play vital roles in both physiological and pathological conditions. Abnormal changes in Ca^{2+} or pH typically cause cell death. TRP channels are involved in Ca^{2+} influx, which affects neuronal and glial functions under normal physiological conditions. However, altered expression of TRP channels can lead to excess Ca^{2+} influx, and intracellular Ca^{2+} overload is maintained due to *ATP2B2*, oxidation, and aging-related downregulation of PMCA, leading to Ca^{2+}-dependent cell death. Alternatively, overexpression of PMCA due to cytoplasmic Ca^{2+} overload causes continuous acidification from inhibition of the pH_i recovery mechanisms by oxidative stress or programmed cell death, resulting in acidification-dependent cell death (**Figure 2**) (Harguindey et al., 2017, 2019). To date, TRP channels have been investigated for their role in NDs. However, targeting TRP channels and PMCA, including Ca^{2+} and pH regulation, as a treatment for NDs requires a deeper understanding of their function in both health and disease. This review describes potential therapeutic targets for NDs by discussing TRP channels and PMCA responsible for the disruption of intracellular Ca^{2+} and pH homeostasis that underpin ND development.

AUTHOR CONTRIBUTIONS

C-KP and YK conceived and supervised the project. S-MH, JL, C-KP, and YK wrote the paper. All authors contributed to the article and approved the submitted version.

REFERENCES

Aarts, M. M., and Tymianski, M. (2005). TRPMs and neuronal cell death. *Pflugers Arch.* 451, 243–249. doi: 10.1007/s00424-005-1439-x

Adachi, N., Kobayashi, T., Takahashi, H., Kawasaki, T., Shirai, Y., Ueyama, T., et al. (2008). Enzymological analysis of mutant protein kinase Cgamma causing spinocerebellar ataxia type 14 and dysfunction in Ca2+ homeostasis. *J. Biol. Chem.* 283, 19854–19863. doi: 10.1074/jbc.M801492200

Akyuva, Y., and Naziroglu, M. (2020). Resveratrol attenuates hypoxia-induced neuronal cell death, inflammation and mitochondrial oxidative stress by modulation of TRPM2 channel. *Sci. Rep.* 10:6449. doi: 10.1038/s41598-020-63577-5

Alavi, M. S., Shamsizadeh, A., Karimi, G., and Roohbakhsh, A. (2020). Transient receptor potential ankyrin 1 (TRPA1)-mediated toxicity: friend or foe? *Toxicol. Mech. Methods* 30, 1–18. doi: 10.1080/15376516.2019.1652872

Annunziato, L., Boscia, F., and Pignataro, G. (2013). Ionic transporter activity in astrocytes, microglia, and oligodendrocytes during brain ischemia. *J. Cereb. Blood Flow Metab.* 33, 969–982. doi: 10.1038/jcbfm.2013.44

Asrar, S., and Aarts, M. (2013). TRPM7, the cytoskeleton and neuronal death. *Channels (Austin)* 7, 6–16. doi: 10.4161/chan.22824

Auer-Grumbach, M., Olschewski, A., Papic, L., Kremer, H., Mcentagart, M. E., Uhrig, S., et al. (2010). Alterations in the ankyrin domain of TRPV4 cause congenital distal SMA, scapuloperoneal SMA and HMSN2C. *Nat. Genet.* 42, 160–164. doi: 10.1038/ng.508

Bagur, R., and Hajnoczky, G. (2017). Intracellular Ca(2+) Sensing: its role in calcium homeostasis and signaling. *Mol. Cell* 66, 780–788. doi: 10.1016/j.molcel.2017.05.028

Balleza-Tapia, H., Crux, S., Andrade-Talavera, Y., Dolz-Gaiton, P., Papadia, D., Chen, G., et al. (2018). TrpV1 receptor activation rescues neuronal function and network gamma oscillations from Abeta-induced impairment in mouse hippocampus *in vitro*. *Elife* 7:37703. doi: 10.7554/eLife.37703.025

Belrose, J. C., and Jackson, M. F. (2018). TRPM2: a candidate therapeutic target for treating neurological diseases. *Acta Pharmacol. Sin.* 39, 722–732. doi: 10.1038/aps.2018.31

Berridge, M. J., Lipp, P., and Bootman, M. D. (2000). The versatility and universality of calcium signalling. *Nat. Rev. Mol. Cell Biol.* 1, 11–21. doi: 10.1038/35036035

Berrocal, M., Caballero-Bermejo, M., Gutierrez-Merino, C., and Mata, A. M. (2019). Methylene blue blocks and reverses the inhibitory effect of tau on PMCA function. *Int. J. Mol. Sci.* 20:3521. doi: 10.3390/ijms20143521

Bezprozvanny, I. B. (2010). Calcium signaling and neurodegeneration. *Acta Naturae* 2, 72–82. doi: 10.32607/20758251-2010-2-1-72-80

Boczek, T., Radzik, T., Ferenc, B., and Zylinska, L. (2019). The puzzling role of neuron-specific PMCA isoforms in the aging process. *Int. J. Mol. Sci.* 20:6338. doi: 10.3390/ijms20246338

Bolcskei, K., Kriszta, G., Saghy, E., Payrits, M., Sipos, E., Vranesics, A., et al. (2018). Behavioural alterations and morphological changes are attenuated by the lack of TRPA1 receptors in the cuprizone-induced demyelination model in mice. *J. Neuroimmunol.* 320, 1–10. doi: 10.1016/j.jneuroim.2018.03.020

Bollimuntha, S., Ebadi, M., and Singh, B. B. (2006). TRPC1 protects human SH-SY5Y cells against salsolinol-induced cytotoxicity by inhibiting apoptosis. *Brain Res.* 1099, 141–149. doi: 10.1016/j.brainres.2006.04.104

Bollimuntha, S., Selvaraj, S., and Singh, B. B. (2011). Emerging roles of canonical TRP channels in neuronal function. *Adv. Exp. Med. Biol.* 704, 573–593. doi: 10.1007/978-94-007-0265-3_31

Bollimuntha, S., Singh, B. B., Shavali, S., Sharma, S. K., and Ebadi, M. (2005). TRPC1-mediated inhibition of 1-methyl-4-phenylpyridinium ion neurotoxicity in human SH-SY5Y neuroblastoma cells. *J. Biol. Chem.* 280, 2132–2140. doi: 10.1074/jbc.M407384200

Bose, T., Cieslar-Pobuda, A., and Wiechec, E. (2015). Role of ion channels in regulating Ca(2)(+) homeostasis during the interplay between immune and cancer cells. *Cell Death Dis.* 6:e1648.

Bosson, A., Paumier, A., Boisseau, S., Jacquier-Sarlin, M., Buisson, A., and Albrieux, M. (2017). TRPA1 channels promote astrocytic Ca(2+) hyperactivity and synaptic dysfunction mediated by oligomeric forms of amyloid-beta peptide. *Mol. Neurodegener.* 12:53. doi: 10.1186/s13024-017-0194-8

Brini, M., Cali, T., Ottolini, D., and Carafoli, E. (2013). The plasma membrane calcium pump in health and disease. *FEBS J.* 280, 5385–5397. doi: 10.1111/febs.12193

Broker-Lai, J., Kollewe, A., Schindeldecker, B., Pohle, J., Nguyen Chi, V., Mathar, I., et al. (2017). Heteromeric channels formed by TRPC1, TRPC4 and TRPC5 define hippocampal synaptic transmission and working memory. *EMBO J.* 36, 2770–2789. doi: 10.15252/embj.201696369

Butenko, O., Dzamba, D., Benesova, J., Honsa, P., Benfenati, V., Rusnakova, V., et al. (2012). The increased activity of TRPV4 channel in the astrocytes of the adult rat hippocampus after cerebral hypoxia/ischemia. *PLoS ONE* 7:e39959. doi: 10.1371/journal.pone.0039959

Cali, T., Lopreiato, R., Shimony, J., Vineyard, M., Frizzarin, M., Zanni, G., et al. (2015). A novel mutation in isoform 3 of the plasma membrane Ca2+ pump impairs cellular Ca2+ homeostasis in a patient with cerebellar ataxia and laminin subunit 1alpha mutations. *J. Biol. Chem.* 290, 16132–16141. doi: 10.1074/jbc.M115.656496

Casey, J. R., Grinstein, S., and Orlowski, J. (2010). Sensors and regulators of intracellular pH. *Nat. Rev. Mol. Cell Biol.* 11, 50–61. doi: 10.1038/nrm2820

Chaste, P., and Leboyer, M. (2012). Autism risk factors: genes, environment, and gene-environment interactions. *Dialogues Clin. Neurosci.* 14, 281–292. doi: 10.31887/DCNS.2012.14.3/pchaste

Chen, D. H., Sul, Y., Weiss, M., Hillel, A., Lipe, H., Wolff, J., et al. (2010). CMT2C with vocal cord paresis associated with short stature and mutations in the TRPV4 gene. *Neurology* 75, 1968–1975. doi: 10.1212/WNL.0b013e3181ffe4bb

Chen, X., Numata, T., Li, M., Mori, Y., Orser, B. A., Jackson, M. F., et al. (2010). The modulation of TRPM7 currents by nafamostat mesilate depends directly upon extracellular concentrations of divalent cations. *Mol. Brain* 3:38. doi: 10.1186/1756-6606-3-38

Chesler, M. (2003). Regulation and modulation of pH in the brain. *Physiol. Rev.* 83, 1183–1221. doi: 10.1152/physrev.00010.2003

Chi, H., Chang, H. Y., and Sang, T. K. (2018). Neuronal cell death mechanisms in major neurodegenerative diseases. *Int. J. Mol. Sci.* 19:3082. doi: 10.3390/ijms19103082

Clement, D., Goodridge, J. P., Grimm, C., Patel, S., and Malmberg, K. J. (2020). TRP channels as interior designers: remodeling the endolysosomal compartment in natural killer cells. *Front. Immunol.* 11:753. doi: 10.3389/fimmu.2020.00753

Coombes, E., Jiang, J., Chu, X. P., Inoue, K., Seeds, J., Branigan, D., et al. (2011). Pathophysiologically relevant levels of hydrogen peroxide induce glutamate-independent neurodegeneration that involves activation of transient receptor potential melastatin 7 channels. *Antioxid. Redox Signal* 14, 1815–1827. doi: 10.1089/ars.2010.3549

Cornillot, M., Giacco, V., and Hamilton, N. B. (2019). The role of TRP channels in white matter function and ischaemia. *Neurosci. Lett.* 690, 202–209. doi: 10.1016/j.neulet.2018.10.042

Cross, J. L., Meloni, B. P., Bakker, A. J., Lee, S., and Knuckey, N. W. (2010). Modes of neuronal calcium entry and homeostasis following cerebral ischemia. *Stroke Res. Treat.* 2010:316862. doi: 10.4061/2010/316862

Cuomo, O., Vinciguerra, A., Cerullo, P., Anzilotti, S., Brancaccio, P., Bilo, L., et al. (2015). Ionic homeostasis in brain conditioning. *Front. Neurosci.* 9:277. doi: 10.3389/fnins.2015.00277

Dhaka, A., Uzzell, V., Dubin, A. E., Mathur, J., Petrus, M., Bandell, M., et al. (2009). TRPV1 is activated by both acidic and basic pH. *J. Neurosci.* 29, 153–158. doi: 10.1523/JNEUROSCI.4901-08.2009

Douglas, R. M., Xue, J., Chen, J. Y., Haddad, C. G., Alper, S. L., and Haddad, G. G. (2003). Chronic intermittent hypoxia decreases the expression of Na/H exchangers and HCO3-dependent transporters in mouse CNS. *J. Appl. Physiol.* 95, 292–299. doi: 10.1152/japplphysiol.01089.2002

Empson, R. M., Akemann, W., and Knopfel, T. (2010). The role of the calcium transporter protein plasma membrane calcium ATPase PMCA2 in cerebellar Purkinje neuron function. *Funct. Neurol.* 25, 153–158.

Enders, M., Heider, T., Ludwig, A., and Kuerten, S. (2020). Strategies for neuroprotection in multiple sclerosis and the role of calcium. *Int. J. Mol. Sci.* 21:1663. doi: 10.3390/ijms21051663

Fatemi, S. H., Aldinger, K. A., Ashwood, P., Bauman, M. L., Blaha, C. D., Blatt, G. J., et al. (2012). Consensus paper: pathological role of the cerebellum in autism. *Cerebellum* 11, 777–807. doi: 10.1007/s12311-012-0355-9

Fernandes, E. S., Fernandes, M. A., and Keeble, J. E. (2012). The functions of TRPA1 and TRPV1: moving away from sensory nerves. *Br. J. Pharmacol.* 166, 510–521. doi: 10.1111/j.1476-5381.2012.01851.x

Fonfria, E., Marshall, I. C., Boyfield, I., Skaper, S. D., Hughes, J. P., Owen, D. E., et al. (2005). Amyloid beta-peptide(1-42) and hydrogen peroxide-induced toxicity are mediated by TRPM2 in rat primary striatal cultures. *J. Neurochem.* 95, 715–723. doi: 10.1111/j.1471-4159.2005.03396.x

Fowler, M. A., Sidiropoulou, K., Ozkan, E. D., Phillips, C. W., and Cooper, D. C. (2007). Corticolimbic expression of TRPC4 and TRPC5 channels in the rodent brain. *PLoS ONE* 2:e573. doi: 10.1371/journal.pone.0000573

Fresu, L., Dehpour, A., Genazzani, A. A., Carafoli, E., and Guerini, D. (1999). Plasma membrane calcium ATPase isoforms in astrocytes. *Glia* 28, 150–155. doi: 10.1002/(SICI)1098-1136(199911)28:2<150::AID-GLIA6>3.0.CO;2-7

Fu, M., Xie, Z., and Zuo, H. (2009). TRPV1: a potential target for antiepileptogenesis. *Med. Hypotheses* 73, 100–102. doi: 10.1016/j.mehy.2009.01.005

Gees, M., Colsoul, B., and Nilius, B. (2010). The role of transient receptor potential cation channels in Ca2+ signaling. *Cold Spring Harb. Perspect. Biol.* 2:a003962. doi: 10.1101/cshperspect.a003962

Gibson, H. E., Edwards, J. G., Page, R. S., Van Hook, M. J., and Kauer, J. A. (2008). TRPV1 channels mediate long-term depression at synapses on hippocampal interneurons. *Neuron* 57, 746–759. doi: 10.1016/j.neuron.2007.12.027

Gilbert, J., and Man, H. Y. (2017). Fundamental elements in autism: from neurogenesis and neurite growth to synaptic plasticity. *Front. Cell. Neurosci.* 11:359. doi: 10.3389/fncel.2017.00359

Gleichmann, M., and Mattson, M. P. (2011). Neuronal calcium homeostasis and dysregulation. *Antioxid. Redox Signal* 14, 1261–1273. doi: 10.1089/ars.2010.3386

Hajieva, P., Baeken, M. W., and Moosmann, B. (2018). The role of Plasma Membrane Calcium ATPases (PMCAs) in neurodegenerative disorders. *Neurosci. Lett.* 663, 29–38. doi: 10.1016/j.neulet.2017.09.033

Hamakawa, H., Murashita, J., Yamada, N., Inubushi, T., Kato, N., and Kato, T. (2004). Reduced intracellular pH in the basal ganglia and whole brain measured by 31P-MRS in bipolar disorder. *Psychiatry Clin. Neurosci.* 58, 82–88. doi: 10.1111/j.1440-1819.2004.01197.x

Harguindey, S., Polo Orozco, J., Alfarouk, K. O., and Devesa, J. (2019). Hydrogen ion dynamics of cancer and a new molecular, biochemical and metabolic approach to the etiopathogenesis and treatment of brain malignancies. *Int. J. Mol. Sci.* 20:4278. doi: 10.3390/ijms20174278

Harguindey, S., Reshkin, S. J., Orive, G., Arranz, J. L., and Anitua, E. (2007). Growth and trophic factors, pH and the Na+/H+ exchanger in Alzheimer's disease, other neurodegenerative diseases and cancer: new therapeutic possibilities and potential dangers. *Curr. Alzheimer Res.* 4, 53–65. doi: 10.2174/156720507779939841

Harguindey, S., Stanciu, D., Devesa, J., Alfarouk, K., Cardone, R. A., Polo Orozco, J. D., et al. (2017). Cellular acidification as a new approach to cancer treatment and to the understanding and therapeutics of neurodegenerative diseases. *Semin. Cancer Biol.* 43, 157–179. doi: 10.1016/j.semcancer.2017.02.003

Hasan, R., and Zhang, X. (2018). Ca(2+) regulation of TRP ion channels. *Int. J. Mol. Sci.* 19:1256. doi: 10.3390/ijms19041256

Hassan, S., Eldeeb, K., Millns, P. J., Bennett, A. J., Alexander, S. P., and Kendall, D. A. (2014). Cannabidiol enhances microglial phagocytosis via transient receptor potential (TRP) channel activation. *Br. J. Pharmacol.* 171, 2426–2439. doi: 10.1111/bph.12615

Hellmich, U. A., and Gaudet, R. (2014). Structural biology of TRP channels. *Handb. Exp. Pharmacol.* 223, 963–990. doi: 10.1007/978-3-319-05161-1_10

Hentschke, M., Wiemann, M., Hentschke, S., Kurth, I., Hermans-Borgmeyer, I., Seidenbecher, T., et al. (2006). Mice with a targeted disruption of the Cl-/HCO3- exchanger AE3 display a reduced seizure threshold. *Mol. Cell. Biol.* 26, 182–191. doi: 10.1128/MCB.26.1.182-191.2006

Hermosura, M. C., Cui, A. M., Go, R. C., Davenport, B., Shetler, C. M., Heizer, J. W., et al. (2008). Altered functional properties of a TRPM2 variant in Guamanian ALS and PD. *Proc. Natl. Acad. Sci. U. S. A.* 105, 18029–18034. doi: 10.1073/pnas.0808218105

Hermosura, M. C., Nayakanti, H., Dorovkov, M. V., Calderon, F. R., Ryazanov, A. G., Haymer, D. S., et al. (2005). A TRPM7 variant shows altered sensitivity to magnesium that may contribute to the pathogenesis of two Guamanian neurodegenerative disorders. *Proc. Natl. Acad. Sci. U. S. A.* 102, 11510–11515. doi: 10.1073/pnas.0505149102

Ho, K. W., Lambert, W. S., and Calkins, D. J. (2014). Activation of the TRPV1 cation channel contributes to stress-induced astrocyte migration. *Glia* 62, 1435–1451. doi: 10.1002/glia.22691

Ho, K. W., Ward, N. J., and Calkins, D. J. (2012). TRPV1: a stress response protein in the central nervous system. *Am. J. Neurodegener. Dis.* 1, 1–14.

Hong, C., Jeong, B., Park, H. J., Chung, J. Y., Lee, J. E., Kim, J., et al. (2020). TRP channels as emerging therapeutic targets for neurodegenerative diseases. *Front. Physiol.* 11:238. doi: 10.3389/fphys.2020.00238

Hong, C., Seo, H., Kwak, M., Jeon, J., Jang, J., Jeong, E. M., et al. (2015). Increased TRPC5 glutathionylation contributes to striatal neuron loss in Huntington's disease. *Brain* 138, 3030–3047. doi: 10.1093/brain/awv188

Huang, J., Du, W., Yao, H., and Wang, Y. (2011). "TRPC channels in neuronal survival," in *TRP Channels,* ed M. X. Zhu (Boca Raton, FL: CRC Press/Taylor & Francis), 1–23.

Huang, S., Turlova, E., Li, F., Bao, M. H., Szeto, V., Wong, R., et al. (2017). Transient receptor potential melastatin 2 channels (TRPM2) mediate neonatal hypoxic-ischemic brain injury in mice. *Exp. Neurol.* 296, 32–40. doi: 10.1016/j.expneurol.2017.06.023

Huang, Y., Fliegert, R., Guse, A. H., Lu, W., and Du, J. (2020). A structural overview of the ion channels of the TRPM family. *Cell Calcium* 85:102111. doi: 10.1016/j.ceca.2019.102111

Hwang, S. M., Koo, N. Y., Jin, M., Davies, A. J., Chun, G. S., Choi, S. Y., et al. (2011). Intracellular acidification is associated with changes in free cytosolic calcium and inhibition of action potentials in rat trigeminal ganglion. *J. Biol. Chem.* 286, 1719–1729. doi: 10.1074/jbc.M109.090951

Jardin, I., Lopez, J. J., Diez, R., Sanchez-Collado, J., Cantonero, C., Albarran, L., et al. (2017). TRPs in pain sensation. *Front. Physiol.* 8:392. doi: 10.3389/fphys.2017.00392

Jiang, L., Bechtel, M. D., Galeva, N. A., Williams, T. D., Michaelis, E. K., and Michaelis, M. L. (2012). Decreases in plasma membrane Ca(2)(+)-ATPase in brain synaptic membrane rafts from aged rats. *J. Neurochem.* 123, 689–699. doi: 10.1111/j.1471-4159.2012.07918.x

Kaczmarek, J. S., Riccio, A., and Clapham, D. E. (2012). Calpain cleaves and activates the TRPC5 channel to participate in semaphorin 3A-induced neuronal growth cone collapse. *Proc. Natl. Acad. Sci. U. S. A.* 109, 7888–7892. doi: 10.1073/pnas.1205869109

Kaneko, S., Kawakami, S., Hara, Y., Wakamori, M., Itoh, E., Minami, T., et al. (2006). A critical role of TRPM2 in neuronal cell death by hydrogen peroxide. *J. Pharmacol. Sci.* 101, 66–76. doi: 10.1254/jphs.FP0060128

Kaneko, Y., and Szallasi, A. (2014). Transient receptor potential (TRP) channels: a clinical perspective. *Br. J. Pharmacol.* 171, 2474–2507. doi: 10.1111/bph.12414

Kato, T., Murashita, J., Kamiya, A., Shioiri, T., Kato, N., and Inubushi, T. (1998). Decreased brain intracellular pH measured by 31P-MRS in bipolar disorder: a confirmation in drug-free patients and correlation with white matter hyperintensity. *Eur. Arch. Psychiatry Clin. Neurosci.* 248, 301–306. doi: 10.1007/s004060050054

Kawamoto, E. M., Vivar, C., and Camandola, S. (2012). Physiology and pathology of calcium signaling in the brain. *Front. Pharmacol.* 3:61. doi: 10.3389/fphar.2012.00061

Kim, S. R., Bok, E., Chung, Y. C., Chung, E. S., and Jin, B. K. (2008). Interactions between CB(1) receptors and TRPV1 channels mediated by 12-HPETE are cytotoxic to mesencephalic dopaminergic neurons. *Br. J. Pharmacol.* 155, 253–264. doi: 10.1038/bjp.2008.246

Kim, S. R., Kim, S. U., Oh, U., and Jin, B. K. (2006). Transient receptor potential vanilloid subtype 1 mediates microglial cell death *in vivo* and *in vitro* via Ca2+-mediated mitochondrial damage and cytochrome c release. *J. Immunol.* 177, 4322–4329. doi: 10.4049/jimmunol.177.7.4322

Kim, S. R., Lee, D. Y., Chung, E. S., Oh, U. T., Kim, S. U., and Jin, B. K. (2005). Transient receptor potential vanilloid subtype 1 mediates cell death of mesencephalic dopaminergic neurons *in vivo* and *in vitro. J. Neurosci.* 25, 662–671. doi: 10.1523/JNEUROSCI.4166-04.2005

Kip, S. N., Gray, N. W., Burette, A., Canbay, A., Weinberg, R. J., and Strehler, E. E. (2006). Changes in the expression of plasma membrane calcium extrusion systems during the maturation of hippocampal neurons. *Hippocampus* 16, 20–34. doi: 10.1002/hipo.20129

Klein, C. J., Shi, Y., Fecto, F., Donaghy, M., Nicholson, G., Mcentagart, M. E., et al. (2011). TRPV4 mutations and cytotoxic hypercalcemia in axonal Charcot-Marie-Tooth neuropathies. *Neurology* 76, 887–894. doi: 10.1212/WNL.0b013e31820f2de3

Kumar, A., Bodhinathan, K., and Foster, T. C. (2009). Susceptibility to calcium dysregulation during brain aging. *Front. Aging Neurosci.* 1:2. doi: 10.3389/neuro.24.002.2009

Kumar, P., Kumar, D., Jha, S. K., Jha, N. K., and Ambasta, R. K. (2016). Ion channels in neurological disorders. *Adv. Protein Chem. Struct. Biol.* 103, 97–136. doi: 10.1016/bs.apcsb.2015.10.006

Kurnellas, M. P., Lee, A. K., Szczepanowski, K., and Elkabes, S. (2007). Role of plasma membrane calcium ATPase isoform 2 in neuronal function in the cerebellum and spinal cord. *Ann. N. Y. Acad. Sci.* 1099, 287–291. doi: 10.1196/annals.1387.025

Landoure, G., Zdebik, A. A., Martinez, T. L., Burnett, B. G., Stanescu, H. C., Inada, H., et al. (2010). Mutations in TRPV4 cause Charcot-Marie-Tooth disease type 2C. *Nat. Genet.* 42, 170–174. doi: 10.1038/ng.512

Lastres-Becker, I., De Miguel, R., De Petrocellis, L., Makriyannis, A., Di Marzo, V., and Fernandez-Ruiz, J. (2003). Compounds acting at the endocannabinoid and/or endovanilloid systems reduce hyperkinesia in a rat model of Huntington's disease. *J. Neurochem.* 84, 1097–1109. doi: 10.1046/j.1471-4159.2003.01595.x

Lee, K. I., Lee, H. T., Lin, H. C., Tsay, H. J., Tsai, F. C., Shyue, S. K., et al. (2016). Role of transient receptor potential ankyrin 1 channels in Alzheimer's disease. *J. Neuroinflammation* 13:92. doi: 10.1186/s12974-016-0557-z

Lee, T. H., Lee, J. G., Yon, J. M., Oh, K. W., Baek, I. J., Nahm, S. S., et al. (2011). Capsaicin prevents kainic acid-induced epileptogenesis in mice. *Neurochem. Int.* 58, 634–640. doi: 10.1016/j.neuint.2011.01.027

Lessard, C. B., Lussier, M. P., Cayouette, S., Bourque, G., and Boulay, G. (2005). The overexpression of presenilin2 and Alzheimer's-disease-linked presenilin2 variants influences TRPC6-enhanced Ca2+ entry into HEK293 cells. *Cell. Signal* 17, 437–445. doi: 10.1016/j.cellsig.2004.09.005

Li, H. B., Mao, R. R., Zhang, J. C., Yang, Y., Cao, J., and Xu, L. (2008). Antistress effect of TRPV1 channel on synaptic plasticity and spatial memory. *Biol. Psychiatry* 64, 286–292. doi: 10.1016/j.biopsych.2008.02.020

Li, W., Calfa, G., Larimore, J., and Pozzo-Miller, L. (2012). Activity-dependent BDNF release and TRPC signaling is impaired in hippocampal neurons of Mecp2 mutant mice. *Proc. Natl. Acad. Sci. U. S. A.* 109, 17087–17092. doi: 10.1073/pnas.1205271109

Liedtke, W., and Friedman, J. M. (2003). Abnormal osmotic regulation in trpv4-/- mice. *Proc. Natl. Acad. Sci. U. S. A.* 100, 13698–13703. doi: 10.1073/pnas.1735416100

Liu, N., Wu, J., Chen, Y., and Zhao, J. (2020). Channels that cooperate with TRPV4 in the brain. *J. Mol. Neurosci.* 70, 1812–1820. doi: 10.1007/s12031-020-01574-z

Liu, N., Zhuang, Y., Zhou, Z., Zhao, J., Chen, Q., and Zheng, J. (2017). NF-kappaB dependent up-regulation of TRPC6 by Abeta in BV-2 microglia cells increases COX-2 expression and contributes to hippocampus neuron damage. *Neurosci. Lett.* 651, 1–8. doi: 10.1016/j.neulet.2017.04.056

Logashina, Y. A., Korolkova, Y. V., Kozlov, S. A., and Andreev, Y. A. (2019). TRPA1 channel as a regulator of neurogenic inflammation and pain: structure, function, role in pathophysiology, and therapeutic potential of ligands. *Biochemistry Mosc.* 84, 101–118. doi: 10.1134/S00062979190 20020

Lu, R., He, Q., and Wang, J. (2017). TRPC channels and Alzheimer's disease. *Adv. Exp. Med. Biol.* 976, 73–83. doi: 10.1007/978-94-024-1088-4_7

Luo, L., Song, S., Ezenwukwa, C. C., Jalali, S., Sun, B., and Sun, D. (2020). Ion channels and transporters in microglial function in physiology and brain diseases. *Neurochem. Int.* 142:104925. doi: 10.1016/j.neuint.2020.104925

Majdi, A., Mahmoudi, J., Sadigh-Eteghad, S., Golzari, S. E., Sabermarouf, B., and Reyhani-Rad, S. (2016). Permissive role of cytosolic pH acidification in neurodegeneration: a closer look at its causes and consequences. *J. Neurosci. Res.* 94, 879–887. doi: 10.1002/jnr.23757

Maklad, A., Sharma, A., and Azimi, I. (2019). Calcium signaling in brain cancers: roles and therapeutic targeting. *Cancers* 11:145. doi: 10.3390/cancers11020145

Mandal, P. K., Akolkar, H., and Tripathi, M. (2012). Mapping of hippocampal pH and neurochemicals from *in vivo* multi-voxel 31P study in healthy normal young male/female, mild cognitive impairment, and Alzheimer's disease. *J. Alzheimers Dis.* 31, S75–86. doi: 10.3233/JAD-2012-120166

Marambaud, P., Dreses-Werringloer, U., and Vingtdeux, V. (2009). Calcium signaling in neurodegeneration. *Mol. Neurodegener.* 4:20. doi: 10.1186/1750-1326-4-20

Mazzitelli, L. R., and Adamo, H. P. (2014). Hyperactivation of the human plasma membrane Ca2+ pump PMCA h4xb by mutation of Glu99 to Lys. *J. Biol. Chem.* 289, 10761–10768. doi: 10.1074/jbc.M113.535583

Mickle, A. D., Shepherd, A. J., and Mohapatra, D. P. (2015). Sensory TRP channels: the key transducers of nociception and pain. *Prog. Mol. Biol. Transl. Sci.* 131, 73–118. doi: 10.1016/bs.pmbts.2015.01.002

Minke, B. (2006). TRP channels and Ca2+ signaling. *Cell Calcium* 40, 261–275. doi: 10.1016/j.ceca.2006.05.002

Mizoguchi, Y., Kato, T. A., Seki, Y., Ohgidani, M., Sagata, N., Horikawa, H., et al. (2014). Brain-derived neurotrophic factor (BDNF) induces sustained intracellular Ca2+ elevation through the up-regulation of surface transient receptor potential 3 (TRPC3) channels in rodent microglia. *J. Biol. Chem.* 289, 18549–18555. doi: 10.1074/jbc.M114.555334

Moran, M. M. (2018). TRP channels as potential drug targets. *Annu. Rev. Pharmacol. Toxicol.* 58, 309–330. doi: 10.1146/annurev-pharmtox-010617-052832

Moran, M. M., Xu, H., and Clapham, D. E. (2004). TRP ion channels in the nervous system. *Curr. Opin. Neurobiol.* 14, 362–369. doi: 10.1016/j.conb.2004.05.003

Morelli, M. B., Amantini, C., Liberati, S., Santoni, M., and Nabissi, M. (2013). TRP channels: new potential therapeutic approaches in CNS neuropathies. *CNS Neurol. Disord. Drug Targets* 12, 274–293. doi: 10.2174/18715273113129990056

Neuner, S. M., Wilmott, L. A., Hope, K. A., Hoffmann, B., Chong, J. A., Abramowitz, J., et al. (2015). TRPC3 channels critically regulate hippocampal excitability and contextual fear memory. *Behav. Brain Res.* 281, 69–77. doi: 10.1016/j.bbr.2014.12.018

Nikoletopoulou, V., and Tavernarakis, N. (2012). Calcium homeostasis in aging neurons. *Front. Genet.* 3:200. doi: 10.3389/fgene.2012.00200

Nilius, B. (2007). TRP channels in disease. *Biochim. Biophys. Acta* 1772, 805–812. doi: 10.1016/j.bbadis.2007.02.002

Nilius, B., and Owsianik, G. (2011). The transient receptor potential family of ion channels. *Genome Biol.* 12:218. doi: 10.1186/gb-2011-12-3-218

Nilius, B., Prenen, J., and Owsianik, G. (2011). Irritating channels: the case of TRPA1. *J. Physiol.* 589, 1543–1549. doi: 10.1113/jphysiol.2010.200717

Nishida, M., Kuwahara, K., Kozai, D., Sakaguchi, R., and Mori, Y. (2015). "TRP channels: their function and potentiality as drug targets," in *Innovative Medicine: Basic Research and Development,* eds K. Nakao, N. Minato, and S. Uemoto (Tokyo: Springer), 195–218. doi: 10.1007/978-4-431-55651-0_17

Oakes, M., Law, W. J., and Komuniecki, R. (2019). Cannabinoids stimulate the trp channel-dependent release of both serotonin and dopamine to modulate behavior in *C. elegans*. *J. Neurosci.* 39, 4142–4152. doi: 10.1523/JNEUROSCI.2371-18.2019

Ostapchenko, V. G., Chen, M., Guzman, M. S., Xie, Y. F., Lavine, N., Fan, J., et al. (2015). The Transient Receptor Potential Melastatin 2 (TRPM2) channel contributes to beta-amyloid oligomer-related neurotoxicity and memory impairment. *J. Neurosci.* 35, 15157–15169. doi: 10.1523/JNEUROSCI.4081-14.2015

Parker, M. D., and Boron, W. F. (2013). The divergence, actions, roles, and relatives of sodium-coupled bicarbonate transporters. *Physiol. Rev.* 93, 803–959. doi: 10.1152/physrev.00023.2012

Piacentini, R., Gangitano, C., Ceccariglia, S., Del Fa, A., Azzena, G. B., Michetti, F., et al. (2008). Dysregulation of intracellular calcium homeostasis is responsible for neuronal death in an experimental model of selective hippocampal degeneration induced by trimethyltin. *J. Neurochem.* 105, 2109–2121. doi: 10.1111/j.1471-4159.2008.05297.x

Popugaeva, E., Pchitskaya, E., and Bezprozvanny, I. (2017). Dysregulation of neuronal calcium homeostasis in Alzheimer's disease - a therapeutic opportunity? *Biochem. Biophys. Res. Commun.* 483, 998–1004. doi: 10.1016/j.bbrc.2016.09.053

Pottorf, W. J. II, Johanns, T. M., Derrington, S. M., Strehler, E. E., Enyedi, A., and Thayer, S. A. (2006). Glutamate-induced protease-mediated loss of plasma membrane Ca2+ pump activity in rat hippocampal neurons. *J. Neurochem.* 98, 1646–1656. doi: 10.1111/j.1471-4159.2006.04063.x

Rakers, C., Schmid, M., and Petzold, G. C. (2017). TRPV4 channels contribute to calcium transients in astrocytes and neurons during peri-infarct depolarizations in a stroke model. *Glia* 65, 1550–1561. doi: 10.1002/glia.23183

Riccio, A., Medhurst, A. D., Mattei, C., Kelsell, R. E., Calver, A. R., Randall, A. D., et al. (2002). mRNA distribution analysis of human TRPC family in CNS and peripheral tissues. *Brain Res. Mol. Brain Res.* 109, 95–104. doi: 10.1016/S0169-328X(02)00527-2

Ronco, V., Grolla, A. A., Glasnov, T. N., Canonico, P. L., Verkhratsky, A., Genazzani, A. A., et al. (2014). Differential deregulation of astrocytic calcium signalling by amyloid-beta, TNFalpha, IL-1beta and LPS. *Cell Calcium* 55, 219–229. doi: 10.1016/j.ceca.2014.02.016

Rosker, C., Graziani, A., Lukas, M., Eder, P., Zhu, M. X., Romanin, C., et al. (2004). Ca(2+) signaling by TRPC3 involves Na(+) entry and local coupling to the Na(+)/Ca(2+) exchanger. *J. Biol. Chem.* 279, 13696–13704. doi: 10.1074/jbc.M308108200

Ruffin, V. A., Salameh, A. I., Boron, W. F., and Parker, M. D. (2014). Intracellular pH regulation by acid-base transporters in mammalian neurons. *Front. Physiol.* 5:43. doi: 10.3389/fphys.2014.00043

Ryazanova, L. V., Rondon, L. J., Zierler, S., Hu, Z., Galli, J., Yamaguchi, T. P., et al. (2010). TRPM7 is essential for Mg(2+) homeostasis in mammals. *Nat. Commun.* 1:109. doi: 10.1038/ncomms1108

Saghy, E., Sipos, E., Acs, P., Bolcskei, K., Pohoczky, K., Kemeny, A., et al. (2016). TRPA1 deficiency is protective in cuprizone-induced demyelination-a new target against oligodendrocyte apoptosis. *Glia* 64, 2166–2180. doi: 10.1002/glia.23051

Samanta, A., Hughes, T. E. T., and Moiseenkova-Bell, V. Y. (2018). Transient receptor potential (TRP) channels. *Subcell. Biochem.* 87, 141–165. doi: 10.1007/978-981-10-7757-9_6

Sawamura, S., Shirakawa, H., Nakagawa, T., Mori, Y., and Kaneko, S. (2017). "TRP channels in the brain: what are they there for?," in *Neurobiology of TRP Channels,* ed T. L. R. Emir (Boca Raton, FL: CRC Press), 295–322. doi: 10.4324/9781315152837-16

Schmiege, P., Fine, M., and Li, X. (2018). The regulatory mechanism of mammalian TRPMLs revealed by cryo-EM. *FEBS J.* 285, 2579–2585. doi: 10.1111/febs.14443

Selvaraj, S., Sun, Y., and Singh, B. B. (2010). TRPC channels and their implication in neurological diseases. *CNS Neurol. Disord. Drug Targets* 9, 94–104. doi: 10.2174/187152710790966650

Selvaraj, S., Sun, Y., Watt, J. A., Wang, S., Lei, S., Birnbaumer, L., et al. (2012). Neurotoxin-induced ER stress in mouse dopaminergic neurons involves downregulation of TRPC1 and inhibition of AKT/mTOR signaling. *J. Clin. Invest.* 122, 1354–1367. doi: 10.1172/JCI61332

Selvaraj, S., Watt, J. A., and Singh, B. B. (2009). TRPC1 inhibits apoptotic cell degeneration induced by dopaminergic neurotoxin MPTP/MPP(+). *Cell Calcium* 46, 209–218. doi: 10.1016/j.ceca.2009.07.008

Shigetomi, E., Tong, X., Kwan, K. Y., Corey, D. P., and Khakh, B. S. (2011). TRPA1 channels regulate astrocyte resting calcium and inhibitory synapse efficacy through GAT-3. *Nat. Neurosci.* 15, 70–80. doi: 10.1038/nn.3000

Shin, H. Y., Hong, Y. H., Jang, S. S., Chae, H. G., Paek, S. L., Moon, H. E., et al. (2010). A role of canonical transient receptor potential 5 channel in neuronal differentiation from A2B5 neural progenitor cells. *PLoS ONE* 5:e10359. doi: 10.1371/journal.pone.0010359

Shirakawa, H., Yamaoka, T., Sanpei, K., Sasaoka, H., Nakagawa, T., and Kaneko, S. (2008). TRPV1 stimulation triggers apoptotic cell death of rat cortical neurons. *Biochem. Biophys. Res. Commun.* 377, 1211–1215. doi: 10.1016/j.bbrc.2008.10.152

Siddiqui, T., Lively, S., Ferreira, R., Wong, R., and Schlichter, L. C. (2014). Expression and contributions of TRPM7 and KCa2.3/SK3 channels to the increased migration and invasion of microglia in anti-inflammatory activation states. *PLoS ONE* 9:e106087. doi: 10.1371/journal.pone.0106087

Sinning, A., and Hubner, C.A. (2013). Minireview: pH and synaptic transmission. *FEBS Lett.* 587, 1923–1928.

Sita, G., Hrelia, P., Graziosi, A., Ravegnini, G., and Morroni, F. (2018). TRPM2 in the brain: role in health and disease. *Cells* 7:82. doi: 10.3390/cells7070082

Slanzi, A., Iannoto, G., Rossi, B., Zenaro, E., and Constantin, G. (2020). *In vitro* models of neurodegenerative diseases. *Front. Cell Dev. Biol.* 8:328. doi: 10.3389/fcell.2020.00328

Smaili, S., Hirata, H., Ureshino, R., Monteforte, P. T., Morales, A. P., Muler, M. L., et al. (2009). Calcium and cell death signaling in neurodegeneration and aging. *An. Acad. Bras. Cienc.* 81, 467–475. doi: 10.1590/S0001-37652009000300011

Smits, J. J., Oostrik, J., Beynon, A. J., Kant, S. G., De Koning Gans, P. a. M., et al. (2019). *De novo* and inherited loss-of-function variants of ATP2B2 are associated with rapidly progressive hearing impairment. *Hum. Genet.* 138, 61–72. doi: 10.1007/s00439-018-1965-1

Song, J., Lee, J. H., Lee, S. H., Park, K. A., Lee, W. T., and Lee, J. E. (2013). TRPV1 activation in primary cortical neurons induces calcium-dependent programmed cell death. *Exp. Neurobiol.* 22, 51–57. doi: 10.5607/en.2013.22.1.51

Song, S., Luo, L., Sun, B., and Sun, D. (2020). Roles of glial ion transporters in brain diseases. *Glia* 68, 472–494. doi: 10.1002/glia.23699

Sprenkle, N. T., Sims, S. G., Sanchez, C. L., and Meares, G. P. (2017). Endoplasmic reticulum stress and inflammation in the central nervous system. *Mol. Neurodegener.* 12:42. doi: 10.1186/s13024-017-0183-y

Stafford, N., Wilson, C., Oceandy, D., Neyses, L., and Cartwright, E. J. (2017). The plasma membrane calcium ATPases and their role as major new players in human disease. *Physiol. Rev.* 97, 1089–1125. doi: 10.1152/physrev.00028.2016

Startek, J. B., Boonen, B., Talavera, K., and Meseguer, V. (2019). TRP channels as sensors of chemically-induced changes in cell membrane mechanical properties. *Int. J. Mol. Sci.* 20:371. doi: 10.3390/ijms20020371

Stauffer, T. P., Guerini, D., and Carafoli, E. (1995). Tissue distribution of the four gene products of the plasma membrane Ca2+ pump. A study using specific antibodies. *J. Biol. Chem.* 270, 12184–12190. doi: 10.1074/jbc.270.20.12184

Strehler, E. E., Caride, A. J., Filoteo, A. G., Xiong, Y., Penniston, J. T., and Enyedi, A. (2007). Plasma membrane Ca2+ ATPases as dynamic regulators of cellular calcium handling. *Ann. N. Y. Acad. Sci.* 1099, 226–236. doi: 10.1196/annals.1387.023

Strehler, E. E., and Thayer, S. A. (2018). Evidence for a role of plasma membrane calcium pumps in neurodegenerative disease: recent developments. *Neurosci. Lett.* 663, 39–47. doi: 10.1016/j.neulet.2017.08.035

Tai, C., Hines, D. J., Choi, H. B., and Macvicar, B. A. (2011). Plasma membrane insertion of TRPC5 channels contributes to the cholinergic plateau potential in hippocampal CA1 pyramidal neurons. *Hippocampus* 21, 958–967. doi: 10.1002/hipo.20807

Tedeschi, V., Petrozziello, T., Sisalli, M. J., Boscia, F., Canzoniero, L. M. T., and Secondo, A. (2019). The activation of Mucolipin TRP channel 1 (TRPML1) protects motor neurons from L-BMAA neurotoxicity by promoting autophagic clearance. *Sci. Rep.* 9:10743. doi: 10.1038/s41598-019-46708-5

Thapak, P., Vaidya, B., Joshi, H. C., Singh, J. N., and Sharma, S. S. (2020). Therapeutic potential of pharmacological agents targeting TRP channels in CNS disorders. *Pharmacol. Res.* 159:105026. doi: 10.1016/j.phrs.2020.105026

Tyrtyshnaia, A. A., Lysenko, L. V., Madamba, F., Manzhulo, I. V., Khotimchenko, M. Y., and Kleschevnikov, A. M. (2016). Acute neuroinflammation provokes intracellular acidification in mouse hippocampus. *J. Neuroinflammation* 13:283. doi: 10.1186/s12974-016-0747-8

Vale-Gonzalez, C., Alfonso, A., Sunol, C., Vieytes, M. R., and Botana, L. M. (2006). Role of the plasma membrane calcium adenosine triphosphatase on domoate-induced intracellular acidification in primary cultures of cerebelar granule cells. *J. Neurosci. Res.* 84, 326–337. doi: 10.1002/jnr.20878

Venkatachalam, K., and Montell, C. (2007). TRP channels. *Annu. Rev. Biochem.* 76, 387–417. doi: 10.1146/annurev.biochem.75.103004.142819

Vennekens, R., Menigoz, A., and Nilius, B. (2012). TRPs in the brain. *Rev. Physiol. Biochem. Pharmacol.* 163, 27–64. doi: 10.1007/112_2012_8

Verkhratsky, A., Reyes, R. C., and Parpura, V. (2014). TRP channels coordinate ion signalling in astroglia. *Rev. Physiol. Biochem. Pharmacol.* 166, 1–22. doi: 10.1007/112_2013_15

Villereal, M. L. (2006). Mechanism and functional significance of TRPC channel multimerization. *Semin. Cell Dev. Biol.* 17, 618–629. doi: 10.1016/j.semcdb.2006.10.010

Von Spiczak, S., Muhle, H., Helbig, I., De Kovel, C. G., Hampe, J., Gaus, V., et al. (2010). Association study of TRPC4 as a candidate gene for generalized epilepsy with photosensitivity. *Neuromolecular Med.* 12, 292–299. doi: 10.1007/s12017-010-8122-x

Wang, H., Cheng, X., Tian, J., Xiao, Y., Tian, T., Xu, F., et al. (2020). TRPC channels: structure, function, regulation and recent advances in small molecular probes. *Pharmacol. Ther.* 209:107497. doi: 10.1016/j.pharmthera.2020.107497

Wang, J., Jackson, M. F., and Xie, Y. F. (2016). Glia and TRPM2 channels in plasticity of central nervous system and Alzheimer's diseases. *Neural Plast.* 2016:1680905. doi: 10.1155/2016/1680905

Wang, J., Lu, R., Yang, J., Li, H., He, Z., Jing, N., et al. (2015). TRPC6 specifically interacts with APP to inhibit its cleavage by gamma-secretase and reduce Abeta production. *Nat. Commun.* 6:8876. doi: 10.1038/ncomms9876

Wang, M., Bianchi, R., Chuang, S. C., Zhao, W., and Wong, R. K. (2007). Group I metabotropic glutamate receptor-dependent TRPC channel trafficking in hippocampal neurons. *J. Neurochem.* 101, 411–421. doi: 10.1111/j.1471-4159.2006.04377.x

Wang, Z., Zhou, L., An, D., Xu, W., Wu, C., Sha, S., et al. (2019). TRPV4-induced inflammatory response is involved in neuronal death in pilocarpine model of temporal lobe epilepsy in mice. *Cell Death Dis.* 10:386. doi: 10.1038/s41419-019-1691-1

Wong, M. M. K., Hoekstra, S. D., Vowles, J., Watson, L. M., Fuller, G., Nemeth, A. H., et al. (2018). Neurodegeneration in SCA14 is associated with increased PKCgamma kinase activity, mislocalization and aggregation. *Acta Neuropathol. Commun.* 6:99. doi: 10.1186/s40478-018-0600-7

Woolums, B. M., Mccray, B. A., Sung, H., Tabuchi, M., Sullivan, J. M., Ruppell, K. T., et al. (2020). TRPV4 disrupts mitochondrial transport and causes axonal degeneration via a CaMKII-dependent elevation of intracellular Ca(2). *Nat. Commun.* 11:2679. doi: 10.1038/s41467-020-16411-5

Wu, D., Huang, W., Richardson, P. M., Priestley, J. V., and Liu, M. (2008). TRPC4 in rat dorsal root ganglion neurons is increased after nerve injury and is necessary for neurite outgrowth. *J. Biol. Chem.* 283, 416–426. doi: 10.1074/jbc.M703177200

Wu, X., Zagranichnaya, T. K., Gurda, G. T., Eves, E. M., and Villereal, M. L. (2004). A TRPC1/TRPC3-mediated increase in store-operated calcium entry is required for differentiation of H19-7 hippocampal neuronal cells. *J. Biol. Chem.* 279, 43392–43402. doi: 10.1074/jbc.M408959200

Xiong, Z. G., Pignataro, G., Li, M., Chang, S. Y., and Simon, R. P. (2008). Acid-sensing ion channels (ASICs) as pharmacological targets for neurodegenerative diseases. *Curr. Opin. Pharmacol.* 8, 25–32. doi: 10.1016/j.coph.2007.09.001

Yamamoto, S., Wajima, T., Hara, Y., Nishida, M., and Mori, Y. (2007). Transient receptor potential channels in Alzheimer's disease. *Biochim. Biophys. Acta* 1772, 958–967. doi: 10.1016/j.bbadis.2007.03.006

Yamamoto, T., Swietach, P., Rossini, A., Loh, S. H., Vaughan-Jones, R. D., and Spitzer, K. W. (2005). Functional diversity of electrogenic Na+-HCO3-cotransport in ventricular myocytes from rat, rabbit and guinea pig. *J. Physiol.* 562, 455–475. doi: 10.1113/jphysiol.2004.071068

Yang, H., and Li, S. (2016). Transient Receptor Potential Ankyrin 1 (TRPA1) channel and neurogenic inflammation in pathogenesis of asthma. *Med. Sci. Monit.* 22, 2917–2923. doi: 10.12659/MSM.896557

Yang, W., Liu, J., Zheng, F., Jia, M., Zhao, L., Lu, T., et al. (2013). The evidence for association of ATP2B2 polymorphisms with autism in Chinese Han population. *PLoS ONE* 8:e61021. doi: 10.1371/journal.pone.0061021

Zaidi, A. (2010). Plasma membrane Ca-ATPases: targets of oxidative stress in brain aging and neurodegeneration. *World J. Biol. Chem.* 1, 271–280. doi: 10.4331/wjbc.v1.i9.271

Zaidi, A., Adewale, M., Mclean, L., and Ramlow, P. (2018). The plasma membrane calcium pumps-the old and the new. *Neurosci. Lett.* 663, 12–17. doi: 10.1016/j.neulet.2017.09.066

Zanni, G., Cali, T., Kalscheuer, V. M., Ottolini, D., Barresi, S., Lebrun, N., et al. (2012). Mutation of plasma membrane Ca2+ ATPase isoform 3 in a family with X-linked congenital cerebellar ataxia impairs Ca2+ homeostasis. *Proc. Natl. Acad. Sci. U. S. A.* 109, 14514–14519. doi: 10.1073/pnas.1207488109

Zeng, Z., Leng, T., Feng, X., Sun, H., Inoue, K., Zhu, L., et al. (2015). Silencing TRPM7 in mouse cortical astrocytes impairs cell proliferation and migration via ERK and JNK signaling pathways. *PLoS ONE* 10:e0119912. doi: 10.1371/journal.pone.0119912

Zhai, K., Liskova, A., Kubatka, P., and Busselberg, D. (2020). Calcium entry through TRPV1: a potential target for the regulation of proliferation and apoptosis in cancerous and healthy cells. *Int. J. Mol. Sci.* 21:4177. doi: 10.3390/ijms21114177

Zhang, E., and Liao, P. (2015). Brain transient receptor potential channels and stroke. *J. Neurosci. Res.* 93, 1165–1183. doi: 10.1002/jnr.23529

Zhao, H., Carney, K. E., Falgoust, L., Pan, J. W., Sun, D., and Zhang, Z. (2016). Emerging roles of Na(+)/H(+) exchangers in epilepsy and developmental brain disorders. *Prog. Neurobiol.* 138–140, 19–35. doi: 10.1016/j.pneurobio.2016.02.002

Zheng, J. (2013). Molecular mechanism of TRP channels. *Compr. Physiol.* 3, 221–242. doi: 10.1002/cphy.c120001

Zundorf, G., and Reiser, G. (2011). Calcium dysregulation and homeostasis of neural calcium in the molecular mechanisms of neurodegenerative diseases provide multiple targets for neuroprotection. *Antioxid. Redox Signal* 14, 1275–1288. doi: 10.1089/ars.2010.3359

6

TRP Channels in Brain Tumors

Giorgia Chinigò[1,2], Hélène Castel[3,4], Oana Chever[3,4] and Dimitra Gkika[5,6]**

[1] Laboratory of Cell Physiology, Department of Life Sciences, Univ. Lille, Inserm, U1003 – PHYCEL, University of Lille, Lille, France, [2] Laboratory of Cellular and Molecular Angiogenesis, Department of Life Sciences and Systems Biology, University of Torino, Turin, Italy, [3] UNIROUEN, Inserm U1239, DC2N, Normandie Université, Rouen, France, [4] Institute for Research and Innovation in Biomedicine, Rouen, France, [5] CNRS, Inserm, CHU Lille, Centre Oscar Lambret, UMR 9020-UMR 1277-Canther-Cancer Heterogeneity, Plasticity and Resistance to Therapies, University of Lille, Lille, France, [6] Institut Universitaire de France, Paris, France

***Correspondence:**
Giorgia Chinigò
giorgia.chinigo@unito.it
Dimitra Gkika
dimitra.gkika@univ-lille.fr

Malignant glioma including glioblastoma (GBM) is the most common group of primary brain tumors. Despite standard optimized treatment consisting of extensive resection followed by radiotherapy/concomitant and adjuvant therapy, GBM remains one of the most aggressive human cancers. GBM is a typical example of intra-heterogeneity modeled by different micro-environmental situations, one of the main causes of resistance to conventional treatments. The resistance to treatment is associated with angiogenesis, hypoxic and necrotic tumor areas while heterogeneity would accumulate during glioma cell invasion, supporting recurrence. These complex mechanisms require a focus on potential new molecular actors to consider new treatment options for gliomas. Among emerging and underexplored targets, transient receptor potential (TRP) channels belonging to a superfamily of non-selective cation channels which play critical roles in the responses to a number of external stimuli from the external environment were found to be related to cancer development, including glioma. Here, we discuss the potential as biological markers of diagnosis and prognosis of TRPC6, TRPM8, TRPV4, or TRPV1/V2 being associated with glioma patient overall survival. TRPs-inducing common or distinct mechanisms associated with their Ca^{2+}-channel permeability and/or kinase function were detailed as involving miRNA or secondary effector signaling cascades in turn controlling proliferation, cell cycle, apoptotic pathways, DNA repair, resistance to treatment as well as migration/invasion. These recent observations of the key role played by TRPs such as TRPC6 in GBM growth and invasiveness, TRPV2 in proliferation and glioma-stem cell differentiation and TRPM2 as channel carriers of cytotoxic chemotherapy within glioma cells, should offer new directions for innovation in treatment strategies of high-grade glioma as GBM to overcome high resistance and recurrence.

Keywords: ion channel, TRP channel, brain tumor, glioma, glioblastoma

INTRODUCTION

Malignant gliomas are the most prevalent group of primary brain tumors in adults, with an incidence of 8.9 cases per 100,000 persons/year in the US (Ostrom et al., 2015, 2017). Glioblastoma (GBM) remains one of the most aggressive human cancers. Glial tumors or glioma represent a wide spectrum of malignancies including grades II and III oligodendroglioma, grades II and III astrocytoma and glioblastoma from initial classification based on anatomocytopathological criteria related to the morphotypic characteristics and numerous cytonuclear atypologies, accompanied by anaplasia for high-grade glioma (GBM, grade IV) (Louis et al., 2007; Miller and Perry, 2007). The diagnosis of GBM was based on the presence of vascular micro-proliferations signs of intense vascularization, associated with zones of necrosis delimited by a hypoxic pseudopalissadic cellular zone, evidencing important intra-tumoral heterogeneity (Karsy et al., 2012; Alifieris and Trafalis, 2015). Now, brain tumors and glioma are classified according to the histomolecular classification recently published by the World Health Organization (WHO) (Louis et al., 2016), which represents a major clinical improvement for both diagnosis and treatments, as well as patient prognosis. The aim was to implement the histopathological classification with the following molecular signatures: first including the mutation in the isocitrate dehydrogenase1/2 (IDH1/2mut) and/or the co-deletion 1p/19q associated with oligodendroglioma or mutation of TP53; second the l'α-thalassemia mental retardation syndrome X-linked (ATX) or amplification of the epidermal growth factor receptor (EGFR) were associated with GBM IDHwt; finally the hypermethylation of the O6-methyl guanine-DNA methyl transferase (MGMT) promoter constitutes an important parameter of the GBM aggressiveness (Louis et al., 2016).

Despite these molecular attempts to stratify glioma patients with the objective to allow personalization of the treatments, the median survival of GBM patients currently ranges from 15 to 17 months, despite a safe maximal surgical resection, radiation/concomitant and adjuvant alkylating-based chemotherapy by temozolomide (TMZ) (Stupp et al., 2005, 2009; Wen and Brandes, 2009). However, more than 95% of GBM recur in the margin of the resection cavity, an area in which glioma tumor cells acting as a tumor reservoir are found (Giese et al., 2003). This invasiveness associated with X-ray and/or intrinsic or acquired chemoresistance of the glioma cells and the presence of an intrinsic or acquired blood-brain barrier (BBB), limit the effectiveness and/or the delivery of anti-neoplastic agents and justify the development of new strategies. In agreement, over the last decade, despite very important advances in the field of targeted therapy, none of them, e.g., drug/antibody or combination of small molecule inhibitors, has been shown to be more effective than TMZ or capable of increasing the efficacy of standard therapy in patients with primary or recurrent GBM (Stepanenko and Chekhonin, 2018), and no curative treatment is currently identified in GBM. This failure may be explained at least in part by the intratumoral heterogeneity which is a conserved consequence of the GBM micro-environment (Prabhu et al., 2017), referring to the physico-chemical characteristics and matrices interacting with the tumor. Indeed, the GBM heterogeneity is tightly related to angiogenic and hypoxic features as well as invasive processes, thus future strategies should consider targeting mechanisms associated with resistance and invasion. In particular, Watkins et al. (2014) showed that GBM cells can thus control the regulation of vascular tone, *via* the release of K^+ through K^+ channels activated in response to Ca^{2+}, leading to an adaptation of cell volume to facilitate their invasion.

Transient receptor potential (TRP) channels are a superfamily of cationic tetrameric channels, mostly permeable to Ca^{2+}, involved in various physiological functions, and for the most part sustain calcium homeostasis and calcium signaling. Calcium-dependent mechanisms determine several aspects of brain tumor cell homeostasis including survival, proliferation, invasion or treatment resistance, making TRP channels putative potent modulators of tumorigenesis and glioma progression. Approximately 30 TRPs have been identified and are classified into TRPA (ankyrin family), TRPC (canonical family), TRPM (melastatin family), TRPN (NomPC family), TRPML (mucolipin family), TRPP (polycystin family), and TRPV (vanilloid family) (Li, 2017). These cationic channels have been shown to be gated by many physical or chemical stimuli (temperature, membrane potential, pH, hormones, vitamins ...). TRP channels are expressed in various excitable and non-excitable cell types and are present in many organs, including brain, heart, liver, lung, kidney, spleen, muscle, skin, pancreas (Venkatachalam and Montell, 2007). Since a decade, TRP channels have attracted much interest in the cancer field and tumorigenesis. Activities of TRP channels have been linked to cell growth, survival or migration, being involved in a plethora of cancers, especially for TRPC, TRPM, and TRPV (Prevarskaya et al., 2007; Gkika and Prevarskaya, 2009; Fiorio Pla and Gkika, 2013). Recent research unravels the role of some TRP channels in glioma growth and progression or glioma stem-like cell fate determination. In this review, we will mainly focus on a new class of molecular players, TRP channels emerging in gliomas and for which we will develop three aspects: (i) the expression profile and use as clinical markers; (ii) the molecular mechanisms through which they act; and (iii) their potential use in therapeutics.

TRANSIENT RECEPTOR POTENTIAL (TRP) EXPRESSION PROFILE AND PUTATIVE BIOMARKERS

Changes in expression of TRP channels have been related to cancer development and progression, thus making them valuable diagnostic and/or prognostic markers in several tumor types, including glioma. Furthermore, a strong correlation between clinical-pathological findings and mRNA and/or protein expression of different TRPs has been recently provided. For instance, mRNA encoding TRPC1, TRPC6, TRPM7, TRPM8, TRPV4, and TRPML2 appeared up-regulated in GBM tumor specimens in comparison with normal tissues and their expression was found to increase with glioma tumor grade with the highest mRNA level found in GBM patient samples (Ding et al., 2010; Alptekin et al., 2015). These findings are consistent with a pro-tumorigenic role of these channels in glioma progression and aggressiveness, as described in more detail in the next paragraph. According to a qPCR screening of 33 GBM patient tumors, additional mRNA-encoding TRP channels including TRPM2, TRPM3, TRPV1, TRPV2 showed significantly higher expression levels in GBM compared with control normal brain tissues (Alptekin et al., 2015). However, other studies reported opposite results, more consistent with an anti-tumorigenic function of these channels, as confirmed by several experimental data (Amantini et al., 2007; Nabissi et al., 2010; Ying et al., 2013; Morelli et al., 2019). These discrepancies could be due to the relatively low number of patients considered in the first study (Alptekin et al., 2015), which may not be very representative enough while further investigations should now be reconsidered in light of the new molecular GBM patient stratification and the methylome.

Among more than 20 TRP channels investigated, TRPM8 showed the highest mRNA upregulation in GBM as compared with normal brain tissue (Alptekin et al., 2015; Zeng et al., 2019), suggesting a pivotal function of TRPM8 in gliomagenesis. Moreover, TRPM8 expression in human GBM specimens and established GBM cell lines was found to be up-regulated at both mRNA and protein level to a variable extent (Klumpp et al., 2017) and to be significantly correlated with worse patient overall survival (Zeng et al., 2019). Interestingly, it was previously reported that TRPM8 is a primary androgen-responsive gene since its promoter is located downstream an androgen response elements (AREs) to which androgen receptor (AR) may bind once activated by androgens thus promoting TRPM8 expression (Bidaux et al., 2005; Asuthkar et al., 2015). Therefore, TRPM8 overexpression in high-grade glioma might be associated with the documented upregulation of AR in GBM (Yu et al., 2015). Moreover, it has been recently found that AR may also directly regulate TRPM8 channel activity via protein-protein interaction and/or TRPM8 phosphorylation, further accentuating the close TRPM8-androgens relationship (Grolez et al., 2019a; Gkika et al., 2020). Similarly to TRPM8, TRPV4 has been shown to positively correlate with glioma progression, since high levels of TRPV4 gene and protein expression were associated with a poorer patient prognosis (Ou-yang et al., 2018). Thus, TRPM8 and TRPV4 may be currently considered promising biomarkers accompanying aggressiveness of glioma and signature of GBM while constituting potential therapeutic targets for future treatment options. TRPML2 expression was also detected in normal astrocytes and neural stem/progenitor cells and to be up-regulated at both mRNA and protein level in glioma to a variable extent, increasing with the pathological grade (Morelli et al., 2016). Such observation was linked to the up-regulation of the transcriptional activator of the TRPML-2 gene Paired box 5 (PAX5) (Valadez and Cuajungco, 2015) found in human astrocytoma and correlated with malignancy and pathological grade of glioma (Stuart et al., 1995).

Moreover, the loss of TRPM3, TRPV1, TRPV2, and TRPML1 expression has been proposed as a negative prognostic marker for GBM patients, because of their significant and progressive down-regulation as the tumor grade increases. For instance, a study focusing on the role of miR-204 in high-grade glioma cell lines has revealed a significant down-regulation of TRPM3, due to the hypermethylation of its promoter (Ying et al., 2013). Interestingly, miR-204 is an intronic miRNA located between exons 7 and 8 of the TRPM3 gene and its loss in glioma, due to the high methylation of its host gene TRPM3, is associated with an enhancement in cell migration and cellular stemness (Ying et al., 2013) questioning the direct role of TRPM3 and the indirect regulatory functions of miR-204 *via* its target genes. Consistently, restoration of miR-204 in LN382T and SNB19 cells orthotopically xenografted in the brains of nude mice suppressed tumorigenesis and invasiveness and increased animal survival (Ying et al., 2013). Taken together, these findings might suggest a potential tumor-suppressive function of TRPM3 in glioma, but further studies are required to clarify its involvement in cancer development and/or progression and to establish whether TRPM3 and miR-204 might cooperate with each other in the pathogenesis of gliomas. Concerning TRPV1 and TRPV2, the preventing role in gliomagenesis and tumor progression has been more clearly established and characterized (see next paragraph). First, TRPV1 and TRPV2 genes and protein expression appeared inversely correlated with glioma grade, showing an almost undetectable level in GBM (Amantini et al., 2007; Nabissi et al., 2010; Morelli et al., 2016). In particular, a study performed by Nabissi and coworkers has shown that GBM and glioma stem-like cells (GSC) selectively express the TRPV1 5′-untranslated region (5′UTR) variant three ($TRPV1_{v3}$), one of the four variants resulting from alternative first exon splicing (Nabissi et al., 2016). The 5′UTR can generate different transcripts encoding the same protein but characterized by different stability and translation efficacy (Audic and Hartley, 2004; Gebauer and Hentze, 2004; Hinnebusch et al., 2016) and $TRPV1_{v3}$ is the most stable TRPV1 5′UTR transcript. In GBM, the mRNA expression of the unique $TRPV1_{v3}$ variant correlates with the patient's survival, suggesting that its loss or low mRNA expression may represent a potential marker of poor prognosis in GBM patients (Nabissi et al., 2016). Similarly, the clinical relevance of the overexpression of TRPV2 in GBM was confirmed through the analysis of the TRPV2-interactome based signature using a systematic proteomics and computational analysis approach (Doñate-Macián et al., 2018), predicting GBM patient overall survival. Indeed, high TRPV2 interactome protein expression was correlated with tumor progression, recurrence, TMZ-resistance and a poor prognosis (Doñate-Macián et al., 2018). Finally, also TRPML1 might have a potential role as a negative prognostic marker for GBM patients (Morelli et al., 2019) since TRPML1 mRNA down-regulation or loss strongly correlates with reduced overall survival in GBM patients. However, additional studies are needed in order to further investigate the relationship between TRPML1 expression and lower glioma grades (Morelli et al., 2019). However, TRPML1 expression at mRNA and protein levels displayed variability within patient samples and its subcellular localization may also be distinct since TRPML1 is mainly expressed in the late endosome/lysosome of normal cells while found in endolysosomes and as dot spots in the nuclear cell compartment in glioma cells (Morelli et al., 2019). The mechanisms underlying this nuclear localization in tumor cells and the effects of this specific localization are not completely characterized, although it has been shown that TRPML1 is able to bind DNA somehow and thus, it might affect the transcription of some genes involved in tumor progression (Morelli et al., 2019).

Together, these studies highlight that some TRPM, TRPV, and/or TRPML channels overexpressed in glioma should be considered as predictive and specific biomarkers of high-grade glioma and GBM, and through changes in their permeability to cations they may play a role in GBM aggressiveness.

MOLECULAR MECHANISMS OF TRP CHANNELS ACTION

Transient receptor potential channels have revealed a direct involvement in determining many hallmarks of glioma and GBM (**Table 1**), including some typical histological cellular abnormalities (Bomben and Sontheimer, 2008), its relentless growth, and its intrinsic severe aggressiveness due to its high capability to diffuse into the non-neoplastic brain parenchyma, which contributes to treatments resistance and bad prognosis (Demuth and Berens, 2004; Schwartzbaum et al., 2006; Liu et al., 2018). TRP channels may exert both anti-tumorigenic and pro-tumorigenic functions in gliomas and the main TRPs-mediated signaling pathways associated with gliomas progression are schematically summarized in **Figure 1**. Most of the TRP channels involved in gliomagenesis and tumor progression were found to affect more than one cellular process related to carcinogenesis. In this chapter, we will therefore discuss the molecular mechanisms by which each TRP affects cancer cell behavior, subgrouping them into subfamilies.

Canonical TRPs

It has been suggested that TRPC channels-relayed mechanisms may contribute to some of the most common histopathological hallmarks of GBM such as nuclear atypia and enlarged cell shape (Bomben and Sontheimer, 2008). Glioma cell lines and surgical patient-derived tumors have revealed the expression of four TRP channels belonging to the TRP canonical subfamily that are TRPC1, TRPC3, TRPC5, and TRPC6. Further investigations on their role in glioma cells have suggested an involvement of these channels in a Ca^{2+} influx pathway impacting cellular growth. More specifically, it has been shown that TRPC channels contribute to the resting conductance of glioma cells while their acute pharmacological inhibition with SKF96365 increased membrane resistance of glioma cells and caused a transient hyperpolarization followed by a sustain depolarization of the cells' membrane (Bomben and Sontheimer, 2008). Additionally, chronic application of the TRPC inhibitor SKF96365 (from 0 to 5 days) would lead to an almost complete growth arrest at the G_2/M phase of GBM D54MG cell cycle, as revealed by FACS analysis (Bomben and Sontheimer, 2008). In most cases the blockage of the cell cycle during the G_2/M transition leads to cell death (Stark and Taylor, 2006), or in the particular case of D54MG cells, TRPC inhibition was accompanied by a continued growth exhibiting multinuclear and enlarged cells due to incomplete cytokinesis. This phenotype might render impossible a dynamic adaptation of the cell volume to invade the brain parenchyma, through the narrow extracellular brain spaces compatible with less recurrence.

Glioma cells display a depolarized resting membrane potential around −30 mV. Some TRPC channels are opened at rest and contribute to this membrane potentials (Bomben and Sontheimer, 2008). Activation of TRPC channels can also lead to membrane potentials fluctuations by various ways. First of all, TRPC channels are non-selective cation channels and they directly depolarize cells following activation. In addition, TRP channels are functionally coupled with other ion channels, so their activation can indirectly lead to depolarizations or hyperpolarizations, depending on the channels involved (Gees et al., 2010). In particular, major conductances of glioma cells are mediated by Ca^{2+}-activated K^+ channels (Ransom et al., 2001) and Cl^- channels such as ClC3 or ClC2 (Mcferrin and Sontheimer, 2006), which both are modulated by TRPC channels. Glioma cells do express many types of channels and transporters (Cuddapah and Sontheimer, 2011; Molenaar, 2011), which are sensitive to membrane potential fluctuations. Furthermore, glioma cells have been shown to display electrical activities similar to Na^+ spikes, which are sustained by TTX-sensitive voltage-gated Na^+ channels (Bordey and Sontheimer, 1998). Thus, TRPC channels may impact many voltage-dependent cellular processes and modulate electrical behavior of glioma cells.

Among the TRPCs, TRPC1, and TRPC6 are those for which the mechanism of action has been best characterized in human malignant glioma. For instance, TRPC1 was found to act on several hallmarks of cancer, including growth, cell cycle and migration. Interestingly, all the TRPC1 effects on glioma cell behavior strictly resulted from lipid regulation, e.g., in some cases the channel activity is directly affected by lipids [phosphatidylinositol-(4,5)-bisphosphate PIP_2, phosphoinositides, diacylglycerol, cholesterol, etc.] localized on the plasma membrane, in other cases, it can be by signaling pathways which lead to the production of specific lipids such as sphingolipids. It has been shown that the loss of TRPC1-mediated Ca^{2+} influx upon pharmacological inhibition or constitutive/inducible shRNA silencing, is associated with reduced cell proliferation and incomplete cell division, thus resulting in multinucleated cells similar to those found in patient biopsies (Bomben and Sontheimer, 2010). The important role of TRPC1 in glioma cell division has been also confirmed *in vivo* through a shRNA knockdown approach on a flank GBM cell tumor model: TRPC1 downregulation led to a significant decrease in tumor size, most likely impairing calcium signaling during cytokinesis (late M-phase) (Bomben and Sontheimer, 2010). TRPC1 has also revealed a role in controlling glioma cell migration. In particular, it has been shown that TRPC1 is essential for chemotactic migration in human malignant gliomas in response to chemoattractant growth factors like epidermal growth factor (EGF) and platelet-derived growth factor (PDGF) which affect TRPC1 activity through different signaling pathways (Bomben et al., 2011; Lepannetier et al., 2016). Stimulation with EGF was associated with a re-localization of TRPC1 channel at the leading edge of migrating D54MG glioma cells within lipid rafts, specialized membrane microdomains enriched in cholesterol and sphingolipids (Mollinedo and Gajate, 2015). In agreement, it has been shown that both TRPC1 channel activity and lipid raft integrity were required for gliomas chemotaxis (Bomben et al., 2011). Moreover, the disruption of lipid rafts by depletion of cholesterol not only affected chemotaxis but also impaired TRPC currents in whole-cell recordings and decreased store-operated Ca^{2+} entry (SOCE), confirming a direct interplay between lipid rafts and TRPC1 channels and localized Ca^{2+} rise in regulating the chemotactic movement of

TABLE 1 | TRP channels expression and functionality in gliomas/glioblastomas.

Channel	Expression: Healthy	Expression: Tumor progression	Biological effect	Mechanism	Potential therapeutic tools	References
TRPC1	Yes	↑	Cell growth (+)	↑ Cytokinesis	TRPC1/SPK/PI3K inhibitors	Bomben and Sontheimer, 2008; Bomben and Sontheimer, 2010
			Cell migration (+)	↑Chemotaxis		Bomben et al., 2011; Lepannetier et al., 2016
TRPC6	Low	↑	Cell growth (+)	→ NFAT	TRPC6/NFAT inhibitors	Chigurupati et al., 2010; Ding et al., 2010
			Cell migration (+)	→ RhoA		Chigurupati et al., 2010
			Angiogenesis (+)	→ NFAT		
			Radioresistance (+)	↑ G_2/M (Cdc25C)		Ding et al., 2010
TRPM2	Yes	↑	Cell death (+)	↑ ROS-induced Ca^{2+} influx	TRPM2 gene insertion (+ Se and DXT)	Ishii et al., 2007; Ertilav et al., 2019
TRPM3	Yes	↑/↓	n.d.	n.d.	n.d.	Ying et al., 2013; Alptekin et al., 2015
TRPM7	Yes	↑	Cell growth (+)	↑ STAT3/Notch	TRPM7/STAT3/Notch/ ALDH1 inhibitors miR-28-5p	Liu et al., 2014; Wan et al., 2019
				⊣miR-28-5p ⊣ Rap1b		
			Cell invasion (+)	⊣miR-28-5p ⊣ Rap1b		Wan et al., 2019
			Stem cell renewal and differentiation (+)	STAT3-ALDH1 ↑		Liu et al., 2014
TRPM8	Yes	↑	Cell migration (+)	↑ BK channels RTK signaling		Wondergem et al., 2008; Wondergem and Bartley, 2009; Klumpp et al., 2017
		(2 different isoforms)	Cell growth (+)	→ BK channels → CaMKII ⊣cdc25C ⊣ cdc2 MAPK signaling		Klumpp et al., 2017; Zeng et al., 2019
			Cell death (–)	MAPK signaling		Klumpp et al., 2017; Zeng et al., 2019
			Radioresistance (+)	Supporting DNA repair and cell cycle upon genotoxic stress		Klumpp et al., 2017
TRPV1	Yes	↓	Apoptosis (+)	→ p38 MAPK		Amantini et al., 2007
				↑ ER stress (ATF3)		Stock et al., 2012
TRPV2	Yes	↓	Cell proliferation (–)	ERK signaling		Nabissi et al., 2010; Morelli et al., 2012
			Apoptosis (+)	Fas signaling		Nabissi et al., 2010
			Cell differentiation (+)	↑ GFAP and β_{III}-tubulin expression ↑ Aml-1 a (PI3K/AKT pathway)	CBD	Morelli et al., 2012; Nabissi et al., 2015
			Drug sensitivity (+)	↑ drug uptake ↑ drug-mediated apoptotic pathway	CBD + TMZ/BCNU/ DOXO	Nabissi et al., 2013, 2015

(Continued)

TABLE 1 | Continued

Channel	Expression		Biological effect	Mechanism	Potential therapeutic tools	References
	Healthy	Tumor progression				
TRPV4	Yes	↑	Cell migration (+)	AKT/Rac1 signaling	TRPV4 inhibitors (HC-067047)	Ou-yang et al., 2018
TRPA1	n.d.	n.d.	Cell apoptosis (+)	↑ mitochondrial stress	TRPA1 activators	Deveci et al., 2019
TRPML1	Yes	↓	Cell apoptosis (+) Autophagy (+)			Morelli et al., 2019
TRPML2	Yes	↑	Cell proliferation (+) Cell apoptosis (–)	PI3K/AKT – ERK 1/2 signaling		Morelli et al., 2016

Abbreviations: +, increase; –, decrease; ↑, increment; ↓, reduction; →, activation; ⊣, inhibition. SPK, sphingosine kinase; PI3K, phosphoinositide-3 kinase; NFAT, nuclear factor of activated T-cells; Se, selenium; DXT, docetaxel; STAT3, signal transducer and activator of transcription 3; miR-28-5p, miRNA 28-5p; ALDH1, aldehyde dehydrogenase1; BK, large-conductance Ca^{2+}-activated K^+ membrane ion channels; RTK, Met receptor tyrosine kinase; CaMKII, Ca^{2+}/calmodulin-dependent protein kinase II; Cdc25C, M-phase inducer phosphatase 3; Cdc2, subunit of the M phase-promoting factor; MAPK, mitogen-activated protein kinase; ATF3, transcription factor-3; CBD, cannabidiol; ERK, extracellular signal-regulated kinase 1/2; GFAP, glial fibrillary acidic protein; Aml-1 a, acute myeloid leukemia variant a; AKT, protein kinase B; TMZ, temozolomide; BCNU, carmustine; DOXO, doxorubicin. n.d., not determined.

glioma cells (Bomben et al., 2011). It must be noted that TRPC pharmacological inhibition through non-selective inhibitors caused an almost complete loss of chemotactic migration but TRPC1 knockdown through shRNA compromised directional migration but did not eliminate it and did not affect non-directional motility. This suggests TRPC1 specific implication in chemotactic migration and the potential implication of other TRPC channels in migration processes (Bomben et al., 2011). As shown by a more recent study by Lepannetier et al. (2016), lipids are not only important for the regulation of TRPC1 at the membrane level, but also through their signaling. The authors shed light on another store-independent mechanism by which TRPC1 may be activated and thus affect cell migration in GBM. In particular, they have shown that PDGF may induce the translocation of TRPC1 from the cytosolic compartment to the front of migrating cells through a mechanism requiring the phosphoinositide-3 kinase (PI3K) and at the same time induces the production of the lipid second messenger sphingosine-1-P (S1P) which in turn, activates TRPC1-mediated Ca^{2+} entry. Indeed, the PDGF-induced Ca^{2+} influx through TRPC1 can be partially inhibited by pretreatment of the cells with a specific inhibitor of the sphingosine kinase (SPK) producing S1P (Lepannetier et al., 2016). However, whether S1P directly or indirectly triggers TRPC1-mediated and store-independent entry of Ca^{2+} channel remains to be clarified (Lepannetier et al., 2016). In any case, it has been well established that both TRPC1 targeting to the leading edge of lamellipodia and its activation by S1P are essential in regulating PDGF-induced chemotaxis in U251 glioblastoma cells (Lepannetier et al., 2016).

Another member of the TRPC subfamily specifically implicated in glioma progression is TRPC6. Indeed, TRPC6 was found to affect different hallmarks of GBM including tumor growth, cell survival, invasiveness and angiogenesis (Chigurupati et al., 2010; Ding et al., 2010). More specifically, it has been demonstrated that under hypoxia, which is one of the main characteristics of GBM aggressiveness, invasion and resistance to treatment (Flynn et al., 2008), Notch1 activation consequently led to TRPC6 upregulation in primary GBM samples and cell lines (Chigurupati et al., 2010). Indeed, the inhibition/silencing of TRPC6 was associated with a reduction in glioma growth, invasion and angiogenesis. This Notch1-mediated induction of TRPC6 expression in hypoxic U373 cell line was subtype-specific, since other members of the TRPC subfamily were unaffected, indicating that TRPC6 is primarily responsible for the hypoxia-induced sustained increase in the intracellular Ca^{2+} concentration. Additionally, it has been proven that TRPC6 is essential for GBM cell survival, since its downregulation not only suppressed cell growth *in vitro* and reduced tumor volume *in vivo*, but also impaired clonogenic ability, induced cell cycle arrest at the G_2/M phase, and enhanced the antiproliferative effect of ionizing radiation.

An accelerated G_2 phase progression may lead to an impaired DNA damage checkpoint and thus to an enhanced genomic instability, explaining the TRPC6 association with enhanced glioma cell malignancy. Mechanistically, TRPC6 effects on cell proliferation, tumor growth and angiogenesis seemed to be directly mediated by the Ca^{2+}-induced activation of the

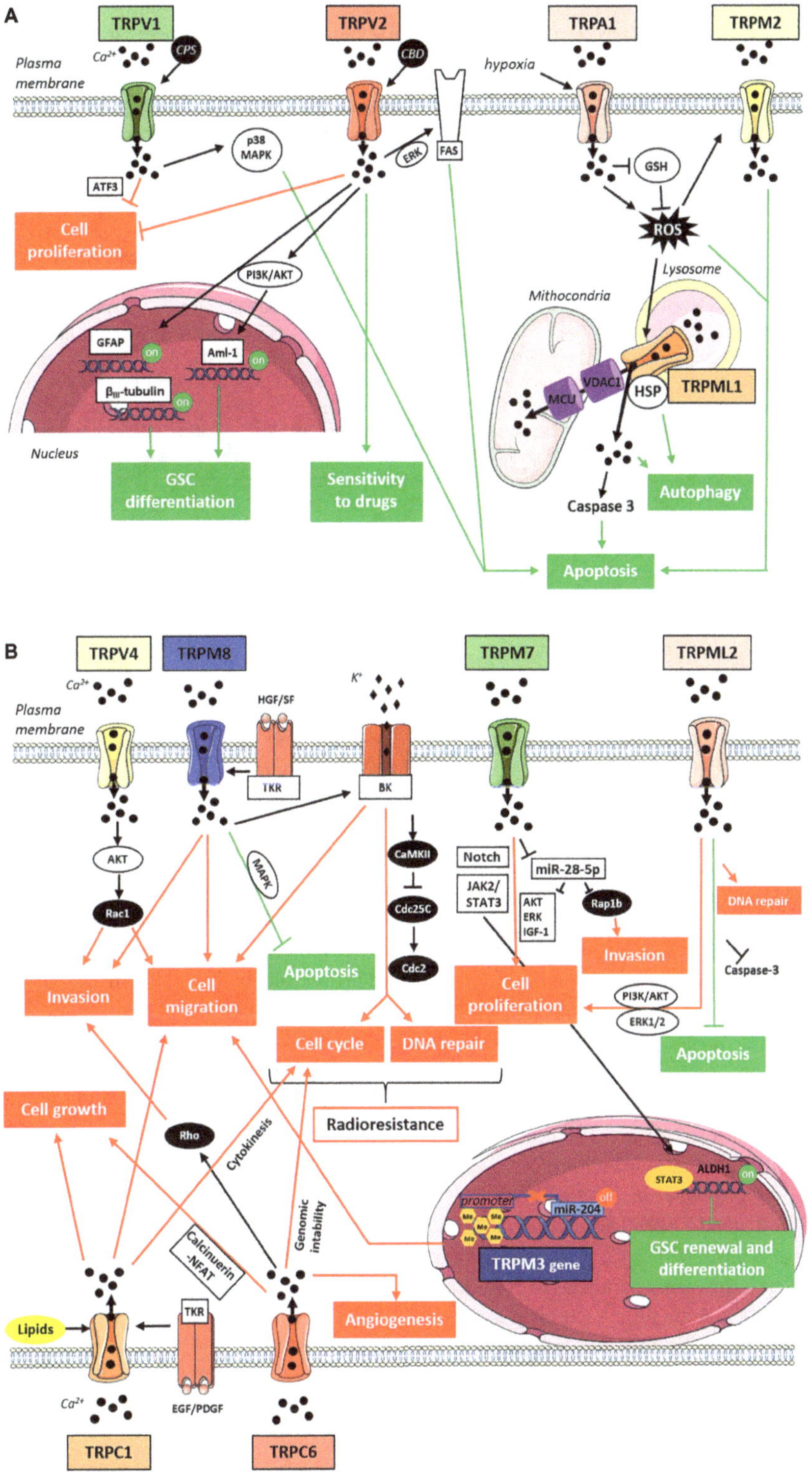

FIGURE 1 | TRPs-mediated signaling pathways in gliomas. **(A)** Anti-tumorigenic TRPs-mediated signaling pathways in gliomas. Cartoon depicting TRP channels signaling pathways suppressing gliomas progression through the inhibition of pro-tumorigenic pathways (in red) and/or the activation of anti-tumorigenic signaling pathways (in green). TRPM2 and TRPML1 upon ROS activation promote cell apoptosis through an increase in oxidative stress and intracellular Ca^{2+} concentration; due to its localization on the lysosomal membrane TRPML1 may also mediates the autophagic cell death pathway through the interaction with HSP; TRPA1 under hypoxia promotes apoptosis inducing ROS formation and inhibiting antioxidants such as GSH; TRPV1 upon stimulation with CPS triggers the apoptotic pathway through p38 MAPK and reduces glioma expansion via ER pathway in a ATF3-dependent manner; TRPV2 reduces cell proliferation and enhances the Fas-induced

(Continued)

FIGURE 1 | Continued
apoptosis in an ERK-dependent manner; TRPV2 also acts on cell differentiation since its overexpression is associated with GFAP and βIII-tubulin increased expression and its activation by CBD promotes Aml-1 up-regulation via PI3K/AKT pathway; finally, TRPV2 activation by CBD can improve cell sensitivity to chemotherapeutic agents favoring drug uptake. **(D)** Pro-tumorigenic TRPs-mediated signaling pathways in gliomas. Cartoon depicting TRP channels signaling pathways promoting gliomas progression through the activation of pro-tumorigenic pathways (in red) and/or the inhibition of anti-tumorigenic signaling pathways (in green). TRPC1 affects cell growth and cell proliferation mainly promoting cytokinesis in response to lipid activation, whereas upon stimulation with growth factors it induces chemotactic migration; TRPC6 affects cell proliferation, tumor growth and angiogenesis likely through the Ca^{2+}-induced activation of the calcineurin-NFAT pathway, whereas TRPC6 effects on cell migration might rather involve Rho activation and subsequent actin cytoskeleton rearrangements; TRPV4 promotes cell migration and tumor invasiveness through the AKT-mediated Rac1 activation; TRPM8 supports glioma progression by inhibiting apoptosis through MAPK pathway and impairing the cell cycle through the activation of BK channels and the subsequent CaMKII-mediated inhibition of phosphatases like Cdc25C and Cdc2; TRPM8 effects on cell migration/invasion are also associated with BK channels activation and the function of TRPM8 in aggressiveness and resistance to treatment may also be potentiated by TKR-mediated HGF/SF stimulation; TRPM7 increases glioma cell proliferation and invasion through the down-regulation of miR-28-5p and the subsequent up-regulation of oncogenic signaling pathways involving AKT, ERK, IGF-1 and Rap1b; TRPM7 effects on glioma proliferation may also be mediated by Notch and/or JAK2/STAT3 signaling pathways and through the activation of STAT3; TRPM7 might also be involved in GSC renewal and differentiation thanks to the up-regulation of the well-known GSC marker ALDH1; the hypermethylation of TRPM3 promoter through the down-regulation of miR-204 enhances cell migration; TRPML2 enhances cell proliferation and slows down apoptosis improving DNA repair and inhibiting Caspase 3 likely through PI3K/AKT and ERK1/2 pathways. Abbreviations: ROS, reactive oxygen species; HSP, heat shock proteins; GSH, glutathione; CPS, capsaicin; ATF3, transcription factor-3; CBD, cannabidiol; GFAP, glial fibrillary acidic protein; Aml-1, acute myeloid leukemia transcription factors; PI3K, phosphoinositide 3-kinases; AKT, protein-kinase B; HGF/SF, hepatocyte growth factor/scatter factor; EGF, epidermal growth factor; PDGF, platelet-derived growth factor; TKR, tyrosine kinase receptor; NFAT, nuclear factor of activated T-cells; MAPK, mitogen-activated protein kinase; BK, big potassium channels; CaMKII, Ca^{2+}/calmodulin-dependent protein kinase II; Cdc25C and Cdc2, cell division cycle proteins; JAK2, janus kinase 2; STAT3, signal transducer and activator of transcription 3; ERK, extracellular signal-regulated kinases; IGF-1, insulin-like growth factor-1; GSC, glioma stem cells; ALDH1, aldehyde dehydrogenase 1.

calcineurin-NFAT pathway (Chigurupati et al., 2010), whereas TRPC6 effects on cell migration might rather involve Rho activation and subsequent actin cytoskeleton rearrangements (Singh et al., 2007). Together, these data stress a possible role of TRPC6 as a promising therapeutic target in the treatment of human GBM (Chigurupati et al., 2010; Ding et al., 2010).

Melastatin TRPs

Four TRP melastatin subfamily members, TRPM2, TRPM3, TRPM7, and TRPM8, have been implicated in glioma cell growth, proliferation and migration. Among them, TRPM2 and TRPM3 would exert anti-tumorigenic effects, while TRPM7 and TRPM8 may contribute to glioma malignancy.

TRPM2 is known for its role as a sensor of oxidative stress and inductor of necrotic cell death upon activation by reactive oxygen species (ROS) (Naziroğlu and Lückhoff, 2008; Takahashi et al., 2011). TRPM2 expression likely induced no effect on cell proliferation, migration and invasion. But in A172 human GBM cells the transfection with TRPM2 channels increased cell death induced by H_2O_2 in a Ca^{2+}-dependent manner (Ishii et al., 2007) and in human GBM (DBTRG) cells, TRPM2 activation led to an increase in oxidative stress and intracellular Ca^{2+} concentration, thus promoting GBM cell death through apoptosis (Ertilav et al., 2019). Concerning TRPM3, which is the most recently described melastatin subfamily member, Its roles and action mechanisms were only recently investigated (Zamudio-Bulcock et al., 2011). Like TRPM2, TRPM3 may show a protective role in glioma probably via the miR-204 regulation (Ying et al., 2013), but its function needs further studies.

TRPM7 also controls glioma progression through miRNA regulation in GBM cells with subsequent effects on cell proliferation and invasion (Wan et al., 2019). More specifically, TRPM7 expression can be associated with a decreased production of miR-28-5p, a tumor suppressor inhibiting the expression of oncogenic signaling pathways involving protein-kinase B (AKT) (Xiao et al., 2018), ERK (Liu et al., 2016), and IGF-1 (Shi and Teng, 2015). Accordingly, the downregulation of miR-28-5p caused a significant increase in glioma cell proliferation and invasion. Among miR-28-5p targets, expression of Rap1b appeared as being positively correlated with TRPM7 in GBM and was up-regulated in tumor samples due to the suppression of the repressing role of miR-28-5p (Wan et al., 2019). This miR-28-5p/Rap1b axis shown in gliomagenesis is not the exclusive signaling route in which TRPM7 acts on GBM progression. Indeed, TRPM7 may also regulate the Notch pathway (Liu et al., 2014), recently shown as linked with Rap1b signaling and integrin-mediated cell adhesion in hematopoietic stem cells (Rho et al., 2019). This can be connected with the role of TRPM7 on cell proliferation, migration and invasion in glioma cells and GSCs through the upregulation of JAK2/STAT3 and/or Notch signaling pathways (Liu et al., 2014). Moreover, TRPM7 was found to activate STAT3, which in turn binds to the aldehyde dehydrogenase1 (ALDH1) promoter upregulating the expression of this well-known GSC marker involved in many pathways maintaining stem cell-like state (Rasper et al., 2010), when expanded as spheroids (Liu et al., 2014). Since ALDH1 is functionally involved in self-protection, differentiation, expansion and proliferation (Choudhary et al., 2005; Ma and Allan, 2011), this potentially means that TRPM7 is not only implicated in proliferation, migration and invasion, but also in GSC renewal and differentiation. This has to be put into the context that TRPM7 channel exhibits an intrinsic kinase activity, thus supporting that TRPM7 effects on glioma cell growth are mediated by its channel activity while cell migration and invasion required its kinase domain (Wan et al., 2019). The discovery of different cellular and molecular targets affecting gliomas development and progression through their modulation by TRPM7 provides key insights for the development of novel therapeutic agents for glioma treatments.

TRPM8 was found to affect the rate of GBM cell migration by mediating a significant increase in intracellular Ca^{2+}

concentration upon stimulation with specific agonists such as menthol and icilin (Wondergem et al., 2008; Wondergem and Bartley, 2009; Klumpp et al., 2017). It has been shown that TRPM8 activation by icilin leads to a significant increase in the migration speed and chemotaxis of GBM cells and, consistently, TRPM8 downregulation by RNA interference as well as TRPM8 inhibition by the specific channel blocker BCTC [*N*-(4-tertiarybutylphenyl)-4-(3-cholorphyridin-2-yl)tet rahydropyrazine-1(2H)-carbox-amide] reduces cell migration rate and decreases transfilter chemotaxis (Klumpp et al., 2017). One of the possible mechanisms through which TRPM8-mediated Ca^{2+} influx may affect cell migration in glioma is by the activation of the large-conductance Ca^{2+}-activated K^+ ion channels (BK channels) (Wondergem and Bartley, 2009). BK channels contribute to maintaining the plasma membrane ionic fluxes essential to support cell shrinkage-driven cell migration (Mcferrin and Sontheimer, 2006). Interestingly, BK overexpression was detected in human glioma cells (Ransom and Sontheimer, 2001) and pharmacological inhibition of BK channels was shown to abolish the menthol-stimulated Ca^{2+} influx within the cell cytoplasm and cell migration suggesting a key role of TRPM8. TRPM8 activation by agonists has been shown to increase the open probability of single BK channels (Wondergem and Bartley, 2009; Klumpp et al., 2017). In agreement, ionizing radiation, known to induce the migration through a Ca^{2+}-mediated activation of BK channels (Steinle et al., 2011; Edalat et al., 2016), has been shown to activate and upregulate TRPM8-mediated Ca^{2+} influx in glioma cells (Klumpp et al., 2017), thus confirming a direct and reciprocal interplay between these two channel families in the control of GBM migration. The function of TRPM8 in aggressiveness and resistance to treatment was suggested by the potentiating impact of hepatocyte growth factor/scatter factor (HGF/SF), a multifunctional effector of cells expressing the Met tyrosine kinase receptor (TKR), on TRPM8-induced Ca^{2+} homeostasis and cell migration. This evidence suggests that TRPM8 might converge to a common HGF/SF and cMET, known to play a role in malignancy of solid tumors including glioma (Laterra et al., 1997; Birchmeier et al., 2003; Wondergem et al., 2008), signaling pathway leading to migration/invasion. An enhancement in the invasion rate of human GBM cells has also been associated with TRPM8 overexpression (Zeng et al., 2019). However, DBTRG cells would express two different variants of TRPM8 (Wondergem et al., 2008) as revealed in Western blot showing a molecular band at 130–140 kDa in the plasma membrane-enriched fraction and consistent with the molecular weight of TRPM8 full-length isoform (Peier et al., 2002), and a second molecular band at 95–100 kDa in microsome- and membrane-enriched fractions more consistent with a truncated TRPM8 splice variant expressed in the endoplasmic reticulum (ER) (Bidaux et al., 2007). The observed greater increase in menthol-induced Ca^{2+} influx among migrating cells compared with non-migrating cells (Wondergem et al., 2008), likely indicates that only migrating cells express full-length TRPM8 protein within the plasma membrane. However, these results have to be taken with caution in a future context of drug therapy, since TRPM8 was shown to have an anti-migratory activity in other cancers including prostate cancer and may play a role in the tumoral and tumor-derived endothelial cells (Gkika et al., 2010, 2015; Genova et al., 2017; Grolez et al., 2019b). TRPM8 contribution to GBM progression was found to go far beyond its effects on cell migration and invasion, significantly affecting other determinant processes such as cell cycle, cell survival and radioresistance (Klumpp et al., 2017; Zeng et al., 2019). Indeed, it has been proven that TRPM8 inhibition or knockdown impaired the cell cycle, triggered apoptotic cell death and attenuated DNA repair and clonogenic survival (Klumpp et al., 2017). A recent study by Zeng et al. (2019) have suggested an involvement of the mitogen-activated protein kinase (MAPK) signaling pathway in TRPM8-mediated effects on cell proliferation and apoptosis, since the expression of the channel was associated with the expression levels of important regulators of these pathways, including extracellular signal-regulated kinase (ERK), cyclin D1 and the apoptosis-related protein Bcl-2 in human glioma cells. Moreover, it has been shown that TRPM8 signaling directly regulates the cell cycle, contributing to S phase progression and mitosis. These effects on glioma's cell cycle are most likely mediated by intracellular signaling pathways involving the Ca^{2+}/calmodulin-dependent protein kinase II (CaMKII) and some Cdc phosphatases like Cdc25C and Cdc2, which control entry into, and progression through, various phases of the cell cycle (Klumpp et al., 2017). More specifically, the TRPM8-mediated Ca^{2+} entry, through the activation of BK channels, may increase the CaMKII activity, which in turn inhibits the Cdc2 subunit of the mitosis-promoting factor likely through the inhibitory phosphorylation of the Cdc25C phosphatase (Klumpp et al., 2017). Finally, TRPM8 channel might also modulate proliferation by dynamically control glioma resting potentials levels, which are key regulator of cell cycle. TRPM8 agonists have been shown to increase the Kir4.1 mediated membrane conductances of glioma cells (Ratto et al., 2020). Kir4.1 is an inward rectifier K^+ channel, with an altered pattern of expression in glioma. In astrocytes, it is responsible for high potassium conductance and hyperpolarized membrane potential (Olsen and Sontheimer, 2008). Overexpression of this channel in glioma cell lines D54MG reduces cell proliferation (Higashimori and Sontheimer, 2007). Thus, TRPM8 channel by regulating K^+ resting conductances of glioma cells may exert a regulation of cell cycle transitions. Moreover, TRPM8 has also been found to be a contributor to the genotoxic stress response of GBM upon treatment with ionizing radiation, restoring G_1/S transition and S phase progression to levels of unirradiated cells (Klumpp et al., 2017). Interestingly, it has been found that ionizing radiation stimulated TRPM8 availability both *in vitro* and *in vivo* and that TRPM8 played a role in the re-entry in mitosis and cell division upon radiation-induced G_2/M arrest, since its knockdown resulted in an impaired DNA repair and a decreased survival of irradiated cells (Klumpp et al., 2017). This, combined with the slowdown of apoptosis in irradiated GBM cells, may explain the enhanced radioresistance acquired by GBM cells overexpressing TRPM8, thus stressing that the key interest of targeting TRPM8 alone or in combination with radiotherapy for future treatments of GBM.

Vanilloid TRPs

Some TRP members of the vanilloid family have been related to gliomagenesis and progression. More specifically, TRPV1 and TRPV2 have revealed a protective role in glioma cells by regulating cell proliferation and survival, stem cell differentiation and sensitivity to drugs, whereas TRPV4 was found to increase cancer cell invasiveness.

The anti-tumorigenic functional role of TRPV1 in gliomas, suggested by its marked downregulation or loss in patients with the shortest overall survival, has been investigated and several findings highlighted a role of TRPV1 in the induction of apoptotic cell death signaling in gliomas (Amantini et al., 2007; Stock et al., 2012). Upon exposure to low doses of the TRPV1 specific agonist capsaicin (CPS), the TRPV1-Ca^{2+} may sustain apoptosis in gliomas through the selective activation of p38 MAPK, but not ERK MAPK (Amantini et al., 2007). More in detail, it has been shown that CPS-mediated TRPV1 activation leads to reduced cell viability, DNA fragmentation, externalization of phosphatidylserine on the outer layer of the plasma membrane, mitochondrial transmembrane potential dissipation, and caspase 3 activation (Amantini et al., 2007). Moreover, TRPV1 translation in GBM was found to be sensitive to interferon-gamma (INF-γ) and to the well-known autophagic inducer rapamycin (Rap), suggesting a link between TRPV1 channel and autophagy often related to pro-survival in tumors including GBM (Galluzzi et al., 2015) but also in migration (Coly et al., 2017). This biological effect might be achieved by the TRPV1-mediated induction of apoptosis previously reported in GBM cells (Amantini et al., 2007).

One of the mechanisms through which the brain, especially in the juvenile phase, can protect itself against high-grade astrocytoma (HGAs) involves the activation of TRPV1 by neural precursor cells (NPCs), known to show extensive tropism for brain tumors (Mayor et al., 2001). Interestingly, NPCs accumulate at HGA especially in the context of the juvenile brain, exhibiting a high proliferative activity in the stem cell niche (Walzlein et al., 2008), and can release tumor-suppressive factors, such as endovanilloids able to activate TRPV1 expressed by HGA cells (Stock et al., 2012). The activation of the latter would trigger astrocytoma cell death through the ER pathway in a transcription factor-3 (ATF3)-dependent manner, thus reducing glioma expansion mostly in young brain (Stock et al., 2012). In light of these data, the inverse correlation between TRPV1 expression and glioma grade from I to III and the reduced or lost TRPV1 expression found in GBM patients is most likely a mechanism by which tumor cells may evade anti-proliferative and pro-apoptotic signals. This hypothesis is also supported by the finding that TRPV1 is also downregulated in GSCs (Stock et al., 2012), whose resistance to cytotoxic therapies and to pro-apoptotic signals is accepted (Bao et al., 2006a). Furthermore, the induction of GSCs differentiation was accompanied by TRPV1$_{\nu3}$ expression at a similar level than found in low-grade glioma, thus confirming a protective role of this channel against aggressiveness (Nabissi et al., 2016).

TRPV2 exerts its anti-tumorigenic function on gliomas through the regulation of several signaling pathways involved in cell proliferation and survival, stem cell differentiation and sensitivity to drugs. Physiologically, the triggering of TRPV2 by agonists/activators such as growth factors, hormones and cannabinoids led to TRPV2 translocation from the endosome to the plasma membrane, where it mediates several pathways associated with cell proliferation and cell death (Liberati et al., 2014). Thus, loss or alterations of TRPV2 expression in cancer cells results in an impairment of these processes, as shown in prostate tumor-derived endothelial cells (Bernardini et al., 2019) and gliomas (Liberati et al., 2014). In gliomas, it has been shown that TRPV2 reduced cell proliferation and increased cell sensitivity to Fas-induced apoptosis in an ERK-dependent manner (Nabissi et al., 2010). Consistently, enhanced cell growth and rescuing from apoptotic cell death was observed when TRPV2 was silencing in U87MG GBM cells. In contrast, TRPV2 upregulation in MZC primary glioma cells, by inducing Fas overexpression led to reduced viability and increased spontaneous as well as Fas-induced apoptosis (Nabissi et al., 2010). Similar findings were also described in GSCs, whose proliferation appeared strongly impaired by TRPV2 pharmacological inhibition or knocking down (Morelli et al., 2012). In GSCs, TRPV2 acts also on differentiation (Morelli et al., 2012; Nabissi et al., 2015). More specifically, TRPV2 overexpression was associated with glial fibrillary acidic protein (GFAP) and β_{III}-tubulin increased expression, thus promoting a glial phenotype differentiation while inhibiting GSCs proliferation both *in vitro* and *in vivo*. In agreement, TRPV2 silencing or inhibition during differentiation impaired differentiation and reduced GFAP and β_{III}-tubulin expression (Morelli et al., 2012). Moreover, TRPV2 activation through cannabidiol (CBD) was found to trigger GSCs differentiation activating the autophagic process, in addition to inhibiting GSCs proliferation and clonogenic capability (Nabissi et al., 2015). More specifically, it has been observed that CBD, through the TRPV2-mediated activation of the PI3K/AKT pathway, upregulated the expression of acute myeloid leukemia (Aml-1) transcription factors, known for their pivotal role in GBM proliferation and differentiation. Furthermore, it has also been shown that the spliced variant Aml-1 a, upregulated during GSCs differentiation, directly influenced the expression of TRPV2 by binding its gene promoter (Nabissi et al., 2015), thus establishing a positive feedback circuit, which on the whole caused glial differentiation.

Conversely to TRPV1 and TRPV2, TRPV4 has revealed a pivotal role in promoting glioma progression (Ou-yang et al., 2018). In particular, the tumorigenic potential of TRPV4 comes from its critical involvement in glioma cell migration and invasion. Indeed, it has been demonstrated that TRPV4-mediated Ca^{2+} influx upon stimulation with the selective agonist GSK1016790 A, is able to promote cell migration of glioma cells (Ou-yang et al., 2018), a similar mechanism previously reported in breast cancer (Lee et al., 2017). It was established that TRPV4 effects on cell migration are relayed by phosphorylation of AKT (P-AKT) and activation of Rac1 (Ou-yang et al., 2018), a member of the Rho GTPases family known for its central role in cytoskeleton remodeling, cell motility and cell adhesion as well as for its involvement in the enhanced migration of several tumor types including GBM, colon, colorectal and ovarian cancer (Guo et al., 2015; Guéguinou et al., 2016; Qin et al., 2017; Zhou et al., 2018). Accordingly, TRPV4 blockade, induced by the specific TRPV4 inhibitor HC-067047, was found to decrease motility and invasiveness of U87 glioma cells through a P-AKT and Rac1 signaling pathway (Ou-yang et al., 2018).

Mucolipin TRPs

The two TRP members of mucolipin subfamily have revealed opposite effects on glioma carcinogenesis.

TRPML1 showed a protective role against glioma progression. Indeed, it has been shown that TRPML1 activation by its specific agonist MK6-83 reduced T98 and U251 cell line viability and increased caspase 3-dependent apoptosis. Accordingly, TRPML1 silencing or pharmacological inhibition restored cell viability suppressing the Ca^{2+} influx responsible for apoptosis induction. Furthermore, TRPML1 may also mediate the autophagic cell death pathway, upon cell treatment with the ROS inducer carbonyl cyanide *m*-chlorophenylhydrazone (CCCP) (Morelli et al., 2019). Indeed, high ROS levels may trigger a TRPML1-mediated lysosomal Ca^{2+} release and the subsequent enhancement of autophagy (Zhang et al., 2016b). Accordingly, TRPML1 silencing or inhibition by sphingomyelin pre-treatment reverted CCCP effects (Morelli et al., 2019). In this context, it has also been demonstrated that TRPML1, through a large intraluminal loop between its first and second transmembrane domains, may interact with chaperone-mediated autophagy-related proteins such as the heat shock proteins Hsc70, and Hsp40 (Venugopal et al., 2009). Therefore, TRPML1 may exert its cytotoxic effects through two different pathways, e.g., (i) it can act as a ROS sensor on the lysosomal membrane and attenuate oxidative cell stress through an autophagy-dependent negative-feedback mechanism (Zhang et al., 2016a; Morelli et al., 2019) or (ii) it may trigger Ca^{2+} release but no ROS production upon direct activation by its specific agonist, thus inducing apoptosis (Morelli et al., 2019). Moreover, the important role of TRPML1 in controlling intracellular Ca^{2+} homeostasis has been further corroborated by the recent finding of a functional localization of TRPML1 at the so-called "mitochondria-lysosome contact sites" where it mediates a calcium flux from lysosomes to mitochondria adjuvanted by VDAC and MCU on the outer and inner mitochondrial membranes, respectively (Peng et al., 2020). Consequently, TRPML1 functions go beyond the regulation of lysosomal dynamics and function and, through the control of mitochondrial Ca^{2+} dynamics, can affect other Ca^{2+}-dependent mitochondrial functions, including oxidative phosphorylation, motility, and ROS signaling (Peng et al., 2020).

Conversely to TRPML1, the other member of the mucolipin family, TRPML2, has revealed a pro-tumorigenic function in glioma progression. Indeed, it has been shown that TRPML2 enhanced glioma cell survival and proliferation (Morelli et al., 2016). More in detail, TRPML2 suppression leads to impaired cell cycle, reduced cell viability and decreased proliferation (Morelli et al., 2016). In addition, its knocking-down was found to induce apoptosis by increasing DNA damage, Ser139 H2AX phosphorylation and caspase-3 activation (Morelli et al., 2016). TRPML2 effects on tumor progression are probably mediated by PI3K/AKT and ERK1/2 pathways, since these pathways remained inactivated in TRPML2-silenced cells (Morelli et al., 2016). Thus, TRPML2 might also be an interesting therapeutic target to control GBM cell survival and proliferation.

THERAPEUTIC TARGETING

Considering the altered expression and the great contribution given by TRP channels to the establishment and progression of glioma, they may be considered very promising new therapeutic molecular targets against which novel drug compounds must be developed. One of the main advantages provided by most TRPs is their accessibility from the extracellular side, which makes them efficient targetable sites via administration of specific TRPs inhibitors or blockers when these channels are overexpressed in high-grade glioma. For instance, some of the TRPC channels by interfering with cytokinesis pathways would be promising targets for the development of drugs able to interfere with the almost unrestrained growth of gliomas, making tumors more susceptible to surgical removal or focal radiotherapy. Moreover, the low specificity of some TRPC modulators might allow to achieve a higher antitumor effect, through the simultaneous triggering of more than one channel. The progressive understanding of the molecular mechanism underlying TRPC function in glioma has also provided opportunities and arguments in favor of small molecule targeted therapies. Through studies concerning TRPC1 and its specific pharmacological inhibition, the key option by inhibiting SPK or PI3K inhibitors is once again here confirmed to attempt controlling GBM growth and invasiveness. Among TRPC channels, great potential as a promising new candidate for GBM treatment comes from TRPC6. Among TRP, TRPC6 is to date the only one being implicated in GBM angiogenesis suggesting that specific TRPC6 inhibitors could simultaneously target both cancer progression and vascularization, thereby improving the efficacy of standard (radio-chemotherapy) options. The barely detectable TRPC6 expression in normal glial cells should limit the potential side effects on normal glial cells. But a possible impact of TRPC6 blockade on neurons must be considered in regards to the central role of TRPC6 in neuronal functions (Tai et al., 2008; Zhou et al., 2008; Kim et al., 2017). A possible strategy to overcome this problem might be the use of viral vectors as a drug delivery system toward glioma cells since adenovirus may target glioma cells more efficiently than neurons (Ding et al., 2010).

As recurrence is due to migration and invasion (and resistance to treatment), pharmacological inhibition of TRPV4 might represent a potential new therapeutic approach in GBM treatment to control migratory and invasive capabilities of GBM cells (Ou-yang et al., 2018). One of the mechanisms through which tumor cells are able to sustain a prolonged survival is by the inhibition of apoptotic pathways (Thompson, 1995). In this context, TRPA1 has been recently proposed as a new potential therapeutic target in GBM treatment. Indeed, TRPA1 is a ROS-sensitive cation channel and can subsequently be activated by hypoxia-induced oxidative stress (Naziroğlu, 2012; Takahashi et al., 2018). It has been shown that TRPA1 activation following cobalt chloride ($CoCl_2$) treatment with the aim to mimic hypoxia, may increase apoptosis, inflammation and oxidative effects on DBTRG cells (Deveci et al., 2019). More specifically, TRPA1-mediated Ca^{2+} entry was associated with an enhancement of ROS production and mitochondrial membrane depolarization (JC-1). Moreover, TRPA1 activation leads to increased levels of Annexin V, cytokines IL-1β and IL-18, and caspase 3 and 9 and decreased levels of thiol cycle antioxidants (GSH and GSH-Px) (Deveci et al., 2019). These effects were shown attenuated by α-lipoic acid (ALA) treatment, a physiological source of energy for cells which may exert both anti- and pro-oxidant functions (Moini et al., 2002). In glioma cells under hypoxia, ALA likely acts as an antioxidant agent, upregulating GSH and GSH-Px and down-regulating mitochondrial ROS production, thus blocking TRPA1-mediated induction of apoptotic cell death (Deveci et al., 2019). This suggests that targeting and activating TRPA1 or targeting TRPV1 in glioma exhibiting such expression, can restore apoptotic signaling and might provide new insights for the development of alternative therapies against glioma progression.

Besides being potential anti-tumor targets, TRP channels should play a role as "drug carriers" in cancer therapy, facilitating *via* the central pore chemotherapy drug uptake thus improving the efficacy of cancer therapies. For instance, TRPV2 activation by CBD can sensitize GBM cells to chemotherapeutic agents currently used, e.g., TMZ, carmustine (BCNU) and doxorubicin (DOXO) (Nabissi et al., 2013, 2015). The CBD-induced TRPV2 activation was found to increase GSCs sensitivity to cytotoxic effects of alkylating agents like BCNU favoring drug uptake (Nabissi et al., 2013), in synergy with the Ca^{2+}-dependent triggering of apoptotic cell death, a mechanism not found in normal astrocytes (Nabissi et al., 2015). Specifically, by using the natural red fluorescent DOXO, it has been demonstrated that TRPV2 overexpression in MZC glioma cells markedly increased DOXO uptake in a Ca^{2+}-dependent manner, since Ca^{2+} chelation by EGTA completely inhibited the CBD-induced TRPV2-mediated increase of DOXO-positive cells (Nabissi et al., 2013). Similar findings were also observed in hepatocellular carcinoma in which TRPV2 activation by CBD or 2-APB (Aminoethoxydiphenyl borate) was found to improve DOXO permeation into tumor cells, thus corroborating an intriguing role of TRPV2 in increasing tumor cell sensitivity to chemotherapy drugs (Neumann-Raizel et al., 2019). Taking into account other evidence on the role of TRP channels as "drug carriers" thanks to the permeation of chemotherapy agents into the cell through their pore domain (Santoni and Farfariello, 2011), it is reasonable to speculate that the activation of TRPV2 channel may cause a conformational change in the pore helix structure, which allow for intracellular non-specific chemotherapy uptake (Nabissi et al., 2013), opening the route for combinatorial co-administration of TRPV2 specific agonist CBD and lower chemotherapeutic doses to overcome the high resistance of GBM and GSCs to chemotherapeutic agents. In this context, recent developments on the role of the so-called "pore turret," i.e., the region of the extracellular ring that connects the S5 helix to the pore helix, in controlling the upper gate of some TRP channels including TRPV2 (Dosey et al., 2019) have provided new insights into the role of TRPV2 as a drug target to reduce GBM chemoresistance. Indeed, the well-defined pore turret, in addition to allowing the coupling between the lower gate and the upper gate in response to intracellular stimuli stabilizing a fully open unliganded channel, represents a possible and interesting binding site for extracellular modulators through which it may affect channel activity allowing the passage through the plasma membrane of partially hydrophilic molecules which otherwise could not enter the cell (Dosey et al., 2019).

With a view to looking ahead, some data indicate that TRP channels may constitute targets of gene therapy. It has been recently shown that TRPM2 can promote cell death (Ertilav et al., 2019). Therefore, TRPM2 might represent a good candidate for gene therapy to be used for instance in combination with γ-radiation and/or chemotherapeutic agents to improve the effectiveness of GBM treatments. Preliminary observations indicate that Selenium (Se) tested on GBM cells resistant to Docetaxel (DTX) may improve the apoptotic efficacy of DTX through the activation of TRPM2 by oxidative stress (Ertilav et al., 2019). The cytotoxic effect of DTX likely comes from the formation of excessive mitochondrial ROS and Ca^{2+} influx into the cells which causes DNA damage by triggering hyperactivation of the DNA nick sensor PARP, thus leading to NAD+ and ATP depletion and subsequent apoptotic cell death (Ertilav et al., 2019). In this case, Se, in particular, stimulated oxidative stress production in the mitochondria, which in turn activated a TRPM2-mediated Ca^{2+} influx, thus supporting and enhancing the same Ca^{2+}-dependent apoptotic pathway induced by DTX and other chemotherapeutic agents, as seen also in other tumor types (Hazane-Puch et al., 2016; Çetin et al., 2017). Overall the combination and synergistic activity of Se and DTX in GBM expressing TRPM2 might offer a new option for adjuvant chemotherapy as treatment of GBM.

FUTURE PERSPECTIVES

Increasing understanding of the signaling pathways involved in tumorigenesis has made it possible to identify a wide range of molecular targets involved in self-renewal and proliferation, angiogenesis but also in invasion of GBM cells. A number of therapeutic strategies have therefore been developed during the last decade and few of them have proven to be effective, even though anti-angiogenic treatments appear to be able to provide a 6 months delay for GBM patients before recurrence. It is, therefore, necessary to identify other therapeutic targets that can be combined with anti-angiogenic, cytotoxic, DNA repair inhibitors and/or immunotherapy strategies. In this context, targeting the activity of factors or components expressed by glioma cells themselves and by other cell types of the micro-environment would also be promising. It has also to be considered that main RNAseq and/or transcriptomic databases were constituted by means of the glioma tumor bulk composed of the different populations of GBM cells and other constituents such as endothelial cells, pericytes, reactive astrocytes, macrophages (M1 and/or M2), microglial, neurons, and potentially lymphocytes, depending on the level of heterogeneity GBM subgroup. New potential family targets, expressed at the plasma membrane and involved in survival, GSC differentiation, angiogenesis and invasion, constitute a choice option. TRP channels not systematically ubiquitously expressed, potentially playing pleiotropic mechanisms and being overexpressed in pathologic situations such as hypoxia in glioma cells deserve to be more explored, especially since they could be also expressed by other cell types belonging to the tumor micro-environment.

For instance, a direct involvement of TRP channels in vascular endothelial growth factor (VEGF) signaling pathways affecting brain neovascularization and tumor growth it has been proven. GCSs positive for CD133 (human prominin-1/AC 133) not only are capable of self-renewal and proliferation, but also possess the capability to secrete high levels of VEGF (Bao et al., 2006b; Yao et al., 2008), known to play a crucial role in endothelial cell recruitment and angiogenesis of malignant human gliomas (Fischer et al., 2005; Bian et al., 2006). In GSCs isolated from U87 cell line the production of VEGF and the angiogenic CXCL8 (chemokine interleukin-8) by tumor cells appeared to be mediated by a G protein-coupled receptor named formylpeptide receptor (FPR) which, upon activation, induces directional migration, growth and angiogenic factors production through a Ca^{2+} mobilization. Although a direct involvement of TRPs in this Ca^{2+}-mediated mechanism has not been highlighted, a GCPR-TRP axis in many signaling pathways is nowadays well established (Veldhuis et al., 2015). Moreover, an interesting crosstalk between TRPM8, TRPV1 and the VEFG receptor (VEGFR) it has been recently characterized in uveal melanoma, suggesting a good potential for TRPM8 as a pharmacological target for blocking brain neovascularization and tumor growth (Walcher et al., 2018). Indeed, it has been demonstrated that in different cell types including corneal epithelial and endothelial cells (Lucius et al., 2016) and uveal melanoma cells (Walcher et al., 2018) the activation of TRPM8 inhibits the VEGF transactivation of TRPV1 and the consequent pro-tumorigenic effects mediated by the VEGFR. These findings further highlighted the central role played by TRPs interactions with other TRP channels, other channels families like that of BK channels, and the GCPRs, in affecting signaling pathways directly involved in carcinogenesis and brain tumor progression. Moreover, they strongly sustain the possible TRPs application in anti-angiogenic therapy.

However, to date, to the best of our knowledge TRPC6 is the only TRP channel directly implicated in GBM angiogenesis. TRPC6 has been found to play a key role in promoting GBM growth, angiogenesis and invasion under hypoxia through Notch1 (Chigurupati et al., 2010). TRPC6 knockdown or NFAT inhibition has been shown to reduce the number of branch points and thus impair the ability of the hypoxic U373MG to induce endothelial cell tube formation *in vitro*, suggesting a role of TRPC6 in the "vascular mimicry" played by glioma cells (Chigurupati et al., 2010).

Other TRPs among those previously described to have a function in gliomas, such as TRPM2, TRPM7, TRPV2, and TRPV4 have also been found in brain vasculature, thus suggesting a possible double function for these channels in affecting glioma progression (Hatano et al., 2013; Pires and Earley, 2017; Ouyang et al., 2018; Luo et al., 2019) and contributing to GBM angiogenesis. Regarding TRPA1 and TRPC3 not likely described in glioma, some studies highlighted their involvement in other brain vasculature diseases, exerting a protective role against ischemic damage, controlling vasodilation in brain endothelial cells (Sullivan et al., 2016; Pires and Earley, 2018). TRPC3, when overexpressed, would lead to an increase in the BBB permeability, leading to vasogenic edema formation (Ryu et al., 2013).

CONCLUSION

Taken together all these data suggest a key role of some TRP channels in high-grade glioma development and angiogenesis. The current activators or inhibitors directed against these channels should provide lead compounds and knowledge for future research in the design of drugs targeting simultaneously glioma cells and key components of the micro-environment such as abnormal tumoral vascularization.

AUTHOR CONTRIBUTIONS

DG and HC provided a rational of the study. GC performed an in-depth analysis of the roles of TRP channels in inducing glioma behavior and generated a preliminary draft. GC, HC, OC, and DG performed the literature searches and contributed to writing and editing of the content. All the authors contributed to the article and approved the submitted version.

REFERENCES

Alifieris, C., and Trafalis, D. T. (2015). Glioblastoma multiforme: pathogenesis and treatment. *Pharmacol. Ther.* 152, 63–82. doi: 10.1016/j.pharmthera.2015.05.005

Alptekin, M., Eroglu, S., Tutar, E., Sencan, S., Geyik, M. A., Ulasli, M., et al. (2015). Gene expressions of TRP channels in glioblastoma multiforme and relation with survival. *Tumor Biol.* 36, 9209–9213. doi: 10.1007/s13277-015-3577-x

Amantini, C., Mosca, M., Nabissi, M., Lucciarini, R., Caprodossi, S., Arcella, A., et al. (2007). Capsaicin-induced apoptosis of glioma cells is mediated by

TRPV1 vanilloid receptor and requires p38 MAPK activation. *J. Neurochem.* 102, 977–990. doi: 10.1111/j.1471-4159.2007.04582.x

Asuthkar, S., Velpula, K. K., Elustondo, P. A., and Demirkhanyan, L. (2015). TRPM8 channel as a novel molecular target in androgen- regulated prostate cancer cells. *Oncotarget* 6, 17221–17236.

Audic, Y., and Hartley, R. S. (2004). Post-transcriptional regulation in cancer. *Biol. Cell* 96, 479–498. doi: 10.1016/j.biolcel.2004.05.002

Bao, S., Wu, Q., Mclendon, R. E., Hao, Y., Shi, Q., Hjelmeland, A. B., et al. (2006a). Glioma stem cells promote radioresistance by preferential activation of the DNA damage response. *Nature* 444, 756–760. doi: 10.1038/nature05236

Bao, S., Wu, Q., Sathornsumetee, S., Hao, Y., Li, Z., Hjelmeland, A. B., et al. (2006b). Stem cell-like glioma cells promote tumor angiogenesis through vascular endothelial growth factor. *Cancer Res.* 66, 7843–7848. doi: 10.1158/0008-5472.CAN-06-1010

Bernardini, M., Brossa, A., Chinigo, G., Grolez, G. P., Trimaglio, G., Allart, L., et al. (2019). Transient receptor potential channel expression signatures in tumor-derived endothelial cells: functional roles in prostate cancer angiogenesis. *Cancers* 11:956.

Bian, X. W., Jiang, X. F., Chen, J. H., Bai, J. S., Dai, C., Wang, Q. L., et al. (2006). Increased angiogenic capabilities of endothelial cells from microvessels of malignant human gliomas. *Int. Immunopharmacol.* 6, 90–99. doi: 10.1016/j.intimp.2005.08.004

Bidaux, G., Flourakis, M., Thebault, S., Zholos, A., Beck, B., Gkika, D., et al. (2007). Prostate cell differentiation status determines transient receptor potential melastatin member 8 channel subcellular localization and function. *J. Clin. Invest.* 117, 1647–1657. doi: 10.1172/JCI30168

Bidaux, G., Roudbaraki, M., Merle, C., Crépin, A., Delcourt, P., Slomianny, C., et al. (2005). Evidence for specific TRPM8 expression in human prostate secretory epithelial cells: functional androgen receptor requirement. *Endocr. Relat. Cancer* 12, 367–382. doi: 10.1677/erc.1.00969

Birchmeier, C., Birchmeier, W., Gherardi, E., and Vande Woude, G. F. (2003). Met, metastasis, motility and more. *Nat. Rev. Mol, Cell Biol.* 4, 915–925. doi: 10.1038/nrm1261

Bomben, V. C., and Sontheimer, H. (2010). Disruption of transient receptor potential canonical channel 1 causes incomplete cytokinesis and slows the growth of human malignant gliomas. *Glia* 58, 1145–1156. doi: 10.1038/jid.2014.371

Bomben, V. C., and Sontheimer, H. W. (2008). Inhibition of transient receptor potential canonical channels impairs cytokinesis in human malignant gliomas. *Cell Prolif.* 41, 98–121. doi: 10.1111/j.1365-2184.2007.00504.x

Bomben, V. C., Turner, K. L., Barclay, T. C., and Sontheimer, H. (2011). Transient receptor potential canonical channels are essential for chemotactic migration of human malignant gliomas. *J. Cell Physiol.* 226, 1879–1888. doi: 10.1161/CIRCULATIONAHA.110.956839

Bordey, A., and Sontheimer, H. (1998). Electrophysiological properties of human astrocytic tumor cells in situ: enigma of spiking glial cells. *J. Neurophysiol.* 79, 2782–2793. doi: 10.1152/jn.1998.79.5.2782

Çetin, E. S., Nazıroğlu, M., Çiğ, B., Övey, ŸS., and Aslan, P. (2017). Selenium potentiates the anticancer effect of cisplatin against oxidative stress and calcium ion signaling-induced intracellular toxicity in MCF-7 breast cancer cells: involvement of the TRPV1 channel. *J. Recept. Signal. Transduct. Res.* 37, 84–93. doi: 10.3109/10799893.2016.1160931

Chigurupati, S., Venkataraman, R., Barrera, D., Naganathan, A., Madan, M., Paul, L., et al. (2010). Receptor channel TRPC6 is a key mediator of notch-driven glioblastoma growth and invasiveness. *Cancer Res.* 6, 418–428. doi: 10.1158/0008-5472.CAN-09-2654

Choudhary, S., Xiao, T., Vergara, L. A., Srivastava, S., Nees, D., Piatigorsky, J., et al. (2005). Role of aldehyde dehydrogenase isozymes in the defense of rat lens and human lens epithelial cells against oxidative stress. *Invest. Ophthalmol. Vis. Sci.* 46, 259–267. doi: 10.1167/iovs.04-0120

Coly, P. M., Gandolfo, P., Castel, H., and Morin, F. (2017). The autophagy machinery: a new player in chemotactic cell migration. *Front. Neurosci.* 11:78. doi: 10.3389/fnins.2017.00078

Cuddapah, V. A., and Sontheimer, H. (2011). Ion channels and tranporters in cancer. 2. Ion channels and the control of cancer cell migration. *Am. J. Physiol. Cell Physiol.* 301, C541–C549. doi: 10.1152/ajpcell.00102.2011

Demuth, T., and Berens, M. E. (2004). Molecular mechanisms of glioma cell migration and invasion. *J. Neurooncol.* 70, 217–228.

Deveci, H. A., Akyuva, Y., Nur, G., and Nazıroğlu, M. (2019). Alpha lipoic acid attenuates hypoxia-induced apoptosis, inflammation and mitochondrial oxidative stress via inhibition of TRPA1 channel in human glioblastoma cell line. *Biomed. Pharmacother.* 111, 292–304. doi: 10.1016/j.biopha.2018.12.077

Ding, X., He, Z., Zhou, K., Cheng, J., Yao, H., Lu, D., et al. (2010). Essential role of TRPC6 channels in G2/M phase transition and development of human glioma. *J. Natl. Cancer Inst.* 102, 1052–1068. doi: 10.1093/jnci/djq217

Doñate-Macián, P., Gómez, A., Dégano, I. R., and Perálvarez-Marín, A. (2018). A TRPV2 interactome-based signature for prognosis in glioblastoma patients. *Oncotarget* 9, 18400–18409. doi: 10.18632/oncotarget.24843

Dosey, T. L., Wang, Z., Fan, G., Zhang, Z., Serysheva, I. I., Chiu, W., et al. (2019). Structures of TRPV2 in distinct conformations provide insight into role of the pore turret. *Nat. Struct. Mol. Biol.* 26, 40–49. doi: 10.1038/s41594-018-0168-8. Structures

Edalat, L., Stegen, B., Klumpp, L., Haehl, E., Schilbach, K., Lukowski, R., et al. (2016). BK K + channel blockade inhibits radiation-induced migration/brain infiltration of glioblastoma cells. *Oncotarget* 7, 14259–14278.

Ertilav, K., Nazıroğlu, M., Ataizi, Z. S., and Braidy, N. (2019). Selenium enhances the apoptotic efficacy of docetaxel through activation of TRPM2 channel in DBTRG glioblastoma cells. *Neurotox. Res.* 35, 797–808. doi: 10.1007/s12640-019-0009-5

Fiorio Pla, A., and Gkika, D. (2013). Emerging role of TRP channels in cell migration: from tumor vascularization to metastasis. *Front. Physiol.* 4:311. doi: 10.3389/fphys.2013.00311

Fischer, I., Gagner, J. P., Law, M., Newcomb, E. W., and Zagzag, D. (2005). Angiogenesis in gliomas: biology and molecular pathophysiology. *Brain Pathol.* 15, 297–310. doi: 10.1111/j.1750-3639.2005.tb00115.x

Flynn, J. R., Wang, L., Gillespie, D. L., Stoddard, G. J., Reid, J. K., Owens, J., et al. (2008).). Hypoxia-regulated protein expression, patient characteristics, and preoperative imaging as predictors of survival in adults with glioblastoma multiforme. *Cancer* 113, 1032–1042.

Galluzzi, L., Pietrocola, F., Bravo-San Pedro, J. M., Amaravadi, R. K., Baehrecke, E. H., Cecconi, F., et al. (2015). Autophagy in malignant transformation and cancer progression. *EMBO J.* 34, 856–880. doi: 10.15252/embj.201490784

Gebauer, F., and Hentze, M. W. (2004). Molecular mechanisms of translational control. *Nat. Rev. Mol. Cell Biol.* 5, 827–835. doi: 10.1038/nrm1488

Gees, M., Colsoul, B., and Nilius, B. (2010). The role of transient receptor potential cation channels in Ca2+ signaling. *Cold Spring Harbor Perspect. Biol.* 2, 1–32. doi: 10.1101/cshperspect.a003962

Genova, T., Grolez, G. P., Camillo, C., Bernardini, M., Bokhobza, A., Richard, E., et al. (2017). TRPM8 inhibits endothelial cell migration via a nonchannel function by trapping the small GTPase Rap1. *J. Cell Biol.* 216, 2107–2130. doi: 10.1083/jcb.201506024

Giese, A., Bjerkvig, R., Berens, M. E., and Westphal, M. (2003). Cost of migration: invasion of malignant gliomas and implications for treatment. *J. Clin. Oncol.* 21, 1624–1636. doi: 10.1200/JCO.2003.05.063

Gkika, D., Flourakis, M., Lemonnier, L., and Prevarskaya, N. (2010). PSA reduces prostate cancer cell motility by stimulating TRPM8 activity and plasma membrane expression. *Oncogene* 29, 4611–4616. doi: 10.1038/onc.2010.210

Gkika, D., Lemonnier, L., Shapovalov, G., Gordienko, D., Poux, C., Bernardini, M., et al. (2015). TRP channel-associated factors are a novel protein family that regulates TRPM8 trafficking and activity. *J. Cell Biol.* 208, 89–107. doi: 10.1083/jcb.201402076

Gkika, D., Lolignier, S., Grolez, G. P., Bavencoffe, A., Shapovalov, G., Gordienko, D., et al. (2020). Testosterone-androgen receptor: the steroid link inhibiting TRPM8-mediated cold sensitivity. *FASEB J.* 34, 7483–7499. doi: 10.1096/fj.201902270R

Gkika, D., and Prevarskaya, N. (2009). Molecular mechanisms of TRP regulation in tumor growth and metastasis. *Biochim. Biophys. Acta* 1793, 953–958. doi: 10.1016/j.bbamcr.2008.11.010

Grolez, G. P., Gordiendko, D. V., Clarisse, M., Hammadi, M., Desruelles, E., Fromont, G., et al. (2019a). TRPM8-androgen receptor association within lipid rafts promotes prostate cancer cell migration. *Cell Death Dis.* 10:652. doi: 10.1038/s41419-019-1891-8

Grolez, G. P., Hammadi, M., Barras, A., Gordienko, D., Slomianny, C., Völkel, P., et al. (2019b). Encapsulation of a TRPM8 Agonist, WS12, in lipid nanocapsules potentiates PC3 prostate cancer cell migration inhibition through channel activation. *Sci. Rep.* 9, 1–15. doi: 10.1038/s41598-019-44452-4

Guéguinou, M., Harnois, T., Crottes, D., Uguen, A., Deliot, N., Gambade, A., et al. (2016). SK3/TRPC1/Orai1 complex regulates SOCE-dependent colon cancer cell migration: a novel opportunity to modulate anti- EGFR mAb action by the alkyl-lipid Ohmline. *Oncotarget* 7, 36168–36184. doi: 10.18632/oncotarget.8786

Guo, Y., Kenney, S. R., Muller, C. Y., Adams, S., Rutledge, T., Romero, E., et al. (2015). R-ketorolac targets Cdc42 and Rac1 and alters ovarian cancer cell behaviors critical for invasion and metastasis. *Mol. Cancer Ther.* 14, 2215–2227. doi: 10.1158/1535-7163.MCT-15-0419

Hatano, N., Suzuki, H., Itoh, Y., and Muraki, K. (2013). TRPV4 partially participates in proliferation of human brain capillary endothelial cells. *Life Sci.* 92, 317–324. doi: 10.1016/j.lfs.2013.01.002

Hazane-Puch, F., Arnaud, J., Trocmé, C., Faure, P., Laporte, F., and Champelovier, P. (2016). Sodium selenite decreased HDAC activity, cell proliferation and induced apoptosis in three human glioblastoma cells. *Anticancer Agents Med. Chem.* 16, 490–500.

Higashimori, H., and Sontheimer, H. (2007). Role of Kir4.1 channels in growth control of glia. *Glia* 55, 1668–1679. doi: 10.1002/glia.20574

Hinnebusch, A. G., Ivanov, I. P., and Sonenberg, N. (2016). Translational control by 5′-untranslated regions of eukaryotic mRNAs. *Science* 352, 1413–1416. doi: 10.1126/science.aad9868

Ishii, M., Oyama, A., Hagiwara, T., Miyazaki, A., Mori, Y., Kiuchi, Y., et al. (2007). Facilitation of H2O2 -induced A172 human glioblastoma cell death by insertion of oxidative stress-sensitive TRPM2 channels. *Anticancer Res.* 27, 3987–3992.

Karsy, M., Gelbman, M., Shah, P., Balumbu, O., Moy, F., and Arslan, E. (2012). Established and emerging variants of glioblastoma multiforme: review of morphological and molecular features. *Folia Neuropathol.* 50, 301–321. doi: 10.5114/fn.2012.32361

Kim, J. E., Park, J. Y., and Kang, T. C. (2017). TRPC6-mediated ERK1/2 activation regulates neuronal excitability via subcellular Kv4.3 localization in the rat hippocampus. *Front. Cell. Neurosci.* 11:413. doi: 10.3389/fncel.2017.00413

Klumpp, D., Frank, S. C., Klumpp, L., Sezgin, E. C., Eckert, M., Edalat, L., et al. (2017). TRPM8 is required for survival and radioresistance of glioblastoma cells. *Oncotarget* 8, 95896–95913. doi: 10.18632/oncotarget.21436

Laterra, J., Rosen, E., Nam, M., Ranganathan, S., Fielding, K., and Johnston, P. (1997). Scatter Factor/Hepatocyte growth factor expression enhances human glioblastoma tumorigenicity and growth. *Biochem. Biophys. Res. Commun.* 235, 743–747.

Lee, W. H., Choong, L. Y., Jin, T. H., Mon, N. N., Chong, S., Liew, C. S., et al. (2017). TRPV4 plays a role in breast cancer cell migration via Ca2+-dependent activation of AKT and downregulation of E-cadherin cell cortex protein. *Oncogenesis* 6:e338. doi: 10.1038/oncsis.2017.39

Lepannetier, S., Zanou, N., Yerna, X., Emeriau, N., Dufour, I., Masquelier, J., et al. (2016). Sphingosine-1-phosphate-activated TRPC1 channel controls chemotaxis of glioblastoma cells. *Cell Calcium* 60, 373–383. doi: 10.1016/j.ceca.2016.09.002

Li, H. (2017). "TRP channel classification," in *Transient Receptor Potential Canonical Channels and Brain Diseases Advances in Experimental Medicine and Biology*, ed. Y. Wang (Dordrecht: Springer Netherlands), 1–8. doi: 10.1007/978-94-024-1088-4_1

Liberati, S., Morelli, M. B., Amantini, C., Santoni, M., Nabissi, M., Cardinali, C., et al. (2014). Advances in transient receptor potential vanilloid-2 channel expression and function in tumor growth and progression. *Curr. Protein Pept. Sci.* 15, 732–737.

Liu, C., Chang, C., Hsueh, K., Su, H., and Chiou, T. (2018). Migration/Invasion of malignant gliomas and implications for therapeutic treatment. *Int. J. Mol. Sci.* 19:1115. doi: 10.3390/ijms19041115

Liu, J., Liu, X. U., Liu, Y., Sun, Y. N., Li, S., and Li, C. M. (2016). MicroRNA 28-5p regulates ATP-binding cassette transporter A1 via inhibiting extracellular signal-regulated kinase 2. *Mol. Med. Rep.* 13, 433–440. doi: 10.3892/mmr.2015.4563

Liu, M., Inoue, K., Leng, T., Guo, S., and Xiong, Z. (2014). TRPM7 channels regulate glioma stem cell through STAT3 and Notch signaling pathways. *Cell. Signal.* 26, 2773–2781. doi: 10.1016/j.cellsig.2014.08.020

Louis, D. N., Ohgaki, H., Wiestler, O. D., Cavenee, W. K., Burger, P. C., Jouvet, A., et al. (2007). The 2007 WHO classification of tumours of the central nervous system. *Acta Neuropathol.* 114, 97–109. doi: 10.1007/s00401-007-0243-4

Louis, D. N., Perry, A., Reifenberger, G., von Deimling, A., Figarella-Branger, D., Cavenee, W. K., et al. (2016). The 2016 World Health Organization classification of tumors of the central nervous system: a summary. *Acta Neuropathol.* 131, 803–820. doi: 10.1007/s00401-016-1545-1

Lucius, A., Khajavi, N., Reinach, P. S., Köhrle, J., Dhandapani, P., Huimann, P., et al. (2016). 3-Iodothyronamine increases transient receptor potential melastatin channel 8 (TRPM8) activity in immortalized human corneal epithelial cells. *Cell. Signal.* 28, 136–147. doi: 10.1016/j.cellsig.2015.12.005

Luo, H., Rossi, E., Saubamea, B., Chasseigneaux, S., Cochois, V., Choublier, N., et al. (2019). Cannabidiol increases proliferation, migration, tubulogenesis, and integrity of human brain endothelial cells through TRPV2 activation. *Mol. Pharm.* 16, 1312–1326. doi: 10.1021/acs.molpharmaceut.8b01252

Ma, I., and Allan, A. L. (2011). the role of human aldehyde dehydrogenase in normal and cancer stem cells. *Stem Cell Rev. Rep.* 7, 292–306. doi: 10.1007/s12015-010-9208-4

Mayor, U., Johnson, C. M., Daggett, V., Brown, A., Nikolai, G., Bower, K. A., et al. (2001). Neural stem cells display extensive tropism for pathology in adult brain: evidence from intracranial gliomas. *PNAS* 97, 12846–12851.

Mcferrin, M. B., and Sontheimer, H. (2006). A role for ion channels in glioma cell invasion. *Neuron Glia Biol.* 2, 39–49.

Miller, C. R., and Perry, A. (2007). Glioblastoma. *Arch. Pathol. Lab. Med.* 131, 397–406.

Moini, H., Packer, L., and Saris, N. E. L. (2002). Antioxidant and prooxidant activities of α-lipoic acid and dihydrolipoic acid. *Toxicol. Appl. Pharmacol.* 182, 84–90. doi: 10.1006/taap.2002.9437

Molenaar, R. J. (2011). Ion channels in glioblastoma. *ISRN Neurol.* 2011, 1–7. doi: 10.5402/2011/590249

Mollinedo, F., and Gajate, C. (2015). Advances in biological regulation lipid rafts as major platforms for signaling regulation in cancer. *Adv. Biol. Regul.* 57, 130–146. doi: 10.1016/j.jbior.2014.10.003

Morelli, M. B., Amantini, C., Tomassoni, D., Nabissi, M., Arcella, A., and Santoni, G. (2019). Transient receptor potential mucolipin-1 channels in glioblastoma: role in patient's survival. *Cancers* 11:525. doi: 10.3390/cancers11040525

Morelli, M. B., Nabissi, M., Amantini, C., Farfariello, V., Ricci-Vitiani, L., Di Martino, S., et al. (2012). The transient receptor potential vanilloid-2 cation channel impairs glioblastoma stem-like cell proliferation and promotes differentiation. *Int. J. Cancer* 131, 1067–1077. doi: 10.1002/ijc.27588

Morelli, M. B., Nabissi, M., Amantini, C., Tomassoni, D., Rossi, F., Cardinali, C., et al. (2016). Overexpression of transient receptor potential mucolipin-2 ion channels in gliomas: role in tumor growth and progression. *Oncotarget* 7, 43654–43668. doi: 10.18632/oncotarget.9661

Nabissi, M., Morelli, M. B., Amantini, C., Farfariello, V., Ricci-Vitiani, L., Caprodossi, S., et al. (2010). TRPV2 channel negatively controls glioma cell proliferation and resistance to Fas-induced apoptosis in ERK-dependent manner. *Carcinogenesis* 31, 794–803. doi: 10.1093/carcin/bgq019

Nabissi, M., Morelli, M. B., Amantini, C., Liberati, S., Santoni, M., Ricci-Vitiani, L., et al. (2015). Cannabidiol stimulates AML-1a-dependent glial differentiation and inhibits glioma stem-like cells proliferation by inducing autophagy in a TRPV2-dependent manner. *Int. J. Cancer* 137, 1855–1869. doi: 10.1002/ijc.29573

Nabissi, M., Morelli, M. B., Arcella, A., Cardinali, C., Santoni, M., Bernardini, G., et al. (2016). Post-transcriptional regulation of 5'-untranslated regions of human transient receptor potential vanilloid type-1 (TRPV-1) channels: role in the survival of glioma patients. *Oncotarget* 7, 81541–81554. doi: 10.18632/oncotarget.13132

Nabissi, M., Morelli, M. B., Santoni, M., and Santoni, G. (2013). Triggering of the TRPV2 channel by cannabidiol sensitizes glioblastoma cells to cytotoxic chemotherapeutic agents. *Carcinogenesis* 34, 48–57. doi: 10.1093/carcin/bgs328

Naziroğlu, M., and Lückhoff, A. (2008). Effects of antioxidants on calcium influx through TRPM2 channels in transfected cells activated by hydrogen peroxide ☆. *J. Neurol. Sci.* 270, 152–158. doi: 10.1016/j.jns.2008.03.003

Naziroğlu, M. (2012). Molecular role of catalase on oxidative stress-induced Ca2 signaling and TRP cation channel activation in nervous system. *J. Recept. Signal Transduct.* 32, 134–141. doi: 10.3109/10799893.2012.672994

Neumann-Raizel, H., Shilo, A., Lev, S., Mogilevsky, M., Katz, B., Shneor, D., et al. (2019). 2-APB and CBD-mediated targeting of charged cytotoxic compounds into tumor cells suggests the involvement of TRPV2 channels. *Front. Pharmacol.* 10:1198. doi: 10.3389/fphar.2019.01198

Olsen, M. L., and Sontheimer, H. (2008). Functional implications for Kir4.1 channels in glial biology: from K + buffering to cell differentiation. *J. Neurochem.* 107, 589–601. doi: 10.1111/j.1471-4159.2008.05615.x

Ostrom, Q. T., Gittleman, H., Fulop, J., Liu, M., Blanda, R., Kromer, C., et al. (2015). CBTRUS statistical report: primary brain and central nervous system tumors diagnosed in the United States in 2008-2012. *Neuro Oncol.* 17, iv1–iv62. doi: 10.1093/neuonc/nov189

Ostrom, Q. T., Gittleman, H., Liao, P., Vecchione-Koval, T., Wolinsky, Y., Kruchko, C., et al. (2017). CBTRUS statistical report: primary brain and other central nervous system tumors diagnosed in the United States in 2010–2014. *Neuro Oncol.* 19, v1–v88. doi: 10.1093/neuonc/nox158

Ou-yang, Q., Li, B., Xu, M., and Liang, H. (2018). TRPV4 promotes the migration and invasion of glioma cells via AKT/Rac1 signaling. *Biochem. Biophys. Res. Commun.* 503, 876–881. doi: 10.1016/j.bbrc.2018.06.090

Peier, A. M., Moqrich, A., Hergarden, A. C., Reeve, A. J., Andersson, D. A., Story, G. M., et al. (2002). A TRP channel that senses cold stimuli and menthol. *Cell* 108, 705–715.

Peng, W., Wong, Y. C., and Krainc, D. (2020). Mitochondria-lysosome contacts regulate mitochondrial Ca2+ dynamics via lysosomal TRPML1. *Proc. Natl. Acad. Sci. U.S.A.* 117, 19266–19275. doi: 10.1073/pnas.2003236117

Pires, P. W., and Earley, S. (2017). Redox regulation of transient receptor potential channels in the endothelium. *Microcirculation* 24:10.1111/micc.12329. doi: 10.1016/j.physbeh.2017.03.040

Pires, P. W., and Earley, S. (2018). Neuroprotective effects of trpa1 channels in the cerebral endothelium following ischemic stroke. *eLife* 7, 1–29. doi: 10.7554/eLife.35316

Prabhu, A., Kesarwani, P., Kant, S., Graham, S. F., and Chinnaiyan, P. (2017). Histologically defined intratumoral sequencing uncovers evolutionary cues into conserved molecular events driving gliomagenesis. *Neuro Oncol.* 19, 1599–1606. doi: 10.1093/neuonc/nox100

Prevarskaya, N., Zhang, L., and Barritt, G. (2007). TRP channels in cancer. *Biochim. Biophys. Acta Mol. Basis Dis.* 1772, 937–946. doi: 10.1016/j.bbadis.2007.05.006

Qin, W., Xiaofeng, R., Jiangchuan, D., Yu, C., and Juan, Y. (2017). MiR-142 inhibits the migration and invasion of glioma by targeting Rac1. *Oncol. Rep.* 38, 1543–1550. doi: 10.3892/or.2017.5816

Ransom, C. B., O'Neal, J. T., and Sontheimer, H. (2001). Volume-activated chloride currents contribute to the resting conductance and invasive migration of human glioma cells. *J. Neurosci.* 21, 7674–7683. doi: 10.1523/jneurosci.21-19-07674.2001

Ransom, C. B., and Sontheimer, H. (2001). BK channels in human glioma cells. *J. Neurophysiol.* 85, 790–803.

Rasper, M., Schafer, A., Piontek, G., Teufel, J., Brockhoff, G., Ringel, F., et al. (2010). Aldehyde dehydrogenase 1 positive glioblastoma cells show brain tumor stem cell capacity. *Neuro Oncol.* 12, 1024–1033.

Ratto, D., Ferrari, B., Roda, E., Brandalise, F., Siciliani, S., De Luca, F., et al. (2020). Squaring the circle: a new study of inward and outward-rectifying potassium currents in U251 GBM cells. *Cell. Mol. Neurobiol.* 40, 813–828. doi: 10.1007/s10571-019-00776-3

Rho, S., Kobayashi, I., Rho, S., Kobayashi, I., Oguri-nakamura, E., Ando, K., et al. (2019). Rap1b promotes notch-signal-mediated hematopoietic stem cell development by enhancing integrin-mediated cell adhesion. *Dev. Cell* 49, 681.e6–696.e6. doi: 10.1016/j.devcel.2019.03.023

Ryu, H. J., Kim, J. E., Kim, Y. J., Kim, J. Y., Kim, W. Il, Choi, S. Y., et al. (2013). Endothelial transient receptor potential conical channel (TRPC)-3 activation induces vasogenic edema formation in the rat piriform cortex following status epilepticus. *Cel. Mol. Neurobiol.* 33, 575–585. doi: 10.1007/s10571-013-9931-x

Santoni, G., and Farfariello, V. (2011). TRP channels and cancer: new targets for diagnosis and chemotherapy. *Endocr. Metab. Immune Disord. Drug Targets* 11, 54–67. doi: 10.2174/187153011794982068

Schwartzbaum, J. A., Fisher, J. L., Aldape, K. D., and Wrensch, M. (2006). Epidemiology and molecular pathology of glioma. *Nat. Clin. Pract. Neurol.* 2, 494–503.

Shi, X., and Teng, F. (2015). Down-regulated miR-28-5p in human hepatocellular carcinoma correlated with tumor proliferation and migration by targeting. *Mol. Cell. Biochem.* 408, 283–293. doi: 10.1007/s11010-015-2506-z

Singh, I., Knezevic, N., Ahmmed, G. U., Kini, V., Malik, A. B., and Mehta, D. (2007). Gαq -TRPC6-mediated Ca 2+ Entry Induces RhoA activation and resultant endothelial cell shape change in response to thrombin. *J. Biol. Chem.* 282, 7833–7843. doi: 10.1074/jbc.M608288200

Stark, G. R., and Taylor, W. R. (2006). Control of the G2/M transition. *Mol. Biotechnol.* 32, 227–248. doi: 10.1385/MB:32:3:227

Steinle, M., Palme, D., Misovic, M., Rudner, J., Dittmann, K., Lukowski, R., et al. (2011). Ionizing radiation induces migration of glioblastoma cells by activating BK K + channels. *Radiother. Oncol.* 101, 122–126. doi: 10.1016/j.radonc.2011.05.069

Stepanenko, A. A., and Chekhonin, V. P. (2018). Recent advances in oncolytic virotherapy and immunotherapy for glioblastoma: a glimmer of hope in the search for an effective therapy? *Cancers* 10:492. doi: 10.3390/cancers10120492

Stock, K., Kumar, J., Synowitz, M., Petrosino, S., Imperatore, R., Smith, E. S. J., et al. (2012). Neural precursor cells induce cell death of high-grade astrocytomas through stimulation of TRPV1. *Nat. Med.* 18, 1232–1238. doi: 10.1038/nm.2827

Stuart, E. T., Kioussi, C., Gruss, P., and Aguzzi, A. (1995). PAX5 expression correlates with increasing malignancy in human astrocytomas. *Clin. Cancer Res.* 1, 207–214.

Stupp, R., Hegi, M. E., Mason, W. P., van den Bent, M. J., Taphoorn, M. J. B., Janzer, R. C., et al. (2009). Effects of radiotherapy with concomitant and adjuvant temozolomide versus radiotherapy alone on survival in glioblastoma in a randomised phase III study: 5-year analysis of the EORTC-NCIC trial. *Lancet. Oncol.* 10, 459–466. doi: 10.1016/S1470-2045(09)70025-7

Stupp, R., Mason, W. P., van den Bent, M. J., Weller, M., Fisher, B., Taphoorn, M. J. B., et al. (2005). Radiotherapy plus concomitant and adjuvant temozolomide for glioblastoma. *N. Engl. J. Med.* 352, 987–996. doi: 10.1056/NEJMoa043330

Sullivan, M. N., Gonzales, A. L., Pires, P. W., Bruhl, A., Leo, M. D., Li, W., et al. (2016). Oxygen species promote cerebral artery dilation. *Sci. Signal.* 8, 1–26. doi: 10.1126/scisignal.2005659.Localized

Tai, Y., Feng, S., Ge, R., Du, W., Zhang, X., He, Z., et al. (2008). TRPC6 channels promote dendritic growth via the CaMKIV-CREB pathway. *J. Cell Sci.* 121, 2301–2307. doi: 10.1242/jcs.026906

Takahashi, N., Chen, H. Y., Harris, I. S., Stover, D. G., Selfors, L. M., Bronson, R. T., et al. (2018). Cancer cells co-opt the neuronal redox-sensing channel TRPA1 to promote oxidative-stress tolerance. *Cancer Cell* 33, 985.e7–1003.e7. doi: 10.1016/j.ccell.2018.05.001

Takahashi, N., Kozai, D., Kobayashi, R., Ebert, M., and Mori, Y. (2011). Cell calcium roles of TRPM2 in oxidative stress. *Cell Calcium* 50, 279–287. doi: 10.1016/j.ceca.2011.04.006

Thompson, C. B. (1995). Apoptosis in the pathogenesis and treatment of disease. *Science* 267, 1456–1462.

Valadez, J. A., and Cuajungco, M. P. (2015). PAX5 is the transcriptional activator of mucolipin-2 (MCOLN2) gene. *Gene* 555, 194–202. doi: 10.1016/j.gene.2014.11.003

Veldhuis, N. A., Poole, D. P., Grace, M., McIntyre, P., and Bunnett, N. W. (2015). The g protein–coupled receptor–transient receptor potential channel axis: molecular insights for targeting disorders of sensation and inflammation. *Pharmacol. Rev.* 67, 36–73. doi: 10.1124/pr.114.009555

Venkatachalam, K., and Montell, C. (2007). TRP channels. *Annu. Rev. Biochem.* 76, 387–417. doi: 10.1146/annurev.biochem.75.103004.142819

Venugopal, B., Mesires, N. T., Kennedy, J. C., Curcio-Morelli, C., Laplante, J. M., Dice, J. F., et al. (2009). Chaperone-mediated autophagy is defective in mucolipidosis type IV. *J. Cell. Physiol.* 219, 344–353. doi: 10.1002/jcp.21676

Walcher, L., Budde, C., Böhm, A., Reinach, P. S., Dhandapani, P., Ljubojevic, N., et al. (2018). Induced transactivation of TRPV1 in human uveal melanoma cells. *Front. Pharmacol.* 9:1234. doi: 10.3389/fphar.2018.01234

Walzlein, J.-H., Synowitz, M., Engels, B., Markovic, D. S., Gabrusiewicz, K., Nikolaev, E., et al. (2008). Antitumorigenic response of neural precursors depends on subventricular proliferation and age. *Stem Cells* 26, 2945–2954. doi: 10.1634/stemcells.2008-0307

Wan, J., Guo, A. A., Chowdhury, I., and Guo, S. (2019). TRPM7 induces mechanistic target of rap1b through the downregulation of miR-28-5p in glioma proliferation and invasion. *Front. Oncol.* 9:1413. doi: 10.3389/fonc.2019.01413

Watkins, S., Robel, S., Kimbrough, I. F., Robert, S. M., Ellis-Davies, G., and Sontheimer, H. (2014). Disruption of astrocyte–vascular coupling and the blood–brain barrier by invading glioma cells. *Nat. Commun.* 5, 1–15. doi: 10.1038/ncomms5196

Wen, P. Y., and Brandes, A. A. (2009). Treatment of recurrent high-grade gliomas. *Curr. Opin. Neurol.* 22, 657–664. doi: 10.1097/WCO.0b013e32833229e3

Wondergem, R., and Bartley, J. W. (2009). Menthol increases human glioblastoma intracellular Ca2+, BK channel activity and cell migration. *J. Biomed. Sci.* 16, 1–7. doi: 10.1186/1423-0127-16-90

Wondergem, R., Ecay, T. W., Mahieu, F., Owsianik, G., and Nilius, B. (2008). Biochemical and biophysical research communications HGF/SF and menthol increase human glioblastoma cell calcium and migration. *Biochem. Biophys. Res. Commun.* 372, 210–215. doi: 10.1016/j.bbrc.2008.05.032

Xiao, F., Cheng, Z., Wang, P., Gong, B., Huang, H., Xing, Y., et al. (2018). MicroRNA-28-5p inhibits the migration and invasion of gastric cancer cells by suppressing AKT phosphorylation. *Oncol. Lett.* 15, 9777–9785. doi: 10.3892/ol.2018.8603

Yao, X. H., Ping, Y.-F., Chen, J.-H., Xu, C.-P., Chen, D.-L., Zhang, R., et al. (2008). Glioblastoma stem cells produce vascular endothelial growth factor by activation of a G-protein coupled formylpeptide receptor FPR. *J. Pathol.* 215, 369–376. doi: 10.1002/path.2356.Glioblastoma

Ying, Z., Li, Y., Wu, J., Zhu, X., Yang, Y., Tian, H., et al. (2013). Loss of miR-204 expression enhances glioma migration and stem cell-like phenotype. *Cancer Res.* 73, 990–1000. doi: 10.1158/0008-5472.CAN-12-2895

Yu, X., Jiang, Y., Wei, W., and Cong, P. (2015). Androgen receptor signaling regulates growth of glioblastoma multiforme in men. *Tumour. Biol.* 36, 967–972. doi: 10.1007/s13277-014-2709-z

Zamudio-Bulcock, P. A., Everett, J., Harteneck, C., and Valenzuela, C. F. (2011). Activation of steroid-sensitive TRPM3 channels potentiates glutamatergic transmission at cerebellar purkinje neurons from developing rats. *Neurochem. J.* 119, 474–485. doi: 10.1111/j.1471-4159.2011.07441.x

Zeng, J., Wu, Y., Zhuang, S., Qin, L., Hua, S., Mungur, R., et al. (2019). Identification of the role of TRPM8 in glioblastoma and its effect on proliferation, apoptosis and invasion of the U251 human glioblastoma cell line. *Oncol. Rep.* 42, 1517–1526. doi: 10.3892/or.2019.7260

Zhang, X., Cheng, X., Yu, L., Yang, J., Calvo, R., Patnaik, S., et al. (2016a). MCOLN1 is a ROS sensor in lysosomes that regulates autophagy. *Nat. Commun.* 7:12109. doi: 10.1038/ncomms12109

Zhang, X., Yu, L., and Xu, H. (2016b). Lysosome calcium in ROS regulation of autophagy. *Autophagy* 12, 1954–1955. doi: 10.1080/15548627.2016.1212787

Zhou, J., Du, W., Zhou, K., Tai, Y., Yao, H., Jia, Y., et al. (2008). Critical role of TRPC6 channels in the formation of excitatory synapses. *Nat. Neurosci.* 11, 741–743. doi: 10.1038/nn.2127

Zhou, K., Rao, J., Zhou, Z., Zhou, Z. H., Yao, X. H., Wu, F., et al. (2018). RAC1-GTP promotes epithelial-mesenchymal transition and invasion of colorectal cancer by activation of STAT3. *Lab. Invest.* 98, 989–998. doi: 10.1038/s41374-018-0071-2

7

TRP Channels Regulation of Rho GTPases in Brain Context and Diseases

Boris Lavanderos[1,2†], Ian Silva[1,2†], Pablo Cruz[1,2†], Octavio Orellana-Serradell[1,2], María Paz Saldías[1,2] and Oscar Cerda[1,2,3]*

[1] Program of Cellular and Molecular Biology, Institute of Biomedical Sciences, Faculty of Medicine, Universidad de Chile, Santiago, Chile, [2] Millennium Nucleus of Ion Channel-Associated Diseases (MiNICAD), Santiago, Chile, [3] The Wound Repair, Treatment and Health (WoRTH) Initiative, Santiago, Chile

***Correspondence:**
Oscar Cerda
oscarcerda@uchile.cl

† These authors have contributed equally to this work

Neurological and neuropsychiatric disorders are mediated by several pathophysiological mechanisms, including developmental and degenerative abnormalities caused primarily by disturbances in cell migration, structural plasticity of the synapse, and blood-vessel barrier function. In this context, critical pathways involved in the pathogenesis of these diseases are related to structural, scaffolding, and enzymatic activity-bearing proteins, which participate in Ca^{2+}- and Ras Homologs (Rho) GTPases-mediated signaling. Rho GTPases are GDP/GTP binding proteins that regulate the cytoskeletal structure, cellular protrusion, and migration. These proteins cycle between GTP-bound (active) and GDP-bound (inactive) states due to their intrinsic GTPase activity and their dynamic regulation by GEFs, GAPs, and GDIs. One of the most important upstream inputs that modulate Rho GTPases activity is Ca^{2+} signaling, positioning ion channels as pivotal molecular entities for Rho GTPases regulation. Multiple non-selective cationic channels belonging to the Transient Receptor Potential (TRP) family participate in cytoskeletal-dependent processes through Ca^{2+}-mediated modulation of Rho GTPases. Moreover, these ion channels have a role in several neuropathological events such as neuronal cell death, brain tumor progression and strokes. Although Rho GTPases-dependent pathways have been extensively studied, how they converge with TRP channels in the development or progression of neuropathologies is poorly understood. Herein, we review recent evidence and insights that link TRP channels activity to downstream Rho GTPase signaling or modulation. Moreover, using the TRIP database, we establish associations between possible mediators of Rho GTPase signaling with TRP ion channels. As such, we propose mechanisms that might explain the TRP-dependent modulation of Rho GTPases as possible pathways participating in the emergence or maintenance of neuropathological conditions.

Keywords: TRP channels, Rho GTPases, actin cytoskeleton, TRP interactome, GEFs, GAPs

INTRODUCTION

Neurological diseases encompass broad pathophysiological events, characterized by alterations such as hypo- or hyper-connectivity of synapses, tumoral growth, and loss of neuronal networks (Forrest et al., 2018; La Rosa et al., 2020; Liu Y. et al., 2020). Nevertheless, in most of the cases the precise cellular and molecular mechanisms involved in the pathogenesis of these disorders have not been fully described. Ion channels have been widely described as pivotal molecular entities that contribute to brain physiology and are associated to the development of various brain diseases, thus emerging as highly potential pharmacological targets (Bagal et al., 2013). Several members of the TRP ion channel family play key roles in the regulation of cellular and tissue structures, such as membrane protrusions, synapses, endothelial barriers and glial architecture (Goswami and Hucho, 2007; Goswami et al., 2007a; Gorse et al., 2018; Zhao et al., 2018; Cornillot et al., 2019), whose abnormal activity is intimately linked to neurodevelopmental and neurodegenerative disorders (Morelli et al., 2013). Despite that, how TRP channels participate in brain physiology and brain-affecting diseases is still not fully understood. The concerted activity of Rho GTPases has been described as a signaling node that governs structural maintenance and dynamic changes of cell architecture, mainly through the control and integration of cytoskeleton rearrangements and membrane trafficking. Similarly to TRP channels, Rho GTPases command neurophysiological processes such as dendritic spines morphology, axon cone growth, glial cells migration, blood-brain barrier permeability and vascular tone (Wu et al., 2005; Stankiewicz and Linseman, 2014; Pennucci et al., 2019). Thus, coordinated TRP channels and Rho GTPases activity might be a conserved mechanism for the modulation of changes in physiological and pathophysiological contexts.

Rho GTPases in Actin-Based Processes in Brain

Ras Homologs (Rho) proteins are a family of small GTPases belonging to the Ras superfamily. Since the discovery of the first Rho protein (Madaule and Axel, 1985), twenty members have been identified in mammals, currently grouped in 8 subfamilies (Vega and Ridley, 2008). These proteins cycle between an "*active*" GTP-bound state, and an "*inactive*" GDP-bound state. The basis for the cyclic activity of Rho GTPases lies in 3 regulators: (1) Guanine Exchange Factor (GEF) proteins, which catalyze swapping of GDP to GTP, allowing the transition of Rho proteins into their "*active*" state; (2) GTPases-Activating Proteins (GAP), which increase the intrinsic GTPase activity of the guanosine nucleotide-binding protein, promoting GTP hydrolysis and leading to the "*inactive*" state (Bos et al., 2007); and (3) Guanine Dissociation Inhibitors (GDI), which sequester the inactive form of Rho GTPases to prevent their activation by GEFs (Dovas and Couchman, 2005) (**Figure 1**).

Rho GTPases are crucial for the regulation of the actin cytoskeleton (Rottner et al., 2017) and processes involving cellular motility such as contractility, migration, and membrane protrusions (Machacek et al., 2009). RhoA, Rac1 and Cdc42 are the most studied and distinguished members of this family (Ridley and Hall, 1992; Ridley et al., 1992; Wedlich-Soldner et al., 2003). In neurons, actin cytoskeleton remodeling is essential for several processes including neuronal growth (Marsh and Letourneau, 1984), dendrite development and synapse formation (Sin et al., 2002). These events are indispensable for proper establishment and plasticity of brain circuits. Thus, neurons require accurate actin cytoskeleton regulation, which in turn depends on the fine spatiotemporal and coordinated control of Rho GTPases activity (Murakoshi et al., 2011). Accordingly, the modulation of Rho GTPases has been described to occur in a time/length scale of minutes/micrometers (Pertz, 2010). Canonically, Rac1 activation facilitates the formation of dendritic spines (Luo et al., 1996) and membrane ruffles, while RhoA inhibits these processes and promotes spine shortening (Tashiro, 2000). Moreover, while Glutamate-promoted Cdc42 activity is confined to stimulated dendritic spines, active RhoA spreads along the dendrites (Murakoshi et al., 2011). Thus, spatiotemporal regulation of Rho GTPases is a key point in spine structural plasticity (Hedrick et al., 2016). In addition to their role in neurons, Rho GTPases also play pivotal functions on brain vessels and glial cells. For instance, Rho GTPases regulate contractility and permeability of endothelial brain vessels (Kutcher et al., 2007; Kruse et al., 2019), as well as coordinate different morphological changes on glial cells (reviewed in Zeug et al., 2018). Therefore, these proteins are an essential component for maintaining brain homeostasis and deregulation of their activity lead to several neurological pathologies (Huang et al., 2017).

The precise coordination of Rho GTPases activity highly depends on GEFs, GDIs and GAPs defined by establishing differential protein–protein interactions (PPIs) of Rho GTPases and their modulators. For instance, Rac1 regulation is mediated by selective association with other proteins such as Tiam1 (Rac-GEF), Bcr (Rac-GAP) (Um et al., 2014), and Vilse (Rac-GAP) (Lim et al., 2014). Moreover, RhoA activity is regulated by the interaction of Graf1c (RhoA-GAP) with the tyrosine kinase Pyk2 in postsynaptic neurons, resulting in spine retraction (Lee et al., 2019). Furthermore, Rho GEFs that contain the PDZ-domain interact with lysophosphatidic acid, which promotes RhoA activation (Yamada et al., 2005). Hence, GAP and GEF differential localization and/or interactions are crucial elements for the spatiotemporal regulation of Rho GTPases. Consistently, mutations on these proteins (GAP/GEF) lead to several congenital malformations or developmental neuropathologies (O'Brien et al., 2000; Bai et al., 2015; Pengelly et al., 2016). In this context, the existence of over 70 GEFs and over 70 GAPs adds a further level of complexity in the regulation of Rho GTPases (Müller et al., 2020). In line with this, GEFs and GAPs are tightly regulated by protein interaction partners, second messengers such as Ca^{2+}, and posttranslational modifications (PTM) such as phosphorylations (Bos et al., 2007) (**Figure 1**).

Rho GTPases are also modulated by posttranslational modifications (PTMs). Prenylation of the carboxyl-terminal is the most frequent modification, which entails the addition of a 15- or 20- carbon isoprenoid to a cysteine residue immersed in a *CAAX* motif (Roberts et al., 2008; Reddy et al., 2020). This PTM causes Rho GTPase targeting to the plasma membrane (Hodge and Ridley, 2016), leading to GTP-bound Rho GTPases interaction with their effectors and regulators (Reddy et al., 2020). Moreover, several Rho GTPases phosphorylations, ubiquitylation, sumoylation, and their differential upstream enzymes and outcomes have been reported (extensively reviewed in Hodge and Ridley, 2016).

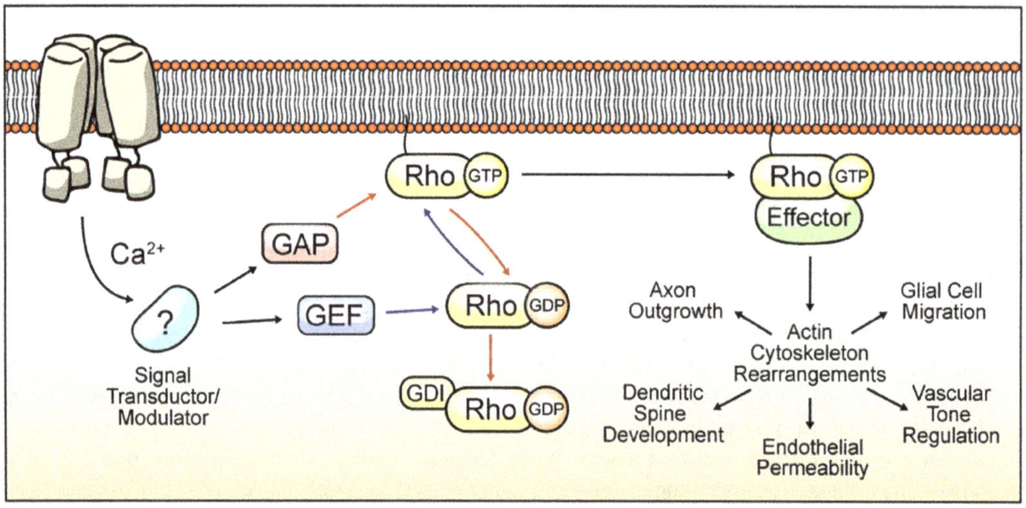

FIGURE 1 | Cyclic Rho GTPase modulation, functions, and TRP channel-mediated regulation hypothesis. Rho GTPases cycle between an active form bound to GTP (blue arrows) and an inactive form that is attached to GDP (red arrows). Binding to guanosine nucleotide is induced by GEF proteins. GAP proteins promote GTPase activity, and GDI proteins preclude GDP exchange to GTP. The active state of Rho GTPase promotes the rearrangement of the actin cytoskeleton by the modulation of several effectors. The actin cytoskeleton mediates multiple processes depending on the cell types. In neurons, axon outgrowth and dendritic spine dynamics regulation. In brain vasculature, Rho GTPases regulate endothelial permeability and vascular tone regulation. Rho GTPases regulates migration in glial cells. TRP channels-mediated Ca^{2+} influx regulates signal transductors/modulators, leading to changes in GAP, GEF, or GDI activity, thus promoting Rho GTPases activation/inactivation and actin cytoskeleton regulation.

The activity of several Rho GTPases is linked to depolarization and Ca^{2+} influx in neurons (Hirata et al., 1992; Szászi et al., 2005). This Ca^{2+} influx is related to Voltage-gated Ca^{2+} Channels (VGCCs), although intracellular Ca^{2+} reservoirs and Store-Operated Ca^{2+} Entry (SOCE) also might have an important role in the activation of Rho GTPases as has been widely reported (Jin et al., 2005; Saneyoshi and Hayashi, 2012; Bollimuntha et al., 2017). In this context, most of the mechanisms described involved in Ca^{2+}-dependent Rho GTPase modulation rely on Calmodulin (CaM) and Calmodulin-dependent Kinases (CaMKs) as transductors of Ca^{2+} signals through the regulation of GEFs, GAPs, and GDIs. For example, neurotrophins induce intracellular long-range Ca^{2+} waves, increasing RhoA activity during axon formation (Takano et al., 2017). Interestingly, Ca^{2+} waves promote CaMKI activation, leading to recruitment and interaction with GEF-H1, promoting RhoA activation (Takano et al., 2017). Also, CaMKII phosphorylates GEFs and GAPs of Rac1 and Cdc42, such as the Rac1 GEF Tiam1, and RICS, a Cdc42/Rac1 GAP (Okabe et al., 2003). CaMKII-dependent phosphorylation of the Rac1 GEF Kalirin-7 promotes cytoskeleton rearrangement and leads to the plasticity of dendritic spines (Xie et al., 2007).

In this context, the correlation between local/broad Ca^{2+} signals and the activation of different Rho GTPases is an interesting issue, but the molecular entities responsible for these Ca^{2+} signals have not been fully identified. TRP channels are implicated in a myriad of cellular processes associated with actin-based events in migratory cells, through the regulation of Rho GTPases activity (Canales et al., 2019). These channels also play an important role in brain physiology (Dussor et al., 2014; Zeng et al., 2016). As such, TRP channels might serve as key hubs for signaling transduction related to Rho GTPases activities, regulating several features of brain function and architecture.

TRP CHANNELS

The TRP ion channel family comprises six subfamilies of non-selective cationic channels in mammals, corresponding to TRPA, TRPC, TRPM, TRPML, TRPP, and TRPV (Clapham et al., 2001). All members present six transmembrane domains (S1 – S6) and cytoplasmic amino- and carboxyl-terminal segments of varying length, and a pore-loop between S5 and S6 domains (**Table 1**) (Hellmich and Gaudet, 2014). The first identified TRP channel in mammals was named as classical or canonical (TRPC). The remaining subfamilies have been named depending on the designation of the first identified member of the respective subfamily, which relies on activation properties, function and/or featured domains (Montell, 2005; Venkatachalam and Montell, 2007).

Transient receptor potential channels can be activated by multiple stimuli, such as temperature, pH changes, and membrane mechanical stress (Clapham, 2003). Moreover, the activity of these channels can be modulated by PIP_2 (Nilius et al., 2008; Rohacs, 2014), PTMs such as phosphorylation (Cerda et al., 2015; Xu et al., 2019; Liu X. et al., 2020) and interacting proteins (Singh et al., 2002; Zhu, 2005; Cho et al., 2014; Rivas et al., 2020). Monomers can form heterotetrameric functional channels with distinctive properties in relation with their homotetrameric counterparts (Chubanov et al., 2004; Ma et al., 2011; Kim et al., 2019). Heteromultimerization can occur not only among members of the same TRP subfamily but

TABLE 1 | TRPA, TRPC, TRPV, TRPM and TRPML channels features.

TRP subfamily	Size	$P_{Ca}{}^{2+}/P_{Na}{}^{+}$	Domains N-term	Domains C-term	Phosphoinositides-Binding	Localization
TRPA	~1000 aa	0.8–1.4	Ankyrin-repeats	TRP-box-like motif Inositol phosphate binding region Coiled-coil region	PIP_2 – Activation	Plasma Membrane
TRPC	<1000 aa	0.5 – 9	Ankyrin-repeats Coiled-coil regions	TRP-box motif Calmodulin-binding CIRB domains PDZ domains	PIP_2-Activation/Inhibition	Plasma Membrane
TRPV	<900 aa	1 - >100	Ankyrin-repeats	TRP-box motif Calmodulin-binding	PIP_2 – Activation/Inhibition PG-Activation (V1) PI-Activation (V1) PS-Activation (V1)	Plasma Membrane
TRPM	<1500 aa	0.5–10 (Except M4/5 which have <0.05)	Melastatin family channel homology region	TRP-box motif Coiled-Coil region Nudix (M2) Kinase (M6/7)	PIP_2 – Activation	Plasma Membrane Melanosomes (M1)
TRPML	<600 aa	~1	–	EF-Hand motifs	PIP_2 – Activation	Endolysosome vesicles

also with those of different subfamilies (Ma et al., 2011). These features and the wide expression of these channels in multiple tissues and cell types, grant a high level of complexity to their role in diverse physiological and pathophysiological processes (Venkatachalam and Montell, 2007). In this context, several TRP channels are implicated in cellular processes related to central nervous system (CNS) functioning such as the modulation of neuronal excitability (Mickle et al., 2016; Hong et al., 2020b), maturation or establishment of subcellular structures such as dendrites (Tai et al., 2008), excitatory synapses (Zhou et al., 2008), axonal outgrowth (Jang et al., 2014), frontal cortex postnatal development (Riquelme et al., 2018) and brain blood flow regulation (Earley et al., 2004; Cornillot et al., 2019). Also, current evidence suggests that TRP channels could regulate downstream processes such as gene expression or more lasting effects, like Long Term Potentiation (LTP). Hence, it is not surprising to find CNS pathophysiological conditions associated with TRP channels activity (**Table 2**). TRP channels have been associated to stroke (Zhang and Liao, 2015), CNS ischemia-reperfusion damage (Gauden et al., 2007; Chen et al., 2017; Leiva-Salcedo et al., 2017), status epilepticus (Kim et al., 2013; Phelan et al., 2017), Alzheimer's and Parkinson's diseases (Zhang et al., 2013; Hong et al., 2020b), and progression of neoplasms of neuronal (Chen et al., 2014; Middelbeek et al., 2015) or glial (Lepannetier et al., 2016; Ou-Yang et al., 2018) origin.

Several reports suggest a role for TRP channels on Rho GTPases regulation. In this context, interactome maps based on different Protein–Protein Interaction databases suggest associations between TRP channels with Rho GTPases-related proteins. For instance, the TRIP database, a curated database from individual studies that report protein interactions with TRP channels, provides insightful information regarding the TRP-Rho GTPase interactions (Shin et al., 2011). Other general interactome databases such as BioGRID (Oughtred et al., 2019) and BioPlex (Schweppe et al., 2018), generated from high-throughput interactome datasets and curated individual studies, complement these interactions. The resulting interactome map reveals that the TRP-interacting proteins network reveals several Rho GTPases-related regulators, such as Src, PLC-γ1, Akt, PKC and the GTPase Gαq (Shin et al., 2011) (**Figure 2**). In this context, the activity or expression of TRPC3 (Kitajima et al., 2011; Numaga-Tomita et al., 2016), TRPC5 (Tian et al., 2010) TRPC6 (Singh et al., 2007; Tian et al., 2010), TRPM4 (Cáceres et al., 2015), TRPM7 (Su et al., 2011), TRPV1 (Li J. et al., 2015; Li et al., 2015a), and TRPV4 (Ou-Yang et al., 2018; Zhao et al., 2018) increase the activity of several Rho GTPases (**Table 3**). Also, there is evidence showing that TRPM8 (Sun et al., 2014), TRPV2 (Laragione et al., 2019), and TRPV4 (Thoppil et al., 2016) channels inhibit Rho GTPases (**Table 3**). These opposite effects could rely on multiple mechanisms that give versatility to Ca^{2+} signals-dependent responses such as specific localization in membrane subdomains or cellular substructures of the channels, leading to differential and dynamic interactions with Ca^{2+}-regulated proteins that might modulate Rho GTPases. This regulation might occur *via* activation of Ca^{2+}-dependent kinases proteins such as PKC and CaM kinases, leading to direct regulatory phosphorylations on Rho GTPases (Hodge and Ridley, 2016). Despite the above, the elevated number of GAPs and GEFs (Müller et al., 2020) and the diverse outcomes on cytoskeleton rearrangement elicited by TRP channels (Kuipers et al., 2012; Canales et al., 2019) might point to an indirect TRP channels-dependent regulation of Rho GTPases through these modulators (GEFs and GAPs).

In the following sections, based on established and inferred interactions, we will discuss and hypothesize possible mechanisms for TRP channels participation *via* Rho GTPases in different neuropathologies.

TRPC Channels

TRPC is the founding subfamily of the mammalian TRP channel family, since the first TRP channel found in mammals was named "canonical" owing to its similarities to the TRP channel from *Drosophila* (Montell and Rubin, 1989; Clapham et al., 2001). The mammalian TRPC subfamily can be divided into two subgroups based on the percentage of identity between their sequences: (1) TRPC1/TRPC2/TRPC4/TRPC6 and (2) TRPC3/TRPC6/TRPC7.

TABLE 2 | TRP channels-associated pathologies and possible Rho GTPases-dependent mechanisms.

TRP Channel	TRP Channel activity deregulation-associated disease	Possible Rho GTPase-dependent mechanism for TRP channel role in disease
TRPC3	Mwk phenotype (Wu et al., 2019), Cerebellar ataxia (Dulneva et al., 2015)	Aberrant spine remodeling/morphology due to deregulation of CaMKII/Tiam1 axis
TRPC5	Substance abuse (Pomrenze et al., 2013) – Excitotoxicity (Phelan et al., 2013)	Rac1 and DR-2-mediated regulation of RhoA
TRPC6	Glioma (Ding et al., 2010). AD (Lessard et al., 2005; Feng, 2017)	Glioma: Promotion of FAK activation, cell proliferation and migration AD: Loss of TRPC6 expression leads to the activation of Rac1, promoting the amyloidogenic pathway
TRPV1	AD (Balleza-Tapia et al., 2018; Du et al., 2020), Glioblastoma (Nabissi et al., 2016)	AD: Protective effect due to induction of axonal filopodia or dendritic spines Glioblastoma:Increment of cell invasion through RhoA activity
TRPV2	Possible participation in neurodegenerative processes	Rac1/RhoA-mediated neuritogenesis and tubulogenesis modulation
TRPV4	ICH, TBI (Zhao et al., 2018), AD (Zhang et al., 2013)	RhoA-mediated endothelial dilation and vascular tone regulation
	Glioma progression (Ou-Yang et al., 2018)	Increased cell migration due to enhanced Rac1 activity
TRPM4	IS (Leiva-Salcedo et al., 2017; Chen et al., 2019), glutamatergic toxicity (Schattling et al., 2012), SCI (Gerzanich et al., 2009)	Rac1-mediated induction of NADPH oxidase and ROS production
TRPM7	IS (Chen et al., 2015), Neuroblastoma (Middelbeek et al., 2015)	IS: RhoA upregulation and subsequent induction of cell death. Neuroblastoma: RhoA-dependent cytoskeleton remodeling Endothelial Barrier disruption
TRPM8	Migraines (Gavva et al., 2019; Ling et al., 2019), Glioblastoma (Zeng et al., 2019)	Regulation of cerebral arterial vasodilation
TRPML1	Mucolipidosis type IV (Bargal et al., 2000)	Control of Rho GTPases-dependent membrane trafficking

ICH, intracerebral hemorrage; IS, ischemic stroke; TBI, traumatic brain injury; SCI, spinal cord injury; AD, Alzheimer's disease.

Of note, TRPC2 is a pseudogene in *Homo sapiens* (Wang et al., 2020). These channels can heteromultimerize with members of the corresponding (TRPC) or other sub-families, which yields functional non-selective ion channels with a wide range of relative P_{Ca}/P_{Na} (**Table 1**) (Chen et al., 2020). All these channels are responsive to GPCR/RTK-induced PLC activation (Wang et al., 2020). Some members also respond to ER-Ca^{2+} stores depletion *via* STIM1, such as TRPC1, TRPC3, TRPC4, and TRPC5 (Yuan et al., 2007; Lee et al., 2014). Moreover, TRPC channels activity is regulated by $PIP(4,5)_2$ and PIP_2-derivates such as DAG, IP3, PI(4)P and PI. Structurally, TRPC channels are composed by intracellular N-terminal and C-terminal domains, and six membrane-spanning domains. Expression of TRPC channels has been reported in various tissues, such as kidney, salivary glands, hippocampus, pancreatic β cells, heart, and vascular smooth muscle, and therefore participate in a wide variety of physiological processes (Chen et al., 2020).

TRPC3

TRPC3 channels are characterized by their coupling to tyrosine kinase and G protein coupled receptors activation, acting as mediators of Ca^{2+} signals induced by these receptors (Ambudkar and Ong, 2007). TRPC3 channels are especially abundant in the brain, mainly in the cerebellum, caudate nucleus, putamen and striatum (Riccio et al., 2002). These channels participate in Purkinje cells physiology in the cerebellum (Hartmann et al., 2008). Indeed, mGluR1 promotes TRPC3-dependent rises of local Ca^{2+} signals, leading to slow membrane depolarization at Purkinje cells dendrites (Hartmann et al., 2008). Accordingly, changes in the expression or mutations of TRPC3 gene cause detrimental consequences on motor functions such as the 'Moonwalker' (Mwk) phenotype (Wu et al., 2019). Mice with Mwk phenotypes display gait and limb incoordination (Becker, 2017). Interestingly, TRPC3 upregulation in Mwk animals impairs the development of dendrites (Becker et al., 2009). Furthermore, the mutant variant R672H of the human TRPC3 gene leads to cerebellar ataxia (Dulneva et al., 2015). Consequently, TRPC3 activity deregulation might induce structural alterations during the progress of cerebellar ataxia by modulating dendrite development.

There is not a direct evidence for TRPC3-mediated regulation of Rho GTPases in neurons or brain tissues. Nevertheless, data obtained from other models, as well as TRPC3/Rho GTPases associated pathways, might suggest a functional relationship between these proteins. For instance, BDNF induces Rac1 and Cdc42 activation, but not RhoA, through activation of TrkB receptor (Hedrick et al., 2016). Moreover, BDNF-induced TrkB activation leads to TRPC3 activation, which is necessary to induce spine remodeling (Amaral and Pozzo-Miller, 2007), suggesting that TRPC3 activation might be a mediator for BDNF-dependent activation of Rac1 and Cdc42, although further studies would be needed to confirm this. Interestingly, TRPC3 inhibition in heart mouse model induces a reduction of CaMKII and Rac1 activity (Kitajima et al., 2011). CaMKII-mediated Tiam1 phosphorylation leads in turn to Rac1 activation (Fleming et al., 1999; Buchanan et al., 2000; Tolias et al., 2005). These data suggest that TRPC3 activation by BDNF might induce Tiam1 CaMKII-dependent phosphorylation (**Table 3**), resulting in dendritic spine remodeling by Rac1 activity (**Figure 3**). Furthermore, downstream effectors might include PAK1, since

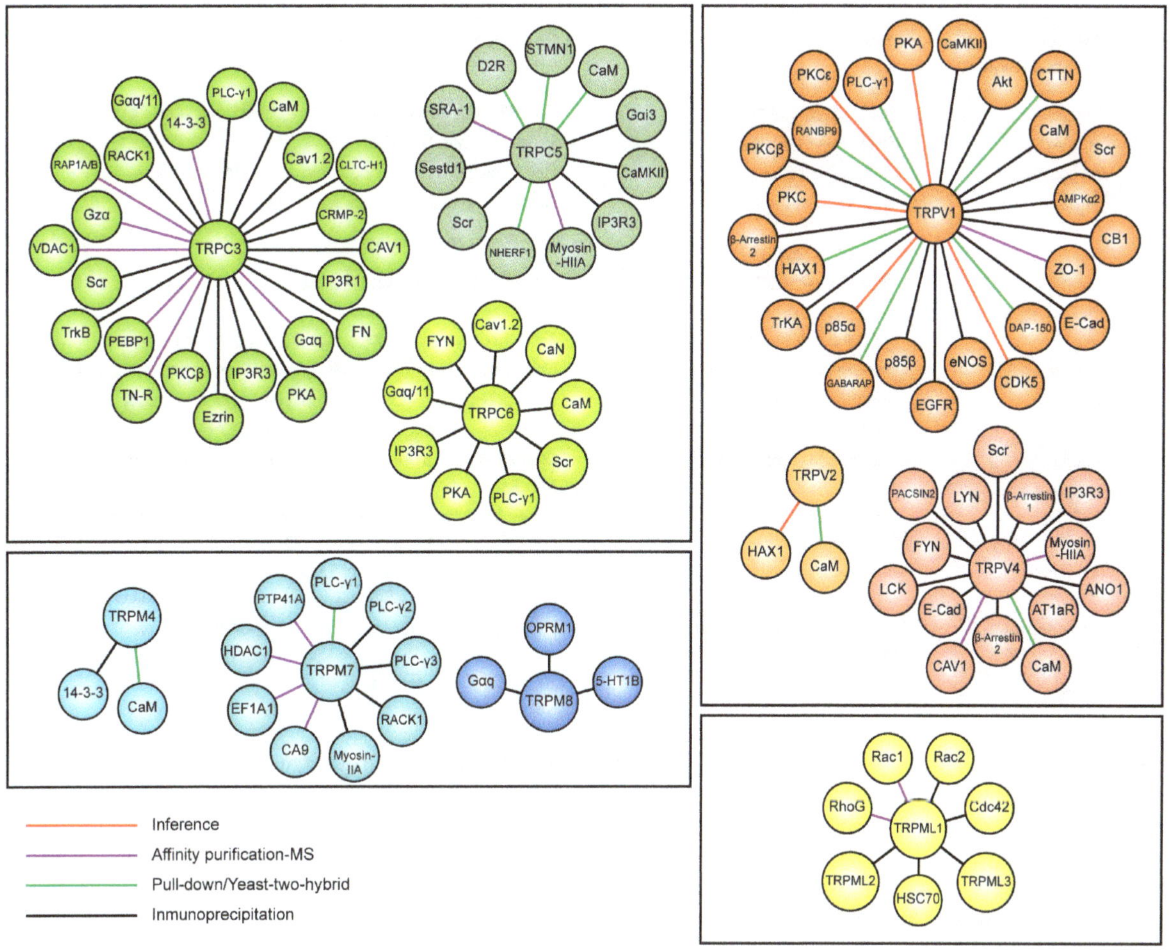

FIGURE 2 | Map of curated TRP ion channel interactors associated with Rho GTPases pathways. Data obtained from the TRIP database showing interactors of TRPC3, TRPC5, TRPC6, TRPV1, TRPV2, TRPV4, TRPM4, TRPM7, TRPM8, and TRPML1. TRP channels members are grouped and color-coded by families.

its activation by Rac1 that leads to actin remodeling through LIMK1 activity (Edwards et al., 1999). Likewise, CaMKII-ß regulates dendritic spine formation in Purkinje cells through a mechanism that involves mGluR1 and PKC activation. This CaMKII-ß-mediated effect requires IP_3R activation (Sugawara et al., 2017). Moreover, CaMKII has an important role in the production of LTP by promoting the insertion of AMPA receptors in the post synaptic region (Lisman et al., 2012). Importantly, our curated search in the TRIP database showed that TRPC3 interacts physically and functionally with the IP_3R isoforms (Kim J.Y. et al., 2006), and also with BDNF receptor TrkB (Li et al., 1999) (**Figure 2**). Thus, we propose that TRPC3 activation by BDNF/TrkB or mGluR1 in Purkinje might elicit spine remodeling through CaMKIIß activation and subsequent Rac1 activation. This proposed pathway could be relevant for pathologies that entail degeneration of neuronal processes. For example, morphology of dendritic spines is heavily altered in conditions of aberrant CaMKII/Tiam1/Rac1 activity, which might collaborate to intellectual disability of patients bearing mutations of the ATRX-encoding gene (Shioda et al., 2011). These data is consistent with a possible role for TRPC3 in this pathology due to the above-mentioned role of this channel in BDNF-dependent spine remodeling, which might open new avenues of studies for novel TRPC3 functions in brain pathophysiology.

TRPC5

TRPC5 is another non-selective cation channel that belongs to the TRPC subfamily. TRPC5 activity is related to many sensorial features such as touch and hearing (Sexton et al., 2016), satiety sensation (Gao et al., 2017), and internal physiological pH chemosensitivity (Cui et al., 2011). TRPC5 regulates neurites length (Greka et al., 2003), neurite outgrowth during neuron differentiation (Heo et al., 2012), neurite retraction (Hui et al., 2006), and axonal outgrowth (Oda et al., 2020). Moreover, several studies link the function of TRPC5 to dynamic behavioral processes that are tightly related to structural changes in synapsis, such as fear (Riccio et al., 2009), addictive behavior (Pomrenze et al., 2013), and tolerance to opioids (Chu et al., 2020) (**Table 2**). Thus, TRPC5 activity has been intimately associated to LTP

TABLE 3 | Rho GTPases regulated by TRP channels.

TRP Channel	Effect on Rho GTPase Regulation	Downstream Rho GTPase	Possible mechanism for GTPase modulation by TRP channel
TRPC3	Positive	Rac1 (Kitajima et al., 2011)	CaMKII-induced Rac1 GEF Tiam1 phosphorylation/activation*
TRPC5	Positive	Rac1 (Tian et al., 2010)	Interaction with SESTD1*
	Negative	Rhoa A (Tian et al., 2010)	Rac1 positive modulation, leading to RhoA inhibition*
TRPC6	Positive	RhoA (Singh et al., 2007; Tian et al., 2010; Jiang et al., 2011)	Calcineurin-dependent regulation of RhoA*
	Negative	Rac1 (Tian et al., 2010)	Downregulation of Rac1 GEF Tiam1 by TRPC6-mediated NMDA receptor inhibition*
TRPV1	Positive	RhoA (Li J. et al., 2015; Li et al., 2015a)	TRPV1-mediated Inhibition of AMPA receptor endocytosis*
TRPV2	Negative	Rac1/RhoA (Laragione et al., 2019)	PKA activation by TRPV2-driven cAMP increases, leading to RhoA inhibition*
TRPV4	Positive	RhoA (Zhao et al., 2018)	PKC-dependent RhoA activation (Brain endothelial cells, Zhao et al., 2018)
		Rac1 (Ou-Yang et al., 2018)	Increasing AKT phosphorylation levels (U87 glioma cells, Ou-Yang et al., 2018)
TRPM4	Positive	Rac1 (Cáceres et al., 2015)	Modulation of Ca^{2+} signals – Vm depolarization-dependent phosphatidylserine translocation*
TRPM7	Positive	RhoA, Rac1, CDC42 (Su et al., 2011)	RhoA: Modulation by p116RIP* Rac1: S1P1 activation through Mg^{2+} influx (Endothelial cells [Zhu et al., 2019])
TRPM8	Negative	RhoA (Sun et al., 2014)	Regulation of mitochondrial function and ROS production, leading to modulation of RhoA/ROCK (Vascular Smooth Muscle cells, Xiong et al., 2017)
TRPML1	Undetermined	Possible modulation of Rac1, Rac2, Cdc42 and RhoG	Interaction with Rac1, Rac2, Cdc42 and RhoG*

**Proposed mechanisms.*

modulation (Phelan et al., 2013), suggesting a participation on synaptic plasticity and in turn, on brain physiology and pathophysiology. The morphological changes mediated by TRPC5 overlap with Rho GTPases-dependent signaling, since this has also been related to structural modifications required for memory and learning (Diana et al., 2007). Thus, TRPC5 might promote structural dynamic changes through the modulation of Rho GTPases. Interestingly, enhanced Rac1 activity has been reported upon TRPC5 overexpression (Tian et al., 2010), although, the underlying mechanisms remain unclear. Interestingly, TRPC5 interacts with Rho GTPases modulators, such as SESTD1 (**Figure 2**) (Miehe et al., 2010). SESTD1 is a putative scaffold protein that diminishes dendritic spine density by abolishing the interaction between Rac1 and the Rac-GEF Trio8 (Lee C.C. et al., 2015). Nevertheless, it is not known whether this mechanism could affect the retraction or extension of dendritic spines. In this context, we suggest that SESTD1 interaction with TRPC5 might decrease its available levels to block the Rac1-Trio8 association, causing an indirect TRPC5-dependent increased Rac1 activity. This is consistent with the negative regulatory effect of TRPC5 on neurites growth as discussed above. Rac1 activity promotes the growth of neurites (Woo and Gomez, 2006). Therefore, a possible negative effect of TRPC5 upon neurite extension through Rac1 modulation seems paradoxical. However, it has been recently reported that either hypo or hyperactivity of Rac1 could lead to neuritogenesis impairment, giving arise to intellectual disability (Zamboni et al., 2018). On the other hand, TRPC5 interacts with CaMKII (Puram et al., 2011). This could be relevant since CaMKII is an activator of RhoA and Cdc42, leading to the induction of dendrites growth (Murakoshi et al., 2011). Consistently, TRPC5 promotes dendrite growth through CaMKII activity (He et al., 2012), suggesting that TRPC5 might control this process through CaMKII/RhoA/Cdc42 axis. As mentioned before, CaMKII is important for the production of LTP response (Lisman et al., 2012), which suggests a TRPC5 participation in processes related to memory and learning.

TRPC5 activity is also associated with cell viability. These channels have been proposed to exert either a protective role (Hong et al., 2020a) or promote neuronal loss depending on its PTM status in neurodegenerative disorders such as Huntington's disease (Hong et al., 2015). Moreover, TRPC5 promotes cell death induced by oxidative stress (Park et al., 2019) and excitotoxicity during epileptic seizures (Phelan et al., 2013). Dopamine D2 receptor (D2R) activity has been reported to enhance cell vulnerability by inducing neurite retraction and axon collapse *via* RhoA/ROCK activity (Deyts et al., 2009). TRPC5 interacts with D2R (**Figure 2**) (Hannan et al., 2008) and as such, TRPC5 channels might induce cell death in a RhoA-dependent manner, although this still needs to be determined. Interestingly, Rac1 activity is associated with cell death promotion during oxidative stress caused by neurovascular ischemia (Smith et al., 2017; Karabiyik et al., 2018). Moreover, Rac1 activity might also have a protective role in epileptic excitotoxicity (Posada-Duque et al., 2015). In contrast, RhoA activation has been linked to Ca^{2+}-dependent neuronal loss elicited by excitotoxicity (Semenova et al., 2007). This dichotomy between protective and degenerative roles of Rho GTPases upon ischemic injury has been widely reviewed elsewhere (Posada-Duque et al., 2014). As such, TRPC5 might have a dual participation in both dynamics of protrusive processes and neuronal death. These effects might depend on differential TRPC5-dependent spatiotemporal regulation of Rho

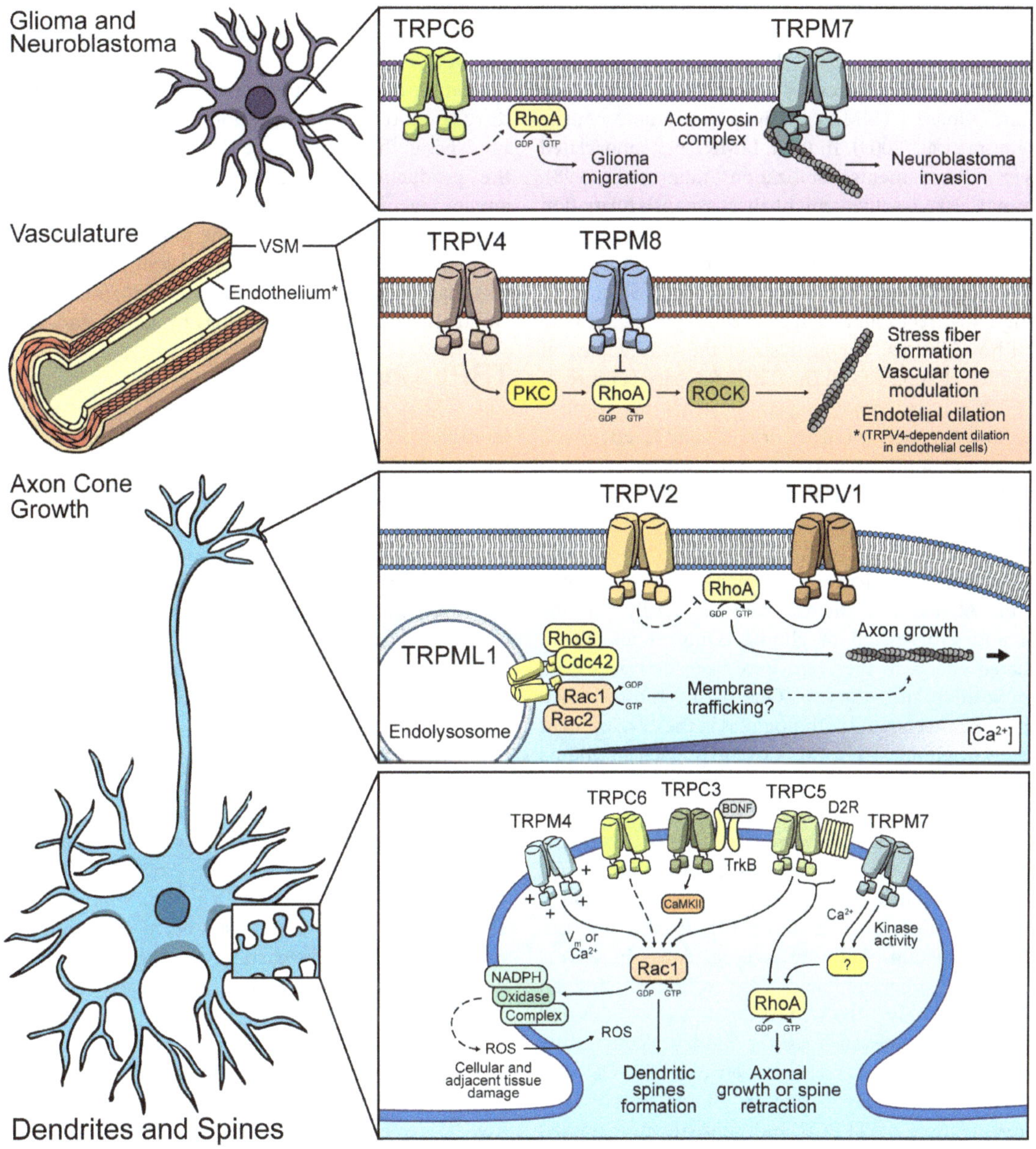

FIGURE 3 | Possible mechanisms of Rho GTPases modulation by TRP channels. Glia and Neuroblastoma: TRPC6 might modulate RhoA in glial cells, thus regulating cell migration. TRPM7 participates in neuroblastoma invasion. Vasculature: TRPV4 and TRPM8 display the opposite effect over RhoA. Both channels modulate vasculature tone. TRPV4 promotes endothelial dilation in a RhoA-dependent fashion. Axon cone: TRPML1-dependent regulation of protein trafficking *via* modulation of Rac1/Cdc42 might occur. TRPV1 promotes RhoA activity and modulates axonal growth. TRPV2 might have an inhibitory role of RhoA. Dendrites and spines: TRPM4, TRPC3, TRPC6, and TRPC5 might induce Rac1 activity, leading to dendritic spines formation. Under ischemic conditions, these channels might have a Rac1-dependent role in ROS production, leading to neuronal cell death. TRPM7 and TRPC5 are proposed to regulate RhoA, favoring the retraction of dendritic spines or axonal growth.

GTPases, a process that could be further analyzed with new tools to study more exactly ion channel-related spatiotemporal events.

TRPC6

TRPC6 shares close sequence and structural homology with TRPC3. TRPC6 can also be modulated by tyrosine kinase receptors and G protein-coupled receptors, being especially sensitive to activation by diacylglycerol (DAG) (Hofmann et al., 1999). TRPC6 is widely expressed in the peripheral nervous system (Riccio et al., 2002). TRPC6 is located in excitatory post-synaptic neurons and regulates the number of spines and spatial learning and memory (Zhou et al., 2008) *via* CaMKIV activation and CREB regulation, promoting both neurite and dendrite growth (Tai et al., 2008; Heiser et al., 2013). The transcription factor CREB is associated with the late phase of LTP. Its activation results in changes in gene expression that promote synapsis development and structural rearrangements (Frey et al., 1993; Nguyen et al., 1994). This suggests that TRPC6 contributes to the late phase of LTP. Interestingly, CaMKIV has been associated with actin cytoskeleton remodeling, since it regulates LIM Kinase 1 (LIMK1) activity to promote neurite growth (Takemura et al., 2009). In turn, LIMK1 phosphorylated cofilin to favor actin filaments stabilization (Yang et al., 1998). This suggests that TRPC6 activity might affect synapsis formation through the CaMKIV-LIMK1-cofilin pathway. Moreover, several reports suggest a protective role for TRPC6 from excitotoxicity by inhibiting NMDA receptor activity (Li et al., 2012; Shen et al., 2013). Although no direct interaction has been reported between TRPC6 and Rho GTPases, our analysis of the curated list of interactors of TRP channels from the TRIP database (**Figure 2**) reveals that TRPC6 interacts with several proteins that regulate Rho GTPases function such as Calcineurin (Ly and Cyert, 2017). Furthermore, several studies report the contribution of TRPC6 in RhoA regulation in non-excitable cells (Singh et al., 2007; Tian et al., 2010).

Similarly to TRPC3, TRPC6 has been involved in different brain disorders such as neuronal damage in stroke, Aβ-production in Alzheimer's disease and especially in the development and progression of glioma (Ding et al., 2010). TRPC6-mediated effects in the brain have been described as a mix between positive and negative. One of the most studied TRPC6-related roles in cerebral pathologies is in the development and progression of gliomas. TRPC6 is overexpressed in glioma samples compared to normal brain tissue. Additionally, its activity is essential for G2/M phase transition and glioma progression (Ding et al., 2010). Moreover, TRPC6 maintains the stability of HIF-1α in glioma cells under hypoxia (Li et al., 2015b) and mediates Notch-Driven glioblastoma growth and invasiveness (Chigurupati et al., 2010). In this context, the RhoA/ROCK signaling pathway is upregulated in glioma cells, promoting cell migration and proliferation (Zohrabian et al., 2009). Interestingly, RhoA/ROCK pathway is activated by TRPC6 in other tissues such as the kidney (Yang et al., 2013), suggesting that this relation between TRPC6 and RhoA/ROCK might also play a role in glioma progression. Moreover, upregulation of TRPC6 and subsequent increased Ca^{2+} influx in podocytes lead to an aberrant activation of focal adhesion kinase (FAK), which is necessary for focal adhesion assembly and disassembly in migratory cells (Nakuluri et al., 2019). RhoA activity can promote the activation of FAK (Al-Koussa et al., 2020), suggesting an additional mechanism for TRPC6-RhoA mediated tumoral progress in glioma (**Figure 3**). Although there are several possible mechanisms for TRPC6-mediated regulation of the RhoA/Rock pathway in glioma progression, this still needs to be confirmed in the context of this neoplastic disease.

As discussed above, TRPC6 also regulates several beneficial processes in the neurons such as survival, synaptogenesis, learning and memory, all of which are altered in Alzheimer's Disease (Feng, 2017). Overexpression of presenilin 2 and/or Alzheimer's-disease-related presenilin 2 variants, decreased TRPC6-mediated Ca^{2+} entry in HEK293 cells (Lessard et al., 2005). Moreover, TRPC6 expression and activity are diminished in neurons from Alzheimer's-disease patients. Also, pharmacological activation of TRPC6 inhibited the elevation of Aβ and phospho-tau in neurons of patients (Tao et al., 2020), indicating a possible protective role of TRPC6 in Alzheimer's-disease. Moreover, upregulation of Rac1 appears to be important in driving the progress of Alzheimer's-disease by promoting the production of the amyloid precursor protein and the amyloidogenic pathway (Aguilar et al., 2017). Importantly, loss of TRPC6 expression leads to the activation of Rac1 in the kidney (Tian et al., 2010), which suggests that the lower expression of this channel observed in the brain of Alzheimer's-disease patients could also promote the pathology by activating Rac1 (**Figure 3**).

TRPV Channels

The TRPV subfamily comprises six members, of which the temperature-sensitive TRPV1 is the founder and the most studied. TRPV1 was first described as an ion channel activated by the vanilloid capsaicin, which explains the name of the subfamily (Caterina et al., 1997, 1999; Güler et al., 2002). The members of the TRPV subfamily share a similar architecture. These channels contain an ankyrin-repeat domain (ARD) and follow six transmembrane helix domains in the amino-terminal region. Cytoplasmatic carboxyl-terminal contains the TRP domain and other binding sites for lipid regulators, all of them with a resolved structure (Yuan, 2019). In addition to the canonical role of TRPV channels in temperature and pain sensing, other functions have been attributed to these channels, wherein the regulation of Rho GTPases emerges. Other characteristics are described in **Table 1** and have been extensively summarized previously (Bevan et al., 2014; Garcia-Elias et al., 2014; Kojima and Nagasawa, 2014).

TRPV1

TRPV1 was the first and most studied member of the vanilloid subfamily of TRP ion channels (Caterina et al., 1997; Benítez-Angeles et al., 2020). TRPV1 can be activated by exogenous agonists such as capsaicin and resiniferatoxin (RTX) (Caterina et al., 1997), as well as high temperature (>42°C), pH and membrane potential changes (Caterina et al., 1997; Piper et al., 1999; Gunthorpe et al., 2000), mechanical forces (Ho et al., 2014), ROS (Starr et al., 2008), arachidonic acid (Chu et al., 2003), and endocannabinoids (Ross, 2003). Initial studies identified TRPV1 in sensory neurons, describing its participation in the regulation of pain transduction. TRPV1 is also expressed in brain cortex, hippocampus, cerebellum, substantia nigra, hypothalamus, midbrain, olfactory bulb and astrocytes (Mezey, 2000; Marinelli et al., 2003; Kim et al., 2005; Kim S.R. et al., 2006; Cavanaugh et al., 2011; Park et al., 2012; Nam et al., 2015). Interestingly, multiple studies associate TRPV1 activity to cytoskeleton remodeling, cellular migration (Ho et al., 2014; Miyake et al., 2015) and cell morphology (Goswami and Hucho, 2007; Goswami et al., 2007b; Li et al., 2015a). For example, mechanical stress-elicited TRPV1-dependent Ca^{2+} signals contribute to astrocyte migration (Ho et al., 2014). Also, mitochondrial TRPV1 enhances microglial cell migration (Miyake et al., 2015). Moreover, TRPV1 localizes in multiple dynamic structures of neurons such as the growth cone, neurites and axonal filopodia, displaying differential roles among these structures. TRPV1 activation results in rapid retraction of growth cones in sensory neurons dependent on microtubule depolymerization (Goswami et al., 2007b). Also, a recent study established that Ca^{2+} influx mediated by TRPV1 is necessary for NGF deprivation-induced axonal degeneration (Johnstone et al., 2019). Interestingly, RhoA activity is necessary for axonal growth cone collapsing and proper polarity establishment for axon guidance (Wu et al., 2005; Loudon et al., 2006). Furthermore, RhoA also controls microtubules protrusion during axonal growth (Dupraz et al., 2019). Importantly, mechanical stress-induced TRPV1 activity participates in guidance during neurite extension of spiral ganglion neurons in a RhoA/ROCK-dependent fashion (**Figure 3**) (Li et al., 2015a). Thus, along with its participation on microtubule dynamics, TRPV1-dependent modulation of RhoA-ROCK might also cooperate in guidance during axonal growth (**Figure 3**). Since Ca^{2+} is crucial for axon specification and outgrowth in CNS neurons (Davare et al., 2009; Nakamuta et al., 2011), these TRPV1-dependent proposed effects might occur in dorsal root ganglion (DRG) and CNS neurons as well, although further studies would be needed to confirm this.

TRPV1 regulates axonal filopodia formation, a key process for axonal branching (Spillane and Gallo, 2014). Interestingly, this process is not dependent on the conductive activity of the channel, but only on its C-terminal domain, which interacts with microtubules (Goswami et al., 2007a). TRPV1-induced filopodia resembles those formed upon ROCK and Myosin II inhibition (Loudon et al., 2006). These data contrast with the role of TRPV1 on the regulation of RhoA since this Rho-GTPase canonically inhibits axonal branching (Spillane and Gallo, 2014). We hypothesize that such discrepancy might be due to the structural features rather than the conductive activity of the TRPV1 channels on axon filopodia initiation, leading to a differential mechanism on cytoskeleton regulation.

The complex role of TRPV1 in the modulation of neuronal structures might be involved in neurodegenerative pathologies such as Alzheimer's disease. Indeed, a protective effect of TRPV1 in Alzheimer's disease has been reported (Balleza-Tapia et al., 2018; Du et al., 2020). One of the proposed mechanisms consists in TRPV1-mediated inhibition of the AMPA receptor endocytosis, which is a key modulator of spine development *via* GEF-H1 (Kim et al., 2004; Kang et al., 2009). Thus, TRPV1-dependent hampering of AMPAR endocytosis might be a putative mechanism for TRPV1 positive modulation of RhoA, thus contributing to the development of Alzheimer's disease (**Table 3**).

TRPV1 has also been proposed as a negative prognosis marker for glioblastoma (Nabissi et al., 2016), in which invasiveness is highly dependent on RhoA activity since it regulates several matrix metalloproteinases in this type of neoplasms (Al-Koussa et al., 2020). Nevertheless, further studies are needed to detail the participation of TRPV1 in the development of neoplastic pathologies associated with neuronal or glial cells in the brain.

TRPV2

TRPV2 is a member of the vanilloid subfamily of TRP ion channels that is activated by high temperatures (>52°C) (Caterina et al., 1999). TRPV2 is also activated by hypoosmolality (Muraki et al., 2003), cell stretching (Sugio et al., 2017) and chemical stimuli such as 2-aminoethoxydiphenyl borate (2-APB) (Hu et al., 2004), cannabinoids (Qin et al., 2008), and probenecid (Bang et al., 2007). TRPV2 is found in DRG neurons (Caterina et al., 1999), trigeminal motor nucleus (Park et al., 2011), hypothalamus and hindbrain regions (Wainwright et al., 2004; Nedungadi et al., 2012), and astrocytes (Shibasaki et al., 2013). TRPV2 localizes in subcellular domains enriched in filamentous actin, such as the growth cone, filopodia, lamellipodia and neurites, where interacts with soluble actin (Yadav and Goswami, 2019). Furthermore, inhibition of TRPV2 produces retraction of the growth cone (Yadav and Goswami, 2019) (unlike TRPV1), while its activation enhances axon outgrowth (Shibasaki et al., 2010) and growth cone motility (Sugio et al., 2017), along with inducing rapid membrane ruffling, changes in lamellipodial and filopodial dynamics, and rapid translocation of leading edges during neuritogenesis (Yadav and Goswami, 2019). Although the downstream signaling pathway of TRPV2 activity has not been elucidated yet, TRPV2 induces an increase in the cAMP levels in neurites and their branching points (Yadav and Goswami, 2019). TRPV2-dependent increase of cAMP leads to PKA activation, which inhibits RhoA (**Figure 3**) (Ellerbroek et al., 2003; Oishi et al., 2012). Therefore, the remodeling effect on the actin cytoskeleton by TRPV2 activity might be through modulation of the Rho GTPase family *via* cAMP/PKA (Howe, 2004) (**Table 3**). Given this data, we hypothesize that these mechanisms might lead to a TRPV2-dependent inhibition of the growth cone retraction. Further studies are needed to determine these mechanisms. Furthermore, PKA activates Rac1 (Goto et al., 2011) and Cdc42 (Leemhuis et al., 2004), crucial proteins for the formation of lamellipodia and filopodia, respectively. Moreover, both GTPases activate PAK1 to promote the axonal growth cone (Toriyama et al., 2013). Thus, these Rho GTPases might also be molecular targets that explain the effects of TRPV2 activity on lamellipodia and filopodia dynamics.

TRPV4

TRPV4 is a major regulator of muscle- and endothelium-dependent vascular tone in blood vessels from multiple organs such as the intestine, lungs and brain (White et al., 2016). TRPV4 responds to shear stress and lipids, such as arachidonic acid and epoxyeicosatrienoic (EET) acid (White et al., 2016), which are essential vasoactive substances required for vascular dilation/contraction (Sudhahar et al., 2010). The participation of TRPV4 in the modulation of brain vessels is related to the activity of the channel in endothelial cells (White et al., 2016) and vascular smooth muscle cells (Chan et al., 2019). For instance, chronic cerebral hypoperfusion produces a myogenic tone decrease of brain parenchymal arterioles, an effect that was not observed in $TRPV4^{-/-}$ mice (Chan et al., 2019). Additionally, TRPV4 loss-of-function is associated with diminished endothelial dilation, decreased cerebral perfusion and impaired cognitive function in aged rats (Diaz-Otero et al., 2019). Moreover, TRPV4 promotes PKC-dependent RhoA activation, leading to stress fibers formation during internal cerebral hemorrhage (ICH) in endothelial cells (**Table 2** and **Figure 3**), presumably by ROCK activation and MLCP inhibition (Zhao et al., 2018). TRPV4 inhibition ameliorates damage produced by ICH, suggesting that TRPV4 promotes blood brain barrier disruption in ICH conditions by inducing the formation of endothelial intercellular gaps in a way that involves RhoA activation and stress fiber formation (Zhao et al., 2018). Long-range Ca^{2+} signals caused by Ca^{2+}-Induced Ca^{2+} Release (CICR) induce RhoA activation after neurotrophin-3 treatment (Takano et al., 2017). TRPV4 promotes CICR in neurons in ICH model, most likely by regulating the IP_3R (Shen et al., 2019). Moreover, the interplay between TRPV4 and IP_3R also occurs at astrocytes endfeet, where TRPV4-dependent Ca^{2+} entry induces Ca^{2+} oscillations mediated by IP_3R, leading to neurovascular coupling and vasodilation (Dunn et al., 2013). In this regard, we propose that the propagation of Ca^{2+} waves in these cells might contribute to RhoA's spatiotemporal regulation and subsequent cytoskeleton remodeling.

TRPV4 promotes Rac1 activity in glioblastoma U87 cells leading to increased cell migration through TRPV4-dependent Akt phosphorylation/activation (Ou-Yang et al., 2018) (**Table 3**). Akt activation induces the phosphorylation of the Rac1 GEF Tiam1, which promotes Rac1 activation, driving tumorigenesis (Zhu et al., 2015). In this context, CaMKII has been shown to phosphorylate Akt in ovarian (Gocher et al., 2017) and prostate cancer cells (Schmitt et al., 2012). Thus, local Ca^{2+} signals elicited by these ion channels might promote Ca^{2+}/CaM binding to CaMK II, leading to Akt-mediated Rac1 activation through Tiam1, suggesting participation of TRPV4-mediated Rac1 regulation in glioblastoma progression.

TRPM Channels

Eight members of this subfamily have been identified. These channels have differential ion selectivity between their members. For instance, TRPM4 and TRPM5 are monovalent cationic channels (Launay et al., 2002; Hofmann et al., 2003), while TRPM7 and TRPM8 mediate divalent cationic (Nadler et al., 2001) and non-selective cationic currents (McKemy et al., 2002). TRPM channels share a Melastatin homology region (MHR) domain located at the amino-terminal region, a transmembrane domain similar to other TRP members, and a versatile carboxyl-terminal that varies between the TRPM members. For instance, TRPM7 contains a functional α-kinase domain in the carboxyl-terminal (Nadler et al., 2001), while TRPM4 and TRPM8 possess coiled-coil domains and binding motifs for different regulatory molecules (Fleig and Penner, 2004). The structures of all the TRPM channels discussed in this review have been recently described (Huang et al., 2020). Thus, the TRPM subfamily is a highly versatile subgroup of TRP channels, due to the particular structures and biophysical properties (Fleig and Penner, 2004). TRPM features have been summarized in **Table 1** and extensively reviewed (Fleig and Penner, 2004; Huang et al., 2020).

TRPM4

TRPM4 is activated by intracellular Ca^{2+} increases (Venkatachalam and Montell, 2007), but, unlike other members of the TRP family, TRPM4 (along with TRPM5) is only permeable to monovalent ions. Despite that, TRPM4 regulates Ca^{2+} signals in different cell types, such as fibroblasts (Cáceres et al., 2015), mastocytes (Shimizu et al., 2009), dendritic cells (Barbet et al., 2008), and lymphocytes (Launay et al., 2004). TRPM4 expression has been described in hypothalamus (Teruyama et al., 2011), hippocampal CA1 area (Menigoz et al., 2016), preBötzinger nucleus (Picardo et al., 2019), and medial prefrontal cortex (Riquelme et al., 2018). Interestingly, TRPM4 increases Rac1 activity in MEF cells (Cáceres et al., 2015). Even though, the Ca^{2+}-permeable ion channels regulated by TRPM4 that could explain changes in Ca^{2+} oscillations have not been identified yet, functional association between NMDA receptors and TRPM4 in postsynaptic dendrites of CA1 hippocampal neurons has been shown (Menigoz et al., 2016). Indeed, TRPM4 activity-mediated postsynaptic depolarization allows proper lifting of Mg^{2+} block from the NMDA receptor, leading to an increased Ca^{2+} entry and initiation of LTP (Menigoz et al., 2016). Moreover, glutamatergic excitotoxicity is decreased in TRPM4$^{-/-}$ mice, further suggesting a functional interaction between NMDA and TRPM4 (Schattling et al., 2012). Interestingly, Ca^{2+} entry mediated by NMDA receptors, and subsequent CaMKII-dependent Tiam1 phosphorylation, induces dendritic/spine development (Tolias et al., 2005). Thus, interplay between TRPM4 and NMDA receptors might be important in Rac1-dependent neuronal plasticity. Other possible mechanisms for Rac1 regulation by TRPM4 could be the regulation of local changes in membrane potential. For instance, voltage-gated Na^+ channel Nav1.5 has been proposed to promote Rac1 activity by producing membrane potential depolarization in breast cancer cells (Yang et al., 2020). Nav1.5-induced membrane potential depolarization causes Rac1 activation by promoting local redistribution of phosphatidylserine, an anionic phospholipid to which Rac1 binds, and known to be important for its activation (Finkielstein et al., 2006; Yang et al., 2020). Interestingly, TRPM4 facilitates cellular depolarization in bone marrow-derived mast cells (BMMC) (Vennekens et al., 2007), HeLa (Simon et al., 2010), and HEK293 cells (Fliegert et al., 2007). Thus, local changes in membrane potential mediated by TRPM4 might induce local phospholipid redistribution and Rac1 activation (**Figure 3**).

TRPM4 participates on damage caused by ischemic stroke (Leiva-Salcedo et al., 2017; Chen et al., 2019) and spinal cord injury (Gerzanich et al., 2009). Importantly, TRPM4 inhibition and silencing improves outcome of both spine cord injury (Gerzanich et al., 2009) and ischemic stroke (Loh et al., 2014; Chen et al., 2019). TRPM4 induces cellular swelling leading to neuronal cell death as a consequence of excessive Na^+ influx mediated by these channels (Gerzanich et al., 2009; Simon et al., 2010; Leiva-Salcedo et al., 2017). Interestingly, Rac1 participates in NADPH oxidase assembly (Acevedo and González-Billault, 2018). Moreover, increased activity of Rac1 induces ROS production by promoting the activation of the NADPH catalytic subunit, Nox2 (Stankiewicz and Linseman, 2014). This enzyme has been proposed as a potential ischemic stroke therapeutic target (Zhang et al., 2016). Consistently, Rac1 downregulation, similar to TRPM4 inhibition, leads to a protective effect in the hippocampal CA1 region and cortex in ischemia/stroke models (Raz et al., 2010) and after permanent middle cerebral artery occlusion (Karabiyik et al., 2018). Given that TRPM4 activity might lead to an increase in Rac1 activity, we hypothesize that an additional mechanism by which this channel could collaborate with brain and vascular tissue-damaging, alongside oncotic cell death induction, is by promoting an increase in Nox2-dependent ROS production *via* Rac1 activation (**Figure 3**). Although this mechanism is only inferred, the suggested evidence makes it an interesting possible new approach to understanding TRPM4-mediated GTPase regulation's role in brain neuropathologies.

TRPM7

TRPM7 is a member of the TRP family that permeates both Ca^{2+} and Mg^{2+}. In addition, this channel has an active kinase domain in their carboxyl-terminal domain (Sun et al., 2015). TRPM7 is widely expressed in the human and mouse brain, with reports in animal models showing equivalent levels in neurons, astrocytes and microglia (Ratnam et al., 2018). TRPM7 localizes in the growth cone of hippocampal neurons, restricting the elongation of primary axons (Turlova et al., 2016). Interestingly, TRPM7 associates with several elements of cytoskeletal structures. For instance, mass spectrometry-based analyses revealed the interaction of TRPM7 with actin and α-actinin-1 (Turlova et al., 2016). Moreover, analysis of the TRPM7-associated interactome in neuroblastoma cells (**Figure 2**) identified proteins which were mainly related to the actin cytoskeleton, such as Myosin IIA, Drebrin and the Myosin phosphatase Rho-interacting protein (p116RIP) (Middelbeek et al., 2016). p116RIP is a modulator of the RhoA/ROCK axis (Koga and Ikebe, 2005), a key pathway that promotes invasion and metastasis of tumor cells (O'Connor and Chen, 2013). This suggests a role for TRPM7 in aggressive phenotypes in neuroblastoma cells *via* p116RIP-mediated RhoA/ROCK regulation and subsequent changes in cytoskeleton dynamics. Also, a functional coupling between TRPM7 and RhoA activation dependent on the TRPM7 kinase activity on hepatocellular carcinoma has been shown (Voringer et al., 2020). These data support a TRPM7-mediated RhoA activation involvement in diverse processes such as the inhibition of axonal growth cone and the migratory phenotype of brain tumor cells like neuroblastoma (**Figure 3**).

Several reports suggest that TRPM7 is a key mediator of neuronal death after ischemia/reperfusion episodes. TRPM7 knock-down in CA1 protected neurons from ischemia-induced cell death as well as maintained neuronal morphology and function (Sun et al., 2009). Moreover, TRPM7 blockage by carvacrol prevented brain damage in a mouse hypoxia-ischemia brain injury model (Chen et al., 2015). TRPM7 silencing leads to a decreased activity of RhoA (Su et al., 2011). This might be important in the context of ischemic damage since RhoA is upregulated in the brains of human stroke patients (Brabeck et al., 2003). The RhoA/ROCK pathway is key to determining neuronal cell death following ischemia/reperfusion events (Shin et al., 2008). This suggests that one of the mechanisms by which TRPM7 might be producing its pathological effect after ischemia/reperfusion is through the activation of RhoA. However, further studies into this association will help clarify this suggested relationship and find additional mediators.

Mg^{2+} permeability of TRPM7 is a particularity among the TRP family. A misbalance in the homeostasis of this ion has been involved in several pathological processes in the brain (Sun et al., 2015). TRPM7-mediated increases of Mg^{2+} intracellular concentration promotes endothelial cell proliferation and enhances the endothelial barrier integrity of the brain. This is due to induced cytoskeletal reorganization and expression of tight junction proteins such as VE-cadherin, occludin, and zonula occludens-1 (ZO-1) (Zhu et al., 2019). Interestingly, TRPM7 achieves this through the activation of S1P1, which in turn activates Rac1 (Zhu et al., 2019). This suggests that the TRPM7-mediated Mg^{2+} influx might play an important role in cerebral vasculature pathologies by regulating the S1P1-Rac1 pathway.

TRPM8

TRPM8 is a non-selective cation channel, which preferably permeates Ca^{2+} (McKemy et al., 2002). TRPM8 has a polymodal gating and is activated by cold and different cooling compounds, such as menthol and icilin (McKemy et al., 2002). Several single nucleotide polymorphisms (SNPs) related to the TRPM8 gene are associated with either the risk (Ling et al., 2019) or protection (Gavva et al., 2019) from migraines. Although the exact mechanisms are unknown, a possible mechanism for TRPM8-mediated risk of migraine headaches might be related to this channel's role in vasoconstriction regulation, which has been related to migraine development (Jacobs and Dussor, 2016). Interestingly, TRPM8 activation by menthol promoted vasodilation by inhibiting Ca^{2+} signaling-mediated RhoA/ROCK activation in mesenteric arteries (**Figure 3**) (Sun et al., 2014). In this regard, the RhoA/ROCK axis inhibition might lead to Myosin Light Chain Phosphatase (MLCP) activation and LIM Kinase 1 inhibition, resulting in an inhibition of the contraction of mesenteric arteries (Shimokawa et al., 2016). Furthermore, TRPM8 can function as an ER Ca^{2+} channel, regulating mitochondrial function and ROS production, which activates the RhoA/ROCK pathway (Xiong et al., 2017) (**Table 3**). Thus, TRPM8-dependent vascular tone modulation through the RhoA/ROCK axis regulation might play an important role. These mechanisms might not only be relevant in the development of migraines but also the progress of other cerebral vasogenic events such as reversible vasoconstriction syndromes.

Recent reports have associated alterations in TRPM8 expression with brain-related cancers. Moreover, TRPM8 was significantly overexpressed in glioblastoma tissue samples compared to normal tissue and its expression correlated with worse prognosis and survival in glioblastoma patients (Zeng et al., 2019). Also, TRPM8 was highly expressed in glioblastoma cell lines and its expression correlated with higher invasive and proliferative capacities (Zeng et al., 2019). In this context, TRPM8-mediated regulation of RhoA/ROCK might be responsible for the pro-tumoral effect of TRPM8, as the RhoA/ROCK pathway has been involved in the proliferation and migration of glioblastoma cells (Fortin Ensign et al., 2013). These data support a role for TRPM8 in diverse aspects of brain pathophysiology, including some that are more particular to this channel. Thus, more studies into the exact proteins mediating TRPM8-mediated RhoA/ROCK activation might be interesting to elucidate its precise role.

TRPML1

The Mucolipin-TRP (TRPML) subfamily are monovalent and divalent cation channels with predominant Ca^{2+} permeability (Peng et al., 2020) (see **Table 1**), although other permeabilities has been described to be important in their function (Dong et al., 2008). Contrary to other TRP subfamilies, these channels are particularly located in endolysosomal vesicles (Manzoni et al., 2004). Consistently, TRPML channels are associated with cellular processes such as vesicle trafficking and endolysosomal-dependent degradation pathways (Cheng et al., 2010). Structurally, these channels have full-length subunits of about 600 amino acids, thus being the smaller members of TRP channel subfamily. As to the other TRP channels, these channels have six transmembrane segments with pore-forming regions located between segments S5 and S6. In addition, amino- and carboxyl-terminal regions have cytoplasmatic orientation (Hellmich and Gaudet, 2014). Moreover, these channels have canonical EF-hand domains at their carboxyl-terminal domain, which allows direct Ca^{2+}-dependent activity modulation (Hellmich and Gaudet, 2014). TRPML activity is positively modulated by PIP_2 binding, which drives to channel activation (Dong et al., 2010). Interestingly, the resolved structure of TRPML1 indicates that its unique PIP_2-binding site is distinct to the reported in others TRP channels (Fine et al., 2018) (**Table 1**).

TRPML1 (also called Mucolipin-1) is an intracellular TRP channel located predominantly in endolysosomal membranes (Lee J.H. et al., 2015). Loss-of-function mutations reported in the TRPML1-encoding gene have been linked to a lysosomal storage disorder known as Mucolipidosis type IV (MLIV). This pathology is one of the first described neurological diseases caused by mutations in TRP channels (Bargal et al., 2000). MLIV is characterized by an early neurodevelopmental delay and a late neurodegenerative phenotype that leads to intellectual disability, delayed psychomotor abilities and retinal abnormalities (as described in OMIM #252650). Although the pathophysiological signs are well known, the cellular mechanisms involved in this disease remain unclear. TRPML1 modulates several aspects of membrane trafficking, particularly participating in trafficking of late endosome vesicles, and controlling the size (Cao et al., 2017), function and biogenesis of lysosomes (Wang et al., 2015). Moreover, TRPML1 regulates lysosome fusion with secretory vesicles, increasing exocytosis (Park et al., 2016). Interestingly, not only a disturbance in membrane trafficking but also lipid accumulation and loss of cell viability have been described as hallmarks of MLIV disorder (Wang et al., 2013), suggesting that TRPML1 loss-of-function might contribute in all these pathological alterations. However, detailed mechanisms by which TRPML1 regulates these processes are poorly understood. Rho GTPases are signaling nodes that coordinate membrane trafficking and lipid homeostasis (reviewed in Ridley, 2001; Olayioye et al., 2019). TRPML1 interactome reports (**Figure 2**) might reveal the mechanisms related to the coordination of cellular processes that lead to the neuropathological phenotype observed in MLIV (Krogsaeter et al., 2019). TRPML1 interacts and colocalizes with Rho GTPases, such as Rac1, Rac2, Cdc42 and RhoG (Spooner et al., 2013). Therefore, these data strongly suggest that TRPML1 might regulate the activity of Rho GTPases and, in this manner, control membrane trafficking (**Figure 3**). Thus, regulating TRPML1 activity might be an effective therapeutic approach for the treatment of other neurological disorders where low TRPML1 activity has been reported, such as ALS (Tedeschi et al., 2019), Parkinson disease (Tsunemi et al., 2019), Alzheimer's Disease (Zhang et al., 2017), and Niemann-Pick disease (Shen et al., 2012). Nevertheless, further studies are needed to determine the specific role of TRPML1-dependent Rho GTPases modulation in these neuropathological conditions and the proteins involved in this relationship.

OUTSTANDING QUESTIONS AND FUTURE DIRECTIONS

Despite extensive evidence on the role of the canonical Rho proteins (RhoA/Rac1/Cdc42) in different neuronal processes and their possible modulation by TRP channels activity presented in this work, little is known about other Rho GTPase members. A limited number of studies have shown the participation of RhoF/RhoD (RhoF/Rif, RhoD) (Zanata et al., 2002; Fan et al., 2015) and atypical Rho GTPases (Aspenström et al., 2007) such as Rnd (Rnd1, Rnd2, and Rnd3/RhoE) (Ishikawa et al., 2003, 2006; Heng et al., 2008; Pacary et al., 2013), RhoU/RhoV (Wrch1, Chp/Wrch2) (Alan et al., 2018) and RhoBTB (RhoBTB3 and RhoBTB2) (Ramos et al., 2002) in neuronal processes. However, these proteins play an important role in developmental synaptogenic stage (Ishikawa et al., 2003), growth cone turning and collapse (Zanata et al., 2002), neurite formation (Tian et al., 2017) and retraction (Fan et al., 2015), axon guidance (Alan et al., 2018), cortical neuron migration (Heng et al., 2008; Tian et al., 2017), and neurogenesis (Pacary et al., 2013). Although no studies indicating that TRP channels regulate these Rho GTPase subfamilies, it has been reported that NFAT1c increases RND1 transcription (Suehiro et al., 2014) and rapid activation and translocation of NFAT to the nucleus is promoted by TRPV1 activity in sensory neurons (Kim and Usachev, 2009). Conversely, Rif has been established as a regulator of cytoskeletal rearrangements mediated by semaphorins (Tian et al., 2017). TRPC5 acts downstream of semaphorin signaling to cause neuronal growth cone morphology (Kaczmarek et al., 2012). These antecedents suggest that both TRP channels and atypical Rho GTPase activity could be involved in the different processes mentioned above. However, more studies need to be performed.

Regarding the discussion raised in this review, the TRP family of ion channels and Rho GTPases are functionally linked to each other due to; (1) mutual cellular functions whose deregulation leads to neuropathological phenomena and (2) Rho GTPases activity modulation by TRP channels. However, spatiotemporal features of TRP channel activity, and how these features could regulate Rho GTPase are still not clear.

TRP-associated interactome suggests that these channels associate with different Rho GTPases-related proteins (Shin et al., 2011) (**Figure 2**). This allows us to hypothesize a potential role for TRP channels as transduction hubs, implying local recruitment of Rho GTPases modulators and spatially delimited Rho GTPases activation/inhibition in subcellular structures. Moreover, Rho GTPases are mainly activated by Ca^{2+} signaling in neurons (Saneyoshi and Hayashi, 2012). Ca^{2+}-sensitive proteins such as the Ca^{2+}/CaM complex play an essential role in Rho GTPase activity modulation (Buchanan et al., 2000; Vidal-Quadras et al., 2011). Differential TRP-CaM binding affinities could lead to subtle changes in the local activity of Ca^{2+}/CaM-dependent proteins, such as CaMKs activation and subsequent Rho GTPases modulation (Wayman et al., 2011; Bossuyt and Bers, 2013). Conversely, TRP channels interaction with downstream targets of Rho GTPases suggests that these channels can be regulated by these proteins. Accordingly, Rho GTPases participate in the regulation of TRP channels trafficking and activity (Bezzerides et al., 2004; Puntambekar et al., 2005). Thus, TRP channels can regulate Rho GTPases and *viceversa*, suggesting a regulatory feedback loop between these proteins.

However, our research demonstrates that the relationship between TRP ion channels and Rho GTPases is not always positive (**Figure 3**). For instance, TRPM8 activation induces RhoA inhibition, while other members like TRPM7 and TRPC5 promote the activity of this Rho GTPase. We reasoned that multiple aspects contribute to establishing the relation between the respective TRP channel and Rho GTPase. Interactome and subcellular localization of both proteins and the biophysics properties of the channel might explain these differences. As we reviewed, most of the TRP channels that regulate Rac1 in neuronal context are localized in the same subcellular compartments (**Figure 3**).

Nevertheless, the proposed mechanisms for the regulation of Rac1 are different, which might be due to each TRP channel's differential interacting partners (**Figure 2**). A combination of complementary approaches to obtain a more global picture of the TRP channels-Rho GTPases network is needed to address this. The following section proposes some strategies to understand better the relationship between TRP ion channels and Rho GTPases.

Signaling mechanisms, such as those proposed above, often involve transient PPIs among regulatory components, which might represent a challenge for their identification due to the limited interaction time or low affinity of each interacting partners (Westermarck et al., 2013). Multiple proteomic approaches have emerged as alternatives to overcome these limitations (Bludau and Aebersold, 2020). These novel approaches could provide new possibilities to identify TRP/Rho GTPases PPIs pathways and give hints of the microdomains where these complexes localize.

Rho GTPases regulation by GEF/GAP/GDI is far more complex than a single GEF or GAP regulating only one Rho GTPase. Promiscuous activity has been reported for GEFs and GAPs, modulating more than one Rho GTPase (Bagci et al., 2020), increasing the complexity of the TRP-dependent modulation of these proteins. Proteomic studies may allow identification of GEFs/GAPs and GDIs implicated in Rho GTPases regulation by TRP channels. Complementing these approaches with assays for describing spatiotemporal dynamics will grant a more accurate characterization of the mechanisms involved in the TRP-dependent regulation of Rho GTPases and their role in neuropathological disorders. This will ultimately contribute to the designing of potential new interventions based on the TRP modulation of Rho GTPases. For instance, diverse strategies have been designed to monitor Rho GTPases activity through different means, such as biochemical approaches (Ren et al., 1999) and Förster Resonance Energy Transfer (FRET)-based sensors. The latter provides the possibility of performing *in vivo* tracking of GTPase activity (Kraynov et al., 2000; Pertz et al., 2006) and several authors have reviewed and corroborated its usefulness (Pertz, 2010; Schaefer et al., 2014). Recently, novel techniques to manipulate Rho GTPases have been designed. For instance, light-inducible sensors which promote RhoA (Wagner and Glotzer, 2016; Oakes et al., 2017) and Rac1 (Wu et al., 2009) translocation to the plasma membrane and subsequent activation. These tools might provide local and temporal inducible activation of Rho GTPases. Importantly, the application of these tools to the structures of TRP channels might also serve to define the role of these channels in the local and temporal regulation of Rho GTPases.

Another critical issue to study Rho GTPases regulation by TRP channels is the identification of Ca^{2+} as an intermediary in these pathways. Since local and broad Ca^{2+} waves have a differential effect on the modulation of Rho GTPases, the establishment of the spatiotemporal features of Ca^{2+} dynamics is necessary to strengthen what we know about these mechanisms. In this regard, fluorescent Ca^{2+} indicators derived from organic compounds provide information about the time-scale properties of Ca^{2+} waves but lack in providing accurate spatial information (Russell, 2011). Accordingly, genetically-encoded Ca^{2+} sensors provide an opportunity to study the time-scale and spatial distribution of Ca^{2+} signals, since they have been designed to monitor Ca^{2+} signals from intracellular organelles accurately (Bassett and Monteith, 2017). This approach has been used on neuronal models (Chen et al., 2012; O'Donnell et al., 2016), and even in the whole brain of living animals (Scott et al., 2018). These approaches, combined with biosensors to track the activity of Rho GTPases and its regulators, could provide novel and valuable information about the mechanisms involved in TRP channels-mediated regulation of Rho GTPases in physiological and pathophysiological brain conditions.

CONCLUDING REMARKS

The study of neurological and neuropsychiatric diseases has been linked to tumoral growth, cell death and loss of cellular structures, such as dendritic spines and axonal processes. In this context, ion channels are essential in cell physiology, as the loss- or gain-of-function of these proteins trigger structural abnormalities and neuropathological conditions. TRP channels have emerged as novel candidates for the treatment of numerous CNS-affecting diseases. Thus, further knowledge of the mechanisms by which TRP channels exert their effects on cellular physiology constitutes an outstanding question. Herein, we exposed evidence and shared arguments and ideas that support general mechanisms by which TRP channels might modulate Rho GTPases in the brain. Although the evidence is strong enough to suggest several pathways, further studies are required to confirm the functional nature of these interactions. Future approaches considering quantitative proteomic analysis of TRP channels and Rho GTPases will reveal common partners that could mediate their functional relationship. Moreover, studies incorporating simultaneous analysis of localization, interaction, dynamic activity of Rho GTPases, TRP channels, and or GEFs/GAPs/GDIs will be required to determine the spatiotemporal features of these mechanisms. This new evidence would contribute to designing novel strategies based on the fine-tuning of transduction mechanisms involved in TRP-modulated processes, providing new therapeutic alternatives to overcome neuropathological conditions.

AUTHOR CONTRIBUTIONS

BL, PC, IS, OO-S, MPS, and OC wrote the manuscript. All the authors contributed to the article and approved the submitted version.

ACKNOWLEDGMENTS

We thank Mr. Diego Morales for illustration editing. We are grateful to Dr. Mónica Cáceres for discussion and critical comments on the manuscript.

REFERENCES

Acevedo, A., and González-Billault, C. (2018). Crosstalk between Rac1-mediated actin regulation and ROS production. *Free Radic. Biol. Med.* 116, 101–113. doi: 10.1016/j.freeradbiomed.2018.01.008

Aguilar, B. J., Zhu, Y., and Lu, Q. (2017). Rho GTPases as therapeutic targets in Alzheimer's disease. *Alzheimer's Res. Ther.* 9, 1–10. doi: 10.2174/156800906775471752

Alan, J. K., Robinson, S. K., Magsig, K. L., Demarco, R. S., and Lundquist, E. A. (2018). The atypical rho GTPase CHW-1 Works with SAX-3/Robo To mediate axon guidance in *Caenorhabditis elegans*. *G3 (Bethesda)* 8, 1885–1895. doi: 10.1534/g3.118.200148

Al-Koussa, H., Atat, O. E., Jaafar, L., Tashjian, H., and El-Sibai, M. (2020). The role of rho gtpases in motility and invasion of glioblastoma cells. *Anal. Cell. Pathol.* 2020, 1–9. doi: 10.1155/2020/9274016

Amaral, M. D., and Pozzo-Miller, L. (2007). TRPC3 channels are necessary for brain-derived neurotrophic factor to activate a nonselective cationic current and to induce dendritic spine formation. *J. Neurosci.* 27, 5179–5189. doi: 10.1523/jneurosci.5499-06.2007

Ambudkar, I. S., and Ong, H. L. (2007). Organization and function of TRPC channelosomes. *Pflugers Arch.Eur. J. Physiol.* 455, 187–200. doi: 10.1007/s00424-007-0252-0

Aspenström, P., Ruusala, A., and Pacholsky, D. (2007). Taking Rho GTPases to the next level: the cellular functions of atypical Rho GTPases. *Exp. Cell Res.* 313, 3673–3679. doi: 10.1016/j.yexcr.2007.07.022

Bagal, S. K., Brown, A. D., Cox, P. J., Omoto, K., Owen, R. M., Pryde, D. C., et al. (2013). Ion channels as therapeutic targets: a drug discovery perspective. *J. Med. Chem.* 56, 593–624.

Bagci, H., Sriskandarajah, N., Robert, A., Boulais, J., Elkholi, I. E., Tran, V., et al. (2020). Mapping the proximity interaction network of the Rho-family GTPases reveals signalling pathways and regulatory mechanisms. *Nat. Cell Biol.* 22, 120–134. doi: 10.1038/s41556-019-0438-7

Bai, Y., Xiang, X., Liang, C., and Shi, L. (2015). Regulating Rac in the nervous system: molecular function and disease implication of Rac GEFs and GAPs. *BioMed Res. Int.* 2015:632450.

Balleza-Tapia, H., Crux, S., Andrade-Talavera, Y., Dolz-Gaiton, P., Papadia, D., Chen, G., et al. (2018). TrpV1 receptor activation rescues neuronal function and network gamma oscillations from Aβ-induced impairment in mouse hippocampus in vitro. *eLife* 7, 1–24.

Bang, S., Kim, K. Y., Yoo, S., Lee, S. H., and Hwang, S. W. (2007). Transient receptor potential V2 expressed in sensory neurons is activated by probenecid. *Neurosci. Lett.* 425, 120–125. doi: 10.1016/j.neulet.2007.08.035

Barbet, G. T., Demion, M., Moura, I. C., Serafini, N., Léger, T., Vrtovsnik, F. O., et al. (2008). The calcium-activated nonselective cation channel TRPM4 is essential for the migration but not the maturation of dendritic cells. *Nat. Immunol.* 9, 1148–1156. doi: 10.1038/ni.1648

Bargal, R., Avidan, N., Ben-Asher, E., Olender, Z., Zeigler, M., Frumkin, A., et al. (2000). Identification of the gene causing mucolipidosis type IV. *Nat. Genet.* 26, 118–121. doi: 10.1038/79095

Bassett, J. J., and Monteith, G. R. (2017). Genetically encoded calcium indicators as probes to assess the role of calcium channels in disease and for high-throughput drug discovery. *Adv. Pharmacol.* 79, 141–171. doi: 10.1016/bs.apha.2017.01.001

Becker, E. B. E. (2017). From mice to men: TRPC3 in cerebellar ataxia. *Cerebellum* 16, 877–879. doi: 10.1007/s12311-015-0663-y

Becker, E. B. E., Oliver, P. L., Glitsch, M. D., Banks, G. T., Achillic, F., Hardy, A., et al. (2009). A point mutation in TRPC3 causes abnormal Purkinje cell development and cerebellar ataxia in moonwalker mice. *Proce. Natl. Acad. Sci. U.S.A.* 106, 6706–6711. doi: 10.1073/pnas.0810599106

Benítez-Angeles, M., Morales-Lázaro, S. L., Juárez-González, E., and Rosenbaum, T. (2020). TRPV1: structure, endogenous agonists, and mechanisms. *Int. J. Mol. Sci.* 21, 1–18. doi: 10.1016/b978-0-08-025488-3.50006-4

Bevan, S., Quallo, T., and Andersson, D. A. (2014). TRPV1. *Handb. Exp. Pharmacol.* 222, 207–245.

Bezzerides, V. J., Ramsey, I. S., Kotecha, S., Greka, A., and Clapham, D. E. (2004). Rapid vesicular translocation and insertion of TRP channels. *Nat. Cell Biol.* 6, 709–720. doi: 10.1038/ncb1150

Bludau, I., and Aebersold, R. (2020). Proteomic and interactomic insights into the molecular basis of cell functional diversity. *Nat. Rev. Mol. Cell Biol.* 21, 327–340. doi: 10.1038/s41580-020-0231-2

Bollimuntha, S., Pani, B., and Singh, B. B. (2017). Neurological and motor disorders: neuronal store-operated Ca(2+) signaling: an overview and its function. *Adv. Exp. Med. Biol.* 993, 535–556. doi: 10.1007/978-3-319-57732-6_27

Bos, J., Rehmann, H., and Wittinghofer, A. (2007). GEFs and GAPs: critial elements in the control of small G proteins. *Cell* 129, 865–877. doi: 10.1016/j.cell.2007.05.018

Bossuyt, J., and Bers, D. M. (2013). Visualizing CaMKII and CaM activity: a paradigm of compartmentalized signaling. *J. Mol. Med.* 91, 907–916. doi: 10.1007/s00109-013-1060-y

Brabeck, C., Mittelbronn, M., Bekure, K., Meyermann, R., Schluesener, H. J., and Schwab, J. M. (2003). Effect of focal cerebral infarctions on lesional RhoA and RhoB expression. *Arch. Neurol.* 60, 1245–1249.

Buchanan, F. G., Elliot, C. M., Gibbs, M., and Exton, J. H. (2000). Translocation of the Rac1 guanine nucleotide exchange factor Tiam1 induced by platelet-derived growth factor and lysophosphatidic acid. *J. Biol. Chem.* 275, 9742–9748. doi: 10.1074/jbc.275.13.9742

Cáceres, M., Ortiz, L., Recabarren, T., Romero, A., Colombo, A., Leiva-Salcedo, E. A., et al. (2015). TRPM4 is a novel component of the adhesome required for focal adhesion disassembly, migration and contractility. *PLoS One* 10:e0130540. doi: 10.1371/journal.pone.0130540

Canales, J., Morales, D., Blanco, C., Rivas, J., Diaz, N., Angelopoulos, I., et al. (2019). A tr(i)p to cell migration: new roles of trp channels in mechanotransduction and cancer. *Front. Physiol.* 10:757. doi: 10.3389/fphys.2019.00757

Cao, Q., Yang, Y., Zhong, X. Z., and Dong, X. P. (2017). The lysosomal Ca2+ release channel TRPML1 regulates lysosome size by activating calmodulin. *J. Biol. Chem.* 292, 8424–8435. doi: 10.1074/jbc.m116.772160

Caterina, M. J., Rosen, T. A., Tominaga, M., Brake, A. J., and Julius, D. (1999). A capsaicin-receptor homologue with a high threshold for noxious heat. *Nature* 398, 436–441. doi: 10.1038/18906

Caterina, M. J., Schumacher, M. A., Tominaga, M., Rosen, T. A., Levine, J. D., and Julius, D. (1997). The capsaicin receptor: a heat-activated ion channel in the pain pathway. *Nature* 389, 816–824. doi: 10.1038/39807

Cavanaugh, D. J., Chesler, A. T., Jackson, A. C., Sigal, Y. M., Yamanaka, H., Grant, R., et al. (2011). Trpv1 reporter mice reveal highly restricted brain distribution and functional expression in arteriolar smooth muscle cells. *J. Neurosci.* 31, 5067–5077. doi: 10.1523/jneurosci.6451-10.2011

Cerda, O., Cáceres, M., Park, K. S., Leiva-Salcedo, E. A., Romero, A., Varela, D., et al. (2015). Casein kinase-mediated phosphorylation of serine 839 is necessary for basolateral localization of the Ca2+-activated non-selective cation channel TRPM4. *Pflugers Arch. Eur. J. Physiol.* 467, 1723–1732. doi: 10.1007/s00424-014-1610-3

Chan, S. L., Nelson, M. T., and Cipolla, M. J. (2019). Transient receptor potential vanilloid-4 channels are involved in diminished myogenic tone in brain parenchymal arterioles in response to chronic hypoperfusion in mice. *Acta Physiol.* 225:e13181. doi: 10.1111/apha.13181

Chen, B., Gao, Y., Wei, S., Low, S. W., Ng, G., Yu, D., et al. (2019). TRPM4-specific blocking antibody attenuates reperfusion injury in a rat model of stroke. *Pflugers Arch. Eur. J. Physiol.* 471, 1455–1466. doi: 10.1007/s00424-019-02326-8

Chen, Q., Cichon, J., Wang, W., Qiu, L., Lee, S. J. R., Campbell, N. R., et al. (2012). Imaging neural activity using Thy1-GCaMP transgenic mice. *Neuron* 76, 297–308. doi: 10.1016/j.neuron.2012.07.011

Chen, S. J., Hoffman, N. E., Shanmughapriy, S., Bao, L., Keefer, K., Conrad, K., et al. (2014). A splice variant of the human ion channel TRPM2 modulates neuroblastoma tumor growth through hypoxia-inducible factor (HIF)-1/2α. *J. Biol. Chem.* 289, 36284–36302. doi: 10.1074/jbc.m114.620922

Chen, W., Xu, B., Xiao, A., Liu, L., Fang, X., Liu, R., et al. (2015). TRPM7 inhibitor carvacrol protects brain from neonatal hypoxic-ischemic injury. *Mol. Brain* 8, 1–13.

Chen, X., Lu, M., He, X., Ma, L., Birnbaumer, L., and Liao, Y. (2017). TRPC3/6/7 knockdown protects the brain from cerebral ischemia injury via astrocyte apoptosis inhibition and effects on NF-êB translocation. *Mol.Neurobiol.* 54, 7555–7566. doi: 10.1007/s12035-016-0227-2

Chen, X., Sooch, G., Demaree, I. S., White, F. A., and Obukhov, A. G. (2020). Transient receptor potential canonical (TRPC) channels: then and now. *Cells* 9:E1983.

Cheng, X., Shen, D., Samie, M., and Xu, H. (2010). Mucolipins: intracellular TRPML1-3 channels. *FEBS Lett.* 584, 2013–2021. doi: 10.1016/j.febslet.2009.12.056

Chigurupati, S., Venkataraman, R., Barrera, D., Naganathan, A., Madan, M., Paul, L., et al. (2010). Receptor channel TRPC6 is a key mediator of Notch-driven glioblastoma growth and invasiveness. *Cancer Res.* 70, 418–427. doi: 10.1158/0008-5472.can-09-2654

Cho, C. H., Kim, E., Lee, Y. S., Yarishkin, O., Yoo, J. C., Park, J. Y., et al. (2014). Depletion of 14-3-3γ reduces the surface expression of transient receptor potential melastatin 4b (TRPM4b) Channels and attenuates TRPM4b-mediated glutamate-induced neuronal cell death. *Mol. Brain* 7, 1–12.

Chu, C. J., Huang, S. M., De Petrocellis, L., Bisogno, T., Ewing, S. A., Miller, J. D., et al. (2003). N-oleoyldopamine, a novel endogenous capsaicin-like lipid that produces hyperalgesia. *J. Biol. Chem.* 278, 13633–13639. doi: 10.1074/jbc.m211231200

Chu, W. G., Wang, F. D., Sun, Z. C., Ma, S. B., Wang, X., Han, W. J., et al. (2020). TRPC1/4/5 channels contribute to morphine-induced analgesic tolerance and hyperalgesia by enhancing spinal synaptic potentiation and structural plasticity. *FASEB J.* 34, 8526–8543. doi: 10.1096/fj.202000154rr

Chubanov, V., Waldegger, S., Mederos, Y., Schnitzler, M., Vitzthum, H., Sassen, M. C., et al. (2004). Disruption of TRPM6/TRPM7 complex formation by a mutation in the TRPM6 gene causes hypomagnesemia with secondary hypocalcemia. *Proc.Natl. Acad. Sci. U.S.A.* 101, 2894–2899. doi: 10.1073/pnas.0305252101

Clapham, D. E. (2003). TRP channels as cellular sensors. *Nature* 426, 517–524. doi: 10.1038/nature02196

Clapham, D. E., Runnels, L. W., Strübing, C., and Medical, H. H. (2001). The TRP Ion channel family. *Nat. Rev. Neurosci.* 2, 387–396. doi: 10.1038/35077544

Cornillot, M., Giacco, V., and Hamilton, N. B. (2019). The role of TRP channels in white matter function and ischaemia. *Neurosci. Lett.* 690, 202–209. doi: 10.1016/j.neulet.2018.10.042

Cui, N., Zhang, X., Tadepalli, J. S., Yu, L., Gai, H., Petit, J., et al. (2011). Involvement of TRP channels in the CO2 chemosensitivity of locus coeruleus neurons. *J. Neurophysiol.* 105, 2791–2801. doi: 10.1152/jn.00759.2010

Davare, M. A., Fortin, D. A., Saneyoshi, T., Nygaard, S., Kaech, S., Banker, G., et al. (2009). Transient receptor potential canonical 5 channels activate Ca2+/calmodulin kinase Igamma to promote axon formation in hippocampal neurons. *J. Neurosci.* 29, 9794–9808. doi: 10.1523/jneurosci.1544-09.2009

Deyts, C., Galan-Rodriguez, B., Martin, E., Bouveyron, N., Roze, E., Charvin, D., et al. (2009). Dopamine D2 receptor stimulation potentiates polyQHuntingtin-induced mouse striatal neuron dysfunctions via Rho/ROCK-II activation. *PLoS One* 4:e8287. doi: 10.1371/journal.pone.0008287

Diana, G., Valentini, G., Travaglione, S., Falzano, L., Pieri, M., Zona, C., et al. (2007). Enhancement of learning and memory after activation of cerebral Rho GTPases. *Proc. Natl. Acad. Sci. U.S.A.* 104, 636–641. doi: 10.1073/pnas.0610059104

Diaz-Otero, J. M., Yen, T. C., Ahmad, A., Laimon-Thomson, E., Abolibdeh, B., Kelly, K., et al. (2019). Transient receptor potential vanilloid 4 channels are important regulators of parenchymal arteriole dilation and cognitive function. *Microcirculation* 26, 1–10. doi: 10.1097/01.anes.0000467023.49828.06

Ding, X., He, Z., Zhou, K., Cheng, J., Yao, H., Lu, D., et al. (2010). Essential role of TRPC6 Channels in G2/M phase transition and development of human glioma. *JNCI J. Natl. Cancer Inst.* 102, 1052–1068. doi: 10.1093/jnci/djq217

Dong, X. P., Cheng, X., Mills, E., Delling, M., Wang, F., Kurz, T., et al. (2008). The type IV mucolipidosis-associated protein TRPML1 is an endolysosomal iron release channel. *Nature* 455, 992–996. doi: 10.1038/nature07311

Dong, X. P., Shen, D., Wang, X., Dawson, T., Li, X., Zhang, Q., et al. (2010). PI(3,5)P(2) controls membrane trafficking by direct activation of mucolipin Ca(2+) release channels in the endolysosome. *Nat. Commun.* 1:38.

Dovas, A., and Couchman, J. R. (2005). RhoGDI: multiple functions in the regulation of Rho family GTPase activities. *Biochem. J.* 390, 1–9. doi: 10.1042/bj20050104

Du, Y., Fu, M., Huang, Z., Tian, X., Li, J., Pang, Y., et al. (2020). TRPV1 activation alleviates cognitive and synaptic plasticity impairments through inhibiting AMPAR endocytosis in APP23/PS45 mouse model of AlzheimerΓÇÖs disease. *Aging Cell* 19, 1–12.

Dulneva, A., Lee, S., Oliver, P. L., Di Gleria, K., Kessler, B. M., Davies, K. E., et al. (2015). The mutant Moonwalker TRPC3 channel links calcium signaling to lipid metabolism in the developing cerebellum. *Hum. Mol. Genet.* 24, 4114–4125. doi: 10.1093/hmg/ddv150

Dunn, K. M., Hill-Eubanks, D. C., Liedtke, W. B., and Nelson, M. T. (2013). TRPV4 channels stimulate Ca2+-induced Ca2+ release in astrocytic endfeet and amplify neurovascular coupling responses. *Proc. Natl. Acad. Sci. U.S.A.* 110, 6157–6162. doi: 10.1073/pnas.1216514110

Dupraz, S., Hilton, B. J., Husch, A., Santos, T. E., Coles, C. H., Stern, S., et al. (2019). RhoA controls axon extension independent of specification in the developing brain. *Curr. Biol.* 29, 3874.e9–3886.e9.

Dussor, G., Yan, J., Xie, J. Y., Ossipov, M. H., Dodick, D. W., and Porreca, F. (2014). Targeting TRP channels for novel migraine therapeutics. *ACS Chem. Neurosci.* 5, 1085–1096. doi: 10.1021/cn500083e

Earley, S., Waldron, B. J., and Brayden, J. E. (2004). Critical role for transient receptor potential channel TRPM4 in myogenic constriction of cerebral arteries. *Circ. Res.* 95, 922–929. doi: 10.1161/01.res.0000147311.54833.03

Edwards, D. C., Sanders, L. C., Bokoch, G. M., and Gill, G. N. (1999). Activation of LIM-kinase by Pak1 couples Rac/Cdc42 GTPase signalling to actin cytoskeletal dynamics. *Nat. Cell Biol.* 1, 253–259. doi: 10.1038/12963

Ellerbroek, S. M., Wennerberg, K., and Burridge, K. (2003). Serine phosphorylation negatively regulates RhoA in vivo. *J. Biolo. Chem.* 278, 19023–19031. doi: 10.1074/jbc.m213066200

Fan, L., Yan, H., Pellegrin, S., Morigen, and Mellor, H. (2015). The Rif GTPase regulates cytoskeletal signaling from plexinA4 to promote neurite retraction. *Neurosci. Lett.* 590, 178–183. doi: 10.1016/j.neulet.2015.02.010

Feng, S. (2017). *Transient Receptor Potential Canonical Channels and Brain Diseases*. Berlin: Springer.

Fine, M., Schmiege, P., and Li, X. (2018). Structural basis for PtdInsP(2)-mediated human TRPML1 regulation. *Nat. Commun.* 9:4192.

Finkielstein, C. V., Overduin, M., and Capelluto, D. G. S. (2006). Cell migration and signaling specificity is determined by the phosphatidylserine recognition motif of Rac1. *J. Biol. Chem.* 281, 27317–27326. doi: 10.1074/jbc.m605560200

Fleig, A., and Penner, R. (2004). The TRPM ion channel subfamily: molecular, biophysical and functional features. *Trends Pharmacol. Sci.* 25, 633–639. doi: 10.1016/j.tips.2004.10.004

Fleming, I. N., Elliott, C. M., Buchanan, F. G., Downes, C. P., Exton, J. H., Fleming, T., et al. (1999). Ca 2/Calmodulin-dependent protein kinase II regulates tiam1 by reversible protein phosphorylation * fibroblasts, and that protein kinase C is involved in. *Biochemistry* 274, 12753–12758. doi: 10.1074/jbc.274.18.12753

Fliegert, R., Glassmeier, G. N., Schmid, F., Cornils, K., Genisyuerek, S., Harneit, A., et al. (2007). Modulation of Ca2+ entry and plasma membrane potential by human TRPM4b. *FEBS J.* 274, 704–713. doi: 10.1111/j.1742-4658.2006.05614.x

Forrest, M. P., Parnell, E., and Penzes, P. (2018). Dendritic structural plasticity and neuropsychiatric disease. *Nat. Rev. Neurosci.* 19, 215–234. doi: 10.1038/nrn.2018.16

Fortin Ensign, S. P., Mathews, I. T., Symons, M. H., Berens, M. E., and Tran, N. L. (2013). Implications of Rho GTPase signaling in glioma cell invasion and tumor progression. *Front. Oncol.* 3:241. doi: 10.3389/fonc.2013.00241

Frey, U., Huang, Y. Y., and Kandel, E. R. (1993). Effects of cAMP simulate a late stage of LTP in hippocampal CA1 neurons. *Science* 260, 1661–1664. doi: 10.1126/science.8389057

Gao, Y., Yao, T., Deng, Z., Sohn, J. W., Sun, J., Huang, Y., et al. (2017). TrpC5 mediates acute leptin and serotonin effects via pomc neurons. *Cell Rep.* 18, 583–592. doi: 10.1016/j.celrep.2016.12.072

Garcia-Elias, A., Mrkonjić, S., Jung, C., Pardo-Pastor, C., Vicente, R., and Valverde, M. A. (2014). The TRPV4 channel. *Handb. Exp. Pharmacol.* 222, 293–319.

Gauden, V., Hu, D. E., Kurokawa, T., Sarker, M. H., and Fraser, P. A. (2007). Novel technique for estimating cerebrovascular permeability demonstrates capsazepine protection following ischemia-reperfusion. *Microcirculation* 14, 767–778. doi: 10.1080/10739680701410421

Gavva, N. R., Sandrock, R., Arnold, G. E., Davis, M., Lamas, E., Lindvay, C., et al. (2019). Reduced TRPM8 expression underpins reduced migraine risk and attenuated cold pain sensation in humans. *Scie. Rep.* 9, 1–11.

Gerzanich, V., Woo, S. K., Vennekens, R., Tsymbalyuk, O., Ivanov, A., Geng, Z., et al. (2009). *De novo* expression of Trpm4 initiates secondary hemorrhage in spinal cord injury. *Nat. Med.* 15, 185–191. doi: 10.1038/nm.1899

Gocher, A. M., Azabdaftari, G., Euscher, L. M., Dai, S., Karacosta, L. G., Franke, T. F., et al. (2017). Akt activation by Ca2+/calmodulin-dependent protein kinase kinase 2 (CaMKK2) in ovarian cancer cells. *J. Biol. Chem.* 292, 14188–14204. doi: 10.1074/jbc.m117.778464

Gorse, K. M., Lantzy, M. K., Lee, E. D., and Lafrenaye, A. D. (2018). Transient receptor potential melastatin 4 induces astrocyte swelling but not death after diffuse traumatic brain injury. *J. Neurotr.* 35, 1694–1704. doi: 10.1089/neu.2017.5275

Goswami, C., and Hucho, T. (2007). TRPV1 expression-dependent initiation and regulation of filopodia. *J. Neurochem.* 103, 1319–1333. doi: 10.1111/j.1471-4159.2007.04846.x

Goswami, C., Hucho, T. B., and Hucho, F. (2007a). Identification and characterisation of novel tubulin-binding motifs located within the C-terminus of TRPV1. *J. Neurochem.* 101, 250–262. doi: 10.1111/j.1471-4159.2006.04338.x

Goswami, C., Schmidt, H., and Hucho, F. (2007b). TRPV1 at nerve endings regulates growth cone morphology and movement through cytoskeleton reorganization. *FEBS J.* 274, 760–772. doi: 10.1111/j.1742-4658.2006.05621.x

Goto, A., Hoshino, M., Matsuda, M., and Nakamura, T. (2011). Phosphorylation of STEF/Tiam2 by protein kinase A is critical for Rac1 activation and neurite outgrowth in dibutyryl cAMP-treated PC12D cells. *Mol. Biol. Cell* 22, 1780–1790. doi: 10.1091/mbc.e10-09-0783

Greka, A., Navarro, B., Oancea, E., Duggan, A., and Clapham, D. E. (2003). TRPC5 is a regulator of hippocampal neurite length and growth cone morphology. *Nat. Neurosci.* 6, 837–845. doi: 10.1038/nn1092

Güler, A. D., Lee, H., Iida, T., Shimizu, I., Tominaga, M., and Caterina, M. (2002). Heat-evoked activation of the ion channel. TRPV4. *J. Neurosci.* 22, 6408–6414. doi: 10.1523/jneurosci.22-15-06408.2002

Gunthorpe, M. J., Harries, M. H., Prinjha, R. K., Davis, J. B., and Randall, A. (2000). Voltage- and time-dependent properties of the recombinant rat vanilloid receptor (rVR1). *J. Physiol.* 525, 747–759. doi: 10.1111/j.1469-7793.2000.t01-1-00747.x

Hannan, M. A., Kabbani, N., Paspalas, C. D., and Levenson, R. (2008). Interaction with dopamine D2 receptor enhances expression of transient receptor potential channel 1 at the cell surface. *Biochim. Biophys. Acta Biomembr.* 1778, 974–982. doi: 10.1016/j.bbamem.2008.01.011

Hartmann, J., Dragicevic, E., Adelsberger, H., Henning, H. A., Sumser, M., Abramowitz, J., et al. (2008). TRPC3 channels are required for synaptic transmission and motor coordination. *Neuron* 59, 392–398. doi: 10.1016/j.neuron.2008.06.009

He, Z., Jia, C., Feng, S., Zhou, K., Tai, Y., Bai, X., et al. (2012). TRPC5 channel is the mediator of neurotrophin-3 in regulating dendritic growth via CaMKIIα in rat hippocampal neurons. *J. Neurosci.* 32, 9383–9395. doi: 10.1523/jneurosci.6363-11.2012

Hedrick, N. G., Harward, S. C., Hall, C. E., Murakoshi, H., Mcnamara, J. O., and Yasuda, R. (2016). Rho GTPase complementation underlies BDNF-dependent homo- and heterosynaptic plasticity. *Nature* 538, 104–108. doi: 10.1038/nature19784

Heiser, J. H., Schuwald, A. M., Sillani, G., Ye, L., Müller, W. E., and Leuner, K. (2013). TRPC6 channel-mediated neurite outgrowth in PC12 cells and hippocampal neurons involves activation of RAS/MEK/ERK, PI3K, and CAMKIV signaling. *J. Neurochemi.* 127, 303–313. doi: 10.1111/jnc.12376

Hellmich, U. A., and Gaudet, R. (2014). Structural biology of TRP channels. *Handb. Exp. Pharmacol.* 223, 963–990. doi: 10.1007/978-3-319-05161-1_10

Heng, J. I., Nguyen, L., Castro, D. S., Zimmer, C., Wildner, H., Armant, O., et al. (2008). Neurogenin 2 controls cortical neuron migration through regulation of Rnd2. *Nature* 455, 114–118. doi: 10.1038/nature07198

Heo, D. K., Chung, W. Y., Park, H. W., Yuan, J. P., Lee, M. G., and Kim, J. Y. (2012). Opposite regulatory effects of TRPC1 and TRPC5 on neurite outgrowth in PC12 cells. *Cell. Signall.* 24, 899–906. doi: 10.1016/j.cellsig.2011.12.011

Hirata, K. I., Kikuchi, A., Sasaki, T., Kuroda, S., Kaibuchi, K., Matsuura, Y., et al. (1992). Involvement of rho p21 in the GTP-enhanced calcium ion sensitivity of smooth muscle contraction. *J. Biol. Chem.* 267, 8719–8722.

Ho, K. W., Lambert, W. S., and Calkins, D. J. (2014). Activation of the TRPV1 cation channel contributes to stress-induced astrocyte migration. *Glia* 62, 1435–1451. doi: 10.1002/glia.22691

Hodge, R. G., and Ridley, A. J. (2016). Regulating Rho GTPases and their regulators. *Nat. Rev. Mol. Biol.* 17, 496–510.

Hofmann, T., Chubanov, V., Gudermann, T., and Montell, C. (2003). TRPM5 is a voltage-modulated and Ca(2+)-activated monovalent selective cation channel. *Curr. Biol.* 13, 1153–1158. doi: 10.1016/s0960-9822(03)00431-7

Hofmann, T., Obukhov, A. G., Schaefer, M., Harteneck, C., Gudermann, T., and Schultz, G. N. (1999). Direct activation of human TRPC6 and TRPC3 channels by diacylglycerol. *Nature* 397, 259–263. doi: 10.1038/16711

Hong, C., Choi, S. H., Kwak, M., Jeong, B., Ko, J., Park, H. J., et al. (2020a). TRPC5 channel instability induced by depalmitoylation protects striatal neurons against oxidative stress in Huntington's disease. *Biochim. Biophys. Acta Mol. Cell Res.* 1867, 118620–118620. doi: 10.1016/j.bbamcr.2019.118620

Hong, C., Jeong, B., Park, H. J., Chung, J. Y., Lee, J. E., Kim, J., et al. (2020b). TRP channels as emerging therapeutic targets for neurodegenerative diseases. *Front. Physiol.* 11:238. doi: 10.3389/fphys.2020.00238

Hong, C., Seo, H., Kwak, M., Jeon, J., Jang, J., Jeong, E. M., et al. (2015). Increased TRPC5 glutathionylation contributes to striatal neuron loss in Huntington's disease. *Brain* 138, 3030–3047. doi: 10.1093/brain/awv188

Howe, A. K. (2004). *Regulation of Actin-Based Cell Migration by cAMP/PKA.* Amsterdam: Elsevier.

Hu, H. Z., Gu, Q., Wang, C., Colton, C. K., Tang, J., Kinoshita-Kawada, M., et al. (2004). 2-Aminoethoxydiphenyl borate is a common activator of TRPV1. TRPV2, and TRPV3. *J. Biol. Chem.* 279, 35741–35748. doi: 10.1074/jbc.m404164200

Huang, G. H., Sun, Z. L., Li, H. J., and Feng, D. F. (2017). Rho GTPase-activating proteins: Regulators of Rho GTPase activity in neuronal development and CNS diseases. *Mol. Cell. Neurosci.* 80, 18–31. doi: 10.1016/j.mcn.2017.01.007

Huang, Y., Fliegert, R., Guse, A. H., Lü, W., and Du, J. (2020). A structural overview of the ion channels of the TRPM family. *Cell Calcium* 85:102111. doi: 10.1016/j.ceca.2019.102111

Hui, H., Mchugh, D., Hannan, M., Zeng, F., Xu, S. Z., Khan, S. U. H., et al. (2006). Calcium-sensing mechanism in TRPC5 channels contributing to retardation of neurite outgrowth. *J. Physiol.* 572, 165–172. doi: 10.1113/jphysiol.2005.102889

Ishikawa, Y., Katoh, H., and Negishi, M. (2003). A role of Rnd1 GTPase in dendritic spine formation in hippocampal neurons. *J. Neurosci.* 23, 11065–11072. doi: 10.1523/jneurosci.23-35-11065.2003

Ishikawa, Y., Katoh, H., and Negishi, M. (2006). Small GTPase Rnd1 is involved in neuronal activity-dependent dendritic development in hippocampal neurons. *Neurosci. Lett.* 400, 218–223. doi: 10.1016/j.neulet.2006.02.064

Jacobs, B., and Dussor, G. (2016). Neurovascular contributions to migraine: moving beyond vasodilation. *Neuroscience* 338, 130–144. doi: 10.1016/j.neuroscience.2016.06.012

Jang, Y., Lee, M. H., Lee, J., Jung, J., Lee, S. H., Yang, D. J., et al. (2014). TRPM2 mediates the lysophosphatidic acid-induced neurite retraction in the developing brain. *Pflugers Arch. Eur. J. Physiol.* 466, 1987–1998. doi: 10.1007/s00424-013-1436-4

Jiang, L., Ding, J., Tsai, H., Li, L., Feng, Q., Miao, J., et al. (2011). Over-expressing transient receptor potential cation channel 6 in podocytes induces cytoskeleton rearrangement through increases of intracellular Ca^{2+} and RhoA activation. *Exp. Biol. Med. (Maywood)*, 236, 184–193. doi: 10.1258/ebm.2010.010237

Jin, M., Guan, C. B., Jiang, Y. A., Chen, G., Zhao, C. T., Cui, K., et al. (2005). Ca2+-dependent regulation of rho GTPases triggers turning of nerve growth cones. *J. Neurosci.* 25, 2338–2347. doi: 10.1523/jneurosci.4889-04.2005

Johnstone, A. D., De Léon, A., Unsain, N. Í, Gibon, J., and Barker, P. A. (2019). Developmental axon degeneration requires trpv1-dependent Ca 2+ influx. *eNeuro* 6:ENEURO.0019-19.2019. doi: 10.1523/ENEURO.0019-19.2019

Kaczmarek, J. S., Riccio, A., and Clapham, D. E. (2012). Calpain cleaves and activates the TRPC5 channel to participate in semaphorin 3A-induced neuronal growth cone collapse. *Proc. Natl. Acad. Sci. U.S.A.* 109, 7888–7892. doi: 10.1073/pnas.1205869109

Kang, M. G., Guo, Y., and Huganir, R. L. (2009). AMPA receptor and GEF-H1/Lfc complex regulates dendritic spine development through RhoA signaling cascade. *Proc. Natl. Acad. Sci. U.S.A.* 106, 3549–3554. doi: 10.1073/pnas.0812861106

Karabiyik, C., Fernandes, R., Figueiredo, F. R. Í, Socodato, R., Brakebusch, C., and Lambertsen, K. L. (2018). Neuronal Rho GTPase Rac1 elimination confers neuroprotection in a mouse model of permanent ischemic stroke. *Brain Pathol.* 28, 569–580. doi: 10.1111/bpa.12562

Kim, D. S., Ryu, H. J., Kim, J. E., and Kang, T. C. (2013). The reverse roles of transient receptor potential canonical channel-3 and -6 in neuronal death following pilocarpine-induced status epilepticus. *Cell. Mol. Neurobiol.* 33, 99–109. doi: 10.1007/s10571-012-9875-6

Kim, J., Ko, J., Myeong, J., Kwak, M., Hong, C., and So, I. (2019). TRPC1 as a negative regulator for TRPC4 and TRPC5 channels. *Pflugers Arch. Eur. J. Physiol.* 471, 1045–1053. doi: 10.1007/s00424-019-02289-w

Kim, J. Y., Zeng, W., Kiselyov, K., Yuan, J. P., Dehoff, M. H., Mikoshiba, K., et al. (2006). Homer 1 mediates store- and inositol 1,4,5-trisphosphate receptor-dependent translocation and retrieval of TRPC3 to the plasma membrane. *J. Biol. Chem.* 281, 32540–32549. doi: 10.1074/jbc.m602496200

Kim, S. R., Kim, S. U., Oh, U., and Jin, B. K. (2006). Transient receptor potential vanilloid subtype 1 mediates microglial cell death in vivo and in vitro via Ca 2+ -Mediated mitochondrial damage and cytochrome c release. *J. Immunol.* 177, 4322–4329. doi: 10.4049/jimmunol.177.7.4322

Kim, M. S., and Usachev, Y. M. (2009). Mitochondrial Ca2+ cycling facilitates activation of the transcription factor NFAT in sensory neurons. *J. Neurosci.* 29, 12101–12114. doi: 10.1523/jneurosci.3384-09.2009

Kim, S.-J., Jeon, S., and Shin, E.-Y. (2004). AM PA, not NMDA, activates RhoA GTPases and subsequetly phosphorylates m oesin. *Exp. Mol. Med.* 36, 98–102. doi: 10.1038/emm.2004.14

Kim, S. R., Lee, D. Y., Chung, E. S., Oh, U. T., Kim, S. U., and Jin, B. K. (2005). Transient receptor potential vanilloid subtype 1 mediates cell death of mesencephalic dopaminergic neurons In vivo and In vitro. *J. Neurosci.* 25, 662–671. doi: 10.1523/jneurosci.4166-04.2005

Kitajima, N., Watanabe, K., Morimoto, S., Sato, Y., Kiyonaka, S., Hoshijima, M., et al. (2011). TRPC3-mediated Ca2+ influx contributes to Rac1-mediated production of reactive oxygen species in MLP-deficient mouse hearts. *Biochem. Biophys. Res. Commun.* 409, 108–113. doi: 10.1016/j.bbrc.2011.04.124

Koga, Y., and Ikebe, M. (2005). p116Rip decreases myosin II phosphorylation by activating myosin light chain phosphatase and by inactivating RhoA. *J. Biol. Chem.* 280, 4983–4991. doi: 10.1074/jbc.m410909200

Kojima, I., and Nagasawa, M. (2014). TRPV2. *Handb. Exp. Pharmacol.* 222, 247–272.

Kraynov, V. S., Chamberlain, C., Bokoch, G. M., Schwartz, M. A., Slabaugh, S., and Hahn, K. M. (2000). Localized rac activation dynamics visualized in living cells. *Science* 290, 333–337. doi: 10.1126/science.290.5490.333

Krogsaeter, E. K., Biel, M., Wahl-Schott, C., and Grimm, C. (2019). The protein interaction networks of mucolipins and two-pore channels. *Biochim. Biophys. Acta Mol. Cell Res.* 866, 1111–1123. doi: 10.1016/j.bbamcr.2018.10.020

Kruse, K., Lee, Q. S., Sun, Y., Klomp, J., Yang, X., Huang, F., et al. (2019). N-cadherin signaling via Trio assembles adherens junctions to restrict endothelial permeability. *J. Cell Biol.* 218, 299–316. doi: 10.1083/jcb.201802076

Kuipers, A. J., Middelbeek, J., and Van Leeuwen, F. N. (2012). Mechanoregulation of cytoskeletal dynamics by TRP channels. *Eur. J. Cell Biol.* 91, 834–846. doi: 10.1016/j.ejcb.2012.05.006

Kutcher, M. E., Kolyada, A. Y., Surks, H. K., and Herman, I. M. (2007). Pericyte Rho GTPase mediates both pericyte contractile phenotype and capillary endothelial growth state. *Am. J. Pathol.* 171, 693–701. doi: 10.2353/ajpath.2007.070102

La Rosa, C., Parolisi, R., and Bonfanti, L. (2020). Brain structural plasticity: from adult neurogenesis to immature neurons. *Front. Neurosci.* 14:75. doi: 10.3389/fnins.2020.00075

Laragione, T., Harris, C., and Gulko, P. S. (2019). TRPV2 suppresses Rac1 and RhoA activation and invasion in rheumatoid arthritis fibroblast-like synoviocytes. *Int. Immunopharmacol.* 70, 268–273. doi: 10.1016/j.intimp.2019.02.051

Launay, P., Cheng, H., Srivatsan, S., Penner, R., Fleig, A., and Kinet, J. P. (2004). TRPM4 regulates calcium oscillations after T cell activation. *Science* 306, 1374–1377. doi: 10.1126/science.1098845

Launay, P., Fleig, A., Perraud, A. L., Scharenberg, A. M., Penner, R., and Kinet, J. P. (2002). TRPM4 is a Ca2+-activated nonselective cation channel mediating cell membrane depolarization. *Cell* 109, 397–407. doi: 10.1016/s0092-8674(02)00719-5

Lee, C. C., Huang, C. C., and Hsu, K. S. (2015). The phospholipid-binding protein SESTD1 negatively regulates dendritic spine density by interfering with Rac1-Trio8 signaling pathway. *Scie. Rep.* 5, 1–16.

Lee, J. H., Mcbrayer, M. K., Wolfe, D. M., Haslett, L. J., Kumar, A., Sato, Y., et al. (2015). Presenilin 1 maintains lysosomal Ca2+ Homeostasis via TRPML1 by regulating vATPase-mediated lysosome acidification. *Cell Rep.* 12, 1430–1444. doi: 10.1016/j.celrep.2015.07.050

Lee, K. P., Choi, S., Hong, J. H., Ahuja, M., Graham, S., Ma, R., et al. (2014). Molecular determinants mediating gating of transient receptor potential canonical (TRPC) channels by stromal interaction molecule 1 (STIM1). *J. Biol. Chem.* 289, 6372–6382. doi: 10.1074/jbc.m113.546556

Lee, S., Salazar, S. V., Cox, T. O., and Strittmatter, S. M. (2019). Pyk2 signaling through Graf1 and RhoA GTPase is required for amyloid-beta oligomer-triggered synapse loss. *J. Neurosci.* 39, 1910–1929. doi: 10.1523/jneurosci.2983-18.2018

Leemhuis, J., Boutillier, S., Barth, H., Feuerstein, T. J., Brock, C., Nürnberg, B., et al. (2004). Rho GTPases and phosphoinositide 3-kinase organize formation of branched dendrites. *J. Biol. Chem.* 279, 585–596. doi: 10.1074/jbc.m307066200

Leiva-Salcedo, E. A., Riquelme, D., Cerda, O., and Stutzin, A. S. (2017). TRPM4 activation by chemically- and oxygen deprivation-induced ischemia and reperfusion triggers neuronal death. *Channels* 11, 624–635. doi: 10.1080/19336950.2017.1375072

Lepannetier, S., Zanou, N. G., Yerna, X., Emeriau, N. M., Dufour, I. S., Masquelier, J., et al. (2016). Sphingosine-1-phosphate-activated TRPC1 channel controls chemotaxis of glioblastoma cells. *Cell Calcium* 60, 373–383. doi: 10.1016/j.ceca.2016.09.002

Lessard, C. B., Lussier, M. P., Cayouette, S., Bourque, G. V., and Boulay, G. (2005). The overexpression of presenilin2 and Alzheimer's-disease-linked presenilin2 variants influences TRPC6-enhanced Ca 2+ entry into HEK293 cells. *Cell. Signal.* 17, 437–445. doi: 10.1016/j.cellsig.2004.09.005

Li, H., Huang, J., Du, W., Jia, C., Yao, H., and Wang, Y. (2012). TRPC6 inhibited NMDA receptor activities and protected neurons from ischemic excitotoxicity. *J. Neurochem.* 123, 1010–1018. doi: 10.1111/jnc.12045

Li, H. S., Xu, X. Z., and Montell, C. (1999). Activation of a TRPC3-dependent cation current through the neurotrophin BDNF. *Neuron* 24, 261–273. doi: 10.1016/s0896-6273(00)80838-7

Li, J., Cong, X., Zhang, Y., Xiang, R. L., Mei, M., Yang, N. Y., et al. (2015). ZO-1 and -2 are required for TRPV1-modulated paracellular permeability. *J. Dental Res.* 94, 1748–1756. doi: 10.1177/0022034515609268

Li, S., Tuft, B. W., Xu, L., Polacco, M. A., Clarke, J. C., Guymon, C. A., et al. (2015a). Microtopographical features generated by photopolymerization recruit RhoA/ROCK through TRPV1 to direct cell and neurite growth. *Biomaterials* 53, 95–106. doi: 10.1016/j.biomaterials.2015.02.057

Li, S., Wang, J., Wei, Y., Liu, Y., Ding, X., Dong, B., et al. (2015b). Crucial role of TRPC6 in maintaining the stability of HIF-1α in glioma cells under hypoxia. *J. Cell Sci.* 128, 3317–3329. doi: 10.1242/jcs.173161

Lim, J., Ritt, D. A., Zhou, M., and Morrison, D. K. (2014). The CNK2 scaffold interacts with vilse and modulates rac cycling during spine morphogenesis in hippocampal neurons. *Curr. Biol.* 24, 786–792. doi: 10.1016/j.cub.2014.02.036

Ling, Y. H., Chen, S. P., Fann, C. S. J., Wang, S. J., and Wang, Y. F. (2019). TRPM8 genetic variant is associated with chronic migraine and allodynia. *J. Headache Pain* 20, 1–8.

Lisman, J., Yasuda, R., and Raghavachari, S. (2012). Mechanisms of CaMKII action in long-term potentiation. *Nat. Rev. Neurosci.* 13, 169–182. doi: 10.1038/nrn3192

Liu, X., Yao, X., and Tsang, S. Y. (2020). Post-translational modification and natural mutation of TRPC channels. *Cell* 9:135. doi: 10.3390/cells9010135

Liu, Y., Hu, G., Yu, Y., Jiang, Z., Yang, K., Hu, X., et al. (2020). Structural and functional reorganization within cognitive control network associated with protection of executive function in patients with unilateral frontal gliomas. *Front. Oncol.* 10:794. doi: 10.3389/fonc.2020.00794

Loh, K. P., Ng, G., Yu, C. Y., Fhu, C. K., Yu, D., Vennekens, R., et al. (2014). TRPM4 inhibition promotes angiogenesis after ischemic stroke. *Pflugers Arch. Eur. J. Physiol.* 466, 563–576. doi: 10.1007/s00424-013-1347-4

Loudon, R. P., Silver, L. D., Yee, H. F., and Gallo, G. (2006). RhoA-kinase and myosin II are required for the maintenance of growth cone polarity and guidance by nerve growth factor. *J. Neurobiol.* 66, 847–867. doi: 10.1002/neu.20258

Luo, L., Hensch, T. K., Ackerman, L., Barbel, S., Jan, L. Y., and Jan, Y. N. (1996). Differential effects of the Rac GTPase on Purkinje cell axons and dendritic trunks and spines. *Nature* 379, 837–840. doi: 10.1038/379837a0

Ly, N., and Cyert, M. S. (2017). Calcineurin, the Ca2+-dependent phosphatase, regulates Rga2, a Cdc42 GTPase-activating protein, to modulate pheromone signaling. *Mol. Biol. Cell* 28, 576–586. doi: 10.1091/mbc.e16-06-0432

Ma, X., Cheng, K. T., Wong, C. O., O'neil, R. G., Birnbaumer, L., Ambudkar, I. S., et al. (2011). Heteromeric TRPV4-C1 channels contribute to store-operated Ca2+ entry in vascular endothelial cells. *Cell Calcium* 50, 502–509. doi: 10.1016/j.ceca.2011.08.006

Machacek, M., Hodgson, L., Welch, C., Elliott, H., Pertz, O., Nalbant, P., et al. (2009). Coordination of Rho GTPase activities during cell protrusion. *Nature* 461, 99–103. doi: 10.1038/nature08242

Madaule, P., and Axel, R. (1985). A novel ras-related gene family. *Cell* 41, 31–40. doi: 10.1016/0092-8674(85)90058-3

Manzoni, M., Monti, E., Bresciani, R., Bozzato, A., Barlati, S., Bassi, M. T., et al. (2004). Overexpression of wild-type and mutant mucolipin proteins in mammalian cells: effects on the late endocytic compartment organization. *FEBS Lett.* 567, 219–224. doi: 10.1016/j.febslet.2004.04.080

Marinelli, S., Di Marzo, V., Berretta, N., Matias, I., Maccarrone, M., Bernardi, G., et al. (2003). Presynaptic facilitation of glutamatergic synapses to dopaminergic neurons of the rat substantia nigra by endogenous stimulation of vanilloid receptors. *J. Neurosci.* 23, 3136–3144. doi: 10.1523/jneurosci.23-08-03136.2003

Marsh, L., and Letourneau, P. C. (1984). Growth of neurites without filopodial or lamellipodial activity in the presence of cytochalasin B. *J. Cell Biol.* 99, 2041–2047. doi: 10.1083/jcb.99.6.2041

McKemy, D. D., Neuhausser, W. M., and Julius, D. (2002). Identification of a cold receptor reveals a general role for TRP channels in thermosensation. *Nature* 416, 52–58. doi: 10.1038/nature719

Menigoz, A. L., Ahmed, T., Sabanov, V., Philippaert, K., Pinto, S., Kerselaers, S., et al. (2016). TRPM4-dependent post-synaptic depolarization is essential for the induction of NMDA receptor-dependent LTP in CA1 hippocampal neurons. *Pflugers Arch. Eur. J. Physiol.* 468, 593–607. doi: 10.1007/s00424-015-1764-7

Mezey, E. (2000). Distribution of mRNA for vanilloid receptor subtype 1 (VR1), and VR1-like immunoreactivity, in the central nervous system of the rat and human. *Proc. Natl. Acad. Sci. U.S.A.* 97, 3655–3660. doi: 10.1073/pnas.97.7.3655

Mickle, A. D., Shepherd, A. J., and Mohapatra, D. P. (2016). Nociceptive TRP channels: Sensory detectors and transducers in multiple pain pathologies. *Pharmaceuticals* 9, 1–26.

Middelbeek, J., Visser, D., Henneman, L., Kamermans, A., Kuipers, A. J., Hoogerbrugge, P. M., et al. (2015). TRPM7 maintains progenitor-like features of neuroblastoma cells: Implications for metastasis formation. *Oncotarget* 6, 8760–8776. doi: 10.18632/oncotarget.3315

Middelbeek, J., Vrenken, K., Visser, D., Lasonder, E., Koster, J., Jalink, K., et al. (2016). The TRPM7 interactome defines a cytoskeletal complex linked to neuroblastoma progression. *Eur. J. Cell Biol.* 95, 465–474. doi: 10.1016/j.ejcb.2016.06.008

Miehe, S., Bieberstein, A., Arnould, I., Ihdene, O., Rütten, H., and Strübing, C. (2010). The phospholipid-binding protein SESTD1 is a novel regulator of the transient receptor potential channels TRPC4 and TRPC5. *J. Biol. Chem.* 285, 12426–12434. doi: 10.1074/jbc.m109.068304

Miyake, T., Shirakawa, H., Nakagawa, T., and Kaneko, S. (2015). Activation of mitochondrial transient receptor potential vanilloid 1 channel contributes to microglial migration. *GLIA* 63, 1870–1882. doi: 10.1002/glia.22854

Montell, C. (2005). The TRP superfamily of cation channels. *Sci. STKE* 2005:re3. doi: 10.1126/stke.2722005re3

Montell, C., and Rubin, G. M. (1989). Molecular characterization of the *Drosophila* trp locus: a putative integral membrane protein required for phototransduction. *Neuron* 2, 1313–1323. doi: 10.1016/0896-6273(89)90069-x

Morelli, M. B., Amantini, C., Liberati, S., Santoni, M., and Nabissi, M. (2013). TRP channels: new potential therapeutic approaches in CNS neuropathies. *CNS Neurol. Disord. Drug Targets* 12, 274–293. doi: 10.2174/18715273113129990056

Müller, P. M., Rademacher, J., Bagshaw, R. D., Wortmann, C., Barth, C., Van Unen, J., et al. (2020). Systems analysis of RhoGEF and RhoGAP regulatory proteins reveals spatially organized RAC1 signalling from integrin adhesions. *Nat. Cell Biol.* 22, 498–511. doi: 10.1038/s41556-020-0488-x

Muraki, K., Iwata, Y., Katanosaka, Y., Ito, T., Ohya, S., Shigekawa, M., et al. (2003). TRPV2 is a component of osmotically sensitive cation channels in murine aortic myocytes. *Circ. Res.* 93, 829–838. doi: 10.1161/01.res.0000097263.10220.0c

Murakoshi, H., Wang, H., and Yasuda, R. (2011). Local, persistent activation of Rho GTPases during plasticity of single dendritic spines. *Nature* 472, 100–106. doi: 10.1038/nature09823

Nabissi, M., Morelli, M. B., Arcella, A., Cardinali, C., Santoni, M., Bernardini, G., et al. (2016). Post-transcriptional regulation of 5′-untranslated regions of human transient receptor potential vanilloid type-1 (TRPV-1) channels: role in the survival of glioma patients. *Oncotarget* 7, 81541–81554. doi: 10.18632/oncotarget.13132

Nadler, M. J., Hermosura, M. C., Inabe, K., Perraud, A. L., Zhu, Q., Stokes, A. J., et al. (2001). LTRPC7 is a Mg.ATP-regulated divalent cation channel required for cell viability. *Nature* 411, 590–595. doi: 10.1038/35079092

Nakamuta, S., Funahashi, Y., Namba, T., Arimura, N., Picciotto, M. R., Tokumitsu, H., et al. (2011). Local application of neurotrophins specifies axons through inositol 1,4,5-trisphosphate, calcium, and Ca2+/calmodulin-dependent protein kinases. *Sci. Signal.* 4:ra76. doi: 10.1126/scisignal.2002011

Nakuluri, K., Nishad, R., Mukhi, D., Kumar, S., Nakka, V. P., Kolligundla, L. P., et al. (2019). Cerebral ischemia induces TRPC6 via HIF1α/ZEB2 axis in the glomerular podocytes and contributes to proteinuria. *Sci. Rep.* 9, 17897–17897.

Nam, J. H., Park, E. S., Won, S.-Y., Lee, Y. A., Kim, K. I., Jeong, J. Y., et al. (2015). TRPV1 on astrocytes rescues nigral dopamine neurons in ParkinsonΓÇÖs disease via CNTF. *Brain* 138, 3610–3622. doi: 10.1093/brain/awv297

Nedungadi, T. P., Dutta, M., Bathina, C. S., Caterina, M. J., and Cunningham, J. T. (2012). Expression and distribution of TRPV2 in rat brain. *Exp. Neurol.* 237, 223–237. doi: 10.1016/j.expneurol.2012.06.017

Nguyen, P. V., Abel, T., and Kandel, E. R. (1994). Requirement of a critical period of transcription for induction of a late phase of LTP. *Science* 265, 1104–1107. doi: 10.1126/science.8066450

Nilius, B., Owsianik, G., and Voets, T. (2008). Transient receptor potential channels meet phosphoinositides. *EMBO J.* 27, 2809–2816. doi: 10.1038/emboj.2008.217

Numaga-Tomita, T., Kitajima, N., Kuroda, T., Nishimura, A., Miyano, K., Yasuda, S., et al. (2016). TRPC3-GEF-H1 axis mediates pressure overload-induced cardiac fibrosis. *Sci. Rep.* 6, 1–12. doi: 10.1254/jpssuppl.92.0_1-ss-36

Oakes, P. W., Wagner, E., Brand, C. A., Probst, D., Linke, M., Schwarz, U. S., et al. (2017). Optogenetic control of RhoA reveals zyxin-mediated elasticity of stress fibres. *Nat. Commun.* 8:15817.

O'Brien, S. P., Seipel, K., Medley, Q. G., Bronson, R., Segal, R., and Streuli, M. (2000). Skeletal muscle deformity and neuroanl disorder in Trio exchange factor-deficient mouse embryos. *Proc. Natl. Acad. Sci. U.S.A.* 97, 12074–12078. doi: 10.1073/pnas.97.22.12074

O'Connor, K. L., and Chen, M. (2013). Dynamic functions of RhoA in tumor cell migration and invasion. *Small GTPases* 4, 37–41.

Oda, M., Yamamoto, H., Matsumoto, H., Ishizaki, Y., and Shibasaki, K. (2020). TRPC5 regulates axonal outgrowth in developing retinal ganglion cells. *Lab. Invest.* 100, 297–310. doi: 10.1038/s41374-019-0347-1

O'Donnell, J. C., Jackson, J. G., and Robinson, M. B. (2016). Transient oxygen/glucose deprivation causes a delayed loss of mitochondria and increases spontaneous calcium signaling in astrocytic processes. *J. Neurosci.* 36, 7109–7127. doi: 10.1523/jneurosci.4518-15.2016

Oishi, A., Makita, N., Sato, J., and Iiri, T. (2012). Regulation of RhoA signaling by the cAMP-dependent phosphorylation of RhoGDIα. *J. Biol. Chem.* 287, 38705–38715. doi: 10.1074/jbc.m112.401547

Okabe, T., Nakamura, T., Nishimura, Y. N., Kohu, K., Ohwada, S., Morishita, Y., et al. (2003). RICS, a novel GTPase-activating protein for Cdc42 and Rac1, is involved in the beta-Catenin-N-cadherin and N-methyl-D-aspartate receptor signaling. *J. Biol. Chem.* 278, 9920–9927. doi: 10.1074/jbc.m208872200

Olayioye, M. A., Noll, B., and Hausser, A. (2019). Spatiotemporal control of intracellular membrane trafficking by Rho GTPases. *Cells* 8, 1478–1478. doi: 10.3390/cells8121478

Oughtred, R., Stark, C., Breitkreutz, B. J., Rust, J., Boucher, L., Chang, C., et al. (2019). The BioGRID interaction database: 2019 update. *Nucleic Acids Res.* 47, D529–D541.

Ou-Yang, Q., Li, B., Xu, M., and Liang, H. (2018). TRPV4 promotes the migration and invasion of glioma cells via AKT/Rac1 signaling. *Biochem. Biophys. Re. Commun.* 503, 876–881. doi: 10.1016/j.bbrc.2018.06.090

Pacary, E., Azzarelli, R., and Guillemot, F. (2013). Rnd3 coordinates early steps of cortical neurogenesis through actin-dependent and -independent mechanisms. *Nat. Commun.* 4:1635.

Park, E. S., Kim, S. R., and Jin, B. K. (2012). Transient receptor potential vanilloid subtype 1 contributes to mesencephalic dopaminergic neuronal survival by inhibiting microglia-originated oxidative stress. *Brain Res. Bull.* 89, 92–96. doi: 10.1016/j.brainresbull.2012.07.001

Park, S., Ahuja, M., Kim, M. S., Brailoiu, G. C., Jha, A., Zeng, M., et al. (2016). Fusion of lysosomes with secretory organelles leads to uncontrolled exocytosis in the lysosomal storage disease mucolipidosis type IV. *EMBO Rep.* 17, 266–278. doi: 10.15252/embr.201541542

Park, S. E., Song, J. H., Hong, C., Kim, D. E., Sul, J. W., Kim, T. Y., et al. (2019). Correction to: contribution of zinc-dependent delayed calcium influx via TRPC5 in oxidative neuronal death and its prevention by novel TRPC Antagonist (Molecular Neurobiology, (2019), 56, 4, (2822-2835), 10.1007/s12035-018-1258-7). *Mol. Neurobiol.* 56, 2836–2837. doi: 10.1007/s12035-018-1447-4

Park, U., Vastani, N., Guan, Y., Raja, S. N., Koltzenburg, M., and Caterina, M. J. (2011). TRP vanilloid 2 knock-out mice are susceptible to perinatal lethality but display normal thermal and mechanical nociception. *J. Neurosci.* 31, 11425–11436. doi: 10.1523/jneurosci.1384-09.2011

Peng, W., Wong, Y. C., and Krainc, D. (2020). Mitochondria-lysosome contacts regulate mitochondrial Ca(2+) dynamics via lysosomal TRPML1. *Proc. Natl. Acad. Sci. U.S.A.* 117, 19266–19275. doi: 10.1073/pnas.2003236117

Pengelly, R. J., Greville-Heygate, S., Schmidt, S., Seaby, E. G., Jabalameli, M. R., Mehta, S. G., et al. (2016). Mutations specific to the Rac-GEF domain of TRIO cause intellectual disability and microcephaly. *J. Med. Genet.* 53, 735–742. doi: 10.1136/jmedgenet-2016-103942

Pennucci, R., Gucciardi, I., and De Curtis, I. (2019). Rac1 and Rac3 GTPases differently influence the morphological maturation of dendritic spines in hippocampal neurons. *PLoS One* 14:e0220496. doi: 10.1371/journal.pone.0220496

Pertz, O. (2010). Spatio-temporal Rho GTPase signaling - Where are we now? *J. Cell Sci.* 123, 1841–1850. doi: 10.1242/jcs.064345

Pertz, O., Hodgson, L., Klemke, R. L., and Hahn, K. M. (2006). Spatiotemporal dynamics of RhoA activity in migrating cells. *Nature* 440, 1069–1072. doi: 10.1038/nature04665

Phelan, K. D., Shwe, U. T., Abramowitz, J., Wu, H., Rhee, S. W., Howell, M. D., et al. (2013). Canonical transient receptor channel 5 (TRPC5) and TRPC1/4 contribute to seizure and excitotoxicity by distinct cellular mechanisms. *Mol. Pharmacol.* 83, 429–438. doi: 10.1124/mol.112.082271

Phelan, K. D., Shwe, U. T., Cozart, M. A., Wu, H., Mock, M. M., Abramowitz, J., et al. (2017). TRPC3 channels play a critical role in the theta component of pilocarpine-induced status epilepticus in mice. *Epilepsia* 58, 247–254. doi: 10.1111/epi.13648

Picardo, M. C. D., Sugimura, Y. K., Dorst, K. E., Kallurkar, P. S., Akins, V. T., Ma, X., et al. (2019). Trpm4 ion channels in pre-bötzinger complex interneurons are essential for breathing motor pattern but not rhythm. *PLoS Biol.* 17:e2006094. doi: 10.1371/journal.pbio.2006094

Piper, A. S., Yeats, J. C., Bevan, S., and Docherty, R. J. (1999). A study of the voltage dependence of capsaicin-activated membrane currents in rat sensory neurones before and after acute desensitization. *J. Physiol.* 518, 721–733. doi: 10.1111/j.1469-7793.1999.0721p.x

Pomrenze, M. B., Baratta, M. V., Rasmus, K. C., Cadle, B. A., Nakamura, S., Birnbaumer, L., et al. (2013). Cocaine self-administration in mice with forebrain knock-down of trpc5 ion channels. *F1000Res.* 2:53. doi: 10.12688/f1000research.2-53.v1

Posada-Duque, R. A., Barreto, G. E., and Cardona-Gomez, G. P. (2014). Protection after stroke: cellular effectors of neurovascular unit integrity. *Front. Cell. Neurosci.* 8:231. doi: 10.3389/fncel.2014.00231

Posada-Duque, R. A. S., Palacio-Castañeda, V., and Cardona-Gómez, G. P. (2015). CDK5 knockdown in astrocytes provide neuroprotection as a trophic source via Rac1. *Mol. Cell. Neurosci.* 68, 151–166. doi: 10.1016/j.mcn.2015.07.001

Puntambekar, P., Mukherjea, D., Jajoo, S., and Ramkumar, V. (2005). Essential role of Rac1/NADPH oxidase in nerve growth factor induction of TRPV1 expression. *J. Neurochem.* 95, 1689–1703. doi: 10.1111/j.1471-4159.2005.03518.x

Puram, S. V., Riccio, A., Koirala, S., Ikeuchi, Y., Kim, A. H., Corfas, G., et al. (2011). A TRPC5-regulated calcium signaling pathway controls dendrite patterning in the mammalian brain. *Genes Dev.* 25, 2659–2673. doi: 10.1101/gad.174060.111

Qin, N., Neeper, M. P., Liu, Y., Hutchinson, T. L., Lubin, M. L., and Flores, C. M. (2008). TRPV2 is activated by cannabidiol and mediates CGRP release in cultured rat dorsal root ganglion neurons. *J. Neurosci.* 28, 6231–6238. doi: 10.1523/jneurosci.0504-08.2008

Ramos, S., Khademi, F., Somesh, B. P., and Rivero, F. (2002). Genomic organization and expression profile of the small GTPases of the RhoBTB family in human and mouse. *Gene* 298, 147–157. doi: 10.1016/s0378-1119(02)00980-0

Ratnam, M., Chan, J., Lesani, N., Sidorova-Darmos, E., Eubanks, J. H., and Aarts, M. M. (2018). mRNA expression of transient receptor potential melastatin (TRPM) channels 2 and 7 in perinatal brain development. *Int. J. Dev. Neurosci.* 69, 23–31. doi: 10.1016/j.ijdevneu.2018.05.008

Raz, L., Zhang, Q. G., Zhou, C. F., Han, D., Gulati, P., Yang, L. C., et al. (2010). Role of Rac1 GTPase in NADPH oxidase activation and cognitive impairment following cerebral ischemia in the rat. *PLoS One* 5:e12606. doi: 10.1371/journal.pone.0012606

Reddy, J. M., Raut, N. G. R., Seifert, J. L., and Hynds, D. L. (2020). Regulation of small GTPase prenylation in the nervous system. *Mol. Neurobiol.* 57, 2220–2231. doi: 10.1007/s12035-020-01870-0

Ren, X. D., Kiosses, W. B., and Schwartz, M. A. (1999). Regulation of the small GTP-binding protein Rho by cell adhesion and the cytoskeleton. *EMBO J.* 18, 578–585. doi: 10.1093/emboj/18.3.578

Riccio, A., Li, Y., Moon, J., Kim, K. S., Smith, K. S., Rudolph, U., et al. (2009). Essential role for TRPC5 in amygdala function and fear-related behavior. *Cell* 137, 761–772. doi: 10.1016/s9999-9994(09)00535-2

Riccio, A., Medhurst, A. D., Mattei, C., Kelsell, R. E., Calver, A. R., Randall, A. D., et al. (2002). mRNA distribution analysis of human TRPC family in CNS and peripheral tissues. *Mol. Brain Res.* 109, 95–104. doi: 10.1016/s0169-328x(02)00527-2

Ridley, A. J. (2001). Rho proteins: linking signaling with membrane trafficking. *Traffic* 2, 303–310. doi: 10.1034/j.1600-0854.2001.002005303.x

Ridley, A. J., and Hall, A. (1992). The small GTP-binding protein rho regulates the assembly of focal adhesions and actin stress fibers in response to growth factors. *Cell* 70, 389–399. doi: 10.1016/0092-8674(92)90163-7

Ridley, A. J., Paterson, H. F., Johnston, C. L., Diekmann, D., and Hall, A. (1992). The small GTP-binding protein rac regulates growth factor-induced membrane ruffling. *Cell* 70, 401–410. doi: 10.1016/0092-8674(92)90164-8

Riquelme, D., Silva, I., Philp, A. M., Huidobro-Toro, J. P., Cerda, O., Trimmer, J. S., et al. (2018). Subcellular localization and activity of TRPM4 in medial prefrontal cortex layer 2/3. *Front. Cell. Neurosci.* 12:12. doi: 10.3389/fncel.2018.00012

Rivas, J., Díaz, N., Silva, I., Morales, D., Lavanderos, B., Álvarez, A., et al. (2020). KCTD5, a novel TRPM4-regulatory protein required for cell migration as a new predictor for breast cancer prognosis. *FASEB J.* 34, 7847–7865. doi: 10.1096/fj.201901195rrr

Roberts, P. J., Mitin, N., Keller, P. J., Chenette, E. J., Madigan, J. P., Currin, R. O., et al. (2008). Rho Family GTPase modification and dependence on CAAX motif-signaled posttranslational modification. *J. Biol. Chem.* 283, 25150–25163. doi: 10.1074/jbc.m800882200

Rohacs, T. (2014). Phosphoinositide regulation of TRP channels. *Handb. Exp. Pharmacol.* 223, 1143–1176. doi: 10.1007/978-3-319-05161-1_18

Ross, R. A. (2003). Anandamide and vanilloid TRPV1 receptors. *Br. J. Pharmacol.* 140, 790–801. doi: 10.1038/sj.bjp.0705467

Rottner, K., Faix, J., Bogdan, S., Linder, S., and Kerkhoff, E. (2017). Actin assembly mechanisms at a glance. *J. Cell Sci.* 130, 3427–3435. doi: 10.1242/jcs.206433

Russell, J. T. (2011). Imaging calcium signals in vivo: a powerful tool in physiology and pharmacology. *Br. J. Pharmacol.* 163, 1605–1625. doi: 10.1111/j.1476-5381.2010.00988.x

Saneyoshi, T., and Hayashi, Y. (2012). The ca 2+ and rho gtpase signaling pathways underlying activity-dependent actin remodeling at dendritic spines. *Cytoskeleton* 69, 545–554. doi: 10.1002/cm.21037

Schaefer, A., Reinhard, N. R., and Hordijk, P. L. (2014). Toward understanding RhoGTPase specificity: structure, function and local activation. *Small GTPases* 5:6.

Schattling, B., Steinbach, K., Thies, E., Kruse, M., Menigoz, A., Ufer, F., et al. (2012). TRPM4 cation channel mediates axonal and neuronal degeneration in experimental autoimmune encephalomyelitis and multiple sclerosis. *Nat. Med.* 18, 1805–1811. doi: 10.1038/nm.3015

Schmitt, J. M., Smith, S., Hart, B., and Fletcher, L. (2012). CaM kinase control of AKT and LNCaP cell survival. *J. Cell. Biochem.* 113, 1514–1526.

Schweppe, D. K., Huttlin, E. L., Harper, J. W., and Gygi, S. P. (2018). BioPlex display: an interactive suite for large-scale ap-ms protein-protein interaction data. *J. Proteome Res.* 17, 722–726. doi: 10.1021/acs.jproteome.7b00572

Scott, B. B., Thiberge, S. Y., Guo, C., Tervo, D. G. R., Brody, C. D., Karpova, A. Y., et al. (2018). Imaging cortical dynamics in GCaMP transgenic rats with a head-mounted widefield macroscope. *Neuron* 100, 1045.e9–1058.e9.

Semenova, M. M., Mäki-Hokkonen, A. M. J., Cao, J., Komarovski, V., Forsberg, K. M., Koistinaho, M., et al. (2007). Rho mediates calcium-dependent activation of p38alpha and subsequent excitotoxic cell death. *Nat. Neurosci.* 10, 436–443. doi: 10.1038/nn1869

Sexton, J. E., Desmonds, T., Quick, K., Taylor, R., Abramowitz, J., Forge, A., et al. (2016). The contribution of TRPC1, TRPC3, TRPC5 and TRPC6 to touch and hearing. *Neurosci. Lett.* 610, 36–42. doi: 10.1016/j.neulet.2015.10.052

Shen, D., Wang, X., Li, X., Zhang, X., Yao, Z., Dibble, S., et al. (2012). Lipid storage disorders block lysosomal trafficking by inhibiting a TRP channel and lysosomal calcium release. *Nat. Commun.* 3:731.

Shen, H., Pan, J., Pan, L., and Zhang, N. (2013). TRPC6 inhibited NMDA current in cultured hippocampal neurons. *NeuroMol. Med.* 15, 389–395. doi: 10.1007/s12017-013-8226-1

Shen, J., Tu, L., Chen, D., Tan, T., Wang, Y., and Wang, S. (2019). TRPV4 channels stimulate Ca 2+ -induced Ca 2+ release in mouse neurons and trigger endoplasmic reticulum stress after intracerebral hemorrhage. *Brain Res. Bull.* 146, 143–152. doi: 10.1016/j.brainresbull.2018.11.024

Shibasaki, K., Ishizaki, Y., and Mandadi, S. (2013). Astrocytes express functional TRPV2 ion channels. *Biochem. Biophys. Res. Commun.* 441, 327–332. doi: 10.1016/j.bbrc.2013.10.046

Shibasaki, K., Murayama, N., Ono, K., Ishizaki, Y., and Tominaga, M. (2010). TRPV2 enhances axon outgrowth through its activation by membrane stretch in developing sensory and motor neurons. *J. Neurosci.* 30, 4601–4612. doi: 10.1523/jneurosci.5830-09.2010

Shimizu, T., Owsianik, G., Freichel, M., Flockerzi, V., Nilius, B., and Vennekens, R. (2009). TRPM4 regulates migration of mast cells in mice. *Cell Calcium* 45, 226–232. doi: 10.1016/j.ceca.2008.10.005

Shimokawa, H., Sunamura, S., and Satoh, K. (2016). RhoA/Rho-kinase in the cardiovascular system. *Circ. Res.* 118, 352–366. doi: 10.1161/circresaha.115.306532

Shin, D. M., Kang, J., Ha, J., Kang, H. S., Park, S. C., Kim, I. G., et al. (2008). Cystamine prevents ischemia-reperfusion injury by inhibiting polyamination of RhoA. *Biochem. Biophys. Res. Commun.* 365, 509–514. doi: 10.1016/j.bbrc.2007.11.007

Shin, Y. C., Shin, S. Y., So, I., Kwon, D., and Jeon, J. H. (2011). TRIP Database: a manually curated database of protein-protein interactions for mammalian TRP channels. *Nucleic Acids Res.* 39, 356–361.

Shioda, N., Beppu, H., Fukuda, T., Li, E., Kitajima, I., and Fukunaga, K. (2011). Aberrant calcium/calmodulin-dependent protein kinase II (CaMKII) activity is associated with abnormal dendritic spine morphology in the ATRX mutant mouse brain. *J. Neurosci.* 31, 346–358. doi: 10.1523/jneurosci.4816-10.2011

Simon, F., Leiva-Salcedo, E., Armisén, R., Riveros, A., Cerda, O., Varela, D., et al. (2010). Hydrogen peroxide removes TRPM4 current desensitization conferring increased vulnerability to necrotic cell death. *J. Biol. Chem.* 285, 37150–37158. doi: 10.1074/jbc.m110.155390

Sin, W. C., Haas, K., Ruthazer, E. S., and Cline, H. T. (2002). Dendrite growth increased by visual activity requires NMDA receptor and Rho GTPases. *Nature* 419, 475–480. doi: 10.1038/nature00987

Singh, B. B., Liu, X., Tang, J., Zhu, M. X., and Ambudkar, I. S. (2002). Calmodulin regulates Ca2+-dependent feedback inhibition of store-operated Ca2+ influx by interaction with a site in the C terminus of TrpC1. *Mol. Cell* 9, 739–750. doi: 10.1016/s1097-2765(02)00506-3

Singh, I., Knezevic, N., Ahmmed, G. U., Kini, V., Malik, A. B., and Mehta, D. (2007). Gαq-TRPC6-mediated Ca2+ entry induces RhoA activation and resultant endothelial cell shape change in response to thrombin. *J. Biol. Chem.* 282, 7833–7843. doi: 10.1074/jbc.m608288200

Smith, K. R., Rajgor, D., and Hanley, J. G. (2017). Differential regulation of the Rac1 GTPaseΓÇôactivating protein (GAP) BCR during oxygen/glucose deprivation in hippocampal and cortical neurons. *J. Biol. Chem.* 292, 20173–20183. doi: 10.1074/jbc.m117.796292

Spillane, M., and Gallo, G. (2014). Involvement of Rho-family GTPases in axon branching. *Small GTPases* 5, 37–41.

Spooner, E., Mclaughlin, B. M., Lepow, T., Durns, T. A., Randall, J., Upchurch, C., et al. (2013). Systematic screens for proteins that interact with the mucolipidosis

Type IV protein TRPML1. *PLoS One* 8:e56780. doi: 10.1371/journal.pone.0056780
Stankiewicz, T. R., and Linseman, D. A. (2014). Rho family GTPases: key players in neuronal development, neuronal survival, and neurodegeneration. *Front. Cell. Neurosci.* 8:314. doi: 10.3389/fncel.2014.00314
Starr, A., Graepel, R., Keeble, J., Schmidhuber, S., Clark, N., Grant, A., et al. (2008). A reactive oxygen species-mediated component in neurogenic vasodilatation. *Cardiovasc. Res.* 78, 139–147. doi: 10.1093/cvr/cvn012
Su, L. T., Liu, W., Chen, H. C., González-Pagán, O., Habas, R., and Runnels, L. W. (2011). TRPM7 regulates polarized cell movements. *Biochem. J.* 434, 513–521. doi: 10.1042/bj20101678
Sudhahar, V., Shaw, S., and Imig, J. (2010). Epoxyeicosatrienoic acid analogs and vascular function. *Curr. Med. Chem.* 17, 1181–1190. doi: 10.2174/092986710790827843
Suehiro, J., Kanki, Y., Makihara, C., Schadler, K., Miura, M., Manabe, Y., et al. (2014). Genome-wide approaches reveal functional vascular endothelial growth factor (VEGF)-inducible nuclear factor of activated T cells (NFAT) c1 binding to angiogenesis-related genes in the endothelium. *J. Biol. Chem.* 289, 29044–29059. doi: 10.1074/jbc.m114.555235
Sugawara, T., Hisatsune, C., Miyamoto, H., Ogawa, N., and Mikoshiba, K. (2017). Regulation of spinogenesis in mature Purkinje cells via mGluR/PKC-mediated phosphorylation of CaMKIIbeta. *Proc. Natl. Acad. Sci. U.S.A.* 114, E5256–E5265.
Sugio, S., Nagasawa, M., Kojima, I., Ishizaki, Y., and Shibasaki, K. (2017). Transient receptor potential vanilloid 2 activation by focal mechanical stimulation requires interaction with the actin cytoskeleton and enhances growth cone motility. *FASEB J.* 31, 1368–1381. doi: 10.1096/fj.201600686rr
Sun, H.-S., Jackson, M. F., Martin, L. J., Jansen, K., Teves, L., Cui, H., et al. (2009). Suppression of hippocampal TRPM7 protein prevents delayed neuronal death in brain ischemia. *Nat. Neurosci.* 12, 1300–1307. doi: 10.1038/nn.2395
Sun, J., Yang, T., Wang, P., Ma, S., Zhu, Z., Pu, Y., et al. (2014). Activation of cold-sensing transient receptor potential melastatin subtype 8 antagonizes vasoconstriction and hypertension through attenuating RhoA/Rho kinase pathway. *Hypertension* 63, 1354–1363. doi: 10.1161/hypertensionaha.113.02573
Sun, Y., Sukumaran, P., Schaar, A., and Singh, B. B. (2015). TRPM7 and its role in neurodegenerative diseases. *Channels* 9, 253–261. doi: 10.1080/19336950.2015.1075675
Szászi, I. K., Sirokmány, G., Di Ciano-Oliveira, C., Rotstein, O. D., and Kapus, A. (2005). Depolarization induces Rho-Rho kinase-mediated myosin light chain phosphorylation in kidney tubular cells. *Am. J. Physiol. Cell Physiol.* 289, C673–C685.
Tai, Y., Feng, S., Ge, R., Du, W., Zhang, X., He, Z., et al. (2008). TRPC6 channels promote dendritic growth via the CaMKIV-CREB pathway. *J. Cell Sci.* 121, 2301–2307. doi: 10.1242/jcs.026906
Takano, T., Wu, M., Nakamuta, S., Naoki, H., Ishizawa, N., Namba, T., et al. (2017). Discovery of long-range inhibitory signaling to ensure single axon formation. *Nat. Commun.* 8, 1–17.
Takemura, M., Mishima, T., Wang, Y., Kasahara, J., Fukunaga, K., Ohashi, K., et al. (2009). Ca2+/Calmodulin-dependent protein kinase IV-mediated LIM kinase activation is critical for calcium signal-inducedneurite outgrowth. *J. Biol. Chem.* 284, 28554–28562. doi: 10.1074/jbc.m109.006296
Tao, R., Lu, R., Wang, J., Zeng, S., Zhang, T., Guo, W., et al. (2020). Probing the therapeutic potential of TRPC6 for Alzheimer's disease in live neurons from patient-specific iPSCs. *J. Mol. Cell Biol.* [Epub ahead of print].
Tashiro, A. (2000). Regulation of dendritic spine morphology by the rho family of small GTPases: antagonistic roles of Rac and Rho. *Cereb. Cortex* 10, 927–938. doi: 10.1093/cercor/10.10.927
Tedeschi, V., Petrozziello, T., Sisalli, M. J., Boscia, F., Canzoniero, L. M. T., and Secondo, A. (2019). The activation of Mucolipin TRP channel 1 (TRPML1) protects motor neurons from L-BMAA neurotoxicity by promoting autophagic clearance. *Sci. Rep.* 9, 1–11. doi: 10.1007/s12640-017-9739-4
Teruyama, R., Sakuraba, M., Kurotaki, H., and Armstrong, W. E. (2011). Transient receptor potential channel M4 and M5 in magnocellular cells in rat supraoptic and paraventricular nuclei. *J. Neuroendocrinol.* 23, 1204–1213. doi: 10.1111/j.1365-2826.2011.02211.x
Thoppil, R. J., Cappelli, H. C., Adapala, R. K., Kanugula, A. K., Paruchuri, S., and Thodeti, C. K. (2016). TRPV4 channels regulate tumor angiogenesis via modulation of Rho/Rho kinase pathway. *Oncotarget* 7, 25849–25861. doi: 10.18632/oncotarget.8405
Tian, D., Jacobo, S. M., Billing, D., Rozkalne, A., Gage, S. D., Anagnostou, T., et al. (2010). Antagonistic regulation of actin dynamics and cell motility by TRPC5 and TRPC6 channels. *Sci. Signal.* 3:ra77. doi: 10.1126/scisignal.2001200
Tian, X., Yan, H., Li, J., Wu, S., Wang, J., and Fan, L. (2017). Neurotrophin promotes neurite outgrowth by inhibiting Rif GTPase activation downstream of MAPKs and PI3K signaling. *Int. J. Mol. Sci.* 18:148. doi: 10.3390/ijms18010148
Tolias, K. F., Bikoff, J. B., Burette, A., Paradis, S., Harrar, D., Tavazoie, S., et al. (2005). The Rac1-GEF Tiam1 couples the NMDA receptor to the activity-dependent development of dendritic arbors and spines. *Neuron* 45, 525–538. doi: 10.1016/j.neuron.2005.01.024
Toriyama, M., Kozawa, S., Sakumura, Y., and Inagaki, N. (2013). Conversion of a signal into forces for axon outgrowth through Pak1-mediated shootin1 phosphorylation. *Curr. Biol.* 23, 529–534. doi: 10.1016/j.cub.2013.02.017
Tsunemi, T., Perez-Rosello, T., Ishiguro, Y., Yoroisaka, A., Jeon, S., Hamada, K., et al. (2019). Increased lysosomal exocytosis induced by lysosomal Ca2+ Channel agonists protects human dopaminergic neurons from alpha-synuclein toxicity. *J. Neurosci.* 39, 5760–5772. doi: 10.1523/jneurosci.3085-18.2019
Turlova, E., Bae, C. Y. J., Deurloo, M., Chen, W., Barszczyk, A., Horgen, F. D., et al. (2016). TRPM7 regulates axonal outgrowth and maturation of primary hippocampal neurons. *Mol. Neurobiol.* 53, 595–610.
Um, K., Niu, S., Duman, J. G., Cheng, J. X., Tu, Y. K., Schwechter, B., et al. (2014). Dynamic control of excitatory synapse development by a Rac1 GEF/GAP regulatory complex. *Dev. Cell* 29, 701–715. doi: 10.1016/j.devcel.2014.05.011
Vega, F. M., and Ridley, A. J. (2008). Rho GTPases in cancer cell biology. *FEBS Lett.* 582, 2093–2101. doi: 10.1016/j.febslet.2008.04.039
Venkatachalam, K., and Montell, C. (2007). TRP channels TRP: transient receptor potential. *Annu. Rev. Biochem.* 76, 387–417.
Vennekens, R., Olausson, J., Meissner, M., Bloch, W., Mathar, I., Philipp, S. E., et al. (2007). Increased IgE-dependent mast cell activation and anaphylactic responses in mice lacking the calcium-activated nonselective cation channel TRPM4. *Nat. Immunol.* 8, 312–320. doi: 10.1038/ni1441
Vidal-Quadras, M., Gelabert-Baldrich, M., Soriano-Castell, D., Lladó, A., Rentero, C., Calvo, M., et al. (2011). Rac1 and calmodulin interactions modulate dynamics of ARF6-dependent endocytosis. *Traffic* 12, 1879–1896. doi: 10.1111/j.1600-0854.2011.01274.x
Voringer, S., Schreyer, L., Nadolni, W., Meier, M. A., Woerther, K., Mittermeier, C., et al. (2020). Inhibition of TRPM7 blocks MRTF/SRF-dependent transcriptional and tumorigenic activity. *Oncogene* 39, 2328–2344. doi: 10.1038/s41388-019-1140-8
Wagner, E., and Glotzer, M. (2016). Local RhoA activation induces cytokinetic furrows independent of spindle position and cell cycle stage. *J. Cell Biol.* 213, 641–649. doi: 10.1083/jcb.201603025
Wainwright, A., Rutter, A. R., Seabrook, G. R., Reilly, K., and Oliver, K. R. (2004). Discrete expression of TRPV2 within the hypothalamo-neurohypophysial system: implications for regulatory activity within the hypothalamic-pituitary-adrenal axis. *J. Comp. Neurol.* 474, 24–42. doi: 10.1002/cne.20100
Wang, D., Chan, C. C., Cherry, S., and Hiesinger, P. R. (2013). Membrane trafficking in neuronal maintenance and degeneration. *Cell. Mol. Life Sci.* 70, 2919–2934. doi: 10.1007/s00018-012-1201-4
Wang, H., Cheng, X., Tian, J., Xiao, Y., Tian, T., Xu, F., et al. (2020). TRPC channels: structure, function, regulation and recent advances in small molecular probes. *Pharmacol. Ther.* 209:107497. doi: 10.1016/j.pharmthera.2020.107497
Wang, W., Gao, Q., Yang, M., Zhang, X., Yu, L., Lawas, M., et al. (2015). Up-regulation of lysosomal TRPML1 channels is essential for lysosomal adaptation to nutrient starvation. *Proc. Natl. Acad. Sci. U.S.A.* 112, E1373–E1381.
Wayman, G. A., Tokumitsu, H., Davare, M. A., and Soderling, T. R. (2011). Analysis of CaM-kinase signaling in cells. *Cell Calcium* 50, 1–8. doi: 10.1016/j.ceca.2011.02.007
Wedlich-Soldner, R., Altschuter, S., Wu, L., and Li, R. (2003). Spontaneous cell polarization through actomyosin-based delivery of the Cdc42 GTPase. *Science* 299, 1231–1235. doi: 10.1126/science.1080944
Westermarck, J., Ivaska, J., and Corthals, G. L. (2013). Identification of protein interactions involved in cellular signaling. *Mol. Cell Proteomics* 12, 1752–1763. doi: 10.1074/mcp.r113.027771

White, J. P. M., Cibelli, M., Urban, L., Nilius, B., Mcgeown, J. G., and Nagy, I. (2016). TRPV4: molecular conductor of a diverse orchestra. *Physiol. Rev.* 96, 911–973. doi: 10.1152/physrev.00016.2015

Woo, S., and Gomez, T. M. (2006). Rac1 and RhoA promote neurite outgrowth through formation and stabilization of growth cone point contacts. *J. Neurosci.* 26, 1418–1428. doi: 10.1523/jneurosci.4209-05.2006

Wu, B., Blot, F. B. G. C., Wong, A. B., Osório, C., Adolfs, Y., Pasterkamp, R. J., et al. (2019). TRPC3 is a major contributor to functional heterogeneity of cerebellar Purkinje cells. *eLife* 8, 1–31.

Wu, K. Y., Hengst, U., Cox, L. J., Macosko, E. Z., Jeromin, A., Urquhart, E. R., et al. (2005). Local translation of RhoA regulates growth cone collapse. *Nature* 436, 1020–1024. doi: 10.1038/nature03885

Wu, Y. I., Frey, D., Lungu, O. I., Jaehrig, A., Schlichting, I., Kuhlman, B., et al. (2009). A genetically encoded photoactivatable Rac controls the motility of living cells. *Nature* 461, 104–108. doi: 10.1038/nature 08241

Xie, Z., Srivastava, D. P., Photowala, H., Kai, L., Cahill, M. E., Woolfrey, K. M., et al. (2007). Kalirin-7 controls activity-dependent structural and functional plasticity of dendritic spines. *Neuron* 56, 640–656. doi: 10.1016/j.neuron.2007. 10.005

Xiong, S., Wang, B., Lin, S., Zhang, H., Li, Y., Wei, X., et al. (2017). Activation of transient receptor potential melastatin subtype 8 attenuates cold-induced hypertension through ameliorating vascular mitochondrial dysfunction. *J. Am. Heart Assoc.* 6, 1–17.

Xu, J., Zhang, W., Cui, W., Shi, B., and Wang, H. (2019). PKCα promotes insulin secretion via TRPC1 phosphorylation in INS-1E cells. *Biosci. Biotechnol. Biochem.* 83, 1676–1682. doi: 10.1080/09168451.2019.16 17106

Yadav, M., and Goswami, C. (2019). TRPV2 activation reorganizes actin cytoskeleton, induces neurite initiation and branching by altering cAMP levels. *bioRxiv* [Preprint]. doi: 10.1101/817684

Yamada, T., Ohoka, Y., Kogo, M., and Inagaki, S. (2005). Physical and functional interactions of the lysophosphatidic acid receptors with PDZ domain-containing Rho guanine nucleotide exchange factors (RhoGEFs). *J. Biol. Chem.* 280, 19358–19363. doi: 10.1074/jbc.m414561200

Yang, H., Zhao, B., Liao, C., Zhang, R., Meng, K., Xu, J., et al. (2013). High glucose-induced apoptosis in cultured podocytes involves TRPC6-dependent calcium entry via the RhoA/ROCK pathway. *Biochem. Biophys. Res. Commun.* 434, 394–400. doi: 10.1016/j.bbrc.2013.03.087

Yang, M., James, A. D., Suman, R., Kasprowicz, R., Nelson, M., O'toole, P. J., et al. (2020). Voltage-dependent activation of Rac1 by Nav1.5 channels promotes cell migration. *J. Cell. Physiol.* 235, 3950–3972. doi: 10.1002/jcp. 29290

Yang, N., Higuchi, O., Ohashi, K., Nagata, K., Wada, A., Kangawa, K., et al. (1998). Cofilin phosphorylation by LIM-kinase 1 and its role in Rac-mediated actin reorganization. *Nature* 393, 809–812. doi: 10.1038/31735

Yuan, J. P., Zeng, W., Huang, G. N., Worley, P. F., and Muallem, S. (2007). STIM1 heteromultimerizes TRPC channels to determine their function as store-operated channels. *Nat. Cell Biol.* 9, 636–645. doi: 10.1038/ncb1590

Yuan, P. (2019). Structural biology of thermoTRPV channels. *Cell Calcium* 84:102106. doi: 10.1016/j.ceca.2019.102106

Zamboni, V., Armentano, M., Berto, G., Ciraolo, E., Ghigo, A., Garzotto, D., et al. (2018). Hyperactivity of Rac1-GTPase pathway impairs neuritogenesis of cortical neurons by altering actin dynamics. *Sci. Rep.* 8, 1–16. doi: 10.1155/ 2013/859257

Zanata, S. M., Hovatta, I., Rohm, B., and Püschel, A. W. (2002). Antagonistic effects of Rnd1 and RhoD GTPases regulate receptor activity in Semaphorin 3A-induced cytoskeletal collapse. *J. Neurosci.* 22, 471–477. doi: 10.1523/ jneurosci.22-02-00471.2002

Zeng, C., Tian, F., and Xiao, B. (2016). TRPC channels: prominent candidates of underlying mechanism in neuropsychiatric diseases. *Mol. Neurobiol.* 53, 631–647. doi: 10.1007/s12035-014-9004-2

Zeng, J., Wu, Y., Zhuang, S., Qin, L., Hua, S., Mungur, R., et al. (2019). Identification of the role of TRPM8 in glioblastoma and its effect on proliferation, apoptosis and invasion of the U251 human glioblastoma cell line. *Oncol. Rep.* 42, 1517–1526.

Zeug, A., Müller, F. E., Anders, S., Herde, M. K., Minge, D., Ponimaskin, E., et al. (2018). Control of astrocyte morphology by Rho GTPases. *Brain Res. Bull.* 136, 44–53. doi: 10.1016/j.brainresbull.2017.05.003

Zhang, E., and Liao, P. (2015). Brain transient receptor potential channels and stroke. *J. Neuroscie. Res.* 93, 1165–1183. doi: 10.1002/jnr.23529

Zhang, L., Fang, Y., Cheng, X., Lian, Y., Xu, H., Zeng, Z., et al. (2017). TRPML1 participates in the progression of Alzheimer's Disease by regulating the PPARγ/AMPK/Mtor signalling pathway. *Cell. Physiol. Biochem.* 43, 2446–2456. doi: 10.1159/000484449

Zhang, L., Papadopoulos, P., and Hamel, E. (2013). Endothelial TRPV4 channels mediate dilation of cerebral arteries: impairment and recovery in cerebrovascular pathologies related to Alzheimer's disease. *Bri. J. Pharmacol.* 170, 661–670. doi: 10.1111/bph.12315

Zhang, L., Wu, J., Duan, X., Tian, X., Shen, H., Sun, Q., et al. (2016). NADPH oxidase: a potential target for treatment of stroke. *Oxid. Med. Cell. Longev.* 2016:5026984.

Zhao, H., Zhang, K., Tang, R., Meng, H., Zou, Y., Wu, P., et al. (2018). TRPV4 blockade preserves the blood-brain barrier by inhibiting stress fiber formation in a rat model of intracerebral hemorrhage. *Front. Mol. Neurosci.* 11:97. doi: 10.3389/fnmol.2018.00097

Zhou, J., Du, W., Zhou, K., Tai, Y., Yao, H., Jia, Y., et al. (2008). Critical role of TRPC6 channels in the formation of excitatory synapses. *Nat. Neurosci.* 11, 741–743. doi: 10.1038/nn.2127

Zhu, D., You, J., Zhao, N., and Xu, H. (2019). Magnesium regulates endothelial barrier functions through TRPM7, MagT1, and S1P1. *Adv. Sci.* 6:1901166. doi: 10.1002/advs.201901166

Zhu, G., Fan, Z., Ding, M., Zhang, H., Mu, L., Ding, Y., et al. (2015). An EGFR/PI3K/AKT axis promotes accumulation of the Rac1-GEF Tiam1 that is critical in EGFR-driven tumorigenesis. *Oncogene* 34, 5971–5982. doi: 10.1038/ onc.2015.45

Zhu, M. X. (2005). Multiple roles of calmodulin and other Ca2+-binding proteins in the functional regulation of TRP channels. *Pflugers Arch. Eur. J. Physiol.* 451, 105–115. doi: 10.1007/s00424-005-1427-1

Zohrabian, V. M., Forzani, B., Chau, Z., Murali, R., and Jhanwar-Uniyal, M. (2009). Rho/ROCK and MAPK signaling pathways are involved in glioblastoma cell migration and proliferation. *Anticancer Res.* 29, 119–123.

8

Resolvins: Potent Pain Inhibiting Lipid Mediators via Transient Receptor Potential Regulation

Jueun Roh[1†], Eun Jin Go[1†], Jin-Woo Park[2], Yong Ho Kim[1] and Chul-Kyu Park[1*]*

[1] *Gachon Pain Center and Department of Physiology, College of Medicine, Gachon University, Incheon, South Korea,*
[2] *Department of Periodontology, School of Dentistry, Kyungpook National University, Daegu, South Korea*

Correspondence:
Yong Ho Kim
euro16@gachon.ac.kr
Chul-Kyu Park
pck0708@gachon.ac.kr

[†] These authors have contributed equally to this work

Chronic pain is a serious condition that occurs in the peripheral nervous system (PNS) and the central nervous system (CNS). It is caused by inflammation or nerve damage that induces the release of inflammatory mediators from immune cells and/or protein kinase activation in neuronal cells. Both nervous systems are closely linked; therefore, inflammation or nerve damage in the PNS can affect the CNS (central sensitization). In this process, nociceptive transient receptor potential (TRP) channel activation and expression are increased. As a result, nociceptive neurons are activated, and pain signals to the brain are amplified and prolonged. In other words, suppressing the onset of pain signals in the PNS can suppress pain signals to the CNS. Resolvins, endogenous lipid mediators generated during the resolution phase of acute inflammation, inhibit nociceptive TRP ion channels and alleviate chronic pain. This paper summarizes the effect of resolvins in chronic pain control and discusses future scientific perspectives. Further study on the effect of resolvins on neuropathic pain will expand the scope of pain research.

Keywords: resolvins, TRP channel, pain, inflammatory, neuropathy

INTRODUCTION

The International Association for the Study of Pain defines pain as an unpleasant sensory and emotional experience associated with, or resembling that associated with, actual or potential tissue damage (Raja et al., 2020). Pain is classified into three types according to its cause. First, the pain generated when individuals are exposed to noxious stimuli such as extreme temperatures or sharp objects, is called nociceptive pain. Generally, pain is considered to be a negative feeling that needs to be eliminated, but nociceptive pain is protective and essential. It protects us from being injured by a hostile environment (Scholz and Woolf, 2002; Woolf, 2010). Second, inflammatory pain is caused by activation of the immune system, and it is also protective. Inflammation following tissue injury or infection is characterized by releasing proinflammatory mediators including bradykinin, prostaglandins, nerve growth factors (NGF), proinflammatory cytokines, and chemokines from immune cells. These mediators bind to pain receptors expressed in nociceptors (Woolf, 2010; Lim et al., 2015). Pathological pain is not protective and results from abnormal functioning of the nervous system. This can be categorized into two types depending on the presence of damage; one is neuropathic pain, which occurs after nerve damage; the other is dysfunctional pain, which can occur in the absence of inflammation or nerve damage (Woolf, 2010).

Inflammation and nerve damage can induce neural plasticity that results from changes in the nervous system and reduces the pain threshold. Therefore, inflammatory pain and neuropathic pain are characterized by peripheral nociceptor sensitization, arising from spontaneous nociceptor activity, hyperalgesia, and allodynia. Transient receptor potential (TRP) ion channels that are expressed in nociceptors are persistently activated by inflammatory mediators during the pathological state. TRPV1 and TRPA1 are notable nociceptive TRP ion channels, and activation of these channels can stimulate hyperexcitability of the peripheral nociceptors that transmit pain signaling to the central nervous system (CNS) (Scholz and Woolf, 2002; Patapoutian et al., 2009; Lim et al., 2015; Jardin et al., 2017; Mourot et al., 2018). Inflammatory pain includes pain from a surgical wound or an inflamed joint, while the etiology of neuropathic pain includes diabetes and chemotherapy-related peripheral neuropathy.

Resolvins (RVs) are lipid mediators that are biosynthesized from omega-3 polyunsaturated fatty acids (PUFAs) that are abundant in marine oil. Aspirin/cyclooxygenase-2 (COX-2) and other enzymes convert omega-3 docosahexaenoic acid (DHA) and eicosapentaenoic acid (EPA) to resolvin D and E through multiple mechanisms (Serhan et al., 2002). These lipid mediators are generated during the resolution phase of acute inflammation and not only terminate inflammation but also alleviate pain (Ariel and Serhan, 2007; Xu et al., 2010). The Ji lab found that the resolvin series has an analgesic effect on various types of inflammatory pain models through regulation of TRP channels (Xu et al., 2010; Park et al., 2011b).

This review will highlight TRP channels, with an emphasis on TRPV1 and TRPA1, as therapeutic targets for the resolution of both inflammatory and neuropathic pain using resolvins. To address this, pain and TRP are first described prior to resolvins. At the end, the importance of further study on the role of resolvins in neuropathic pain via TRP regulation is also suggested.

CONNECTIVITY OF PERIPHERAL AND CENTRAL NERVOUS SYSTEMS IN PAIN PATHWAYS

Anatomical Pain Pathway

Primary afferent neurons are pseudounipolar neurons that have one axon from the soma and bidirectional branches at the axon terminals (Amir and Devor, 2003; Gibson and Ma, 2011). The branches project to the peripheral (target organ) and central projection (spinal cord), respectively (Gibson and Ma, 2011), and transduce sensory information (mechanical, thermal, and chemical) from the peripheral to the central nervous system (Hasegawa et al., 2007).

Primary afferent nerve fibers are classified by fiber diameter or myelination and project to distinct laminae in the dorsal horn of the spinal cord. Fiber diameter and myelination are related to conduction velocity. Myelinated Aα and Aβ fibers have a large diameter and fast conduction velocity. Rapidly conducting Aβ fibers conduct proprioception and touch sensations and project to deeper laminae: III, IV, and V. However, studies have revealed that some Aβ fibers also are related to pain regulation (Xu et al., 2015; Tashima et al., 2018; Nagi et al., 2019). While thinly myelinated Aδ fibers and unmyelinated C fibers both have relatively small diameters, the former have faster conduction velocities than do the latter. Aδ fibers conduct touch, pressure, and "first" pain signals to laminae I and V. Slowly conducting C fibers respond to heat and mechanical stimuli and conduct "second" pain related signals to lamina I (peptidergic C fibers) and lamina II (non-peptidergic C fibers) (Julius and Basbaum, 2001; Furue et al., 2004; Basbaum et al., 2009). Unmyelinated C fibers and thinly myelinated Aδ fibers are activated by high-intensity stimuli (Ji and Woolf, 2001). The activation of Aδ fibers evokes sharp and pricking pain, whereas the activation of C fibers evokes a burning sensation (Bishop, 1980).

Different pathways to the brain carry different types of sensory information. Pain and heat signals from C and Aδ fibers in the superficial dorsal horn cross the midline and ascend the spinal cord. Then, sensory information is carried to the brain through the lateral spinothalamic tract (Melzack and Wall, 1962; Basbaum et al., 2009). On the other hand, proprioception and touch signals do not cross the spinal cord but ascend to the brain through the anterior spinothalamic tract (Basbaum et al., 2009).

Central Sensitization

Central sensitization involves the increased responsiveness of nociceptive neurons in the CNS that can be generated from intense and repeated peripheral inputs. Sensitized C-fibers lead to the increased release of neurotransmitters such as glutamate, substance P (SP), calcitonin gene-related peptide (CGRP), and brain-derived neurotrophic factor (BDNF) into central terminals of the spinal cord dorsal horn (postsynaptic). Released neurotransmitters bind to their receptors, including *N*-methyl-D-aspartate receptors (NMDAR), α-Amino-3-hydroxy-5-methyl-4-isoxazolepropionic acid receptors (AMPAR), metabotropic glutamate receptors (mGluR), neurokinin-1 receptors (NK-1R), and tropomyosin receptor kinase (Trk) receptors, on the postsynaptic neurons. These series of processes induce hyperactive/hyperexcited states in the postsynaptic neurons and result in hyperalgesia (an abnormal increase in pain sensitivity from painful stimuli), allodynia (pain caused by non-painful stimuli), and the expansion of the receptive fields of nociceptors (Hylden et al., 1989; Latremoliere and Woolf, 2009; Woolf, 2011). Additionally, peripheral injury can redistribute the central terminals of myelinated afferents and induce pain by non-painful afferents (Woolf et al., 1992; Tashima et al., 2018; Nagi et al., 2019). This process seems similar to peripheral sensitization in so far as it also results in hyperalgesia and allodynia but differs in the range of sites that cause the resulting pain. Peripheral sensitization occurs when nociceptors are exposed to inflammatory mediators and damaged tissue. Consequently, the abnormal pain sensation prompted by peripheral sensitization is limited to inflamed or damaged sites. Hence, this phenomenon can function to protect sites of injury. By contrast, central sensitization can induce pain either in sites where inflammation or injury has already been resolved or without no obvious inflammation or injury.

Intracellular Ca^{2+} is important to initiating central sensitization. Under normal conditions, the pores of NMDARs are blocked by Mg^{2+}. However, glutamates released from presynaptic buds dislodge Mg^{2+} and allow Ca^{2+} to enter the cytosol. Further, activation of the group I mGluRs (mGluR1 and 5) opens the Ca^{2+} channels on the endoplasmic reticulum (ER). Intracellular Ca^{2+} activates protein kinase C (PKC), PKA, and calmodulin-dependent protein kinase II (CaMKII). These kinases phosphorylate ion channels and glutamate receptors, and their properties are rapidly changed. PKC phosphorylates Ser831 on the GluR1 of AMPAR, Ser880 on GluR2, and Ser896 on NR1 of the NMDAR subunit. PKA phosphorylates Ser890 and Ser897 on NR1 and Ser845 on GluR1. CaMKII phosphorylates Ser1303 on NR2B and Ser831 on GluR1 (Suo et al., 2013; Ji et al., 2018). These processes correspond to the early, phosphorylation-dependent phase of central sensitization in which extracellular signal-regulated protein kinase (ERK) is important to sustain central sensitization. The activation of ERK stimulates increases in the transcription of several genes, such as c-*Fos*, NK1, TrkB, and Cox-2, the phosphorylation of NMDAR and Ser616 on Kv4.2, and the insertion of AMPAR into the membrane. Together, these events increase neuronal excitability in the spinal cord (Ji and Woolf, 2001; Pace et al., 2018).

TRP CHANNEL AND PAIN

Unpleasant and painful sensations signal organisms to subsequently avoid these situations, allowing the organisms to survive noxious insults and injuries. Such noxious stimuli are detected by nociceptors, specialized peripheral sensory neurons that send the threatening signals to the spinal cord and the brain. If a stimulus is intense enough to reach the noxious range, ion channels expressed in the nociceptors are activated and generate action potentials. Ion channels called TRP channels are considered to play an important role in transducing noxious thermal, chemical, and mechanical stimuli.

The TRP channels were first discovered in the eyes of a TRP-mutant *Drosophila melanogaster*, where the mutant fly displayed a transient abnormal response to a bright light, while wild type flies showed a sustained response (Cosens and Manning, 1969). Later, TRP channels in mammalian were introduced with an extended protein family comprising more than 30 distinct subtypes (Ramsey et al., 2006). The TRP family can be distinguished into 6 members: TRPV (vanilloid), TRPA (ankyrin), TRPM (melastatin), TRPC (canonical), TRPP (polycystin), and TRPML (mucolipin) (Chung and Caterina, 2007). These TRP families are similar in architecture, having six putative transmembrane domains with cytoplasmic amino and carboxyl termini, although they differ in amino-acid conservation. Among these members of TRP family, at least six subtypes, including TRPV1-4, TRPA1, and TRPM8, are closely related to painful thermal, chemical, and mechanical stimuli evoking nociceptive pain (Patapoutian et al., 2009; Dai, 2016). Intracellular Ca^{2+} concentration increases in response to stimuli that are specific to certain TRP channels, such as Ca^{2+} entry channels (Zheng, 2013). TRP channels also stimulate intracellular signaling pathways (e.g., PKC activity) and cause transcriptional changes, all of which promote the expression and release of pro-inflammatory peptides such as SP and CGRP (Veldhuis et al., 2015). Moreover, G protein-coupled receptors (GPCRs) are located in the plasma membrane along with TRP channels and are responsible for the central transduction of painful signals from the periphery nociceptors. These GPCRs are activated by noxious stimuli from the extracellular environment and control TRP channel activity through several mechanisms, wherein the G-protein subunits stimulate second messenger kinases [e.g., cyclic adenosine monophosphate (cAMP)-dependent protein kinase A, phospholipase C (PLC), PKC] (Veldhuis et al., 2015).

TRPV1 as Thermal Sensor

Transient receptor potential channels specifically related to pain and thermosensation were first suggested when the capsaicin receptor, TRPV1, was cloned from a rodent dorsal root ganglia (DRG) in 1997 and was reported as a non-selective cation channel exhibiting high calcium permeability (Caterina, 2007). TRPV1 is mainly expressed in small diameter neurons in the DRG and trigeminal ganglion (TG). TRPV1 is activated by both noxious heat (≥43°C) and capsaicin, the pungent ingredient of chili peppers, triggering a sensation of burning pain. In addition to capsaicin and noxious heat, TRPV1 is also activated by spider toxin (Siemens et al., 2006) and low pH (protons) (Caterina et al., 1997). Therefore, TRPV1 is defined as a polymodal receptor (Clapham, 2003). Moreover, certain studies revealed that TRPV1-deficient mice had a complete loss of physiological and behavioral responses to capsaicin, along with significant impairment in responses to noxious heat and mechanical stimuli (Caterina et al., 2000; Davis et al., 2000; Bolcskei et al., 2005). However, other studies reported that TRPV1 null mice had no differences in sensitivity to acute noxious heat compared to wild type mice (Davis et al., 2000; Woodbury et al., 2004). This suggests that TRPV1 is not solely responsible for the sensation of noxious heat, indicating the presence of other possible compensatory mechanisms.

TRPA1 as a Chemical and Thermal Sensor

Another non-selective cation channel of the TRP family subtypes, TRPA1, is also found to be critical in nociception. TRPA1 is highly co-expressed with TRPV1 in small-diameter nociceptors in the DRG and TG and can be influenced by TRPV1 (Salas et al., 2009; Staruschenko et al., 2010). TRPA1 is a polymodal receptor, like TRPV1 (Story et al., 2003; Dai et al., 2007). TRPA1 is activated by a variety of noxious stimuli that induce acute painful burning or stinging sensations including chemicals, such as mustard oil (isothiocyanates), garlic (allicin), and cinnamon oil (cinnamaldehyde) (Bandell et al., 2004; Jordt et al., 2004; Bautista et al., 2005; Macpherson et al., 2005). These chemicals are all electrophilic and activate TRPA1 by covalent modification of cysteine residues in the channel, suggesting that the reactivity of such chemicals is not necessarily dependent on its structure (Hinman et al., 2006; Macpherson et al., 2007). In TRPA1 knockout mice studies, those chemicals showed reduced nociceptive pain behavior (Macpherson et al., 2007; McNamara et al., 2007), indicating TRPA1 as a key detector of chemical damage. Additionally, TRPA1 has also been suggested to detect noxious cold stimuli (<15°C) (Story et al., 2003; Sawada et al., 2008), even though studies of TRPA1-deficient mice showed discordant results (Bandell et al., 2004; Jordt et al., 2004; Zurborg et al., 2007; Karashima et al., 2009).

TRP CHANNELS IN INFLAMMATORY PAIN CONDITIONS

Depending on pathological conditions such as inflammation (inflammatory pain) or nerve injury (neuropathic pain), changes occur in the expression of TRP channels and their function, including transcriptional and translational regulation and post-translational alteration (Patapoutian et al., 2009). As mentioned above, inflammatory pain is generated from the activation and sensitization of nociceptive pain signaling in the form of a reduced threshold and an increased responsiveness of nociceptors. Three cellular and molecular mechanisms have been suggested in the development of inflammatory pain involved in TRP channels. First, TRP channel expression increases in the sensory neurons either transcriptionally or post-translationally during inflammation. For instance, the activation of C-C chemokine receptor type 2 (CCR2) by the macrophage inflammatory protein-1α (MIP-1α/CCL3) increases the transcription of TRPV1 and TRPA1 (Jung et al., 2008); i.e., TRPV1 levels in peripheral terminal or nociceptors are increased in order to maintain the inflammatory heat hypersensitivity (Ji et al., 2002). TRPA1 in DRG neurons is also upregulated by peripheral inflammation transcriptionally, leading to inflammatory cold hyperalgesia (Obata et al., 2005). In other words, the increase in expression and the oxidative products from tissue damage and inflammation led to a drastic decrease in the activation threshold, thereby increasing sensitivity to noxious stimuli (via peripheral sensitization) (Hucho and Levine, 2007). Second, translocation of functional TRP channels from the cytoplasm to the plasma membrane is induced following the activation of second-messenger pathways and subsequent post-translational modification (e.g., channel phosphorylation or glycosylation) (Morenilla-Palao et al., 2004; Nguyen et al., 2005; Zhang et al., 2005). Third, channel phosphorylation as a disinhibition mechanism with inflammatory mediators might cause channel structure alteration and functionally enhance the channel sensitivity (Dai et al., 2007). Tumor necrosis factor (TNF)-α increases the frequency, not the amplitude, of spontaneous excitatory postsynaptic currents (sEPSCs) in wild type mice but not in TRPV1 KO mice (Park et al., 2011a). Importantly, studies conducted using knockout mice lacking TRPV1 showed that the development of inflammatory thermal hyperalgesia became defective (Keeble et al., 2005; Barton et al., 2006). This suggests that TRPV1 is a key component of the mechanism in which inflammation causes thermal hyperalgesia and pain hypersensitivity (Caterina et al., 2000; Davis et al., 2000; Bolcskei et al., 2005; Basbaum et al., 2009). In addition to TRPV1, TRPA1-deficient mice studies also showed markedly reduced development of hyperalgesia in response to inflammation-related chemicals that were injected such as formalin and bradykinin (Bautista et al., 2006; McNamara et al., 2007; Andersson et al., 2008).

TRP CHANNELS IN NEUROPATHIC PAIN CONDITIONS

Physiological changes such as increasing the local Ca^{2+} ion concentration in primary sensory neurons or in the spinal cord owing to nerve injury consequently affect signal processing in the CNS, evoking neuropathic pain (Fernyhough and Calcutt, 2010). When neuropathic pain impulses are transmitted from the periphery to the CNS, nociceptive transmitters such as SP are released by exocytosis from the primary sensory terminals in the spinal dorsal horn, where TRP channels are mediated by voltage-dependent Ca^{2+} channels (Verkhratsky and Fernyhough, 2008).

After nerve damage, expression in TRP channel changes dynamically in sensory neurons, and different TRP channels are involved in the management of neuropathic pain. In the spinal nerve section model, the expression of TRPV1 mRNA is reduced in the axotomized ganglia, suggesting loss of trophic support after the injury (Michael and Priestley, 1999). In L5 spinal nerve ligation model, TRPV1, TRPA1, and TRPM8 are upregulated in uninjured L4 somata (Hudson et al., 2001; Obata et al., 2005). It has been suggested that the injured neurons might release growth factors and neurotransmitters into the surrounding region, causing an increase in the excitability of nearby uninjured spared neurons (Fukuoka et al., 2001; Sexton et al., 2014). Vilceanu et al. (2010) revealed that the proportion of TRPV1-expressing DRG neurons was increased and its TRPV1 function was improved after nerve injury induced by spinal nerve ligation (SNL). Moreover, sciatic nerve transection in rats results in up-regulation of TRPV1 at the central terminals of the primary afferent neurons in the spinal cord, increased release of inflammatory neuropeptides such as calcitonin gene-related peptide and SP from the presynaptic central terminals, and enhanced glutamatergic neurotransmission (Kanai et al., 2005; Lappin et al., 2006; Lee and Kim, 2007; Spicarova et al., 2011). Both TRPV1 and TRPA1 are involved in peripheral neuropathy and neuropathic pain induced by chemotherapeutic agents such as cisplatin, oxaliplatin, and paclitaxel. Inhibition of TRPA1 function eliminates mechanical as well as cold allodynia induced by cisplatin and oxaliplatin, which are most commonly used for chemotherapy (Baron, 2009; Nassini et al., 2011; Zhao et al., 2012). Paclitaxel chemotherapy mediates neuropathic pain behaviors by the release of mast cell tryptase to activate the protease-activated receptor 2 (PAR 2), which then sensitizes TRPV1, TRPV4, and TRPA1 via PLC, PKC, and PKA signaling (Chen et al., 2011); it also enhances the TRPV1 mRNA transcripts and TRPV1 protein in small-to-medium diameter DRG neurons (Hara et al., 2013). Additionally, in neuropathic pain induced by a chronic constriction injury model, inhibition of TRPA1 function also diminishes cold allodynia (Hara et al., 2013).

Certain pro-inflammatory lipid mediators [e.g., leukotrienes (LTs) and prostaglandins (PGs)] in the spinal cord reportedly contribute to neuropathic pain. Of interest, a growing evidence has established that microglial activation has emerged as key players in maintaining pain hypersensitivity in the dorsal horn. Together, the activation of microglia induces dramatic changes including an intracellular signaling molecules [e.g., mitogen-activated protein kinases (MAPKs)], leading to increase the production of pro-inflammatory lipid mediators in the microglia. Following peripheral nerve injury, adenosine triphosphate (ATP) is known to be released from the primary afferent central terminals in the spinal cord, and studies have shown that expression of the purinergic P2 (P2X) receptors was upregulated in microglia to be able to detect extracellular ATP in the spinal cord (Tsuda et al., 2003; Ulmann et al., 2008). LTs are a group of lipid mediators derived from arachidonic acid (AA) which is converted into leukotriene A4 (LTA4) via the 5-lipoxygenase (5-LO) pathway in microglia. LTA4 is then enzymatically converted into LTB4 (Noguchi and Okubo, 2011). In the rat model of spared nerve injury (SNI), LTB4 was expressed in both the spinal neurons and microglia along with LTB4 receptor 1 (BLT1), and the BLT1 was expressed in the spinal neurons. The effect of LTs on neuropathic pain behaviors was identified by intrathecal administration of a 5-LO inhibitor that attenuated the mechanical hypersensitivity caused by SNI surgery (Okubo et al., 2010). Okubo and researchers also found that the increase of 5-LO in spinal microglia was reduced on treatment with an p38 MAPK inhibitor, but not mitogen-activated protein kinase (MEK) inhibitor, indicating that the p38 MAPK pathway is crucial in the generation of neuropathic pain (**Figure 1**). While BLT1 binds LTB4 as its agonist, resolvin E1 and E2 are considered as endogenous receptor antagonists for BLT1. A previous study showed that intrathecal pre-treatment of RvE1 attenuated neuropathic pain by modulating microglial activation in the spinal cord (Xu et al., 2013); thus, there may be an association of BLT1 with RvE1 and E2. In the context of AA metabolites, it is also known to be metabolized into the epoxygenase metabolite, 5,6-EET, which directly activates TRPV4 channels (Vriens et al., 2004). However, not all AA-derived mediators have pro-inflammatory action. Lipoxin A4 (LXA4) is an eicosanoid derived from AA through sequential actions of lipoxygenases, 15-LO and 5-LO; it is known to be an agonist for ALX/FPR2, acting as an endogenous "stop" signal in acute inflammation to switch into the resolution phase (Levy et al., 2001). Martini et al. showed that treatment with LXA4 modulated microglial activation and TNF-α release via ALX/FPR2 receptors, thereby reducing neuropathic pain in rodents after spinal cord hemisection (Martini et al., 2016). PG, a pro-inflammatory mediator synthesized from AA by the COX enzyme in microglia, has been identified as another factor in mechanical allodynia in an SNI model. PGH2 is synthesized from AA by the action of COX and serves as a substrate of the prostaglandin synthase enzymes for producing the bioactive prostaglandins, PGE2 and PGD2, which bind to the EP and DP receptors, respectively (Kanda et al., 2013). Like LTB4, p38 activation in spinal microglia induces the release of PGE2 (Ji and Suter, 2007). Nakayama et al. reported an increase in PGE2 concentration and activation of EP1 receptors in the spinal dorsal horn in the late phase after carrageenan-induced mechanical hyperalgesia in rats (Nakayama et al., 2002). Moreover, following peripheral injury, an increase in PGD2 was noted, which was subsequent to the upregulation of COX-1, and the intrathecal injection of DP2 receptor antagonists attenuated the mechanical allodynia (Kanda et al., 2013). The activation of both EP and DP receptor initiate G-protein coupling to increase intracellular concentration of Ca^{2+} or cAMP in the dorsal horn (Jang et al., 2020). Although evidence of the mechanisms of prostaglandin and its receptors have been accumulated, their role in neuropathic pain and the resolution strategy remain unknown.

Moreover, these pathways of pro-inflammatory lipid mediators contributing to neuropathic pathways has not been studied in the context of TRP regulation. Moreover, even though these findings do not involve TRP regulation, LTs and PGs might be implicated in neuropathic pain by acting like G-protein-mediated signal transducers to initiate second messenger systems, which in turn activate TRP channels (**Figure 1**). Interestingly, TRPV1 is found to be upregulated in the spinal cord dorsal horn in the chronic constriction injury (CCI) neuropathic pain model, indicating possible interaction between the receptors mentioned above (Kanai et al., 2005). Further research will contribute identifying the analgesic effect caused by those pro-inflammatory mediators on neuropathic pain.

Transient receptor potential channels are upregulated in order to manage hypersensitivity of both inflammatory and neuropathic pain at the site of inflammation and the remaining intact neurons close to the damaged nerve, respectively. However, different mediators and intracellular mechanisms of TRP channels are involved, depending on what type of pain is occurring. Hence, it is important to elaborate the role of TRP channels in the resolution of different types of pathological pain using resolvin, which will be discussed in detail next.

RESOLVINS (ENDOGENOUS LIPID MEDIATORS) INHIBIT TRP CHANNELS

Lipid Mediators in Resolution of Acute Inflammation

Acute inflammation is a host defense system, and its resolution may serve as a gateway to chronic inflammation. In health status, inflammatory responses are self-limited, with many cell types and tissues involved in initiation and termination of acute inflammation (Serhan, 2007). Tissue injury or infection triggers the release of a train of signals, including damage-associated molecular patterns (DAMPs), pathogen-associated molecular patterns (PAMPs), lipid mediators and chemokines, such as formylmethionyl-leucyl-phenylalanine (fMLP), ATP, high mobility group box-1 (HMGB1), F-actin, N-glycan, LTB4, CCR1 ligands, chemokine (C-X-C motif) ligand (CXCL) 2, and CXCL8, from injury sites (McDonald and Kubes, 2010; Selders et al., 2017; Peiseler and Kubes, 2019; Gong et al., 2020). Neutrophils move through the chemoattractant gradient, while the integrin molecules on neutrophil surface bind to integrin receptors on endothelial cells enabling their infiltration into the tissues. The infiltrated neutrophils remove pathogens via phagocytosis and release reactive oxygen species (ROS), degradative enzymes, microbicidal agents, and neutrophil extracellular traps (Metzemaekers et al., 2020). Neutrophils are the first defender against hazardous invaders, but their high numbers can induce excessive inflammation (Freire and Van Dyke, 2013). Since excessive inflammation is considered to be a component in many chronic diseases, such as vascular diseases, metabolic syndrome, neurological diseases, and many others, proper resolution of acute inflammation is important. (Serhan et al., 2015b). Resolution of acute inflammation was introduced as a passive process following disappearance of the chemoattractant and other chemical mediators, but Dr. Serhan's group uncovered endogenous lipid mediators in inflammatory exudate: resolvins, protectins, and maresins (Serhan et al., 2002; Serhan, 2014). These pro-resolving lipid mediators are often referred to as specialized pro-resolving mediators (SPMs) because they stimulate efferocytosis of polymorphonuclear leukocytes (PMNs) to facilitate complete removal of pathogens, recruit macrophages, attenuate activated neutrophil through NF-κB inhibition, and initiate the resolution phase of acute inflammation (Flower and Perretti, 2005; Lee et al., 2013; Francos-Quijorna et al., 2017; Yurdagul et al., 2017; Rymut et al., 2020).

Biosynthesis of Resolvins

Notable omega-3 fatty acids are alpha-linolenic acid (ALA), EPA, and DHA. In humans, ALA converts to EPA and DHA, but the conversion rate of ALA to EPA is 8–20%, and that to DHA is 0.5–9%, which are very low (Stark et al., 2008).

In vascular endothelial cells, EPA is converted into 18R-hydroperoxy-EPE (18-HpEPE) with aspirin/COX-2 or microbial p450. 18-HpEPE is converted to 5S(6)-epoxy-18-hydroxy-HEPE

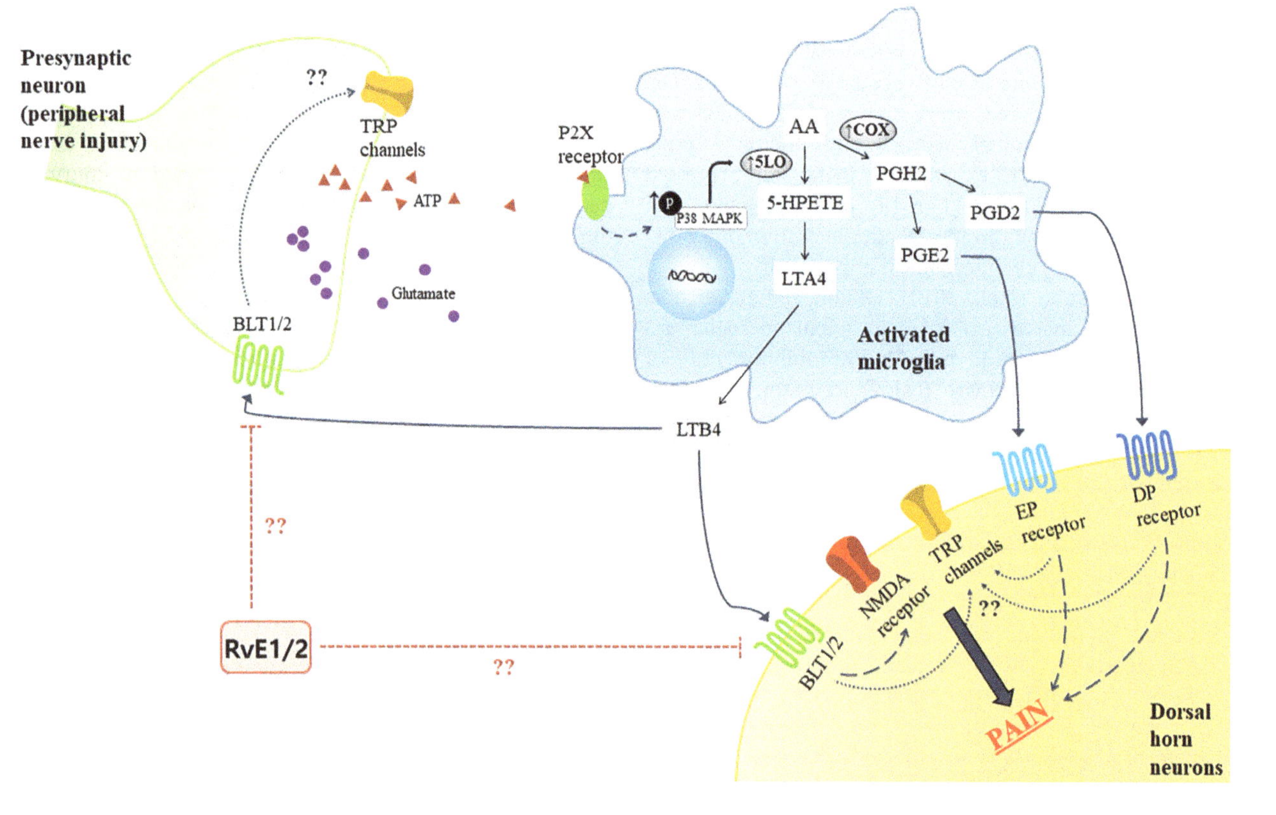

FIGURE 1 | Proposed model for LTs and PGs synthase mechanism from AA in activated microglia by ATP due to peripheral nerve injury, and the receptors in the spinal cord. The activated microglia phosphorylate p38 MAPK, upregulating 5-LO expression. Bioactive LTB4, PGE2, and PGD2 bind to their receptors (BLT1/2, EP and DP receptors, respectively) and evoke pain. The possible analgesic role of RvE1 and E2, which is known to be antagonists of BLT1, and the relationship TRP channel in the presynaptic and spinal dorsal horn neuron are depicted. AA, Arachidonic acid; ATP, adenosine triphosphate; BLT, leukotriene B4 receptor; DP, D-type prostanoid; EP, E-type prostanoid; MAPK, mitogen-activated protein kinases; PG, prostaglandin; PGD, prostaglandin D; PGE, prostaglandin E; RvE1, resolvin E1; RvE2, resolving E2; TRP, transient receptor potential; 5-LO, 5-lipoxygenase.

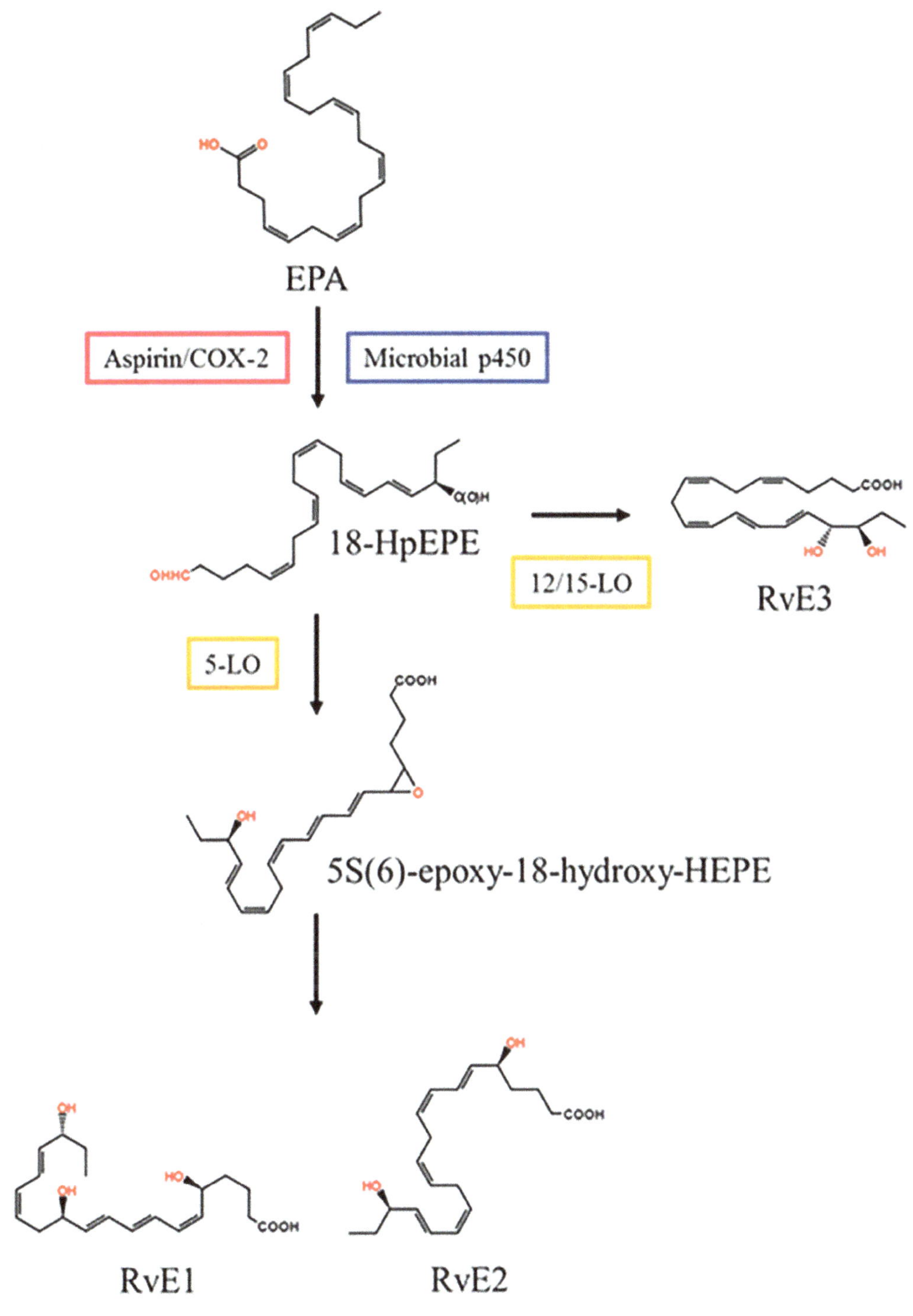

FIGURE 2 | Resolvin E series biosynthetic pathway. EPA is converted into 18-HpEPE. 5S(6)-epoxy-18-hydroxy-HEPE is synthesized from 18-HpEPE with 5-LO and is transformed into RvD1 and RvD2. 18-HpEPE is also transformed into RvD3 by 12/15-LO. EPA, eicosapentaenoic acid; LO, lipoxygenase; RvD, resolvin D; 18-HpEPE, 18R-hydroperoxy-EPE.

with 5- LO in leukocytes and then converted to resolvin E1 via enzymatic hydrolysis or to resolvin E2 via reduction (Serhan et al., 2015a). In eosinophils, 18-HpEPE is also converted to resolvin E3 via 12/15-LO pathways (Isobe et al., 2012) (**Figure 2**).

In exudates, resolvin D series are biosynthesized by PMNs or macrophages. DHA is metabolized to 17-hydroxydocosahexaenoic acid (17-HDHA) via 17-hydroperoxydocosahexaenoic acid through 15-LO (Gleissman et al., 2010). 17-HDHA is converted to resolvin D1, D2, D3, D4,

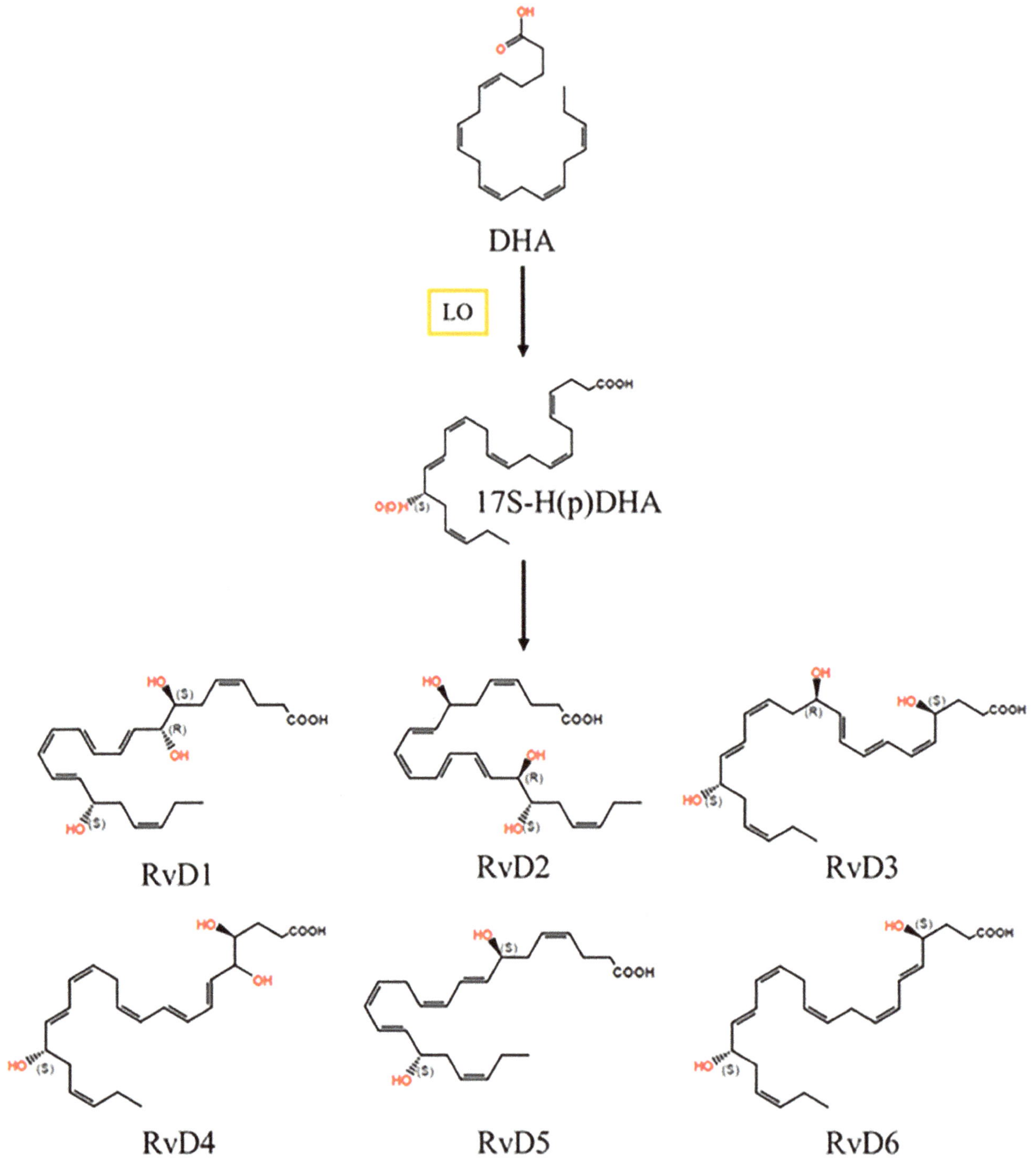

FIGURE 3 | Resolvin D series biosynthetic pathway. DHA is converted into 17S-HpDHA by LO. 17S-HpDHA is further transformed into RvD1, RvD2, RvD3, RvD4, RvD5, and RvD6. DHA, docosahexaenoic acid; LO, lipoxygenase; RvD, resolvin D; 17-hydroperoxydocosahexaenoic acid.

D5, and D6 through epoxidation and 5-LO (**Figure 3**). DHA is also metabolized with aspirin/COX-2, and then the aspirin-triggered resolvin D (AT-RvD) series is formed (Lim et al., 2015; Serhan et al., 2015a; Serhan and Levy, 2018). AT-RvD3 is more potent than resolvin D3 in phagocytosis of 10 and 100 pM zymosan (Dalli et al., 2013).

Since TRP channels are expressed in nociceptors where pain is generated, the roles of TRP channels in mediating pathological pain make them potential therapeutic targets for resolution. Until now, in addition to RvE1 and RvD1/AT-RvD1, more resolving family members have been biosynthesized: RvD2, RvD3, RvD4, and RvD5. RvE1, RvD1, and AT-TvD1 are already well-known agonists that resolve inflammation and inflammation-associated pain by mediating specific GPCRs [e.g., chemerin receptor23 (ChemR23) and GPR32], which are expressed by immune cells, glia cells, and neurons. This, in turn, reduces inflammation, glial activation, and spinal cord synaptic plasticity (Ji et al., 2011). Mounting evidence on resolvins as potent inhibitors for both inflammatory and neuropathic pain will be discussed with recent findings.

Resolvin Receptors

Resolvins can directly act on nociceptors but little is known about how resolvins inhibit TRP channels in neurons. Five GPCRs - ERV/ChemR23, BLT1, ALX/FPR2, DRV1/GPR32, and DRV2/GPR18 - are receptors for resolvin D and E series that play an important role in the modulation of the TRP channels (Pirault and Back, 2018) (**Figure 4**).

ChemR23, resolvin E1 and chemerin receptors (Herova et al., 2015) are co-expressed with TRPV1 in small sized-DRG neurons and in the spinal cord dorsal horn. Activation of chemR23 by resolvin E1 or chemerin blocked capsaicin-evoked spontaneous excitatory postsynaptic current frequency increases via the ERK pathway in the spinal cord dorsal horn, and resolvin E1 also blocked phosphorylation of ERK by capsaicin treatment in DRG neurons (Xu et al., 2010; Park et al., 2011b; Jo et al., 2016). ERK is a member of the mitogen-activated protein kinase superfamily of signaling pathways, an important kinase in painful conditions. In addition to capsaicin, noxious heat, cold, and prick upregulate the pERK intensity in neurons (Ji et al., 1999). In particular, pERK is upregulated in DRG and in the spinal cord in neuropathic pain models of partial sciatic nerve ligation (PSNL), SNL, CCI and diabetes (Seltzer et al., 1990; Song et al., 2005; Liu et al., 2012; Xu et al., 2014; Guo et al., 2019; Wang et al., 2020).

BLT1, LTB4 (agonist), and resolvin E1 (antagonist) receptor are co-expressed with TRPV1 in DRG neurons (Andoh and Kuraishi, 2005; Serhan and Chiang, 2013). LTB4 functions as an agonist and sensitizes TRPV1-mediated Ca^{2+} increase. Although pain behavior in the second phase of the formalin pain model is significantly attenuated in BLT1-KO mice relative to WT mice, no analgesic effect has been observed in the first phase. This is because the first phase is mainly mediated by *TRPA1* and *TRPV1* gene expression, which do not change in the DRG and spinal cords of BLT1-KO mice. Hence, BLT1 may not be involved in mediating the properties of TRPA1 (McNamara et al., 2007; Asahara et al., 2015).

Resolvin D1 inhibits TRPA1, TRPV3, and TRPV4 in heterogeneous systems. FPR2/ALX is a resolvin D1 receptor, but treatment with FPR2/ALX agonists, cathelicidin LL-37 and Trp-Lys-Tyr-Met-Val-Met (WKYMVM), do not affect TRPA1, TPRV3, and TRPV4 inhibition (Bang et al., 2010). However, there is another resolvin D1 receptor, GPR32, that is also activated

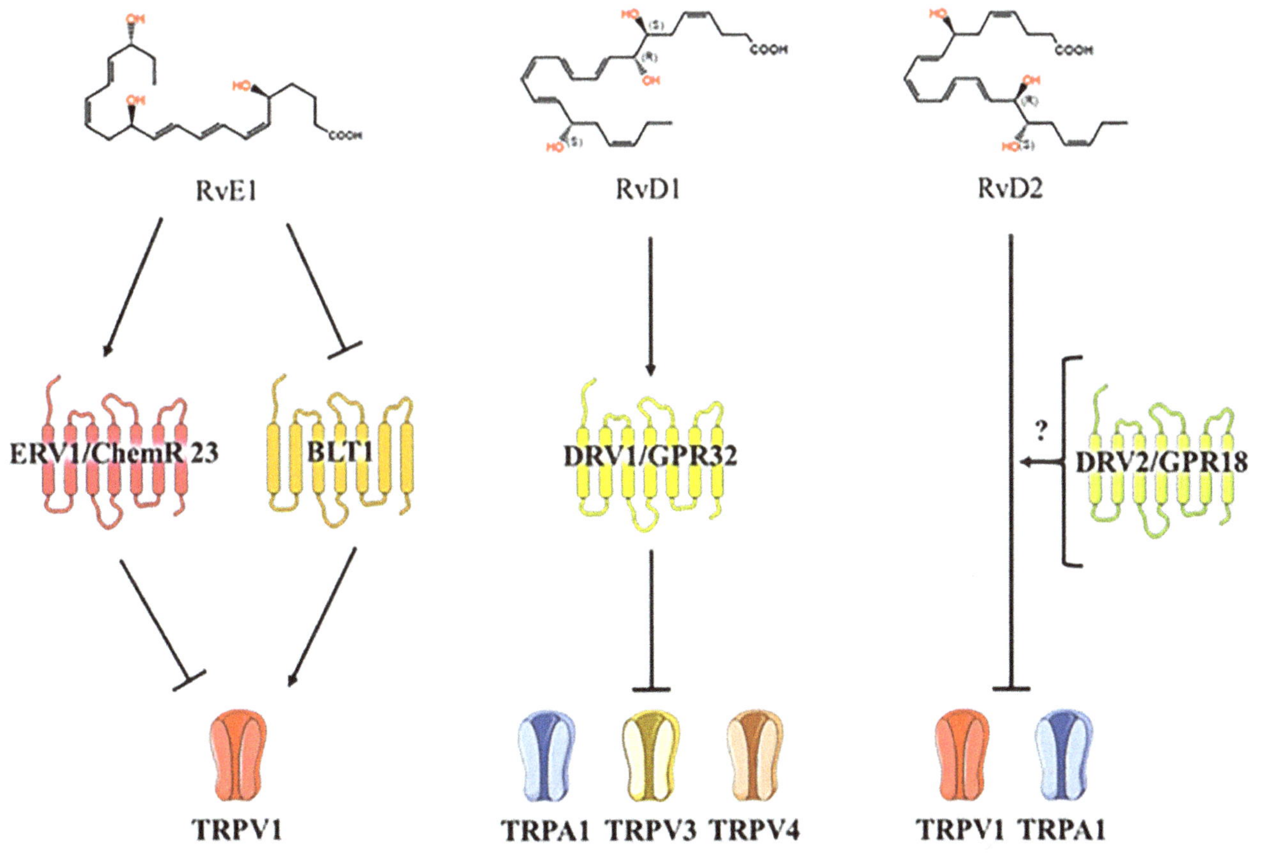

FIGURE 4 | Resolvin series inhibit TRP channels. RvD, resolvin D; TRP, transient receptor potential.

by AT-RvD1. FPR2/ALX and GPR32 are GPCRs that regulate specific microRNAs and their target genes that promote the resolution of acute inflammation (Krishnamoorthy et al., 2012).

Resolvin D2 is known to activate a cell surface GPCR, GPR18/DRV2 (Chiang et al., 2015, 2017). GPR18 is expressed in lumbar DRG and in the spinal cord at a genetic level and under neuropathic conditions; it is also upregulated in the spinal cord (Malek et al., 2016). Resolvin D2 inhibits TRPV1 and TRPA1 activation dose-dependently. Resolvin D2 is ten times more potent than resolvin E1 on TRPV1 inhibition ($IC_{50} = 0.04 \pm 0.01$ and 0.4 ± 0.05, respectively), and it is four times more potent than resolvin D1 on TRPA1 inhibition ($IC_{50} = 0.8 \pm 0.2$ and 3.2 ± 0.05, respectively) (Park et al., 2011b).

RESOLVINS ALLEVIATE CHRONIC PAIN

Resolvins in the Resolution of Inflammatory Pain

Studies have shown that both peripheral (intraplanar) and central (intrathecal) administration of RvE1 and RvD1 reduce inflammatory pain (Bang et al., 2010; Xu et al., 2010; Lima-Garcia et al., 2011; Park et al., 2011b) and postoperative pain (Huang et al., 2011; Wang and Strichartz, 2017) by modulating the activation of TRP channels. Bang et al. reported that pretreatment with RvD1 (20 ng) suppressed pain behaviors induced by intraplanar formalin injection (Bang et al., 2010) and attempted to determine whether activators of the RvD1 receptor (FPR2/ALX) inhibits the effect of TRP channels (TRPV3/4 and A1), however, no such effect was found (Krishnamoorthy et al., 2010). Xu et al. (2010) found that both RvD1 and RvE1 (1–20 ng) suppressed inflammatory pain behaviors induced by formalin, carrageenan, or complete Freund's adjuvant (CFA); they also indicated that the possible mechanism where RvE1 inhibits ERK signaling pathways to block TNF-α induced increased EPSC frequency and NMDAR hyperactivity in spinal dorsal horn neurons. Additionally, an agonist of ChemR23, which was considered to be an RvE1 receptor, also abolished capsaicin-induced increase in sEPSC frequency, implicating the role of RvE1 in mediating TRPV1 activity via ChemR23. Moreover, Park et al. examined RvD2 at very low doses (10 ng) injected intrathecally and found that it prevented spontaneous pain induced by formalin as well as reversed inflammatory pain induced by CFA (Park et al., 2011b). They identified RvD2 as endogenous inhibitors both for TRPV1 and TRPA1, by which RvD2 acts on specific GPCRs. **Table 1** shows a list of the published findings of the resolution effect of resolvins specifically on TRP channels for inflammatory pain.

Resolvins in the Resolution of Neuropathic Pain

While there is mounting research on the analgesic effect of resolvins in inflammatory pain, the role of resolvins in TRP channels to alleviate neuropathic pain is not well known. One study evaluated the analgesic actions of resolvin D-series (D1 to D5) in a TRPA1 and TRPV1 knockout mouse model of chemotherapy-induced peripheral neuropathy induced by paclitaxel (Luo et al., 2019). They found that RvD1 and RvD2 reduced mechanical allodynia in both sexes of TRPV1 and TRPA1 deficient mice, whereas RvD3 and RvD4 had no effects on either sex. Interestingly, RvD5 reduced mechanical allodynia only in male mice but not in female mice, indicating there is a sex dimorphism in pain regulation. Since RvD5 affected the TRPV1 and TRPA1 knockout male mice only, this might implicate the TRP channel in the role of RvD5 to attenuate neuropathic pain in female mice.

TABLE 1 | Analgesic effects of different resolvins in distinctive TRP channels for inflammatory and neuropathic pain.

Research article	Pain type	Resolvin	TRP channel	Results	Potential mechanisms
Bang et al., 2010	Inflammatory	RvD1	TRPA1 TRPV3 TRPV4	↓activities the three TRP channels at nanomolar and micromolar levels ***No effects of FPR2/ALX agonists on the three TRP channels*	
Xu et al., 2010	Inflammatory	RvE1 RvD1	TRPV1	↓EPSC frequency increases induced by capsaicin, with the ChemR23 agonist ↓EPSC frequency increase by TNF-α and NMDAR hyperactivity with RvE1	RvE1 modulates the ERK signaling pathway to abolish TNF-α-evoked NMDA receptor hyperactivity in dorsal horn neurons
Park et al., 2011b	Inflammatory	RvD1 RvD2 RvE1	TRPV1 TRPA1	↓sEPSC increases both TRP channels with RvD2 at extremely low doses (compared to RvD1/E1) ***No effect of RvD2 when GPCRs are blocked*	Distinct mechanisms of the resolvins in regulating TRP channels RvD2 involves specific GPCRs
Luo et al., 2019	Neuropathic (CIPN induced) Inflammatory (**RvD5 only)	RvD1 RvD2 RvD5	*TRPA1* *TRPV1* *(**Knock-out mice)*	↓ neuropathic pain behaviors, with RvD1/D2 ** *only in male mice, with RvD5* ↓inflammatory pain behaviors in male mice only with RvD5	Sex dimorphism of RvD5's analgesia in both pain models

*CFA, complete Freund's adjuvant; CIPN, chemotherapy-induced peripheral neuropathy; EPSC, excitatory postsynaptic current; ERK, extracellular signal-regulated kinase; FPR2/ALX, formyl peptide receptor 2; GPCRs, G-protein coupled receptors; NMDAR, N-methyl-D-aspartic acid receptor; RvE, resolvin E; RvD, resolvin D; TNF-α, tumor necrosis factor-α; TRP, transient receptor potential. ** Indicates supplementary information.*

CONCLUSION: IMPORTANCE OF PAIN RELIEF USING RESOLVINS VIA TRP MODULATION

Opioid and non-opioid analgesic drugs for the treatment acute and chronic pain. Opioids are a type of medications that are used to relieve severe chronic pain. However, as opioid receptors are expressed throughout the entire nervous system and gastrointestinal tract and do not operate on specific pain pathways, their abuse and misuse can induce unexpected physiological and psychological side effects that devastate the lives of the affected individuals and their families. Morphine, one of the most widely prescribed opioid analgesics, increases pain hypersensitivity at low doses (Ghelardini et al., 2015). Morphine-6-glucuronide (M6G), a metabolite of morphine, has more potent analgesic effect than does morphine. However, M6G is dangerous to patients with renal failure and relate to respiratory depression (Lotsch, 2005). For these reasons, several nations and international organizations have thoroughly controlled the prescription and use of opioids (Rosenblum et al., 2008; Rogers et al., 2013). Further, the consequences of opioid use underscore the need to develop non-opioid analgesics and thus minimize the prescription of opioid analgesics.

Non-opioid analgesics include both selective and non-selective cyclooxygenase (COX) inhibitors, as well as well-known non-steroidal anti-inflammatory drugs and acetaminophen. COX contributes to the synthesis of PG, which causes inflammation, pain and fever. Because of this, COX inhibitors are used for antipyretics and antiphlogistics, as well as analgesics (Qureshi and Dua, 2020). However, the administration of COX-2 inhibitors can induce cardiovascular complications (Nussmeier et al., 2005).

Therefore, it is necessary to develop new analgesic targets that are specific to nociceptive neurons. One of the targets is TRP channels that mediate nociception, especially TRPV1. Many models have shown that TRPV1 inhibition reduces chronic pain including inflammatory and neuropathic pain. TRP channels in nerve systems have been emerging targets for pain management, and several TRPV1 antagonists (ABT-102, AMG-517, AZD-1386, DWP-05195, JTS-653, MK-2295, PHE-377 and SB-705498) have already entered clinical trials (Wu et al., 2018). However, TRPV1 antagonists can induce abnormal changes in body temperature (hyperthermia and hypothermia (Gavva et al., 2008; Garami et al., 2018, 2020) or decrease heat sensation (Crutchlow et al., 2009). For these reasons, many TRPV1 antagonists have failed to be developed as painkillers.

Nevertheless, TRPV1 inhibitors are still being discovered. Resolvins, a class of lipid mediators, has been identified in this capacity. Resolvins are produced from omega-3 fatty acids and therefore have a great potential for reducing the incidence of side effects associated with pain management. Further, the fact that resolvins can attenuate powerful type cardiovascular disease enhances its potential as a useful analgesic (Salic et al., 2016; Capo et al., 2018). The analgesic role of resolvins has already been proven at nanomolar levels, resolvins are excellent potential therapeutic targets for pain. However, most current studies of resolvins in an analgesic role have been limited to inflammatory pain. Therefore, more studies on the analgesic effect of resolvins for neuropathic pain are needed.

AUTHOR CONTRIBUTIONS

C-KP and YHK conceived and supervised the project. JR, EJG, J-WP, YHK, and C-KP wrote the manuscript. All authors contributed to the article and approved the submitted version.

REFERENCES

Amir, R., and Devor, M. (2003). Electrical excitability of the soma of sensory neurons is required for spike invasion of the soma, but not for through-conduction. *Biophys. J.* 84, 2181–2191. doi: 10.1016/s0006-3495(03)75024-3

Andersson, D. A., Gentry, C., Moss, S., and Bevan, S. (2008). Transient receptor potential A1 is a sensory receptor for multiple products of oxidative stress. *J. Neurosci.* 28, 2485–2494. doi: 10.1523/jneurosci.5369-07.2008

Andoh, T., and Kuraishi, Y. (2005). Expression of BLT1 leukotriene B4 receptor on the dorsal root ganglion neurons in mice. *Brain Res. Mol. Brain Res* 137, 263–266. doi: 10.1016/j.molbrainres.2005.02.029

Ariel, A., and Serhan, C. N. (2007). Resolvins and protectins in the termination program of acute inflammation. *Trends Immunol.* 28, 176–183. doi: 10.1016/j.it.2007.02.007

Asahara, M., Ito, N., Yokomizo, T., Nakamura, M., Shimizu, T., and Yamada, Y. (2015). The absence of the leukotriene B4 receptor BLT1 attenuates peripheral inflammation and spinal nociceptive processing following intraplantar formalin injury. *Mol. Pain* 11:11.

Bandell, M., Story, G. M., Hwang, S. W., Viswanath, V., Eid, S. R., Petrus, M. J., et al. (2004). Noxious cold ion channel TRPA1 is activated by pungent compounds and bradykinin. *Neuron* 41, 849–857. doi: 10.1016/s0896-6273(04)00150-3

Bang, S., Yoo, S., Yang, T. J., Cho, H., Kim, Y. G., and Hwang, S. W. (2010). Resolvin D1 attenuates activation of sensory transient receptor potential channels leading to multiple anti-nociception. *Br. J. Pharmacol.* 161, 707–720. doi: 10.1111/j.1476-5381.2010.00909.x

Baron, R. (2009). Neuropathic pain: a clinical perspective. *Handb. Exp. Pharmacol.* 2009, 3–30. doi: 10.1007/978-3-540-79090-7_1

Barton, N. J., Mcqueen, D. S., Thomson, D., Gauldie, S. D., Wilson, A. W., Salter, D. M., et al. (2006). Attenuation of experimental arthritis in TRPV1R knockout mice. *Exp. Mol. Pathol.* 81, 166–170. doi: 10.1016/j.yexmp.2006.04.007

Basbaum, A. I., Bautista, D. M., Scherrer, G., and Julius, D. (2009). Cellular and molecular mechanisms of pain. *Cell* 139, 267–284.

Bautista, D. M., Jordt, S. E., Nikai, T., Tsuruda, P. R., Read, A. J., Poblete, J., et al. (2006). TRPA1 mediates the inflammatory actions of environmental irritants and proalgesic agents. *Cell* 124, 1269–1282. doi: 10.1016/j.cell.2006.02.023

Bautista, D. M., Movahed, P., Hinman, A., Axelsson, H. E., Sterner, O., Hogestatt, E. D., et al. (2005). Pungent products from garlic activate the sensory ion channel TRPA1. *Proc. Natl. Acad. Sci. U.S.A.* 102, 12248–12252. doi: 10.1073/pnas.0505356102

Bishop, B. (1980). Pain: its physiology and rationale for management. Part II. Analgesic systems of the CNS. *Phys. Ther.* 60, 21–23. doi: 10.1093/ptj/60.1.21

Bolcskei, K., Helyes, Z., Szabo, A., Sandor, K., Elekes, K., Nemeth, J., et al. (2005). Investigation of the role of TRPV1 receptors in acute and chronic nociceptive processes using gene-deficient mice. *Pain* 117, 368–376. doi: 10.1016/j.pain.2005.06.024

Capo, X., Martorell, M., Busquets-Cortes, C., Tejada, S., Tur, J. A., Pons, A., et al. (2018). Resolvins as proresolving inflammatory mediators in cardiovascular disease. *Eur. J. Med. Chem.* 153, 123–130. doi: 10.1016/j.ejmech.2017.07.018

Caterina, M. J. (2007). Transient receptor potential ion channels as participants in thermosensation and thermoregulation. *Am. J. Physiol. Regul. Integr, Comp. Physiol.* 292, R64–R76.

Caterina, M. J., Leffler, A., Malmberg, A. B., Martin, W. J., Trafton, J., Petersen-Zeitz, K. R., et al. (2000). Impaired nociception and pain sensation in mice lacking the capsaicin receptor. *Science* 288, 306–313. doi: 10.1126/science.288.5464.306

Caterina, M. J., Schumacher, M. A., Tominaga, M., Rosen, T. A., Levine, J. D., and Julius, D. (1997). The capsaicin receptor: a heat-activated ion channel in the pain pathway. *Nature* 389, 816–824. doi: 10.1038/39807

Chen, J., Joshi, S. K., Didomenico, S., Perner, R. J., Mikusa, J. P., Gauvin, D. M., et al. (2011). Selective blockade of TRPA1 channel attenuates pathological pain without altering noxious cold sensation or body temperature regulation. *Pain* 152, 1165–1172. doi: 10.1016/j.pain.2011.01.049

Chiang, N., Dalli, J., Colas, R. A., and Serhan, C. N. (2015). Identification of resolvin D2 receptor mediating resolution of infections and organ protection. *J. Exp. Med.* 212, 1203–1217. doi: 10.1084/jem.20150225

Chiang, N., De La Rosa, X., Libreros, S., and Serhan, C. N. (2017). Novel resolvin D2 receptor axis in infectious inflammation. *J. Immunol.* 198, 842–851. doi: 10.4049/jimmunol.1601650

Chung, M. K., and Caterina, M. J. (2007). TRP channel knockout mice lose their cool. *Neuron* 54, 345–347. doi: 10.1016/j.neuron.2007.04.025

Clapham, D. E. (2003). TRP channels as cellular sensors. *Nature* 426, 517–524. doi: 10.1038/nature02196

Cosens, D. J., and Manning, A. (1969). Abnormal electroretinogram from a Drosophila mutant. *Nature* 224, 285–287. doi: 10.1038/224285a0

Crutchlow, M., Dong, Y., Schulz, V., Von Hoydonck, P., Laethem, T., and Maes, A. (2009). "Pharmacologic inhibition of TRPV1 impairs sensation of potentially injurious heat in healthy subjects. 2009," in *ASCPT 2009 Annual Meeting*, National Harbor, MD, 69.

Dai, Y. (2016). TRPs and pain. *Semin. Immunopathol.* 38, 277–291. doi: 10.1007/s00281-015-0526-0

Dai, Y., Wang, S., Tominaga, M., Yamamoto, S., Fukuoka, T., Higashi, T., et al. (2007). Sensitization of TRPA1 by PAR2 contributes to the sensation of inflammatory pain. *J. Clin. Invest.* 117, 1979–1987. doi: 10.1172/jci30951

Dalli, J., Winkler, J. W., Colas, R. A., Arnardottir, H., Cheng, C. Y., Chiang, N., et al. (2013). Resolvin D3 and aspirin-triggered resolvin D3 are potent immunoresolvents. *Chem. Biol.* 20, 188–201. doi: 10.1016/j.chembiol.2012.11.010

Davis, J. B., Gray, J., Gunthorpe, M. J., Hatcher, J. P., Davey, P. T., Overend, P., et al. (2000). Vanilloid receptor-1 is essential for inflammatory thermal hyperalgesia. *Nature* 405, 183–187.

Fernyhough, P., and Calcutt, N. A. (2010). Abnormal calcium homeostasis in peripheral neuropathies. *Cell Calcium* 47, 130–139. doi: 10.1016/j.ceca.2009.11.008

Flower, R. J., and Perretti, M. (2005). Controlling inflammation: a fat chance? *J. Exp. Med.* 201, 671–674.

Francos-Quijorna, I., Santos-Nogueira, E., Gronert, K., Sullivan, A. B., Kopp, M. A., Brommer, B., et al. (2017). Maresin 1 promotes inflammatory resolution, neuroprotection, and functional neurological recovery after spinal cord injury. *J. Neurosci.* 37, 11731–11743. doi: 10.1523/jneurosci.1395-17.2017

Freire, M. O., and Van Dyke, T. E. (2013). Natural resolution of inflammation. *Periodontol* 2000, 149–164. doi: 10.1111/prd.12034

Fukuoka, T., Kondo, E., Dai, Y., Hashimoto, N., and Noguchi, K. (2001). Brain-derived neurotrophic factor increases in the uninjured dorsal root ganglion neurons in selective spinal nerve ligation model. *J. Neurosci.* 21, 4891–4900. doi: 10.1523/jneurosci.21-13-04891.2001

Furue, H., Katafuchi, T., and Yoshimura, M. (2004). Sensory processing and functional reorganization of sensory transmission under pathological conditions in the spinal dorsal horn. *Neurosci. Res.* 48, 361–368. doi: 10.1016/j.neures.2003.12.005

Garami, A., Pakai, E., Mcdonald, H. A., Reilly, R. M., Gomtsyan, A., Corrigan, J. J., et al. (2018). TRPV1 antagonists that cause hypothermia, instead of hyperthermia, in rodents: compounds' pharmacological profiles, in vivo targets, thermoeffectors recruited and implications for drug development. *Acta Physiol.* 223:e13038. doi: 10.1111/apha.13038

Garami, A., Shimansky, Y. P., Rumbus, Z., Vizin, R. C. L., Farkas, N., Hegyi, J., et al. (2020). Hyperthermia induced by transient receptor potential vanilloid-1 (TRPV1) antagonists in human clinical trials: insights from mathematical modeling and meta-analysis. *Pharmacol. Ther.* 208:107474. doi: 10.1016/j.pharmthera.2020.107474

Gavva, N. R., Treanor, J. J., Garami, A., Fang, L., Surapaneni, S., Akrami, A., et al. (2008). Pharmacological blockade of the vanilloid receptor TRPV1 elicits marked hyperthermia in humans. *Pain* 136, 202–210. doi: 10.1016/j.pain.2008.01.024

Ghelardini, C., Di Cesare Mannelli, L., and Bianchi, E. (2015). The pharmacological basis of opioids. *Clin. Cases Miner Bone Metab.* 12, 219–221.

Gibson, D. A., and Ma, L. (2011). Developmental regulation of axon branching in the vertebrate nervous system. *Development* 138, 183–195. doi: 10.1242/dev.046441

Gleissman, H., Yang, R., Martinod, K., Lindskog, M., Serhan, C. N., Johnsen, J. I., et al. (2010). Docosahexaenoic acid metabolome in neural tumors: identification of cytotoxic intermediates. *Faseb J.* 24, 906–915. doi: 10.1096/fj.09-137919

Gong, T., Liu, L., Jiang, W., and Zhou, R. (2020). DAMP-sensing receptors in sterile inflammation and inflammatory diseases. *Nat. Rev. Immunol.* 20, 95–112. doi: 10.1038/s41577-019-0215-7

Guo, J., Wang, C., Niu, X., Zhou, F., Li, H., and Gao, W. (2019). Effects of resveratrol in the signaling of neuropathic pain involving P2X3 in the dorsal root ganglion of rats. *Acta Neurol. Belg.* 1–8.

Hara, T., Chiba, T., Abe, K., Makabe, A., Ikeno, S., Kawakami, K., et al. (2013). Effect of paclitaxel on transient receptor potential vanilloid 1 in rat dorsal root ganglion. *Pain* 154, 882–889. doi: 10.1016/j.pain.2013.02.023

Hasegawa, H., Abbott, S., Han, B. X., Qi, Y., and Wang, F. (2007). Analyzing somatosensory axon projections with the sensory neuron-specific Advillin gene. *J. Neurosci.* 27, 14404–14414. doi: 10.1523/jneurosci.4908-07.2007

Herova, M., Schmid, M., Gemperle, C., and Hersberger, M. (2015). ChemR23, the receptor for chemerin and resolvin E1, is expressed and functional on M1 but not on M2 macrophages. *J. Immunol.* 194, 2330–2337. doi: 10.4049/jimmunol.1402166

Hinman, A., Chuang, H. H., Bautista, D. M., and Julius, D. (2006). TRP channel activation by reversible covalent modification. *Proc. Natl. Acad. Sci. U.S.A.* 103, 19564–19568. doi: 10.1073/pnas.0609598103

Huang, L., Wang, C. F., Serhan, C. N., and Strichartz, G. (2011). Enduring prevention and transient reduction of postoperative pain by intrathecal resolvin D1. *Pain* 152, 557–565. doi: 10.1016/j.pain.2010.11.021

Hucho, T., and Levine, J. D. (2007). Signaling pathways in sensitization: toward a nociceptor cell biology. *Neuron* 55, 365–376. doi: 10.1016/j.neuron.2007.07.008

Hudson, L. J., Bevan, S., Wotherspoon, G., Gentry, C., Fox, A., and Winter, J. (2001). VR1 protein expression increases in undamaged DRG neurons after partial nerve injury. *Eur. J. Neurosci.* 13, 2105–2114. doi: 10.1046/j.0953-816x.2001.01591.x

Hylden, J. L., Nahin, R. L., Traub, R. J., and Dubner, R. (1989). Expansion of receptive fields of spinal lamina I projection neurons in rats with unilateral adjuvant-induced inflammation: the contribution of dorsal horn mechanisms. *Pain* 37, 229–243. doi: 10.1016/0304-3959(89)90135-8

Isobe, Y., Arita, M., Matsueda, S., Iwamoto, R., Fujihara, T., Nakanishi, H., et al. (2012). Identification and structure determination of novel anti-inflammatory mediator resolvin E3, 17,18-dihydroxyeicosapentaenoic acid. *J. Biol. Chem.* 287, 10525–10534. doi: 10.1074/jbc.m112.340612

Jang, Y., Kim, M., and Hwang, S. W. (2020). Molecular mechanisms underlying the actions of arachidonic acid-derived prostaglandins on peripheral nociception. *J. Neuroinflammation* 17:30.

Jardin, I., Lopez, J. J., Diez, R., Sanchez-Collado, J., Cantonero, C., Albarran, L., et al. (2017). TRPs in pain sensation. *Front. Physiol.* 8:392. doi: 10.3389/fphys.2017.00392

Ji, R. R., Baba, H., Brenner, G. J., and Woolf, C. J. (1999). Nociceptive-specific activation of ERK in spinal neurons contributes to pain hypersensitivity. *Nat. Neurosci.* 2, 1114–1119. doi: 10.1038/16040

Ji, R. R., Nackley, A., Huh, Y., Terrando, N., and Maixner, W. (2018). Neuroinflammation and central sensitization in chronic and widespread pain. *Anesthesiology* 129, 343–366. doi: 10.1097/aln.0000000000002130

Ji, R. R., Samad, T. A., Jin, S. X., Schmoll, R., and Woolf, C. J. (2002). p38 MAPK activation by NGF in primary sensory neurons after inflammation increases TRPV1 levels and maintains heat hyperalgesia. *Neuron* 36, 57–68. doi: 10.1016/s0896-6273(02)00908-x

Ji, R. R., and Suter, M. R. (2007). p38 MAPK, microglial signaling, and neuropathic pain. *Mol. Pain* 3:33.

Ji, R. R., and Woolf, C. J. (2001). Neuronal plasticity and signal transduction in nociceptive neurons: implications for the initiation and maintenance of pathological pain. *Neurobiol. Dis.* 8, 1–10. doi: 10.1006/nbdi.2000.0360

Ji, R. R., Xu, Z. Z., Strichartz, G., and Serhan, C. N. (2011). Emerging roles of resolvins in the resolution of inflammation and pain. *Trends Neurosci.* 34, 599–609. doi: 10.1016/j.tins.2011.08.005

Jo, Y. Y., Lee, J. Y., and Park, C. K. (2016). Resolvin E1 inhibits substance P-Induced potentiation of TRPV1 in primary sensory neurons. *Mediators Inflamm.* 2016:5259321.

Jordt, S. E., Bautista, D. M., Chuang, H. H., Mckemy, D. D., Zygmunt, P. M., Hogestatt, E. D., et al. (2004). Mustard oils and cannabinoids excite sensory nerve fibres through the TRP channel ANKTM1. *Nature* 427, 260–265. doi: 10.1038/nature02282

Julius, D., and Basbaum, A. I. (2001). Molecular mechanisms of nociception. *Nature* 413, 203–210. doi: 10.1038/35093019

Jung, H., Toth, P. T., White, F. A., and Miller, R. J. (2008). Monocyte chemoattractant protein-1 functions as a neuromodulator in dorsal root ganglia neurons. *J. Neurochem.* 104, 254–263.

Kanai, Y., Nakazato, E., Fujiuchi, A., Hara, T., and Imai, A. (2005). Involvement of an increased spinal TRPV1 sensitization through its up-regulation in mechanical allodynia of CCI rats. *Neuropharmacology* 49, 977–984. doi: 10.1016/j.neuropharm.2005.05.003

Kanda, H., Kobayashi, K., Yamanaka, H., and Noguchi, K. (2013). COX-1-dependent prostaglandin D2 in microglia contributes to neuropathic pain via DP2 receptor in spinal neurons. *Glia* 61, 943–956. doi: 10.1002/glia.22487

Karashima, Y., Talavera, K., Everaerts, W., Janssens, A., Kwan, K. Y., Vennekens, R., et al. (2009). TRPA1 acts as a cold sensor in vitro and in vivo. *Proc. Natl. Acad. Sci. U.S.A.* 106, 1273–1278. doi: 10.1073/pnas.0808487106

Keeble, J., Russell, F., Curtis, B., Starr, A., Pinter, E., and Brain, S. D. (2005). Involvement of transient receptor potential vanilloid 1 in the vascular and hyperalgesic components of joint inflammation. *Arthritis Rheum* 52, 3248–3256. doi: 10.1002/art.21297

Krishnamoorthy, S., Recchiuti, A., Chiang, N., Fredman, G., and Serhan, C. N. (2012). Resolvin D1 receptor stereoselectivity and regulation of inflammation and proresolving microRNAs. *Am. J. Pathol.* 180, 2018–2027. doi: 10.1016/j.ajpath.2012.01.028

Krishnamoorthy, S., Recchiuti, A., Chiang, N., Yacoubian, S., Lee, C. H., Yang, R., et al. (2010). Resolvin D1 binds human phagocytes with evidence for proresolving receptors. *Proc. Natl. Acad. Sci. U.S.A.* 107, 1660–1665. doi: 10.1073/pnas.0907342107

Lappin, S. C., Randall, A. D., Gunthorpe, M. J., and Morisset, V. (2006). TRPV1 antagonist, SB-366791, inhibits glutamatergic synaptic transmission in rat spinal dorsal horn following peripheral inflammation. *Eur. J. Pharmacol.* 540, 73–81. doi: 10.1016/j.ejphar.2006.04.046

Latremoliere, A., and Woolf, C. J. (2009). Central sensitization: a generator of pain hypersensitivity by central neural plasticity. *J. Pain* 10, 895–926. doi: 10.1016/j.jpain.2009.06.012

Lee, H. N., Kundu, J. K., Cha, Y. N., and Surh, Y. J. (2013). Resolvin D1 stimulates efferocytosis through p50/p50-mediated suppression of tumor necrosis factor-alpha expression. *J. Cell Sci.* 126, 4037–4047. doi: 10.1242/jcs.131003

Lee, S. E., and Kim, J. H. (2007). Involvement of substance P and calcitonin gene-related peptide in development and maintenance of neuropathic pain from spinal nerve injury model of rat. *Neurosci. Res.* 58, 245–249. doi: 10.1016/j.neures.2007.03.004

Levy, B. D., Clish, C. B., Schmidt, B., Gronert, K., and Serhan, C. N. (2001). Lipid mediator class switching during acute inflammation: signals in resolution. *Nat. Immunol.* 2, 612–619. doi: 10.1038/89759

Lim, J. Y., Park, C. K., and Hwang, S. W. (2015). Biological roles of resolvins and related substances in the resolution of pain. *Biomed. Res. Int.* 2015:830930.

Lima-Garcia, J. F., Dutra, R. C., Da Silva, K., Motta, E. M., Campos, M. M., and Calixto, J. B. (2011). The precursor of resolvin D series and aspirin-triggered resolvin D1 display anti-hyperalgesic properties in adjuvant-induced arthritis in rats. *Br. J. Pharmacol.* 164, 278–293. doi: 10.1111/j.1476-5381.2011.01345.x

Liu, L., Ji, F., Liang, J., He, H., Fu, Y., and Cao, M. (2012). Inhibition by dexmedetomidine of the activation of spinal dorsal horn glias and the intracellular ERK signaling pathway induced by nerve injury. *Brain Res.* 1427, 1–9. doi: 10.1016/j.brainres.2011.08.019

Lotsch, J. (2005). Opioid metabolites. *J/ Pain Symptom. Manag.* 29, S10–S24.

Luo, X., Gu, Y., Tao, X., Serhan, C. N., and Ji, R. R. (2019). Resolvin D5 inhibits neuropathic and inflammatory pain in male but not female mice: distinct actions of D-Series resolvins in chemotherapy-induced peripheral neuropathy. *Front. Pharmacol.* 10:745. doi: 10.3389/fphar.2019.00745

Macpherson, L. J., Geierstanger, B. H., Viswanath, V., Bandell, M., Eid, S. R., Hwang, S., et al. (2005). The pungency of garlic: activation of TRPA1 and TRPV1 in response to allicin. *Curr. Biol.* 15, 929–934. doi: 10.1016/j.cub.2005.04.018

Macpherson, L. J., Xiao, B., Kwan, K. Y., Petrus, M. J., Dubin, A. E., Hwang, S., et al. (2007). An ion channel essential for sensing chemical damage. *J. Neurosci.* 27, 11412–11415. doi: 10.1523/jneurosci.3600-07.2007

Malek, N., Kostrzewa, M., Makuch, W., Pajak, A., Kucharczyk, M., Piscitelli, F., et al. (2016). The multiplicity of spinal AA-5-HT anti-nociceptive action in a rat model of neuropathic pain. *Pharmacol. Res.* 111, 251–263. doi: 10.1016/j.phrs.2016.06.012

Martini, A. C., Berta, T., Forner, S., Chen, G., Bento, A. F., Ji, R. R., et al. (2016). Lipoxin A4 inhibits microglial activation and reduces neuroinflammation and neuropathic pain after spinal cord hemisection. *J. Neuroinflammation* 13:75.

McDonald, B., and Kubes, P. (2010). Chemokines: sirens of neutrophil recruitment-but is it just one song? *Immunity* 33, 148–149. doi: 10.1016/j.immuni.2010.08.006

McNamara, C. R., Mandel-Brehm, J., Bautista, D. M., Siemens, J., Deranian, K. L., Zhao, M., et al. (2007). TRPA1 mediates formalin-induced pain. *Proc. Natl. Acad. Sci. U.S.A.* 104, 13525–13530. doi: 10.1073/pnas.0705924104

Melzack, R., and Wall, P. D. (1962). On the nature of cutaneous sensory mechanisms. *Brain* 85, 331–356. doi: 10.1093/brain/85.2.331

Metzemaekers, M., Gouwy, M., and Proost, P. (2020). Neutrophil chemoattractant receptors in health and disease: double-edged swords. *Cell Mol. Immunol.* 17, 433–450. doi: 10.1038/s41423-020-0412-0

Michael, G. J., and Priestley, J. V. (1999). Differential expression of the mRNA for the vanilloid receptor subtype 1 in cells of the adult rat dorsal root and nodose ganglia and its downregulation by axotomy. *J. Neurosci.* 19, 1844–1854. doi: 10.1523/jneurosci.19-05-01844.1999

Morenilla-Palao, C., Planells-Cases, R., Garcia-Sanz, N., and Ferrer-Montiel, A. (2004). Regulated exocytosis contributes to protein kinase C potentiation of vanilloid receptor activity. *J. Biol. Chem.* 279, 25665–25672. doi: 10.1074/jbc.m311515200

Mourot, A., Herold, C., Kienzler, M. A., and Kramer, R. H. (2018). Understanding and improving photo-control of ion channels in nociceptors with azobenzene photo-switches. *Br. J. Pharmacol.* 175, 2296–2311. doi: 10.1111/bph.13923

Nagi, S. S., Marshall, A. G., Makdani, A., Jarocka, E., Liljencrantz, J., Ridderstrom, M., et al. (2019). An ultrafast system for signaling mechanical pain in human skin. *Sci. Adv.* 5:eaaw1297. doi: 10.1126/sciadv.aaw1297

Nakayama, Y., Omote, K., and Namiki, A. (2002). Role of prostaglandin receptor EP1 in the spinal dorsal horn in carrageenan-induced inflammatory pain. *Anesthesiology* 97, 1254–1262. doi: 10.1097/00000542-200211000-00032

Nassini, R., Gees, M., Harrison, S., De Siena, G., Materazzi, S., Moretto, N., et al. (2011). Oxaliplatin elicits mechanical and cold allodynia in rodents via TRPA1 receptor stimulation. *Pain* 152, 1621–1631. doi: 10.1016/j.pain.2011.02.051

Nguyen, N. L., Van Buren, V., Reimert, R., and Von Garnier, A. (2005). Determination of porosity and flow distribution in packed beds by magnetic resonance imaging. *Magn. Reson. Imaging* 23, 395–396. doi: 10.1016/j.mri.2004.11.061

Noguchi, K., and Okubo, M. (2011). Leukotrienes in nociceptive pathway and neuropathic/inflammatory pain. *Biol. Pharm. Bull.* 34, 1163–1169. doi: 10.1248/bpb.34.1163

Nussmeier, N. A., Whelton, A. A., Brown, M. T., Langford, R. M., Hoeft, A., Parlow, J. L., et al. (2005). Complications of the COX-2 inhibitors parecoxib and valdecoxib after cardiac surgery. *N. Engl. J. Med.* 352, 1081–1091. doi: 10.1056/nejmoa050330

Obata, K., Katsura, H., Mizushima, T., Yamanaka, H., Kobayashi, K., Dai, Y., et al. (2005). TRPA1 induced in sensory neurons contributes to cold hyperalgesia after inflammation and nerve injury. *J. Clin. Invest.* 115, 2393–2401. doi: 10.1172/jci25437

Okubo, M., Yamanaka, H., Kobayashi, K., and Noguchi, K. (2010). Leukotriene synthases and the receptors induced by peripheral nerve injury in the spinal cord contribute to the generation of neuropathic pain. *Glia* 58, 599–610.

Pace, M. C., Passavanti, M. B., De Nardis, L., Bosco, F., Sansone, P., Pota, V., et al. (2018). Nociceptor plasticity: a closer look. *J. Cell Physiol.* 233, 2824–2838. doi: 10.1002/jcp.25993

Park, C. K., Lu, N., Xu, Z. Z., Liu, T., Serhan, C. N., and Ji, R. R. (2011a). Resolving TRPV1- and TNF-alpha-mediated spinal cord synaptic plasticity and inflammatory pain with neuroprotectin D1. *J. Neurosci.* 31, 15072–15085. doi: 10.1523/jneurosci.2443-11.2011

Park, C. K., Xu, Z. Z., Liu, T., Lu, N., Serhan, C. N., and Ji, R. R. (2011b). Resolvin D2 is a potent endogenous inhibitor for transient receptor potential subtype V1/A1, inflammatory pain, and spinal cord synaptic plasticity in mice: distinct roles of resolvin D1. D2, and E1. *J. Neurosci.* 31, 18433–18438. doi: 10.1523/jneurosci.4192-11.2011

Patapoutian, A., Tate, S., and Woolf, C. J. (2009). Transient receptor potential channels: targeting pain at the source. *Nat. Rev. Drug Discov.* 8, 55–68. doi: 10.1038/nrd2757

Peiseler, M., and Kubes, P. (2019). More friend than foe: the emerging role of neutrophils in tissue repair. *J. Clin. Invest.* 129, 2629–2639. doi: 10.1172/jci124616

Pirault, J., and Back, M. (2018). Lipoxin and resolvin receptors transducing the resolution of inflammation in cardiovascular disease. *Front. Pharmacol.* 9:1273. doi: 10.3389/fphar.2018.01273

Qureshi, O., and Dua, A. (2020). *COX Inhibitors*. Treasure Island, FL: StatPearls.

Raja, S. N., Carr, D. B., Cohen, M., Finnerup, N. B., Flor, H., Gibson, S., et al. (2020). The revised international association for the study of pain definition of pain: concepts, challenges, and compromises. *Pain* 161, 1976–1982.

Ramsey, I. S., Delling, M., and Clapham, D. E. (2006). An introduction to TRP channels. *Annu. Rev. Physiol.* 68, 619–647.

Rogers, E., Mehta, S., Shengelia, R., and Reid, M. C. (2013). Four strategies for managing opioid-induced side effects in older adults. *Clin. Geriatr.* 21, 1–14.

Rosenblum, A., Marsch, L. A., Joseph, H., and Portenoy, R. K. (2008). Opioids and the treatment of chronic pain: controversies, current status, and future directions. *Exp. Clin. Psychopharmacol.* 16, 405–416. doi: 10.1037/a0013628

Rymut, N., Heinz, J., Sadhu, S., Hosseini, Z., Riley, C. O., Marinello, M., et al. (2020). Resolvin D1 promotes efferocytosis in aging by limiting senescent cell-induced MerTK cleavage. *FASEB J.* 34, 597–609. doi: 10.1096/fj.201902126r

Salas, M. M., Hargreaves, K. M., and Akopian, A. N. (2009). TRPA1-mediated responses in trigeminal sensory neurons: interaction between TRPA1 and TRPV1. *Eur. J. Neurosci.* 29, 1568–1578. doi: 10.1111/j.1460-9568.2009.06702.x

Salic, K., Morrison, M. C., Verschuren, L., Wielinga, P. Y., Wu, L., Kleemann, R., et al. (2016). Resolvin E1 attenuates atherosclerosis in absence of cholesterol-lowering effects and on top of atorvastatin. *Atherosclerosis* 250, 158–165. doi: 10.1016/j.atherosclerosis.2016.05.001

Sawada, Y., Hosokawa, H., Matsumura, K., and Kobayashi, S. (2008). Activation of transient receptor potential ankyrin 1 by hydrogen peroxide. *Eur. J. Neurosci.* 27, 1131–1142. doi: 10.1111/j.1460-9568.2008.06093.x

Scholz, J., and Woolf, C. J. (2002). Can we conquer pain? *Nat. Neurosci.* 5(Suppl.), 1062–1067. doi: 10.1038/nn942

Selders, G. S., Fetz, A. E., Radic, M. Z., and Bowlin, G. L. (2017). An overview of the role of neutrophils in innate immunity, inflammation and host-biomaterial integration. *Regen. Biomater.* 4, 55–68. doi: 10.1093/rb/rbw041

Seltzer, Z., Dubner, R., and Shir, Y. (1990). A novel behavioral model of neuropathic pain disorders produced in rats by partial sciatic nerve injury. *Pain* 43, 205–218. doi: 10.1016/0304-3959(90)91074-s

Serhan, C. N. (2007). Resolution phase of inflammation: novel endogenous anti-inflammatory and proresolving lipid mediators and pathways. *Annu. Rev. Immunol.* 25, 101–137. doi: 10.1146/annurev.immunol.25.022106.141647

Serhan, C. N. (2014). Pro-resolving lipid mediators are leads for resolution physiology. *Nature* 510, 92–101. doi: 10.1038/nature13479

Serhan, C. N., and Chiang, N. (2013). Resolution phase lipid mediators of inflammation: agonists of resolution. *Curr. Opin. Pharmacol.* 13, 632–640. doi: 10.1016/j.coph.2013.05.012

Serhan, C. N., Chiang, N., Dalli, J., and Levy, B. D. (2015a). Lipid mediators in the resolution of inflammation. *Cold Spring Harbor Perspect. Biol.* 7:a016311.

Serhan, C. N., Chiang, N., and Dalli, J. (2015b). The resolution code of acute inflammation: novel pro-resolving lipid mediators in resolution. *Semin. Immunol.* 27, 200–215. doi: 10.1016/j.smim.2015.03.004

Serhan, C. N., Hong, S., Gronert, K., Colgan, S. P., Devchand, P. R., Mirick, G., et al. (2002). Resolvins: a family of bioactive products of omega-3 fatty acid transformation circuits initiated by aspirin treatment that counter proinflammation signals. *J. Exp. Med.* 196, 1025–1037.

Serhan, C. N., and Levy, B. D. (2018). Resolvins in inflammation: emergence of the pro-resolving superfamily of mediators. *J. Clin. Invest.* 128, 2657–2669. doi: 10.1172/jci97943

Sexton, J. E., Vernon, J., and Wood, J. N. (2014). TRPs and pain. *Handb. Exp. Pharmacol.* 223, 873–897. doi: 10.1007/978-3-319-05161-1_6

Siemens, J., Zhou, S., Piskorowski, R., Nikai, T., Lumpkin, E. A., Basbaum, A. I., et al. (2006). Spider toxins activate the capsaicin receptor to produce inflammatory pain. *Nature* 444, 208–212. doi: 10.1038/nature05285

Song, X. S., Cao, J. L., Xu, Y. B., He, J. H., Zhang, L. C., and Zeng, Y. M. (2005). Activation of ERK/CREB pathway in spinal cord contributes to chronic constrictive injury-induced neuropathic pain in rats. *Acta Pharmacol. Sin.* 26, 789–798. doi: 10.1111/j.1745-7254.2005.00123.x

Spicarova, D., Nerandzic, V., and Palecek, J. (2011). Modulation of spinal cord synaptic activity by tumor necrosis factor alpha in a model of peripheral neuropathy. *J. Neuroinflammation* 8:177. doi: 10.1186/1742-2094-8-177

Stark, A. H., Crawford, M. A., and Reifen, R. (2008). Update on alpha-linolenic acid. *Nutr. Rev.* 66, 326–332. doi: 10.1111/j.1753-4887.2008.00040.x

Staruschenko, A., Jeske, N. A., and Akopian, A. N. (2010). Contribution of TRPV1-TRPA1 interaction to the single channel properties of the TRPA1 channel. *J. Biol. Chem.* 285, 15167–15177. doi: 10.1074/jbc.m110.106153

Story, G. M., Peier, A. M., Reeve, A. J., Eid, S. R., Mosbacher, J., Hricik, T. R., et al. (2003). ANKTM1, a TRP-like channel expressed in nociceptive neurons, is activated by cold temperatures. *Cell* 112, 819–829. doi: 10.1016/s0092-8674(03)00158-2

Suo, Z. W., Fan, Q. Q., Yang, X., and Hu, X. D. (2013). Ca2+ /calmodulin-dependent protein kinase II in spinal dorsal horn contributes to the pain hypersensitivity induced by gamma-aminobutyric acid type a receptor inhibition. *J. Neurosci. Res.* 91, 1473–1482. doi: 10.1002/jnr.23270

Tashima, R., Koga, K., Sekine, M., Kanehisa, K., Kohro, Y., Tominaga, K., et al. (2018). Optogenetic activation of non-nociceptive abeta fibers induces neuropathic pain-like sensory and emotional behaviors after nerve injury in rats. *eNeuro* 5:ENEURO.0450-17.2018. doi: 10.1523/ENEURO.0450-17.2018

Tsuda, M., Shigemoto-Mogami, Y., Koizumi, S., Mizokoshi, A., Kohsaka, S., Salter, M. W., et al. (2003). P2X4 receptors induced in spinal microglia gate tactile allodynia after nerve injury. *Nature* 424, 778–783. doi: 10.1038/nature01786

Ulmann, L., Hatcher, J. P., Hughes, J. P., Chaumont, S., Green, P. J., Conquet, F., et al. (2008). Up-regulation of P2X4 receptors in spinal microglia after peripheral nerve injury mediates BDNF release and neuropathic pain. *J. Neurosci.* 28, 11263–11268. doi: 10.1523/jneurosci.2308-08.2008

Veldhuis, N. A., Poole, D. P., Grace, M., Mcintyre, P., and Bunnett, N. W. (2015). The G protein-coupled receptor-transient receptor potential channel axis: molecular insights for targeting disorders of sensation and inflammation. *Pharmacol. Rev.* 67, 36–73. doi: 10.1124/pr.114.009555

Verkhratsky, A., and Fernyhough, P. (2008). Mitochondrial malfunction and Ca2+ dyshomeostasis drive neuronal pathology in diabetes. *Cell Calcium.* 44, 112–122. doi: 10.1016/j.ceca.2007.11.010

Vilceanu, D., Honore, P., Hogan, Q. H., and Stucky, C. L. (2010). Spinal nerve ligation in mouse upregulates TRPV1 heat function in injured IB4-positive nociceptors. *J. Pain* 11, 588–599. doi: 10.1016/j.jpain.2009.09.018

Vriens, J., Watanabe, H., Janssens, A., Droogmans, G., Voets, T., and Nilius, B. (2004). Cell swelling, heat, and chemical agonists use distinct pathways for the activation of the cation channel TRPV4. *Proc. Natl. Acad. Sci. U.S.A.* 101, 396–401. doi: 10.1073/pnas.0303329101

Wang, J. C., and Strichartz, G. R. (2017). Prevention of chronic post-thoracotomy pain in rats by intrathecal resolvin D1 and D2: effectiveness of perioperative and delayed drug delivery. *J. Pain* 18, 535–545. doi: 10.1016/j.jpain.2016.12.012

Wang, Z., Ling, D., Wu, C., Han, J., and Zhao, Y. (2020). Baicalin prevents the up-regulation of TRPV1 in dorsal root ganglion and attenuates chronic neuropathic pain. *Vet. Med. Sci.* 1–7.

Woodbury, C. J., Zwick, M., Wang, S., Lawson, J. J., Caterina, M. J., Koltzenburg, M., et al. (2004). Nociceptors lacking TRPV1 and TRPV2 have normal heat responses. *J. Neurosci.* 24, 6410–6415. doi: 10.1523/jneurosci.1421-04.2004

Woolf, C. J. (2010). What is this thing called pain? *J. Clin. Invest.* 120, 3742–3744.

Woolf, C. J. (2011). Central sensitization: implications for the diagnosis and treatment of pain. *Pain* 152, S2–S15.

Woolf, C. J., Shortland, P., and Coggeshall, R. E. (1992). Peripheral nerve injury triggers central sprouting of myelinated afferents. *Nature* 355, 75–78. doi: 10.1038/355075a0

Wu, Y., Heymann, H. M., and Gross, E. R. (2018). Non-opioid analgesic use and concerns for impaired organ protection. *Br. J. Anaesth* 120, 403–405. doi: 10.1016/j.bja.2017.11.070

Xu, X., Chen, H., Ling, B. Y., Xu, L., Cao, H., and Zhang, Y. Q. (2014). Extracellular signal-regulated protein kinase activation in spinal cord contributes to pain hypersensitivity in a mouse model of type 2 diabetes. *Neurosci. Bull.* 30, 53–66. doi: 10.1007/s12264-013-1387-y

Xu, Z. Z., Berta, T., and Ji, R. R. (2013). Resolvin E1 inhibits neuropathic pain and spinal cord microglial activation following peripheral nerve injury. *J. Neuroimmune Pharmacol.* 8, 37–41. doi: 10.1007/s11481-012-9394-8

Xu, Z. Z., Kim, Y. H., Bang, S., Zhang, Y., Berta, T., Wang, F., et al. (2015). Inhibition of mechanical allodynia in neuropathic pain by TLR5-mediated A-fiber blockade. *Nat. Med.* 21, 1326–1331. doi: 10.1038/nm.3978

Xu, Z. Z., Zhang, L., Liu, T., Park, J. Y., Berta, T., Yang, R., et al. (2010). Resolvins RvE1 and RvD1 attenuate inflammatory pain via central and peripheral actions. *Nat. Med.* 16, 592–597. doi: 10.1038/nm.2123

Yurdagul, A. Jr., Doran, A. C., Cai, B., Fredman, G., and Tabas, I. A. (2017). Mechanisms and consequences of defective efferocytosis in atherosclerosis. *Front. Cardiovasc. Med.* 4:86. doi: 10.3389/fcvm.2017.00086

Zhang, X., Huang, J., and Mcnaughton, P. A. (2005). NGF rapidly increases membrane expression of TRPV1 heat-gated ion channels. *EMBO J.* 24, 4211–4223. doi: 10.1038/sj.emboj.7600893

Zhao, M., Isami, K., Nakamura, S., Shirakawa, H., Nakagawa, T., and Kaneko, S. (2012). Acute cold hypersensitivity characteristically induced by oxaliplatin is caused by the enhanced responsiveness of TRPA1 in mice. *Mol. Pain* 8:55.

Zheng, J. (2013). Molecular mechanism of TRP channels. *Compr. Physiol.* 3, 221–242.

Zurborg, S., Yurgionas, B., Jira, J. A., Caspani, O., and Heppenstall, P. A. (2007). Direct activation of the ion channel TRPA1 by Ca2+. *Nat. Neurosci.* 10, 277–279. doi: 10.1038/nn1843

9

Activation of TRPV1 by Capsaicin or Heat Drives Changes in 2-Acyl Glycerols and *N*-Acyl Ethanolamines in a Time, Dose and Temperature Dependent Manner

Meera Manchanda, Emma Leishman, Kishan Sangani, Ali Alamri and Heather B. Bradshaw*

Bradshaw Laboratory of Lipid Neuroscience, Indiana University Bloomington, Bloomington, IN, United States

***Correspondence:**
Heather B. Bradshaw
hbbradsh@indiana.edu

Endocannabinoids (eCBs) and transient receptor potential (TRP) channels are associated with thermoregulation; however, there are many gaps in the understanding of how these signaling systems work together in responding to changes in temperature. TRPV1, a calcium-permeable ion channel, is activated by capsaicin, elevated temperature, the eCB Anandamide, and over 15 additional endogenous lipids. There is also evidence for signaling crosstalk between TRPV1 and the eCB receptor, CB_1. We recently found that activation of TRPV1-HEK cells by capsaicin increases the production of the eCB, 2-arachidonoyl glycerol (2-AG), suggesting a molecular link between these receptors. Here, we tested the hypothesis that TRPV1 activation by capsaicin drives regulation of a wider-range of lipid signaling molecules and is time and dose-dependent. We also tested the hypothesis that changes in temperature that drive changes in calcium mobilization in TRPV1-HEK will likewise drive similar changes in lipid signaling molecule regulation. Lipid analysis was conducted by partial purification of methanolic extracts on C18 solid phase extraction columns followed by HPLC/MS/MS. Capsaicin increased the release of 2-acyl glycerols (2-AG, 2-linoleoyl glycerol, 2-oleoyl glycerol), in a concentration- and time-dependent manner, whereas levels of *N*-acyl ethanolamines (NAEs), including Anandamide, were significantly decreased. Analogous changes in 2-acyl glycerols and NAEs were measured upon ramping the temperature from 37 to 45°C. In contrast, opposite effects were measured when analyzing lipids after they were maintained at 27°C and then quickly ramped to 37°C, wherein 2-acyl glycerol levels decreased and NAEs increased. These results provide further evidence that the eCB system and TRPV1 have integrated signaling functions that are associated with the molecular response to temperature variation.

Keywords: TRPV1, lipidomics, thermoregulation, endocannabinoid, anandamide, 2-AG

INTRODUCTION

Temperature, touch, and pain are perceptions resulting from CNS processing of the transduction of stimuli by somatosensory neurons that innervate skin and organs (Lumpkin and Caterina, 2007). Among these sensations and perceptions, understanding of the transduction of temperature and heat remains elusive. It has been hypothesized that a stimulus such as heat may require more than one transduction mechanism for thermoperception to occur (Lumpkin and Caterina, 2007). Thermoregulation is a crucial, homeostatic function that promotes an organism's ability to maintain its core body temperature within a specific range (Hardy, 1961; Hensel, 1973). Changes in the environmental temperature have a more significant and immediate effect on skin temperature, compared to the body's core temperature (Schlader et al., 2011). This characteristic indicates that changes in the core body temperature cannot necessarily serve as the primary thermal signal. A straightforward example is that the human hand has evolved to perceive highly acute stimuli, with the threshold for detecting a change in temperature being $<0.5°C$, even if this is not a noxious change (Stevenson et al., 1999; Frenzel et al., 2012). Therefore, the thermoregulatory responses must be rapid, in order to prevent body core temperature challenges (Nakamura, 2011; Schlader et al., 2011), which suggests rapid modifications of the transduction apparatus by signaling molecules.

Transient receptor potential channels are ubiquitous ligand-gated ion channels, known for their role in the detection and perception of various sensations such as pain, pressure, and temperature (Montell and Rubin, 1989; Caterina et al., 1997; Patapoutian et al., 2003), and are, therefore, involved in many important physiological processes (e.g., perception of various stimuli and maintaining ion homeostasis) (Hansen et al., 2001). Eleven TRP channels have been categorized as temperature-sensitive TRPs. Six out of the eleven channels within this category have highly specific temperature thresholds and are known as thermoreceptor TRPs, or "thermoTRPs" (Montell et al., 2002; McKemy, 2005; Tominaga, 2006; Caterina, 2007). TRPV (vanilloid) cation channels 1–4 are thermoTRP channels that are able to detect thermal stimuli ranging from mild warmth to painfully hot (Clapham, 2003; Caterina, 2007; Nakamura and Morrison, 2008; Sisignano et al., 2014). TRPV1 has a temperature threshold of $\sim42°C$, TRPV2 responds to temperatures $\geq52°C$, and TRPV3 and TRPV4 are responsive to innocuous warmth (~26–$34°C$) (Caterina et al., 1999; Smith et al., 2002; Julius, 2013). ThermoTRP channels exist as membrane proteins that enable ionic mobilization upon stimulation due to a change in temperature (Caterina et al., 1997; Story et al., 2003). If the magnitude of influx is above the threshold, the influx of these ions leads to a temporary depolarization of the cell membrane and initiates a signaling cascade to ultimately allow an organism to perceive that stimulus (Hirst et al., 2006).

The TRPV1 ion channel is the most widely studied receptor of those belonging to the TRPV family. TRPV1 was initially identified in rat dorsal root ganglion (DRG) in 1997, and coined with the name "the capsaicin receptor" (Caterina et al., 1997). These receptors are localized most notably in primary afferent nociceptive neurons in the peripheral nervous system, though they are also expressed in several non-neuronal cell types, along with higher regions of the brain, such as the striatum, hippocampus, midbrain, cerebellum, thalamus, and the hypothalamus (Caterina et al., 1997; Holzer, 2008; Starowicz et al., 2008). The TRPV1 moniker, "the capsaicin receptor," derived from the receptors' sensitivity to capsaicin, the primary pungent ingredient in hot chili peppers that elicits a "burning sensation" upon consumption (Jancso et al., 1977). The "burning pain" perception evoked upon encountering capsaicin led to the theory that, due to receptor activation by capsaicin and subsequent response mechanisms determined by the CNS, capsaicin might be eliciting the perception of pain in a manner similar to the endogenous ligands produced and released upon tissue damage (Bevan and Szolcsanyi, 1990; Caterina and Julius, 2001). This drives that hypothesis that there are endogenous ligands that regulate the function of TRPV1.

The discovery of the cannabinoid receptor 1 (CB_1) lead to the subsequent uncovering of the endocannabinoid (eCB) system. The two most studied signaling molecules within this network are Anandamide (*N*-arachidonoyl ethanolamine; AEA) and 2-arachidonoyl-*sn*-glycerol (2-AG) (Devane et al., 1992; Sugiura et al., 1995). AEA and 2-AG are both derived from membrane phospholipids that contain arachidonic acid and are hypothesized to be produced and released in response to various homeostatic disruptions (Maccarrone et al., 2000). AEA and 2-AG are recognized as lipid signaling molecules that modulate various physiological processes within the nervous system, in part by targeting the cannabinoid receptors, CB_1 and CB_2 (Di Marzo and Maccarrone, 2008). Several other members of the *N*-acyl ethanolamine (NAE) family have been identified and appear to be co-regulated by similar biosynthetic and metabolic pathways as AEA, but are conjugated to other fatty acids, such as docosahexaenoic acid, linoleic acid, oleic acid, stearic acid, or palmitic acid (Movahed et al., 2005; Dalle Carbonare et al., 2008). Although AEA was originally identified as an agonist for cannabinoid receptors, it is also capable of activating specialized, non-cannabinoid receptors, as are some of its congeners (Zygmunt et al., 1999; Smart et al., 2000; Ahern, 2003; Movahed et al., 2005). One example of these "non-cannabinoid" receptors are members of the transient receptor potential (TRP) channel superfamily (Raboune et al., 2014).

N-arachidonoyl ethanolamine (AEA) is a shared ligand between CB_1 and TRPV1, synthesized intracellularly in a PKC-mediated, calcium-dependent manner within the nervous system (Okamoto et al., 2007, 2009; Liu et al., 2008). Although not as potent as capsaicin, AEA is considered a full agonist at human TRPV1, as it displays the same maximal effect as capsaicin when administered exogenously in functional assays (Zygmunt et al., 1999; Smart et al., 2000). Additionally, it has been proposed that the activity of AEA at TRPV1 may be dependent on specific ambient temperatures, in a manner similar to capsaicin (Smart et al., 2000; Sprague et al., 2001). An earlier study suggested that 2-AG may have some effect on TRPV1 activity; but as a modulator of membrane potential, rather than as a driver of calcium mobilization (Zygmunt et al., 2013). As an agonist of CB_1, it is also possible that 2-AG may be involved in the crosstalk between CB_1 and TRPV1, given the widespread tissue types that co-express these two receptors (Woo et al., 2008). Previously, we showed that capsaicin-stimulated TRPV1-transfected HEK cells drive an increase in production of 2-AG, providing further evidence of a molecular signaling link between the two (Leishman et al., 2017).

Here, we test the hypothesis TRPV1 activity plays an important modulatory role in the biosynthesis and metabolism of AEA, 2-AG and related lipids by analyzing their levels in TRPV1-transfected HEK cells stimulated by either capsaicin or by changes in temperature. We show that there are time and dose dependent effects with capsaicin stimulation and that many of these are mirrored with changes in temperature. Specifically, levels of 2-acyl glycerols, including 2-AG, increased and levels of NAEs, including AEA, decreased with increasing levels of capsaicin and temperature. The opposite effect in lipid production was found when TRPV1-HEK cells were cooled to 27°C in that levels of 2-acyl glycerols decreased and NAEs increased. These data provide a novel insight into the signaling mechanisms of TRPV1 activity and how this signaling system is linked to the eCB signaling system through the modulation of eCB endogenous ligands.

MATERIALS AND METHODS

Analysis of Lipids in TRPV1-HEK Cells After Stimulation by 100 nM, 1 μM, and 10 μM Capsaicin

hTRPV1-HEK cells, a kind gift from Merck (Whitehouse Station, NJ, United States), were grown in high-glucose Dulbecco's Modified Eagle's Medium (DMEM) (Thermo Fisher Scientific, Waltham, MA, United States), supplemented with 10% fetal bovine serum (Gibco, Dublin, Ireland), and 1% penicillin/streptomycin antibiotic (Thermo Fisher Scientific), as previously described (Leishman et al., 2017). Stock solutions of capsaicin were prepared in-house in 100% ethanol and stored at −80°C. Solutions of appropriate molarities were made immediately before experimentation in >99% DMSO. For each experiment, TRPV1-HEK cells at approximately 85% confluency were split into 12 individual T-25 cm^2 flasks. For each condition, the cells were gently washed twice with HEPES buffer [HEPES 0.025 mol, NaCl 0.140 mol, KCl 0.0027 mol, $CaCl_2$ 0.0018 mol, $MgCl_2$ 0.0005 mol, NaH_2PO_4 and D-glucose 0.05 mol (Sigma-Aldrich) in DI H_2O (prepared in-house)] that had been pre-warmed to 37°C in a water bath. The cells then incubated at 37°C, 5% CO_2 for 45 min in 4 mL of HEPES buffer. After the 45-min equilibration incubation, the buffer was replaced with 4 mL of the vehicle (0.1% DMSO) or capsaicin-buffer solution. The cells incubated in the capsaicin or vehicle solution for either 1 min or 5 min before lipid extraction was performed. HEPES was used to simulate our calcium-imaging protocols that validated that these cells drive calcium mobilization as previously published (Raboune et al., 2014).

After each flask's incubation period, the buffer solution was collected in a 15 mL centrifuge tube. Then, 2 mL of 100% HPLC-grade methanol (MeOH; Avantor Performance Materials, Inc., Center Valley, PA, United States) was added to the flask. The cells were harvested from the flasks using cell scrapers, and the cell solution gathered was added to the corresponding collected buffer. An additional 2 mL of MeOH was added to the flask to collect any remaining cells, which were also transferred to the 15 mL centrifuge tube. All tubes were spiked with 50 pmols deuterium-labeled *N*-arachidonoyl glycine (d_8NaGly; Cayman Chemical, Ann Arbor, MI, United States), prepared in MeOH, which served as an internal standard. After centrifugation, the supernatants were partially purified using C18 solid phase extraction columns (Agilent, Palo Alto, CA, United States) as previously described (Leishman et al., 2018).

Analysis of Lipids in TRPV1-HEK Cells After Changes in Temperature

60 mm × 15 mm glass petri dishes (Thermo Fisher Scientific) were coated with 50 μg/mL PDL prior to experimentation, to enhance cell adherence. Growth and maintenance of cells was as described above. Cells were grown to 85% confluence before experimentation.

Procedure for Temperature Ramp From 27 to 37°C

Cells in the temperature change condition were washed twice with HEPES-Tyrode buffer that had been pre-warmed to 27°C. The cells then incubated in 4 mL HEPES buffer at room temperature inside a cell culture hood for 45 min. In the hood, the cells were covered by a deep stainless-steel tray, accompanied by a beaker of hot water to provide humidity and assist in maintaining a steady temperature of 27°C, which was monitored by a digital wire probe thermometer. After the 45-min incubation period, each dish was transferred to a digital hot plate that had been pre-warmed to 27°C. The lid for the dish was removed and replaced by foil, which was fit snugly over the dish to ensure minimal heat loss and/or evaporation. A wire probe digital thermometer was positioned under the foil and submerged in the buffer solution approximately 2–3 mm from the cell layer to monitor the temperature change. The probe was situated this close in order to avoid mechanical stimulation, but close enough that the temperature being measured was as close as possible to the cell layer. The hot plate temperature was slowly raised using a manual dial while the temperature read-outs from the plate and the probe were monitored, ensuring a steady increase of 15 ± 2–4 s per degree. On average, it took 2.5 min for the buffer solution in each dish to reach 37°C. Upon reaching 37°C, the dish was removed from the hot plate, and the buffer solution was transferred to a conical tube. Subsequently, 2 mL of 100% HPLC-grade MeOH was added to the dish. The cells were then harvested from the dishes using cell scrapers and the cell solution was added to the tube containing the corresponding buffer solution. An additional 2 mL of MeOH was added to the dish to collect any remaining cells, which were also transferred to the conical tube.

Procedure for Temperature Ramp From 37 to 45°C

TRPV1-HEK cells were washed twice with HEPES buffer that had been pre-warmed to 37°C. The cells were then incubated at 37°C, 5% CO_2 for 45 min in 4 mL of HEPES buffer, to allow for equilibration. After the 45-min incubation period, each dish was removed from the incubator and placed on a digital hot plate that was pre-warmed to 37°C. The lid for the dish was removed and replaced with a piece of aluminum foil. A wire probe digital thermometer was positioned under the foil and submerged in the buffer solution to monitor the temperature change. The hot plate temperature was slowly raised, while the temperature read-outs from the plate and the probe were monitored to ensure a steady increase of 15 ± 2–4 s per degree. On average, it took 2–2.25 min for each plate to reach 45°C. Upon reaching 45°C, the dish was removed from the hot plate and the buffer solution was transferred to a conical tube. Cells were harvested from each dish using HPLC-grade MeOH, as described above.

The cells in the control condition for each temperature ramp group were washed twice with HEPES-Tyrode buffer, which was pre-warmed to 37°C, and were then incubated under standard cell culture incubator conditions in 4 mL HEPES buffer for 45 min. The temperature of the solution in each dish was taken after each 45-min incubation period, to ensure the temperature had been maintained at 37°C, ±1°C. The buffer solution was then transferred to a 15 mL conical centrifuge tube. Cells were harvested from each dish using HPLC-grade MeOH, as described above for the temperature-change condition.

To test the hypothesis that the effects of the change in temperature were dependent on TRPV1 activation, cells were treated with 500 nM of the TRPV1 antagonist, iRTX (iodo-resiniferatoxin) prior to the 45-min incubation period and then the identical procedure as outlined above was performed.

All cell solutions from each condition were spiked with 50 pmols d_8 N-arachidonoyl glycine (NAGly), which served as an internal standard. The spiked samples were

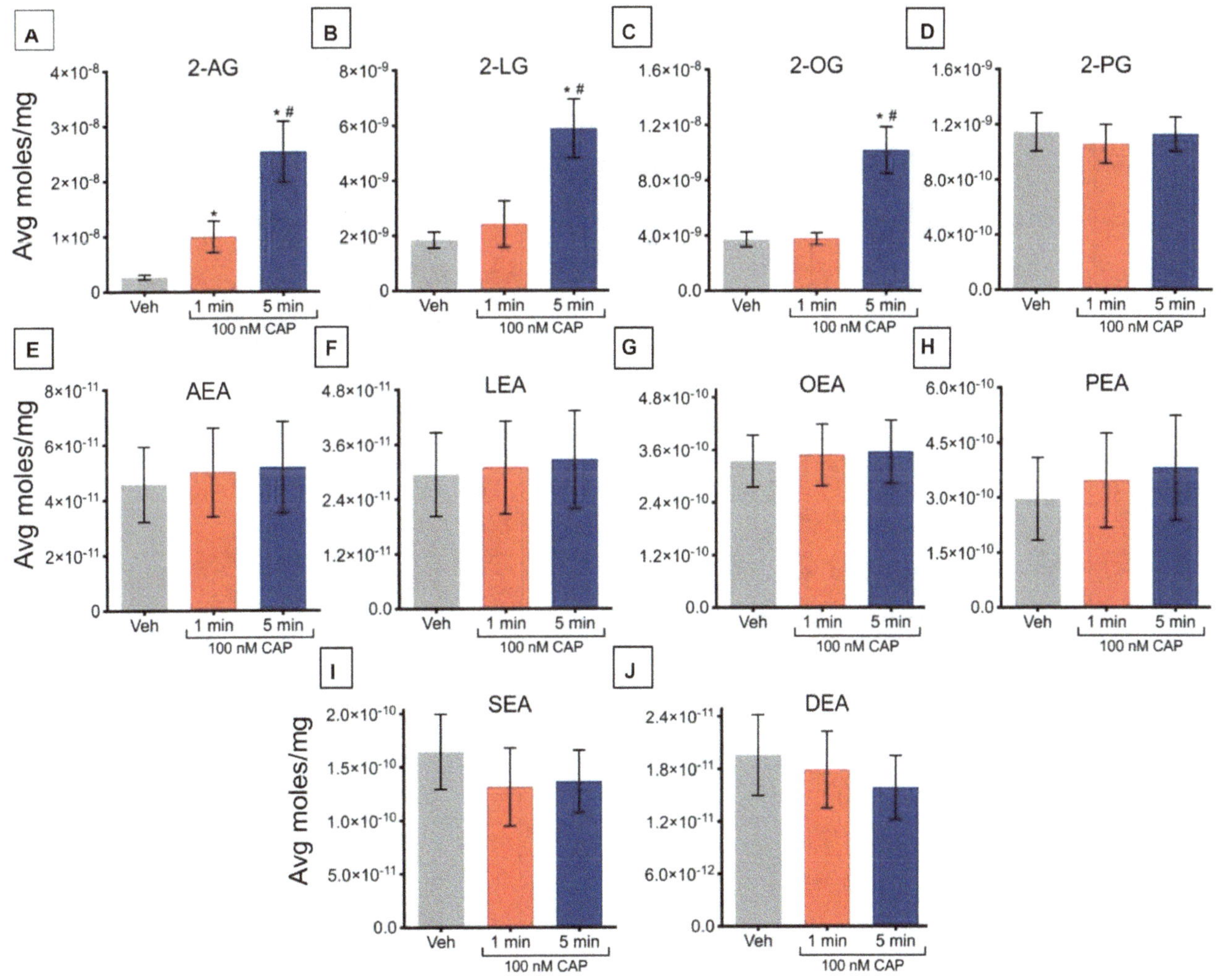

FIGURE 1 | Changes in lipid levels of 2-acyl glycerols **(A–D)** and *N*-acyl ethanolamines **(E–J)** after TRPV1-HEK293 cells incubated in 100 nM capsaicin (CAP) for 1 min or 5 min. Significant changes in lipid levels when comparing capsaicin-induced changes after 1 min or 5 min to vehicle is indicated by * ($p \leq 0.05$). Significant changes in lipid levels when comparing capsaicin-induced changes after 1 min of incubation vs. 5 min of incubation is indicated by # ($p \leq 0.05$). Data were averaged over 12 total data points per condition ($n = 3$ individual experiments) and presented as average moles/mg (y-axis).

centrifuged at 3,000 rpm for 15 min at 24°C. After centrifugation, the supernatants were partially purified using C18 solid phase extraction columns as previously described (Leishman et al., 2018).

HPLC/MS/MS Quantification and Analysis

Analysis of the samples was carried out using an Applied Biosystems API 3000 triple quadrupole mass spectrometer with electrospray ionization (Applied Biosystems Sciex, Foster City, CA, United States) in MRM mode as previously described (Leishman et al., 2017, 2018). Analyst 1.4.2 software (Applied Biosystems) was used to quantify the HPLC/MS/MS data. The software generated chromatograms by determining the retention times of each analyte with a programmed parent ion and a fragmentation ion mass. Quantification of the analytes were calculated by coupling the calibration curves of the synthetic standards and the recovery adjustments, determined by the d_8NAGly standard.

Concentrations of each analyte were reported as moles per gram, after measuring the weights of each dried cell pellet. Recoveries were calculated by measuring the amount of d_8NaGly remaining in each sample after lipid extraction and comparing those values to the recovery standard that represented 100% recovery. IBM SPSS Statistics 23 (IBM, Armonk, NY, United States) was used to determine statistical differences between conditions, implementing one-way ANOVAs. Data comparisons from the capsaicin incubations were made across all three conditions (vehicle, 1-min incubations, and 5 min incubations). A 95% confidence interval was calculated for the means, and statistical significance was defined as $p \leq 0.05$. For temperature experiments, comparisons were made between the vehicle conditions and the heat-challenged conditions using SPSS one-way ANOVAs. A 95% confidence interval was calculated for the means, and statistical significance was defined as $p \leq 0.05$.

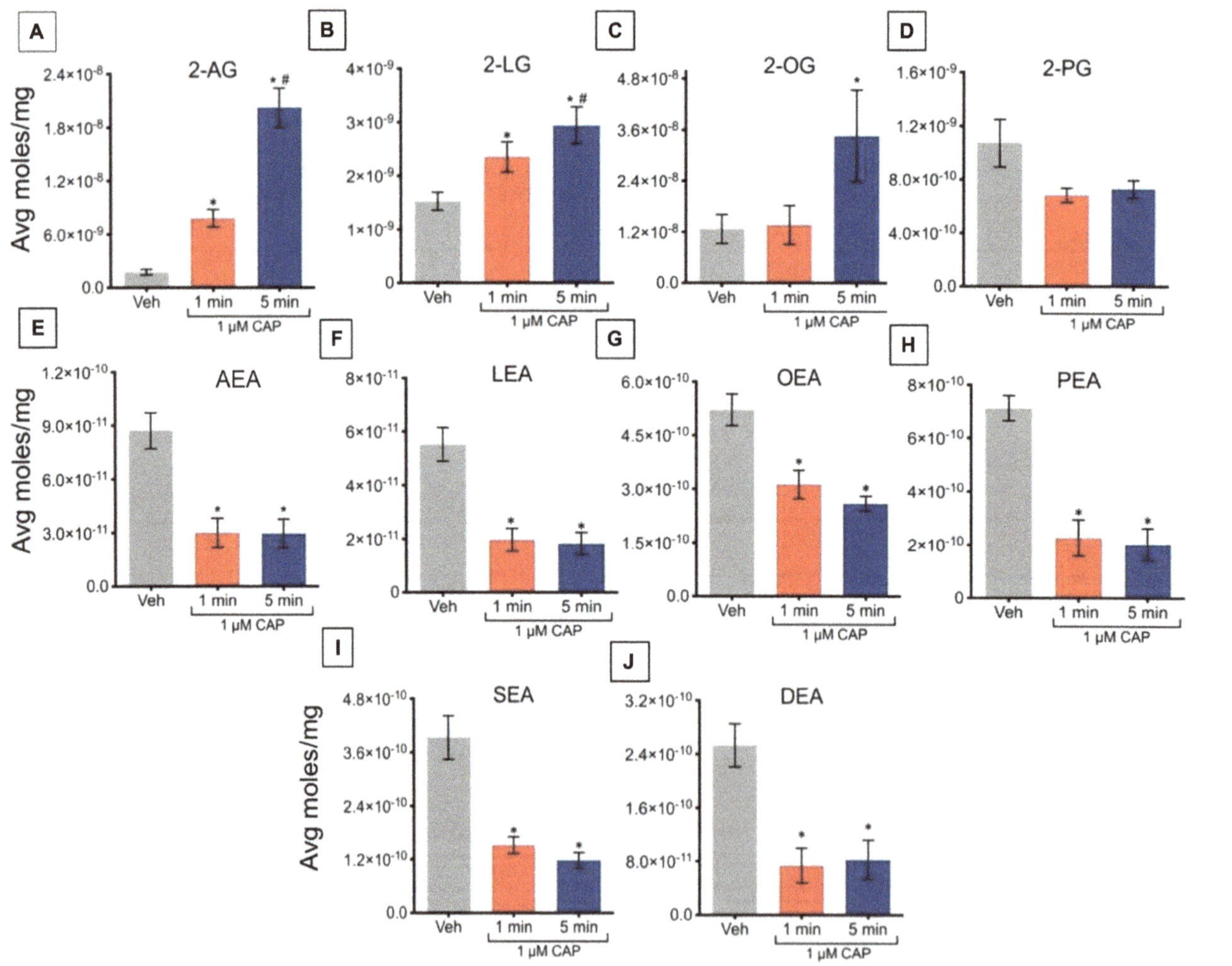

FIGURE 2 | Changes in lipid levels of 2-acyl glycerols **(A–D)** and *N*-acyl ethanolamines **(E–J)** after TRPV1-HEK293 cells incubated in 1 μM capsaicin (CAP) for 1 min or 5 min. Significant changes in lipid levels when comparing capsaicin-induced changes after 1 min or 5 min to vehicle is indicated by * ($p \leq 0.05$). Significant changes in lipid levels when comparing capsaicin-induced changes after 1 min of incubation vs. 5 min of incubation is indicated by # ($p \leq 0.05$). Data were averaged over 8 total data points per condition (n = 2 individual experiments) and presented as average moles/mg (y-axis).

GraphPad Prism 7.0 (GraphPad, San Diego, CA, United States) was used to generate graphs.

RESULTS

Lipidomics Analysis of TRPV1-HEK Cells After Capsaicin Stimulation

The following lipids were detected and analyzed in all samples: 2-arachidonoyl glycerol (2-AG), 2-linoleoyl glycerol (2-LG), 2-oleoyl glycerol (2-OG), 2-palmitoyl glycerol (2-PG), AEA, *N*-linoleoyl ethanolamine (LEA), *N*-oleoyl ethanolamine (OEA), *N*-palmitoyl ethanolamine (PEA), *N*-stearoyl ethanolamine (SEA), and *N*-docosahexaenoyl ethanolamine (DEA). Data are analyzed by time; however, they are presented independently by concentration of capsaicin and not as a direct comparison of concentrations. This is because these are data from independent experiments and not on the same cells, which precludes the ability for reliable direct comparisons of absolute lipid concentrations with capsaicin concentrations.

Capsaicin-Induced Changes in Lipids Levels After TRPV1-HEK Cells Incubated in 100 nM Capsaicin for 1 min or 5 min

Incubation of TRPV1-HEK293 cells with 100 nM capsaicin for 1 min caused a significant increase in 2-AG concentrations but had no significant effect on the other 2-acyl-glycerols measured. Incubation with 100 nM capsaicin for 5 min drove significant increases in 2-AG, 2-LG, and 2-OG, relative to vehicle (**Figures 1A–C**). Levels of 2-AG, 2-LG, and 2-OG were significantly higher after 5 min than after 1 min, indicating that regulation of these lipids may be time-dependent at this

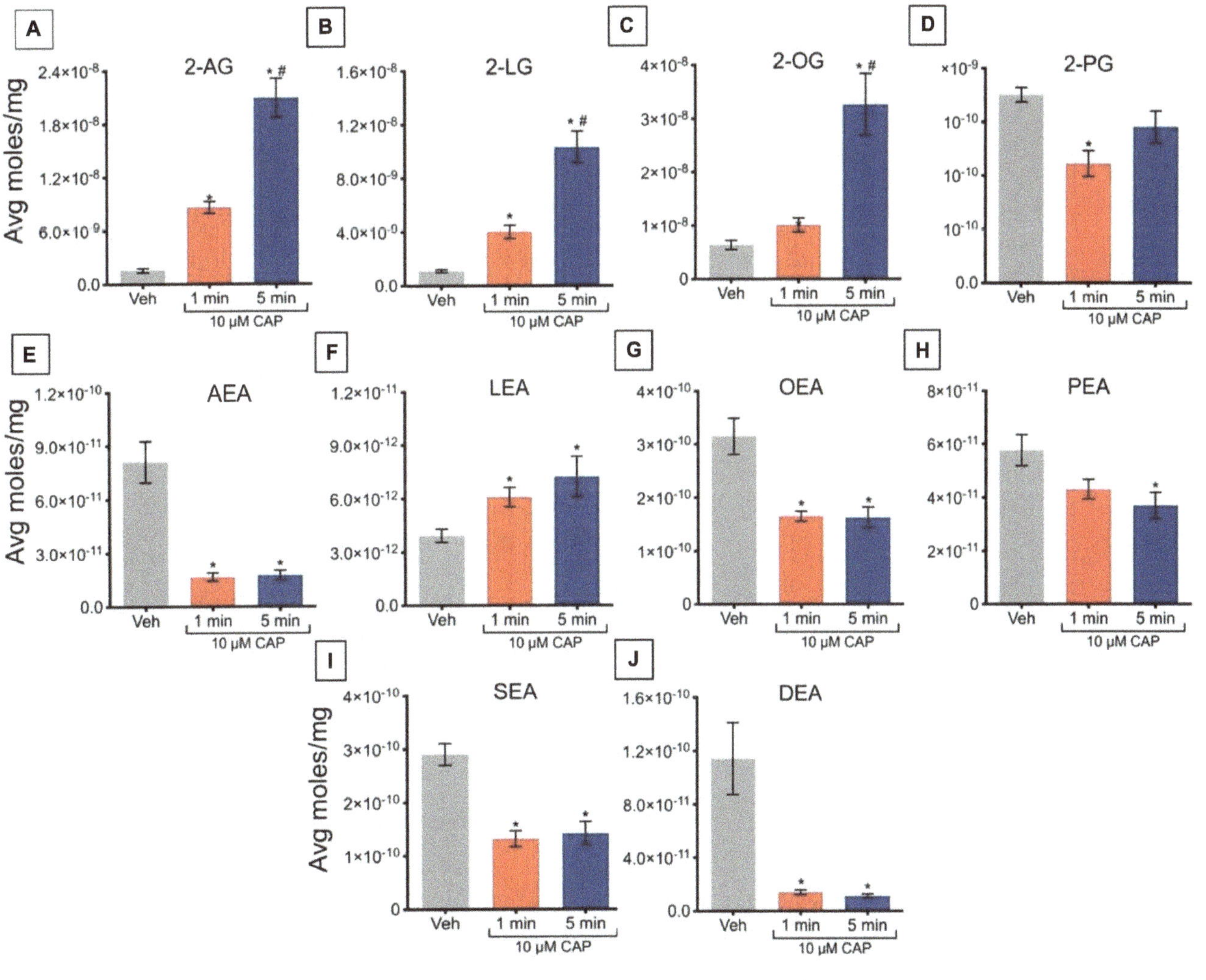

FIGURE 3 | Changes in lipid levels of 2-acyl glycerols **(A–D)** *N*-acyl ethanolamines **(E–J)** after TRPV1-HEK293 cells incubated in 10 μM capsaicin (CAP) for either 1 min or 5 min. Significant changes in lipid levels when comparing capsaicin-induced changes after 1 min or 5 min to vehicle is indicated by * ($p \leq 0.05$). Significant changes in lipid levels when comparing capsaicin-induced changes after 1 min of incubation vs. 5 min of incubation is indicated by # ($p \leq 0.05$). Data depicted in each graph were averaged over 16 total data points per condition (n = 4 individual experiments) and presented as average moles/mg (y-axis).

concentration of capsaicin (**Figures 1A–C**). There were no significant changes seen in levels of 2-PG at both 1 min and 5 min (**Figure 1D**). Likewise, no changes were measured in any of the NAEs at either time point (**Figures 1E–J**).

Capsaicin-Induced Changes in Lipids Levels After TRPV1-HEK Cells Incubated in 1 μM Capsaicin for 1 min or 5 min

Incubation of TRPV1-HEK293 cells with 1 μM capsaicin for 1 min caused a significant increase in levels of 2-AG and 2-LG, relative to vehicle, with no changes in levels of 2-OG or 2-PG (**Figures 2A–D**). Capsaicin incubation for 5 min significantly increased levels of 2-AG, 2-LG, and 2-OG, but not 2-PG, relative to vehicle. The increased levels of 2-AG and 2-LG after 5 min of incubation was significantly higher than levels at 1 min, indicating that regulation of these lipids is time-dependent at this concentration of capsaicin. Incubation of TRPV1-HEK293 cells with 1 μM capsaicin for 1 min and 5 min significantly decreased levels of all NAEs, including the eCB anandamide. In contrast to effects on 2-AG and 2-LG, which were time-dependent, the effects on NAEs were independent of time, showing similar decreases at both time points (**Figures 2E–J**).

Capsaicin-Induced Changes in Lipids Levels After TRPV1-HEK Cells Incubated in 10 μM Capsaicin for 1 min or 5 min

Incubation of TRPV1-HEK293 cells with 10 μM capsaicin for 1 min significantly increased levels of 2-AG, 2-LG, and 2-OG, relative to vehicle (**Figures 3A–C**); however, this incubation significantly decreased levels of 2-PG (**Figure 3D**). At 5 min, levels of 2-AG, 2-LG, and 2-OG remained elevated relative to vehicle, but no significant changes were observed in the levels of 2-PG. Effects on 2-acyl glycerols were time-dependent, with significantly higher levels of 2-AG, 2-LG, and 2-OG after 5 min of incubation versus 1 min. Incubation of TRPV1-HEK293 cells with 10 μM capsaicin for 1 min and 5 min significantly reduced levels of AEA, OEA, SEA, and DEA, relative to vehicle (**Figures 3E,G,I,J**), whereas LEA levels increased relative to vehicle (**Figure 3F**), while levels of PEA remained unchanged (**Figure 3H**). No significant effects of time were detected for

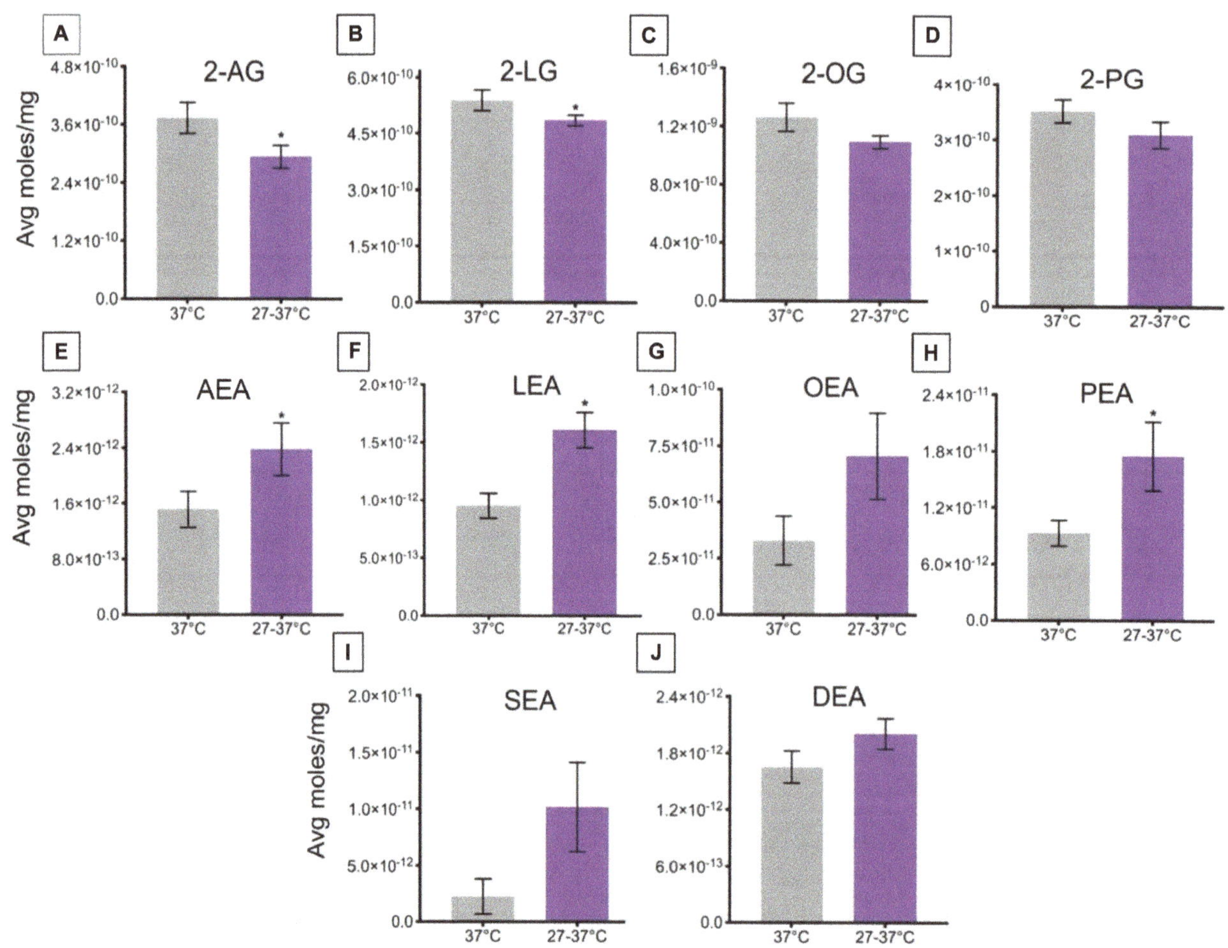

FIGURE 4 | Changes in lipid levels of 2-acyl glycerols **(A–D)** and *N*-acyl ethanolamines **(E–J)** upon an increase in temperature from 27 to 37°C. Significant temperature-induced changes after TRPV1-HEK293 cells were exposed to a change in ambient temperature from 27 to 37°C is indicated by * ($p \leq 0.05$). Data depicted in each graph were averaged over 15 total data points per condition (n = 3 individual experiments) and are presented as average moles/mg (y-axis).

NAEs in these experiments, in that levels of NAEs did not further change at 5 min versus 1 min (**Figures 3E–J**).

Lipidomics Analysis of TRPV1-HEK Cells After Changes in Temperature

Temperature-Induced Changes in Lipid Levels After Change From 27 to 37°C in TRPV1-HEK Cells

A change in ambient temperature to 27°C for 45 min and then a ramp to 37°C over ~2 min caused a significant decrease the levels of 2-AG and 2-LG, relative to controls maintained at a temperature of 37°C (**Figures 4A,B**). Levels of 2-OG and 2-PG were unaffected by this change in temperature (**Figures 4C,D**). This change in temperature drove a significant increase in levels of AEA, LEA, and PEA, relative to a maintained temperature of 37°C (**Figures 4E,F,H**), whereas no significant changes occurred in levels of OEA, SEA, and DEA (**Figures 4G,I,J**).

Temperature-Induced Changes in Lipid Levels After Change From 37 to 45°C in TRPV1-HEK Cells

A change in ambient temperature from 37 to 45°C over ~2.5 min caused a significant increase in levels of 2-AG, 2-LG, and 2-OG (**Figures 5A–C**), whereas there was no significant change in levels of 2-PG (**Figure 5D**). This change in temperature significantly decreased levels of AEA, LEA, and DEA (**Figures 5E,F,J**), whereas the change in temperature caused a significant increase in lipid levels of SEA (**Figure 5I**). No significant changes were measured in levels of OEA or PEA (**Figures 5G,H**).

Temperature-Induced Changes in Lipid Levels After Change From 37°C–45°C in iRTX-Treated TRPV1-HEK Cells

To determine the extent to which TRPV1 activation during heat ramp stimulation drives changes in these lipids the same testing protocol was used on HEK TRPV1 cells with a pre-treatment of 500 nM iRTX, a potent TRPV1 antagonist. **Table 1** shows that there is only one significant change in any of the lipids measured. 2-LG was still significantly increased in the presence of iRTX; however, the magnitude of effect is much reduced. These data support the involvement of TRPV1 in the modulation of these lipids.

DISCUSSION

The detection of ambient temperature is vital for organisms that seek temperatures that are optimal for life, and to avoid any potentially damaging environmental conditions. The activity

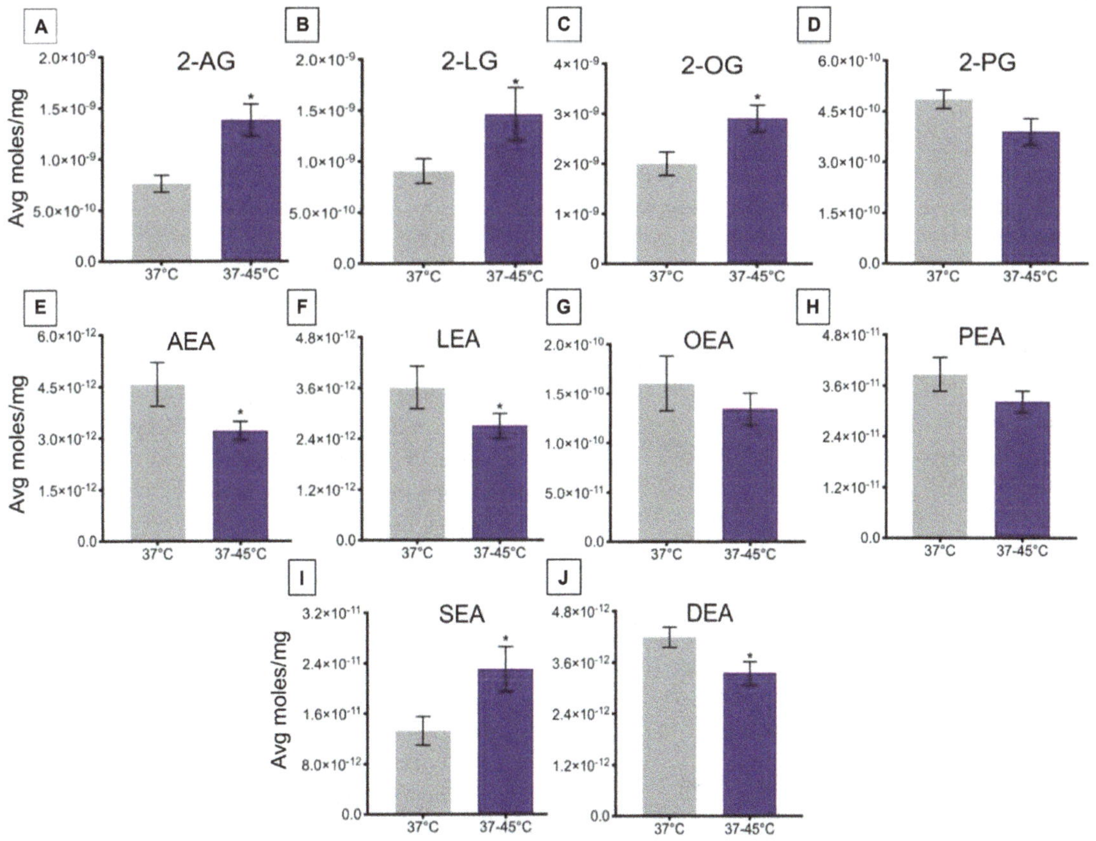

FIGURE 5 | Changes in lipid levels of 2-acyl glycerols **(A–D)** and *N*-acyl ethanolamines **(E–J)** upon an increase in temperature from 37 to 45°C. Significant temperature-induced changes after TRPV1-HEK293 cells were exposed to a change in ambient temperature from 37 to 45°C, is indicated by * ($p \leq 0.05$). Data depicted in each graph were averaged over 15 total data points per condition (n = 3 individual experiments) and are presented as average moles/mg (y-axis).

TABLE 1 | Levels of lipids in HEK-TRPV1 cells after heat ramp from 37–45°C in the presence of the TRPV1 antagonist, iRTX.

	500 nM iRTX	Mean	SEM
2-AG	37°C	3.07E-10	2.25E-11
	37–45°C	3.39E-10	3.40E-11
2-LG	37°C	3.43E-10	2.34E-11
	37–45°C	**4.44E-10**	3.00E-11
2-OG	37°C	5.88E-09	2.45E-10
	37–45°C	6.90E-09	5.22E-10
2-PG	37°C	4.56E-10	3.63E-11
	37–45°C	4.69E-10	3.71E-11
AEA	37°C	7.56E-11	6.31E-12
	37–45°C	6.18E-11	5.26E-12
LEA	37°C	6.53E-10	3.87E-11
	37–45°C	7.40E-10	3.32E-11
OEA	37°C	5.16E-11	4.01E-12
	37–45°C	6.01E-11	3.02E-12
PEA	37°C	2.73E-10	1.87E-11
	37–45°C	3.21E-10	2.04E-11
SEA	37°C	4.04E-10	2.77E-11
	37–45°C	3.56E-10	2.99E-11
DEA	37°C	1.83E-10	1.22E-11
	37–45°C	2.27E-10	2.05E-11

All lipids levels are expressed as mols/gram dried cell pellet weight. Bold indicates $p < 0.05$. See text for abbreviations.

of thermoTRPs facilitates the ability of organisms to adjust other physiological functions and behaviors, upon detecting an environmental cue such as temperature (Castillo et al., 2018). This type of regulation can ensure that prolonged periods of core body temperature elevation or depression are minimized, preserving a hospitable environment for necessary enzymatic reactions to occur (Romanovsky, 2007). As a thermoTRP, a notable characteristic of TRPV1 channels is that they are responsive to exogenous and endogenous chemical stimuli (capsaicin) and physical stimuli, such as heat (Caterina et al., 1997; Clapham, 2003). This characteristic ability to respond to such a range of stimuli categorizes TRPV1 as a polymodal receptor. As a polymodal molecular integrator, TRPV1 has evolved an ability to have several mechanisms/pathways by which it can transduce information gathered from a diverse set of ligands (Julius and Basbaum, 2001; Raboune et al., 2014). Our current data suggests that TRPV1 activation drives changes in eCB and related lipid mediators by both chemical and thermal stimuli. These data presented in this study provide a novel insight into the dynamic molecular signaling systems involved in the thermoregulatory system at the level of TRPV1 activation.

The surprising finding that increases in levels of 2-AG corresponded with decreases in levels of AEA with both capsaicin and heat in a time range of only 1–5 min suggests a potential molecular link in their biosynthesis and/or metabolism. It is a typical assumption when measuring an increase in a signaling molecule to infer that the metabolism has been inhibited. Likewise, there is often the inference of an upregulation in metabolism when the levels of a molecule decrease. The other side of the equation rests with the regulation of the biosynthesis wherein increases in a molecule can denote an upregulation of this biosynthesis process and a downregulation with decreases. Both processes may also be at play in the rapid modulation to a cellular event, especially when two divergent pathways for biosynthesis share a common precursor.

While AEA and 2-AG both contain arachidonic acid (AA), their biosynthetic pathways are not through conjugation of free AA; instead, they are both produced through enzymatic modulation of AA-containing membrane phospholipids (Liu et al., 2008; Okamoto et al., 2009; Leishman et al., 2016; Mock et al., 2020). Three separate synthesis pathways have been hypothesized to generate AEA (Ueda et al., 2013). Each of these pathways require availability of *N*-arachidonoyl-phosphatidylethanolamine (NAPE). NAPE is the product of the membrane phospholipid, phosphatidylethanolamine (PE) through an acyl transfer from phosphatidylcholine (PC) via an *N*-acyl transferase (NAT) enzyme in a calcium-dependent manner (Di Marzo et al., 1994). More recently, the Cravatt group isolated the serine hydrolase PLA2G4E as a specific NAT in CNS tissue that produces the NAPE species that are precursors to NAEs including AEA (Ogura et al., 2016). NAPE-PLD cleaves the NAPE glycerophosphate group via hydrolysis, yielding NAEs (Di Marzo et al., 1994; Leishman et al., 2016). The second pathway first requires conversion of NAPE into lyso-NAPE, which occurs when the two NAPE-specific phospholipases (A1/A2) cleave the molecule into lyso-NAPE and glycerophosphoanandamide. From here, a specific PLD can hydrolyze the intermediate molecule to yield NAEs (Simon and Cravatt, 2006). The third pathway requires the use of a NAPE-specific PLC to cleave NAPE and acquire phospho-NAE. Dephosphorylation of this intermediate using a lipid phosphatate yields NAEs (Liu et al., 2008).

Biosynthesis of 2-AG is like AEA in that both are derived from membrane phospholipids. Diacylglycerols (DAGs) are analogous to NAPEs in that they are likewise generated by multiple pathways (Stella et al., 1997; Sugiura et al., 2006). One of the pathways to generate DAGs is through the hydrolysis of phosphatidic acid (PA), which can be generated from PC enzymatically via phospholipase D (PLD) or phospholipase C (PLC), and a third is through the direct hydrolysis of triacylglycerols (Stella et al., 1997; Sugiura et al., 2006). DAGs are then hydrolyzed via diacylglycerol lipase (DAGL) into monoacylglycerols (MAGs) such as the 2-acyl glycerols including the eCB, 2-AG (Sugiura et al., 2006).

It is important to note that PC is a precursor to both AEA and 2-AG. We hypothesize that the regulation of PC metabolism may be a factor in shunting toward one pathway over the other. The evidence that lower temperatures drive the opposite effect with increases and NEAs and decreases in 2-acyl glycerols further supports this hypothesis. **Figure 6** outlines the specific pathways

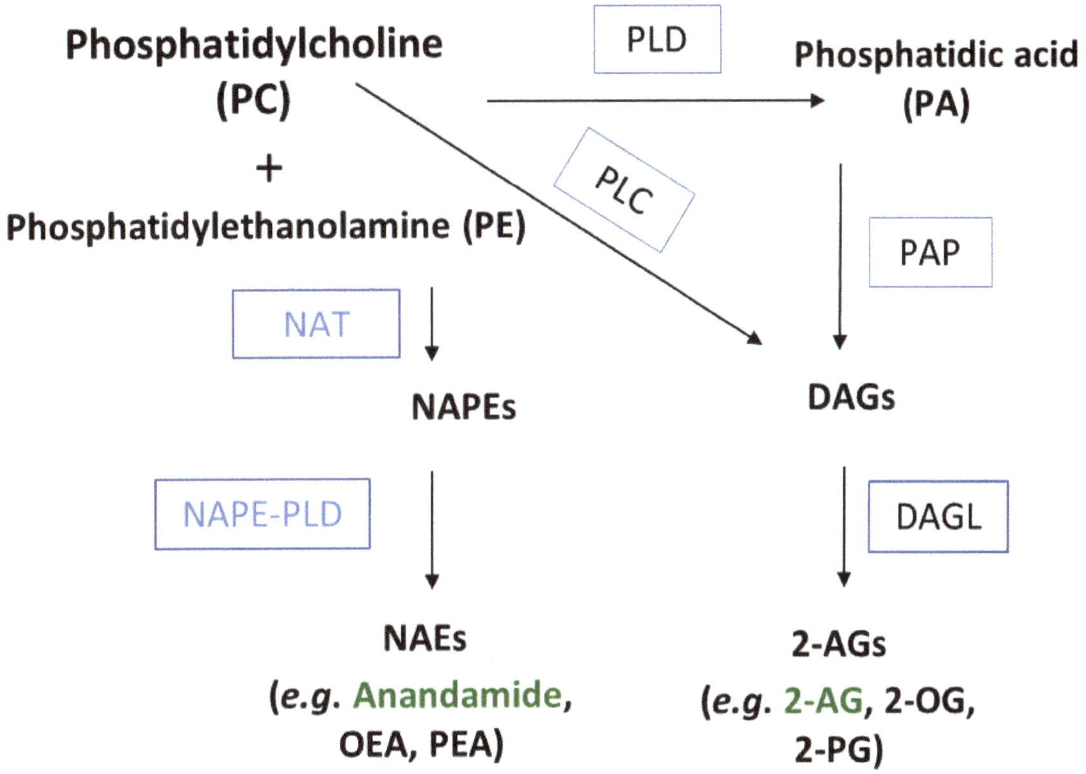

FIGURE 6 | Schematic of NAE and 2-acyl glycerol biosynthesis through a phosphatidylcholine (PC) precursor. Substrates and products in bold black. Enzymes abbreviated in boxes. NAT, N-acyl transferase; PLD, phospholipase D; PLC, phospholipase C; PA, phosphatidic acid; NAPE, N-acyl phosphatidylethanolamine; PAP, phosphatidic acid phosphohydrolase; DAG, diacylglycerol; DAGL, diacylglycerol lipase.

that involve PC in both NAE and 2-acyl glycerol biosynthesis. We hypothesize that TRPV1 activity is driving a shift in the amount of PC being shunted in the PLD pathway toward DAGs, which is creating a precursor deficit for NAPE and then NAE production. As with all hypotheses, this one comes with caveats. While AEA and 2-AG as well as OEA and 2-OG have a very predictable inverse relationship with TRPV1 activity at 1 and 10 μM capsaicin and heat, the linoleoyl derivatives (2-LG and LEA) only show this tight relationship with 1 μM capsaicin and heat. Whereas PEA and 2-PG do not show this same relationship, wherein 2-PG and PEA are less effected by capsaicin and heat overall, but both decrease with 10 μM capsaicin. The standards for 2-stearoyl glycerol and 2-docosahexaenoyl glycerol were not available for analysis during these experiments, so we were unable to ascertain the relationships between the species. However, it is important to note that SEA increased with heat instead of decreased like the rest of the NAEs; therefore, it is likely that there are multiple ways that these signaling molecules are regulated with temperature. What the purpose of these lipid signaling molecules is another important aspect of study for future experiments.

CONCLUSION

Here, we demonstrate that activity of TRPV1 via capsaicin and temperature drives increases in levels of 2-acyl glycerols and decreases in NAEs in a time and dose dependent manner. These novel findings provide a unique insight in the signaling systems involving TPRV1 activity and in lipid signaling molecule regulation by temperature. The data further illustrate that the modulation of intracellular calcium is only one of the many signaling cascades that are relevant to TRPV1 signaling.

AUTHOR CONTRIBUTIONS

MM, KS, and AA performed the TRPV1 HEK cell experiments (MM and KS with capsaicin, MM and AA with temperature). EL performed the mass spectrometric analysis. MM and KS performed the statistical analyses. MM, EL, and HB shared contribution to the manuscript. MM and HB conceived of the idea and developed methods for experimental implementation. All authors contributed to the article and approved the submitted version.

REFERENCES

Ahern, G. P. (2003). Activation of TRPV1 by the satiety factor oleoylethanolamide. *J. Biol. Chem.* 278, 30429–30434. doi: 10.1074/jbc.m305051200

Bevan, S., and Szolcsanyi, J. (1990). Sensory neuron-specific actions of capsaicin: mechanisms and applications. *Trends Pharmacol. Sci.* 11, 330–333.

Castillo, K. I, Diaz-Franulic, J. Canan, Gonzalez-Nilo, F., and Latorre, R. (2018). Thermally activated TRP channels: molecular sensors for temperature detection. *Phys. Biol.* 15:021001. doi: 10.1088/1478-3975/aa9a6f

Caterina, M. J. (2007). Transient receptor potential ion channels as participants in thermosensation and thermoregulation. *Am. J. Physiol. Regul. Integr. Comp. Physiol.* 292, R64–R76.

Caterina, M. J., and Julius, D. (2001). The vanilloid receptor: a molecular gateway to the pain pathway. *Annu. Rev. Neurosci.* 24, 487–517. doi: 10.1146/annurev.neuro.24.1.487

Caterina, M. J., Rosen, T. A., Tominaga, M., Brake, A. J., and Julius, D. (1999). A capsaicin-receptor homologue with a high threshold for noxious heat. *Nature* 398, 436–441. doi: 10.1038/18906

Caterina, M. J., Schumacher, M. A., Tominaga, M., Rosen, T. A., Levine, J. D., and Julius, D. (1997). The capsaicin receptor: a heat-activated ion channel in the pain pathway. *Nature* 389, 816–824. doi: 10.1038/39807

Clapham, D. E. (2003). TRP channels as cellular sensors. *Nature* 426, 517–524. doi: 10.1038/nature02196

Dalle Carbonare, M., Giudice, E. Del, Stecca, A., Colavito, D., Fabris, M., D'Arrigo, A., et al. (2008). A saturated N-acylethanolamine other than N-palmitoyl ethanolamine with anti-inflammatory properties: a neglected story. *J. Neuroendocrinol.* 20, 26–34. doi: 10.1111/j.1365-2826.2008.01689.x

Devane, W. A., Hanus, L., Breuer, A., Pertwee, R. G., Stevenson, L. A., Griffin, G., et al. (1992). Isolation and structure of a brain constituent that binds to the cannabinoid receptor. *Science* 258, 1946–1949. doi: 10.1126/science.1470919

Di Marzo, V., Fontana, A., Cadas, H., Schinelli, S., Cimino, G., Schwartz, J. C., et al. (1994). Formation and inactivation of endogenous cannabinoid anandamide in central neurons. *Nature* 372, 686–691. doi: 10.1038/372686a0

Di Marzo, V., and Maccarrone, M. (2008). FAAH and anandamide: is 2-AG really the odd one out? *Trends Pharmacol. Sci.* 29, 229–233. doi: 10.1016/j.tips.2008.03.001

Frenzel, H., Bohlender, J., Pinsker, K., Wohlleben, B., Tank, J., Lechner, S. G., et al. (2012). A genetic basis for mechanosensory traits in humans. *PLoS Biol.* 10:e1001318. doi: 10.1371/journal.pbio.1001318

Hansen, H. S., Moesgaard, B., Hansen, H. H., and Petersen, G. (2001). When and where are N-acylethanolamine phospholipids and anandamide formed? *World Rev. Nutr. Diet.* 88, 223–227. doi: 10.1159/000059758

Hardy, J. D. (1961). Physiology of temperature regulation. *Physiol. Rev.* 41, 521–606.

Hensel, H. (1973). Neural processes in thermoregulation. *Physiol. Rev.* 53, 948–1017. doi: 10.1152/physrev.1973.53.4.948

Hirst, R. A., Harrison, C., Hirota, K., and Lambert, D. G. (2006). Measurement of [Ca2+]i in whole cell suspensions using fura-2. *Methods Mol. Biol.* 312, 37–45. doi: 10.1007/978-1-62703-086-1_2

Holzer, P. (2008). The pharmacological challenge to tame the transient receptor potential vanilloid-1 (TRPV1) nocisensor. *Br. J. Pharmacol.* 155, 1145–1162. doi: 10.1038/bjp.2008.351

Jancso, G., Kiraly, E., and Jancso-Gabor, A. (1977). Pharmacologically induced selective degeneration of chemosensitive primary sensory neurones. *Nature* 270, 741–743. doi: 10.1038/270741a0

Julius, D. (2013). TRP channels and pain. *Annu. Rev. Cell Dev. Biol.* 29, 355–384.

Julius, D., and Basbaum, A. I. (2001). Molecular mechanisms of nociception. *Nature* 413, 203–210. doi: 10.1038/35093019

Leishman, E., Kunkler, P. E., Manchanda, M., Sangani, K., Stuart, J. M., Oxford, G. S., et al. (2017). Environmental toxin acrolein alters levels of endogenous lipids, including TRP agonists: a potential mechanism for headache driven by TRPA1 activation. *Neurobiol. Pain* 1, 28–36. doi: 10.1016/j.ynpai.2017.03.001

Leishman, E., Mackie, K., Luquet, S., and Bradshaw, H. B. (2016). Lipidomics profile of a NAPE-PLD KO mouse provides evidence of a broader role of this enzyme in lipid metabolism in the brain. *Biochim. Biophys. Acta* 1861, 491–500. doi: 10.1016/j.bbalip.2016.03.003

Leishman, E., Murphy, M., Mackie, K., and Bradshaw, H. B. (2018). Delta(9)-Tetrahydrocannabinol changes the brain lipidome and transcriptome differentially in the adolescent and the adult. *Biochim. Biophys. Acta Mol. Cell Biol. Lipids* 1863, 479–492. doi: 10.1016/j.bbalip.2018.02.001

Liu, J., Wang, L., Harvey-White, J., Huang, B. X., Kim, H. Y., Luquet, S., et al. (2008). Multiple pathways involved in the biosynthesis of anandamide. *Neuropharmacology* 54, 1–7. doi: 10.1016/j.neuropharm.2007.05.020

Lumpkin, E. A., and Caterina, M. J. (2007). Mechanisms of sensory transduction in the skin. *Nature* 445, 858–865. doi: 10.1038/nature05662

Maccarrone, M., Salvati, S., Bari, M., and Finazzi, A. (2000). Anandamide and 2-arachidonoylglycerol inhibit fatty acid amide hydrolase by activating the lipoxygenase pathway of the arachidonate cascade. *Biochem. Biophys. Res. Commun.* 278, 576–583. doi: 10.1006/bbrc.2000.3869

McKemy, D. D. (2005). How cold is it? TRPM8 and TRPA1 in the molecular logic of cold sensation. *Mol. Pain* 1:16.

Mock, E. D., Mustafa, M., Gunduz-Cinar, O., Cinar, R., Petrie, G. N., Kantae, V., et al. (2020). Discovery of a NAPE-PLD inhibitor that modulates emotional behavior in mice. *Nat. Chem. Biol.* 16, 667–675. doi: 10.1038/s41589-020-0528-7

Montell, C., Birnbaumer, L., Flockerzi, V., Bindels, R. J., Bruford, E. A., Caterina, M. J., et al. (2002). A unified nomenclature for the superfamily of TRP cation channels. *Mol. Cell.* 9, 229–231. doi: 10.1016/s1097-2765(02)00448-3

Montell, C., and Rubin, G. M. (1989). Molecular characterization of the *Drosophila* trp locus: a putative integral membrane protein required for phototransduction. *Neuron* 2, 1313–1323. doi: 10.1016/0896-6273(89)90069-x

Movahed, P., Jonsson, B. A., Birnir, B., Wingstrand, J. A., Jorgensen, T. D., Ermund, A., et al. (2005). Endogenous unsaturated C18 N-acylethanolamines are vanilloid receptor (TRPV1) agonists. *J. Biol. Chem.* 280, 38496–38504. doi: 10.1074/jbc.m507429200

Nakamura, K. (2011). Central circuitries for body temperature regulation and fever. *Am. J. Physiol. Regul. Integr. Comp. Physiol.* 301, R1207–R1228.

Nakamura, K., and Morrison, S. F. (2008). A thermosensory pathway that controls body temperature. *Nat. Neurosci.* 11, 62–71. doi: 10.1038/nn2027

Ogura, Y., Parsons, W. H., Kamat, S. S., and Cravatt, B. F. (2016). A calcium-dependent acyltransferase that produces N-acyl phosphatidylethanolamines. *Nat. Chem. Biol.* 12, 669–671. doi: 10.1038/nchembio.2127

Okamoto, Y., Tsuboi, K., and Ueda, N. (2009). Enzymatic formation of anandamide. *Vitam. Horm.* 81, 1–24. doi: 10.1016/s0083-6729(09)81001-7

Okamoto, Y., Wang, J., Morishita, J., and Ueda, N. (2007). Biosynthetic pathways of the endocannabinoid anandamide. *Chem. Biodivers.* 4, 1842–1857. doi: 10.1002/cbdv.200790155

Patapoutian, A., Peier, A. M., Story, G. M., and Viswanath, V. (2003). ThermoTRP channels and beyond: mechanisms of temperature sensation. *Nat. Rev. Neurosci.* 4, 529–539. doi: 10.1038/nrn1141

Raboune, S., Stuart, J. M., Leishman, E., Takacs, S. M., Rhodes, B., Basnet, A., et al. (2014). Novel endogenous N-acyl amides activate TRPV1-4 receptors, BV-2 microglia, and are regulated in brain in an acute model of inflammation. *Front. Cell. Neurosci.* 8:195. doi: 10.3389/fncel.2014.00195

Romanovsky, A. A. (2007). Thermoregulation: some concepts have changed. Functional architecture of the thermoregulatory system. *Am. J. Physiol. Regul. Integr. Comp. Physiol.* 292, R37–R46.

Schlader, Z. J., Simmons, S. E., Stannard, S. R., and Mundel, T. (2011). The independent roles of temperature and thermal perception in the control of human thermoregulatory behavior. *Physiol. Behav.* 103, 217–224. doi: 10.1016/j.physbeh.2011.02.002

Simon, G. M., and Cravatt, B. F. (2006). Endocannabinoid biosynthesis proceeding through glycerophospho-N-acyl ethanolamine and a role for α/β-hydrolase 4 in this pathway. *J. Biol. Chem.* 281, 26465–26472. doi: 10.1074/jbc.m604660200

Sisignano, M., Bennett, D. L., Geisslinger, G., and Scholich, K. (2014). TRP-channels as key integrators of lipid pathways in nociceptive neurons. *Prog. Lipid Res.* 53, 93–107. doi: 10.1016/j.plipres.2013.11.002

Smart, D., Gunthorpe, M. J., Jerman, J. C., Nasir, S., Gray, J., Muir, A. I., et al. (2000). The endogenous lipid anandamide is a full agonist at the human vanilloid receptor (hVR1). *Br. J. Pharmacol.* 129, 227–230. doi: 10.1038/sj.bjp.0703050

Smith, G. D., Gunthorpe, M. J., Kelsell, R. E., Hayes, P. D., Reilly, P., Facer, P., et al. (2002). TRPV3 is a temperature-sensitive vanilloid receptor-like protein. *Nature* 418, 186–190. doi: 10.1038/nature00894

Sprague, J., Harrison, C., Rowbotham, D. J., Smart, D., and Lambert, D. G. (2001). Temperature-dependent activation of recombinant rat vanilloid VR1 receptors expressed in HEK293 cells by capsaicin and anandamide. *Eur. J. Pharmacol.* 423, 121–125. doi: 10.1016/s0014-2999(01)01123-2

Starowicz, K., Cristino, L., and Marzo, V. Di (2008). TRPV1 receptors in the central nervous system: potential for previously unforeseen therapeutic applications. *Curr. Pharm. Des.* 14, 42–54. doi: 10.2174/138161208783330790

Stella, N., Schweitzer, P., and Piomelli, D. (1997). A second endogenous cannabinoid that modulates long-term potentiation. *Nature* 388, 773–778. doi: 10.1038/42015

Stevenson, C. L., Leonard, J. J., and Hall, S. C. (1999). Effect of peptide concentration and temperature on leuprolide stability in dimethyl sulfoxide. *Int. J. Pharm.* 191, 115–129. doi: 10.1016/s0378-5173(99)00289-6

Story, G. M., Peier, A. M., Reeve, A. J., Eid, S. R., Mosbacher, J., Hricik, T. R., et al. (2003). ANKTM1, a TRP-like channel expressed in nociceptive neurons, is activated by cold temperatures. *Cell* 112, 819–829. doi: 10.1016/s0092-8674(03)00158-2

Sugiura, T., Kishimoto, S., Oka, S., and Gokoh, M. (2006). Biochemistry, pharmacology and physiology of 2-arachidonoylglycerol, an endogenous cannabinoid receptor ligand. *Prog. Lipid Res.* 45, 405–446. doi: 10.1016/j.plipres.2006.03.003

Sugiura, T., Kondo, S., Sukagawa, A., Nakane, S., Shinoda, A., Itoh, K., et al. (1995). 2-Arachidonoylglycerol: a possible endogenous cannabinoid receptor ligand in brain. *Biochem. Biophys. Res. Commun.* 215, 89–97.

Tominaga, M. (2006). "20 The Role of TRP Channels in Thermosensation," in *TRP Ion Channel Function in Sensory Transduction and Cellular Signaling Cascades*, eds M. D. Wolfgang and B. Liedtke (Boca Raton, FL: CRC Press), 271. doi: 10.1201/9781420005844.ch20

Ueda, N., Tsuboi, K., and Uyama, T. (2013). Metabolism of endocannabinoids and related N-acylethanolamines: canonical and alternative pathways. *FEBS J.* 280, 1874–1894. doi: 10.1111/febs.12152

Woo, D. H., Jung, S. J., Zhu, M. H., Park, C. K., Kim, Y. H., Oh, S. B., et al. (2008). Direct activation of transient receptor potential vanilloid 1(TRPV1) by diacylglycerol (DAG). *Mol. Pain* 4:42.

Zygmunt, P. M., Ermund, A., Movahed, P., Andersson, D. A., Simonsen, C., Jonsson, B. A., et al. (2013). Monoacylglycerols activate TRPV1–a link between phospholipase C and TRPV1. *PLoS One* 8:e81618. doi: 10.1371/journal.pone.0081618

Zygmunt, P. M., Petersson, J., Andersson, D. A., Chuang, H., Sorgard, M., Marzo, V. Di, et al. (1999). Vanilloid receptors on sensory nerves mediate the vasodilator action of anandamide. *Nature* 400, 452–457. doi: 10.1038/22761

10

TRPV4-Mediated Regulation of the Blood Brain Barrier is Abolished During Inflammation

Sina C. Rosenkranz[1†], Artem Shaposhnykov[1†], Oliver Schnapauff[2], Lisa Epping[3], Vanessa Vieira[1], Karsten Heidermann[1], Benjamin Schattling[1], Volodymyr Tsvilovskyy[4], Wolfgang Liedtke[5], Sven G. Meuth[3], Marc Freichel[4], Mathias Gelderblom[2†] and Manuel A. Friese[1†]*

[1] Institut für Neuroimmunologie und Multiple Sklerose, Universitätsklinikum Hamburg-Eppendorf, Hamburg, Germany, [2] Klinik und Poliklinik für Neurologie, Universitätsklinikum Hamburg-Eppendorf, Hamburg, Germany, [3] Klinik für Neurologie mit Institut für Translationale Neurologie, Universität Münster, Münster, Germany, [4] Pharmakologisches Institut, Universität Heidelberg, Heidelberg, Germany, [5] Departments of Neurology, Anesthesiology and Neurobiology, Duke University Medical Center, Durham, NC, United States

***Correspondence:**
Manuel A. Friese
manuel.friese@zmnh.uni-hamburg.de

† These authors have contributed equally to this work

Blood-brain barrier (BBB) dysfunction is critically involved in determining the extent of several central nervous systems (CNS) pathologies and here in particular neuroinflammatory conditions. Inhibiting BBB breakdown could reduce the level of vasogenic edema and the number of immune cells invading the CNS, thereby counteracting neuronal injury. Transient receptor potential (TRP) channels have an important role as environmental sensors and constitute attractive therapeutic targets that are involved in calcium homeostasis during pathologies of the CNS. Transient receptor potential vanilloid 4 (TRPV4) is a calcium permeable, non-selective cation channel highly expressed in endothelial cells. As it is involved in the regulation of the blood brain barrier permeability and consequently cerebral edema formation, we anticipated a regulatory role of TRPV4 in CNS inflammation and subsequent neuronal damage. Here, we detected an increase in transendothelial resistance in mouse brain microvascular endothelial cells (MbMECs) after treatment with a selective TRPV4 inhibitor. However, this effect was abolished after the addition of IFNγ and TNFα indicating that inflammatory conditions override TRPV4-mediated permeability. Accordingly, we did not observe a protection of *Trpv4*-deficient mice when compared to wildtype controls in a preclinical model of multiple sclerosis, experimental autoimmune encephalomyelitis (EAE), and no differences in infarct sizes following transient middle cerebral artery occlusion (tMCAO), the experimental stroke model, which leads to an acute postischemic inflammatory response. Furthermore, Evans Blue injections did not show differences in alterations of the blood brain barrier (BBB) permeability between genotypes in both animal models. Together, TRPV4 does not regulate brain microvascular endothelial permeability under inflammation.

Keywords: TRPV4, transendothelial resistance, blood brain barrier, experimental autoimmune encephalomyelitis, stroke

INTRODUCTION

The blood-brain barrier (BBB) is responsible for maintaining the separation of the central nervous system (CNS) from the blood and thereby controls the entry of neurotoxic metabolites, ions, pathogens and blood cells (Zhao et al., 2015). The cells of the BBB communicate with cells of the CNS but also with circulating immune cells allowing a tight adaption to maintain the highly regulated CNS internal milieu (Banks, 2016). The major component of the BBB are pericytes, astrocytes and endothelial cells that control the passage of molecules by a crosstalk between tight and adherens junctions (Obermeier et al., 2013; Keaney and Campbell, 2015; Tietz and Engelhardt, 2015).

Diminished BBB integrity results in increased vascular permeability and is essential for the development of cerebral edema (Sweeney et al., 2018). Similarly, a breakdown of the BBB facilitates the entry of immune cells into the CNS and is crucial for neuroinflammation (Man et al., 2007; Bennett et al., 2010; Ransohoff and Engelhardt, 2012). Proinflammatory cytokines evoke an upregulation of cell adhesion molecules on endothelial cells which can bind to integrins on leukocytes and thereby facilitate transendothelial leukocyte migration (Minagar and Alexander, 2003; Keaney and Campbell, 2015). Attenuating BBB permeability reduces the number of invading immune cells and the extent of a subsequent edema, which then ameliorates neuronal loss. Interventional studies in animal models of multiple sclerosis (Göbel et al., 2019; Viñuela-Berni et al., 2020) and stroke (Casas et al., 2017; Pan et al., 2020) where the BBB permeability was decreased as a result of treatment showed improved neurological outcomes. However, until now no clinically approved drug exists, highlighting the need to identify new effective targets.

A promising candidate which is known to regulate the integrity of several endo- and epithelial barriers, is the transient receptor potential vanilloid 4 (TRPV4), which is a calcium-permeable non-selective cation channel and a member of the transient receptor potential (TRP) superfamily of cation channels (Liedtke et al., 2000; Strotmann et al., 2000; Wissenbach et al., 2000). TRP channels play an important role as environmental sensors and constitute an attractive gene family that could be involved in CNS pathologies (Schattling et al., 2012; Gelderblom et al., 2014; Kanju and Liedtke, 2016). *Trpv4* is expressed widely including endothelial cells and astrocytes. TRPV4 is polymodally activated (Nilius et al., 2004; Moore et al., 2018) by multiple extracellular mechanic stimuli such as cellular shear, stretch and cell compression (Michalick and Kuebler, 2020), by osmotic changes (Liedtke et al., 2000; Liedtke, 2005), by thermal cues (Tominaga and Caterina, 2004), by UVB radiation (Moore et al., 2013), by endogenous bioactive lipids such as arachidonic acids metabolites (Watanabe et al., 2003) and others. However, the molecular mechanisms of TRPV4 activation could differ from cell-type to cell-type and are overall not completely understood. In endothelial cells, TRPV4 functions as mechanoreceptor in response to shear stress (Matthews et al., 2010). Upon TRPV4 activation calcium fluxes into the cell and activates calcium-activated potassium channels. This can result in increased barrier permeability (Morty and Kuebler, 2014). It was shown that TRPV4 inhibition prevents and resolves pulmonary edema (Hamanaka et al., 2010; Thorneloe et al., 2012; Michalick et al., 2017), reduces the infarct size in myocardial ischemia (Dong et al., 2017), decreases the vascular endothelial permeability in murine colitis (Matsumoto et al., 2018) and diabetic retinal injury (Arredondo Zamarripa et al., 2017; Ríos et al., 2019). Furthermore, TRPV4 also regulates the integrity of the blood-cerebrospinal fluid barrier (Narita et al., 2015) and TRPV4 inhibition reduced BBB disruption and consecutive edema in a mouse model of intracerebral hemorrhage and thereby ameliorated neurological symptoms (Zhao et al., 2018). These observations imply an important role of TRPV4 in the BBB.

Therefore, modifications of TRPV4 could constitute an attractive therapeutic target in diseases with neuroinflammatory pathways that rely on temporarily impaired BBB integrity for influx of disease-enhancing immune cells. Here we analyzed whether TRPV4 inhibition has an impact on transendothelial resistance under homeostatic and inflammatory conditions and whether deletion of *Trpv4* affects the clinical outcome in mouse models of multiple sclerosis and stroke. We show that inflammation overrules the homeostatic TRPV4-mediated regulation of the BBB, and that *Trpv4* deficiency does not modify the outcome in these disease models.

MATERIALS AND METHODS

Mice

All mice [C57BL/6J wild-type, The Jackson Laboratory; *Trpv4*$^{-/-}$ mice on a C57BL/6J genetic background (Liedtke and Friedman, 2003)] were kept under specific pathogen-free conditions in the central animal facility of the Universitätsklinikum Hamburg-Eppendorf (UKE). Animals were housed in a facility with 55–65% humidity at 24 ± 2°C with a 12-h light/dark cycle and had free access to food and water.

EAE Induction

Mice were anaesthetized with isoflurane 1–2% v/v oxygen and immunized subcutaneously with 200 μg myelin oligodendrocyte glycoprotein 35–55 (MOG_{35-55}) peptide (peptides & elephants) in complete Freund's adjuvant (BD) containing 4 mg ml^{-1} *Mycobacterium tuberculosis* (BD). 200 ng pertussis toxin (Merck) was injected intravenously on the day of immunization and 48 h later. Animals were scored daily for clinical signs by the following system: 0, no clinical deficits; 1, tail weakness; 2, hind limb paresis; 3, partial hind limb paralysis; 3.5, full hind limb paralysis; 4, full hind limb paralysis and forelimb paresis; 5, premorbid or dead. Animals reaching a clinical score ≥ 4 were sacrificed according to the regulations of the Animal Welfare Act. The experimenters were blinded to the genotype until the end of the experiment, including data analysis. Sex- and age-matched adult animals (8–12 weeks of age) were used in all experiments. For *Trpv4*$^{-/-}$ mice and WT controls, three independent EAE experiments were conducted. The data were pooled for final analysis. For analysis of the disease course and weight we only included animals which received a score ≥ 1 until day 20 and survived until day 30. For analysis of onset we included all mice which received a score ≥ 1.

Determination of Blood Brain Barrier Permeability in EAE

BBB integrity was measured at the peak (day 13 after immunization) of EAE (n = 5 per genotype). Mice were intravenously injected with 200 μl of 2% Evans Blue (Millipore Sigma) dissolved in 0.1 M phosphate buffer saline (PBS). 2 h later mice were anesthetized intraperitoneally with 100 μl solution (10 mg ml^{-1} esketamine hydrochloride (Pfizer), 1.6 mg ml^{-1} xylazine hydrochloride (Bayer) dissolved in water) per 10 g of body weight and perfused with PBS. Brain, spinal cord and kidney were resected, dried for 24 h at 50°C and placed into formamide (Sigma) the volume of which was adjusted to the tissue weight. For the complete Evans Blue extraction, samples were incubated 24 h at 55°C. Amount of dye was determined by colorimetric analysis as absorbance coefficient at 610 nm. The data for brains and spinal cords were normalized to the kidneys values (Radu and Chernoff, 2013).

Mouse Tissue Preparation and Histopathology of EAE Mice

Mice were anesthetized intraperitoneally with 100 μl solution (10 mg ml^{-1} esketamine hydrochloride (Pfizer), 1.6 mg ml^{-1} xylazine hydrochloride (Bayer) dissolved in water) per 10 g of body weight. Afterward mice were perfused with 4% paraformaldehyde (PFA) and cervical spinal cord was resected, dehydrated and cast in paraffin. CD3 staining (rabbit IgG, Abcam ab16669) was visualized by the avidin-biotin technique with 3,3-diaminobenzidine according to standard procedures of the UKE Mouse Pathology Facility. The slides were analyzed using a NanoZoomer 2.0-RS digital slide scanner and NDP.view2 software (Hamamatsu). Quantification of infiltrating CD3 cells was done with ImageJ software (NIH), using the same settings across experimental groups.

In vivo Stroke Model

Mice were anesthetized using isoflurane 1–2% v/v oxygen and we injected buprenorphine 0.03 mg/kg body weight intraperitoneally (i.p.) every 12 h for 24 h as analgesia. We conducted transient middle cerebral artery occlusion (tMCAO) for 45 min using the intraluminal filament method (6-0 nylon, Docoll) as described before (Gelderblom et al., 2014). We monitored mice for heart rate, respiratory rate, oxygen saturation, rectal body temperature, and cerebral blood flow by using transcranial temporal laser Doppler technique. Only mice with a sufficient decrease in the ipsilateral laser Doppler flow (below 20 % when compared to the contralateral site) were included in the study, to ensure an appropriate occlusion of the middle cerebral artery. Animals were scored immediately after reawakening and daily for clinical signs by the following system (Bederson Score): 0, no deficit; 1, preferential turning; 2, circling; 3, longitudinal rolling; 4, no movement; 5, death. For *Trpv4*$^{-/-}$ mice and WT controls, two independent stroke experiments were conducted. The data were pooled for final analysis. Mortality did not differ between the groups. To reduce the variability of our outcome parameters caused by sex-differences only male mice (12–16 weeks of age) were used throughout the study.

Analysis of Infarct Size by TTC Staining

Only mice with a Bederson score greater or equal than one after reawakening and a sufficient occlusion of the middle cerebral artery during MCAO as measured by laser Doppler technique were included in stroke size analysis. Mice were sacrificed 3 days after reperfusion using isoflurane and decapitation. Brains were harvested and cut into 1 mm slices (Braintree Scientific, 1 mm) followed by vital staining using 2% (wt/vol) 2,3,5-triphenyl-2-hydroxy-tetrazolium chloride (TTC) in phosphate buffer. We determined infarct volumes blinded for genotype by using NIH ImageJ software.

Determination of Blood Brain Barrier Permeability in Stroke

BBB integrity following stroke was assessed in mice (n = 6 per experimental group) that were intraperitoneally injected with 200 μl of 2% Evans Blue (Millipore Sigma, Cat. No. E2129) dissolved in 0.1 M phosphate buffer saline (PBS) directly after tMCAO. 24 h later mice were processed as described above. We additionally analyzed Evans Blue staining after 72 h of tMCAO.

Primary Endothelial Culture and Transendothelial Electrical Resistance (TEER)

Mouse brain microvascular endothelial cells (MbMECs) were isolated as previously described (Weidenfeller et al., 2005; Ruck et al., 2014) and incubated in a humidified incubator with 5% CO_2 at 37°C. Fresh, puromycin free MbMEC medium was added 4 days after isolation. Two days later, when cells reached confluence, they were harvested by trypsinization and seeded for subsequent TEER experiments onto pre-coated transwell inserts (pore size 0.4 μm; Corning) at 2×10^4 cells per insert. TEER measurements were performed and analyzed using the cellZscope 24-cell module and cellZscope v2.2.2 software, respectively (nanoAnalytics GmbH) as described before (Kuzmanov et al., 2016). Automated TEER and cell layer capacitance (Ccl) measurements were performed every hour for 3 to 4 days until the MbMEC monolayer reached full confluence, as determined by stable Ccl below 1 $\mu F/cm^2$ and TEER at its maximum plateau for at least 6 h. At that time point, MbMECs were either kept naïve or inflammation was induced by addition of 50 U/ml IFNγ and 50 U/ml TNFα. Additionally, either vehicle or GSK2193874 (Sigma), a TRPV4-specific inhibitor, which has been shown to inhibit TRPV4-dependent calcium influx in endothelial cells and exerts potent *in vivo* activity (Thorneloe et al., 2012; Cheung et al., 2017), were applied and TEER measurements were resumed for another 24 h.

Expression Analysis

For analysis of *Trpv4* mRNA expression on MbMECs, total RNA was extracted from naïve MbMECs or MbMECs inflamed for 24 h with 50 U/ml IFNγ and 50 U/ml TNFα by using a Quick RNA Micro Prep Kit (Zymo Research); cDNA was synthesized from 300 ng of total RNA by using a Maxima First Strand cDNA Synthesis Kit (ThermoFisher Scientific), all performed according to the manufacturers' instructions. For quantitative

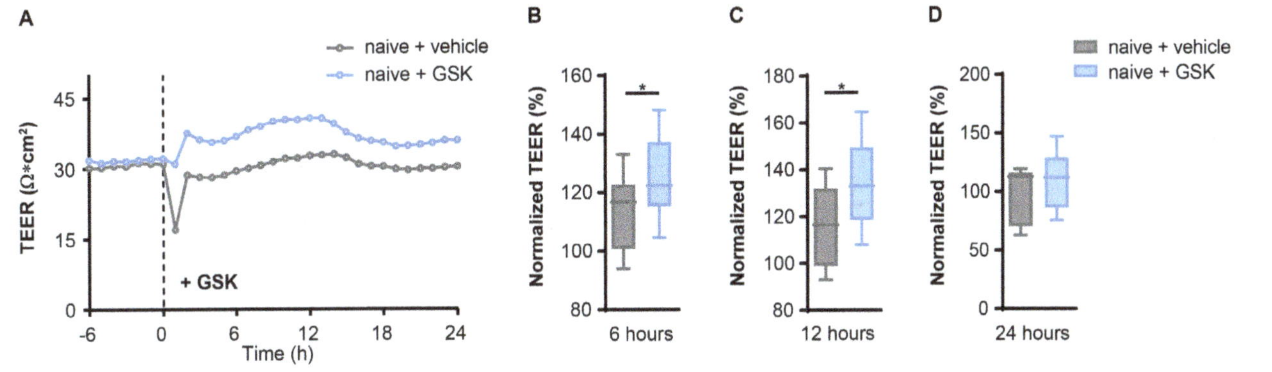

FIGURE 1 | TRPV4 inhibition increases transendothelial electrical resistance (TEER) in mouse brain microvascular endothelial cells (MbMECs) under homeostatic conditions. **(A)** TEER of MbMECs treated with 5 nM of GSK2193874 in comparison to vehicle-treated MbMECs. One representative experiment out of 12 is shown. **(B–D)** Quantification of TEER of MbMECs treated with 5 nM of GSK2193874 (n = 12) in comparison to vehicle treated MbMECs (n = 12) at 6, 12, and 24 h. TEER was normalized to the time-point of GSK treatment (0 h). Data are presented as box plots. Statistical analysis was performed by two-tailed Student's t-test. $^{*}P < 0.05$.

RT-PCR (RT-qPCR), a mouse *Trpv4* TaqMan Gene Expression Assay (Mm00499025_m1) with 18S rRNA as endogenous control was used. RT-qPCR was performed by using the StepOnePlus System (Applied Biosystems). Data were analyzed using the $\Delta\Delta$CT method followed by relative quantification ($2^{-\Delta\Delta CT}$).

Study Approval

All animal care and experimental procedures were performed according to institutional guidelines and conformed to requirements of the German Animal Welfare Act. All animal experiments were approved by the local ethics committee (Behörde für Soziales, Familie, Gesundheit und Verbraucherschutz in Hamburg; G22/13 and 59/17. We conducted all procedures in accordance with the ARRIVE guidelines (Kilkenny et al., 2010).

Statistics

Experimental data were analyzed using Prism 8 software (GraphPad) and are presented as mean values ± SEM. Statistical analyses were performed using the appropriate test indicated in the figure legends. D'Agostino and Pearson test was used to analyze normality. Unless stated otherwise, differences between two experimental groups were determined by unpaired, two-tailed Mann-Whitney or Students t-test. Significant results are indicated by asterisks: $^{*}P < 0.05$.

RESULTS

TRPV4 Inhibition Increases Transendothelial Resistance

First, we validated a regulative role of TRPV4 for BBB permeability. We measured the transendothelial electrical resistance (TEER) of mouse brain microvascular endothelial cells (MbMECs) in the absence and presence of the specific pharmacological TRPV4 inhibitor GSK2193874, which has been previously shown to have potent efficiency in ameliorating lung edema (Thorneloe et al., 2012). Six and 12 h after addition of GSK2193874 we detected a significant increase of the TEER, which was not anymore detectable after 24 h (**Figures 1A–D**). Thus, TRPV4 inhibition by GSK2193874 induces an increased endothelial cell barrier integrity.

Inflammation Overrides TRPV4-Mediated Permeability of the Blood Brain Barrier

Since TRPV4 inhibition leads to an increased resistance in MbMECs, we next investigated whether this could be confirmed under inflammatory conditions. We analyzed TRPV4 functionality after the exposure of tumor necrosis factor-α (TNFα) and interferon-γ (INFγ) that are key cytokines during neuroinflammation (Becher et al., 2017). Notably, in the presence of TNFα and INFγ the observed effect of TEER increase by inhibiting TRPV4 activity under homeostatic conditions was abolished (**Figures 2A–D**).

As changes in cytokine-mediated *Trpv4* expression could be an explanation for the abolished regulation, we next analyzed *Trpv4* expression in MbMECs under the different conditions. Indeed, we observed a significant reduction of *Trpv4* mRNA in MbMECs after exposure to TNFα and INFγ in comparison to homeostatic conditions (**Figure 2E**). We concluded that inflammatory cytokines induce a TRPV4 loss-of-function in MbMECs by attenuating the gene expression of *Trpv4.*

Blood Brain Barrier Permeability in EAE Is Not Altered by TRPV4

As TRPV4 inhibition leads to an increased resistance of endothelial cells, which is abrogated under inflammatory conditions, we next investigated whether TRPV4-mediated BBB regulation is indeed overruled in EAE. For this, we induced EAE in *Trpv4*-deficient ($Trpv4^{-/-}$) mice and compared their disease course to wild-type (WT) controls. We did not see any differences in hallmark clinical phenotypes such as disease onset (**Figure 3A**), disease disability score (**Figure 3B**) or body weight changes (**Supplementary Figure 1A**).

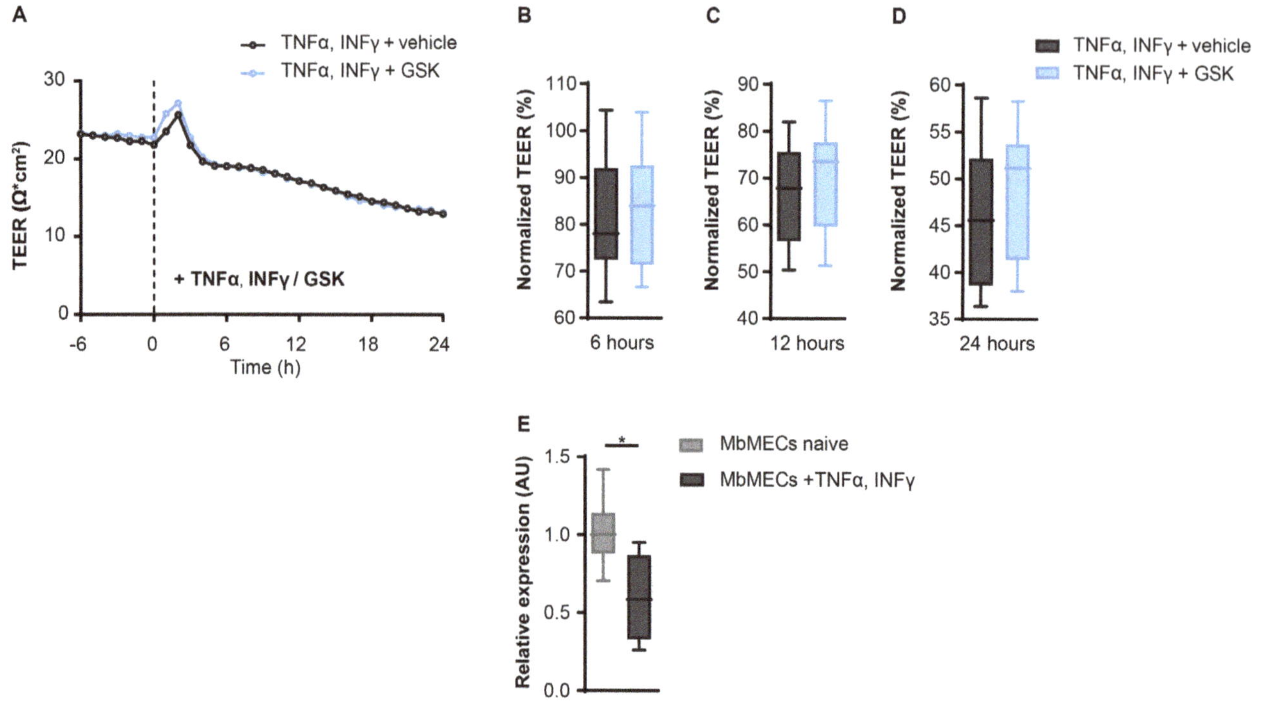

FIGURE 2 | Inflammatory conditions abolish the effect of TRPV4 inhibition on transendothelial electrical resistance (TEER) in mouse brain microvascular endothelial cells (MbMECs). **(A)** TEER of MbMECs treated with 5 nM of GSK2193874 in comparison to vehicle-treated MbMECs, both were exposed to 50 U/ml TNFα and INFγ. One representative experiment out of 14 is shown. **(B–D)** Quantification of TEER of MbMECs treated with 5 nM of GSK2193874 (n = 14) in comparison to vehicle-treated MbMECs (n = 14) at 6, 12, and 24 h, both were exposed to 50 U/ml TNFα and INFγ. TEER was normalized to the time-point of GSK treatment (0 h). **(E)** Relative *Trpv4* mRNA expression assessed by qPCR in MbMECs exposed to 50 U/ml TNFα and INFγ (n = 4) in comparison to homeostatic conditions (n = 8). Data are presented as box plots. Statistical analysis was performed by two-tailed Student's t-test **(A)** and **(B–D)** or two-tailed Mann Whitney test **(E)**. $^{*}P < 0.05$.

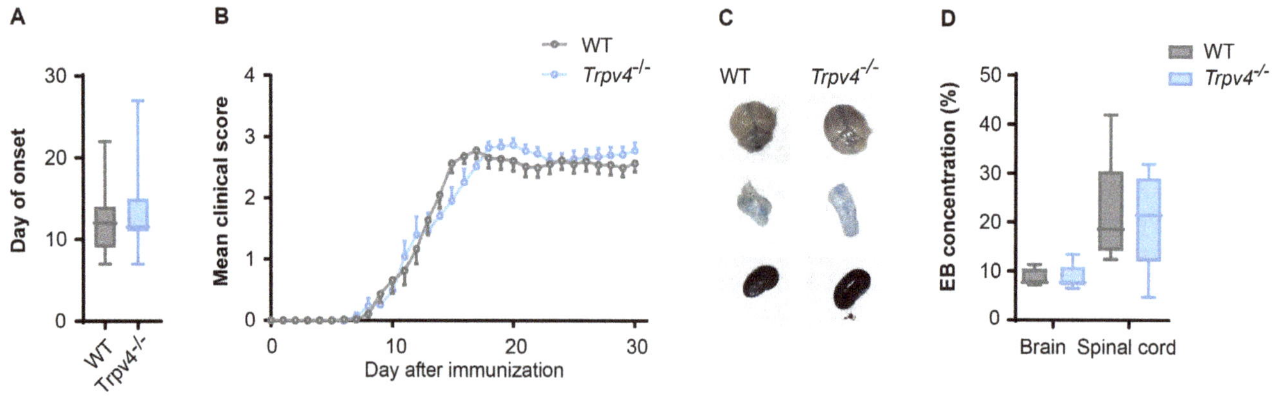

FIGURE 3 | No difference between *Trpv4*$^{-/-}$ mice and WT controls on the disease course and BBB permeability in EAE. **(A)** Day of onset of WT (n = 33) and *Trpv4*$^{-/-}$ mice (n = 32) during the course of EAE. **(B)** Clinical scores of WT (n = 27) and *Trpv4*$^{-/-}$ mice (n = 23) undergoing EAE. **(C)** Evans Blue (EB) quantification in brain and spinal cord of WT (n = 5) and *Trpv4*$^{-/-}$ (n = 5) mice at day 13 after EAE immunization. Evans Blue concentration was normalized to the concentration of the right kidney of the corresponding animal. **(D)** Representative images of brain, spinal cord and kidney of WT- and *Trpv4*$^{-/-}$-EAE mice 2 h after Evans Blue injection. Data in **(A,C)** are presented as box plots, in **(B)** as mean values ± s.e.m. Statistical analysis was performed by two-tailed Student's t-test in **(A)** by two-tailed Mann Whitney test in **(B,C)**.

Additionally, we assessed the BBB permeability by analyzing Evans Blue staining at the peak of disease. As this form of EAE mainly affects the spinal cord we observed higher levels of Evans Blue in the spinal cord than the brain at day 13 after immunization, without detecting a significant difference in the amount of Evans Blue in *Trpv4*$^{-/-}$ mice in

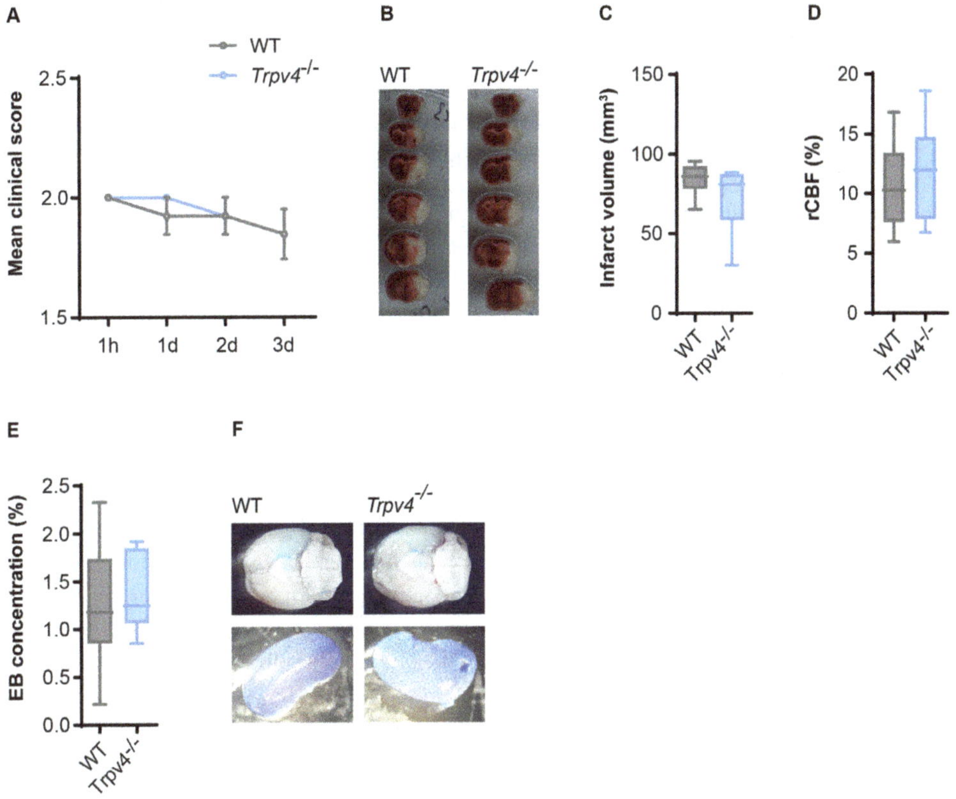

FIGURE 4 | No difference between *Trpv4*$^{-/-}$ mice and WT controls on disease course and BBB permeability in tMCAO. **(A)** Clinical scores of WT (*n* = 13) and *Trpv4*$^{-/-}$ mice (*n* = 13) after tMCAO; h = hours, d = days. **(B)** Representative TTC staining of WT and *Trpv4*$^{-/-}$brains 3 days after tMCAO. **(C)** Quantification of infarct volume of WT (*n* = 8) and *Trpv4*$^{-/-}$ (*n* = 9) 3 days after tMCAO. **(D)** Regional cerebral blood flow (rCBF) of WT (*n* = 13) and *Trpv4*$^{-/-}$ mice (*n* = 13) was measured during occlusion by laser Doppler and normalized to contralateral hemispheres. **(E)** Evans Blue (EB) quantification in brains of WT (*n* = 6) and *Trpv4*$^{-/-}$ (*n* = 6) mice 24 h after tMCAO. Evans Blue concentration was normalized to the concentration of the right kidney of the corresponding animal. **(F)** Representative images of brains and kidneys of WT and *Trpv4*$^{-/-}$ mice 24 h after tMCAO and Evans Blue injection. Data in **(A)** are presented as mean values ± s.e.m, in **(C–E)** as box plots. Statistical analysis was performed by two-tailed Mann Whitney test for (A) and two-tailed Student's *t*-test for **(C–E)**.

comparison to WT mice (**Figures 3C,D**). Moreover, we could not detect any differences in the numbers of infiltrating T cells (**Supplementary Figures 1B,C**).

Blood Brain Barrier Permeability in tMCAO Is Not Altered by TRPV4

Given the absence of a phenotype and a difference in BBB permeability in *Trpv4*$^{-/-}$ mice subjected to EAE, we decided to investigate the effects on experimental stroke, another model with significant impact of BBB disruption on clinical outcome but with more mildly and acute inflammation.

Therefore, we induced cerebral ischemia by tMCAO in *Trpv4*$^{-/-}$ and WT control mice and assessed their infarct sizes and neurological scores. After three days we were not able to detect any differences in the disease score between the two groups (**Figure 4A**) or in the body weight (**Supplementary Figure 2A**). There was also no difference in the volume of infarcted tissue (**Figures 4B,C**). Notably, both genotypes showed the same regional cerebral blood flow in the tMCAO model assessed by laser Doppler (**Figure 4D**) and were not different in physiological parameters (**Supplementary Figures 2B–E**).

Moreover, Evans Blue staining of the brain was assessed 24 h (**Figures 4E,F**) and 72 h (data not shown) after tMCAO, revealing lack of any differences between the two groups.

DISCUSSION

Here we show that TRPV4 inhibition increases endothelial resistance under homeostatic conditions, however, this effect was lost during inflammatory conditions. TRPV4 activation led to a disintegration of tight junctions (Narita et al., 2015) and TRPV4 inhibition decreases the vascular endothelial permeability and thereby counteracts pulmonary edema induced by heart failure (Thorneloe et al., 2012). Our data support these previously established concepts, as we detected a higher TEER in MbMECs after inhibiting TRPV4. Of note, inflammatory cytokines abolished this effect and led to a downregulation of *Trpv4* in MbMECs. Consistently, previous data showed that proinflammatory cytokines (e.g., TNF-α and IL-1β) had inhibitory effects on TRPV4-stimulated transepithelial ion flux and permeability changes in the choroid plexus, whereas anti-inflammatory cytokines (e.g., IL-10 and IL-4) showed no effect (Simpson et al., 2019). However, in this study the cytokines reduced only the functional but not the transcriptional regulation of TRPV4. Thus, it is likely a contribution of transcriptional regulation, alteration of TRPV4 channel function by trafficking and/or post-translational modification, and other complex regulation. Hence, further studies exploring the impact of inflammation on *Trpv4* expression and TRPV4 ion channel function in endothelial cells and their respective barrier are required.

In our study, we were not able to detect any differences in the *Trvp4*-deficient mice in EAE and tMCAO. Immune cell infiltration, microglia activation and increased level of proinflammatory cytokine release into the CNS accounts for the pathogenesis of both disease models (Lopes Pinheiro et al., 2016) but in comparison to EAE with abundant immune cell infiltration into the spinal cord, tMCAO is accompanied by less robust immune cell invasion of the cortex. We could not detect any difference of BBB permeability in *Trvp4*-deficient in comparison to WT control mice in both models.

We conclude that the inflammation overrides the possible protective effects of TRPV4. In line with our data, TRPV4 inhibition showed no protective effect in TNF-α induced sepsis, whereas it does in LPS induced sepsis (Dalsgaard et al., 2016). Therefore, it needs to be further specified which mechanisms and conditions lead to the abolishment of TRPV4 induced regulation of BBB permeability during inflammation.

Our lack of an *in vivo* phenotype might be rooted in several factors so that we are not claiming a decisively confirmed lack of a role of *Trpv4* in the examined animal models. *Trpv4* is also expressed on the other side of the endothelial side of the BBB, in astrocytes, in particular in astrocytic endfeet abutting the capillary (Shibasaki et al., 2007; Benfenati et al., 2011; Dunn et al., 2013; Filosa et al., 2013). Absence of astrocytic TRPV4 could alter the astrocytic contribution to the BBB. In that case the net result of absence of TRPV4 in endothelial cells and astrocytes could be lack of a phenotype in *Trpv4*-deficient mice because of opposite effects. In addition, there are other relevant cell migratory types such as macrophages that also express *Trpv4* and might contribute to the phenotype in various ways (Hamanaka et al., 2010; Scheraga et al., 2016; Michalick and Kuebler, 2020). Importantly, *Trpv4*-deficient mice have a genetically encoded absence of *Trpv4* in all cells at all developmental stages. For critical structures and function such as the BBB, this means compensatory gene expression to back up TRPV4 function might not be unlikely, plus cells that normally express *Trpv4* and have regulated expression of *Trpv4* under stress/injury can have a very different response, which is not directly rooted in absence of TRPV4, but rather in developmental compensation of gene expression. This uncertainty could be further addressed by studies in mice with lineage-specific gene targeting so that the deletion of *Trpv4* can be induced (Moore et al., 2013). Such dedicated studies can be combined with acute application of selective inhibitor molecules with systemic and compartmentalized application.

Beyond *Trpv4* expression in endothelial cells and astrocytes of the BBB, the channel appears to function in multiple roles and multiple lineages of the CNS (Lee and Choe, 2014; Kanju and Liedtke, 2016). For example, in a cuprizone-induced mouse model of demyelination a TRPV4 antagonist, RN-1734, alleviated demyelination and inhibited glial activation (Liu et al., 2018). Intracerebroventricular injection of HC-067047, a specific TRPV4 antagonist, reduced brain infarction 24 h after tMCAO (Jie et al., 2016). It appears therefore puzzling that TRPV4 activation using the selective activator 4α-PDD, induced angiogenesis and neurogenesis and thereby contributed to functional recovery from ischemic stroke in mice (Chen et al., 2017). These could be off-target effects of the different "specific" chemicals, but perhaps could highlight different signaling functions of TRPV4 in different lineages at different phases of ischemic injury of the CNS, characterized by different stages of BBB injury.

In summary, we demonstrate that TRPV4 inhibition leads to an increase of transendothelial resistance under homeostatic conditions, while this effect could not be observed under inflammatory conditions. In our *in vivo* models of EAE and acute cerebral ischemia, *Trpv4*-deficient mice were devoid of a phenotype, especially regarding BBB injury. These results build the foundation for a future quest for the role of TRPV4 in the BBB with focus on relevant constituting and TRPV4-expressing cells such as endothelial cells. However, our data do not support therapeutic TRPV4 channel inhibition in patients with multiple sclerosis or ischemic stroke.

ETHICS STATEMENT

The animal study was reviewed and approved by the Behörde Für Soziales, Familie, Gesundheit und Verbraucherschutz in Hamburg; G22/13 and 59/17.

AUTHOR CONTRIBUTIONS

SR and AS conducted and designed the experiments, analyzed the data, and wrote the manuscript. OS, VV, LE, and KH conducted the experiments and analyzed the data. BS, SM, and MF designed the experiments. WL interpreted the data and wrote the manuscript. MG and MAF designed the experiments, conceived, supervised, and funded the study, and wrote the manuscript. All authors contributed to the article and approved the submitted version.

ACKNOWLEDGMENTS

We thank Annika Ruhl for excellent technical assistance. We thank the professional staff of our animal facility for their dedicated work. We thank the mouse pathology core at the Universitätsklinikum Hamburg-Eppendorf for the histopathology of EAE mice.

REFERENCES

Arredondo Zamarripa, D., Noguez Imm, R., Bautista Cortés, A. M., Vázquez Ruíz, O., Bernardini, M., Fiorio Pla, A., et al. (2017). Dual contribution of TRPV4 antagonism in the regulatory effect of vasoinhibins on blood-retinal barrier permeability: diabetic milieu makes a difference. *Sci. Rep.* 7, 1–16. doi: 10.1038/s41598-017-13621-8

Banks, W. A. (2016). From blood–brain barrier to blood–brain interface: new opportunities for CNS drug delivery. *Nat. Rev. Drug Discov.* 15, 275–292. doi: 10.1038/nrd.2015.21

Becher, B., Spath, S., and Goverman, J. (2017). Cytokine networks in neuroinflammation. *Nat. Rev. Immunol.* 17, 49–59. doi: 10.1038/nri.2016.123

Benfenati, V., Caprini, M., Dovizio, M., Mylonakou, M. N., Ferroni, S., Ottersen, O. P., et al. (2011). An aquaporin-4/transient receptor potential vanilloid 4 (AQP4/TRPV4) complex is essential for cell-volume control in astrocytes. *Proc. Natl. Acad. Sci. U.S.A.* 108, 2563–2568. doi: 10.1073/pnas.1012867108

Bennett, J., Basivireddy, J., Kollar, A., Biron, K. E., Reickmann, P., Jefferies, W. A., et al. (2010). Blood-brain barrier disruption and enhanced vascular permeability in the multiple sclerosis model EAE. *J. Neuroimmunol.* 229, 180–191. doi: 10.1016/j.jneuroim.2010.08.011

Casas, A. I., Geuss, E., Kleikers, P. W. M., Mencl, S., Herrmann, A. M., Buendia, I., et al. (2017). NOX4-dependent neuronal autotoxicity and BBB breakdown explain the superior sensitivity of the brain to ischemic damage. *Proc. Natl. Acad. Sci. U.S.A.* 114, 12315–12320. doi: 10.1073/pnas.1705034114

Chen, C. K., Hsu, P. Y., Wang, T. M., Miao, Z. F., Lin, R. T., and Juo, S. H. H. (2017). TRPV4 activation contributes functional recovery from ischemic stroke via angiogenesis and neurogenesis. *Mol. Neurobiol.* 55, 4127–4135. doi: 10.1007/s12035-017-0625-0

Cheung, M., Bao, W., Behm, D. J., Brooks, C. A., Bury, M. J., Dowdell, S. E., et al. (2017). Discovery of GSK2193874: an orally active, potent, and selective blocker of transient receptor potential vanilloid 4. *ACS Med. Chem. Lett.* 8, 549–554. doi: 10.1021/acsmedchemlett.7b00094

Dalsgaard, T., Sonkusare, S. K., Teuscher, C., Poynter, M. E., and Nelson, M. T. (2016). Pharmacological inhibitors of TRPV4 channels reduce cytokine production, restore endothelial function and increase survival in septic mice. *Sci. Rep.* 6:33841. doi: 10.1038/srep33841

Dong, Q., Li, J., Wu, Q. F., Zhao, N., Qian, C., Ding, D., et al. (2017). Blockage of transient receptor potential vanilloid 4 alleviates myocardial ischemia/reperfusion injury in mice. *Sci. Rep.* 7:42678. doi: 10.1038/srep42678

Dunn, K. M., Hill-Eubanks, D. C., Liedtke, W. B., and Nelson, M. T. (2013). TRPV4 channels stimulate Ca^{2+}-induced Ca^{2+} release in astrocytic endfeet and amplify neurovascular coupling responses. *Proc. Natl. Acad. Sci. U.S.A.* 110, 6157–6162. doi: 10.1073/pnas.1216514110

Filosa, J. A., Yao, X., and Rath, G. (2013). TRPV4 and the regulation of vascular tone. *J. Cardiovasc. Pharmacol.* 61, 113–119. doi: 10.1097/FJC.0b013e318279ba42

Gelderblom, M., Melzer, N., Schattling, B., Göb, E., Hicking, G., Arunachalam, P., et al. (2014). Transient receptor potential melastatin subfamily member 2 cation channel regulates detrimental immune cell invasion in ischemic stroke. *Stroke* 45, 3395–3402. doi: 10.1161/STROKEAHA.114.005836

Göbel, K., Asaridou, C. M., Merker, M., Eichler, S., Herrmann, A. M., Geuß, E., et al. (2019). Plasma kallikrein modulates immune cell trafficking during neuroinflammation via PAR2 and bradykinin release. *Proc. Natl. Acad. Sci. U.S.A.* 116, 271–276. doi: 10.1073/pnas.1810020116

Hamanaka, K., Jian, M.-Y., Townsley, M. I., King, J. A., Liedtke, W., Weber, D. S., et al. (2010). TRPV4 channels augment macrophage activation and ventilator-induced lung injury. *Am. J. Physiol. Lung Cell. Mol. Physiol.* 299, L353–L362. doi: 10.1152/ajplung.00315.2009

Jie, P., Lu, Z., Hong, Z., Li, L., Zhou, L., Li, Y., et al. (2016). Activation of transient receptor potential vanilloid 4 is involved in neuronal injury in middle cerebral artery occlusion in mice. *Mol. Neurobiol.* 53, 8–17. doi: 10.1007/s12035-014-8992-2

Kanju, P., and Liedtke, W. (2016). Pleiotropic function of TRPV4 ion channels in the central nervous system. *Exp. Physiol.* 101, 1472–1476. doi: 10.1113/EP085790

Keaney, J., and Campbell, M. (2015). The dynamic blood-brain barrier. *FEBS J.* 282, 4067–4079. doi: 10.1111/febs.13412

Kilkenny, C., Browne, W. J., Cuthill, I. C., Emerson, M., and Altman, D. G. (2010). Improving bioscience research reporting: the ARRIVE guidelines for reporting animal research. *PLoS Biol.* 8:e1000412. doi: 10.1371/journal.pbio.1000412

Kuzmanov, I., Herrmann, A. M., Galla, H. J., Meuth, S. G., Wiendl, H., and Klotz, L. (2016). An in vitro model of the blood-brain barrier using impedance spectroscopy: a focus on T cell-endothelial cell interaction. *J. Vis. Exp.* 2016:54925. doi: 10.3791/54592

Lee, J. C., and Choe, S. Y. (2014). Age-related changes in the distribution of transient receptor potential vanilloid 4 channel (TRPV4) in the central nervous system of rats. *J. Mol. Histol.* 45, 497–505. doi: 10.1007/s10735-014-9578-z

Liedtke, W. (2005). TRPV4 plays an evolutionary conserved role in the transduction of osmotic and mechanical stimuli in live animals. *J. Physiol.* 567, 53–58. doi: 10.1113/jphysiol.2005.088963

Liedtke, W., Choe, Y., Martí-Renom, M. A., Bell, A. M., Denis, C. S., Šali, A., et al. (2000). Vanilloid receptor-related osmotically activated channel (VR-OAC), a candidate vertebrate osmoreceptor. *Cell* 103, 525–535. doi: 10.1016/S0092-8674(00)00143-4

Liedtke, W., and Friedman, J. M. (2003). Abnormal osmotic regulation in trpv4–/- mice. *Proc. Natl. Acad. Sci. U S.A.* 100, 13698–13703. doi: 10.1073/pnas.1735416100

Liu, M., Liu, X., Wang, L., Wang, Y., Dong, F., Wu, J., et al. (2018). TRPV4 inhibition improved myelination and reduced glia reactivity and inflammation in a cuprizone-induced mouse model of demyelination. *Front. Cell. Neurosci.* 12:392. doi: 10.3389/fncel.2018.00392

Lopes Pinheiro, M. A., Kooij, G., Mizee, M. R., Kamermans, A., Enzmann, G., Lyck, R., et al. (2016). Immune cell trafficking across the barriers of the central nervous system in multiple sclerosis and stroke. *Biochim. Biophys. Acta Mol. Basis Dis.* 1862, 461–471. doi: 10.1016/J.BBADIS.2015.10.018

Man, S., Ubogu, E. E., and Ransohoff, R. M. (2007). Inflammatory cell migration into the central nervous system: a few new twists on an old tale. *Brain Pathol.* 17, 243–250. doi: 10.1111/j.1750-3639.2007.00067.x

Matsumoto, K., Yamaba, R., Inoue, K., Utsumi, D., Tsukahara, T., Amagase, K., et al. (2018). Transient receptor potential vanilloid 4 channel regulates vascular endothelial permeability during colonic inflammation in dextran sulphate sodium-induced murine colitis. *Br. J. Pharmacol.* 175, 84–99. doi: 10.1111/bph.14072

Matthews, B. D., Thodeti, C. K., Tytell, J. D., Mammoto, A., Overby, D. R., and Ingber, D. E. (2010). Ultra-rapid activation of TRPV4 ion channels by mechanicalforces applied to cell surface β1 integrins. *Integr Biol* 2, 435–442. doi: 10.1039/c0ib00034e

Michalick, L., Erfinanda, L., Weichelt, U., Van der Giet, M., Liedtke, W., and Kuebler, W. M. (2017). Transient receptor potential vanilloid 4 and serum glucocorticoid-regulated kinase 1 are critical mediators of lung injury in overventilated mice. *Anesthesiology* 126, 300–311. doi: 10.1097/ALN.0000000000001443

Michalick, L., and Kuebler, W. M. (2020). TRPV4—A Missing Link Between Mechanosensation and Immunity. *Front. Immunol.* 11:9. doi: 10.3389/fimmu.2020.00413

Minagar, A., and Alexander, J. S. (2003). Blood-brain barrier disruption in multiple sclerosis. *Mult. Scler. J.* 9, 540–549. doi: 10.1191/1352458503ms965oa

Moore, C., Cevikbas, F., Pasolli, H. A., Chen, Y., Kong, W., Kempkes, C., et al. (2013). UVB radiation generates sunburn pain and affects skin by activating epidermal TRPV4 ion channels and triggering endothelin-1 signaling. *Proc. Natl. Acad. Sci. U.S.A.* 110, E3225–E3234. doi: 10.1073/pnas.1312933110

Moore, C., Gupta, R., Jordt, S. E., Chen, Y., and Liedtke, W. B. (2018). Regulation of Pain and Itch by TRP Channels. *Neurosci. Bull.* 34, 120–142. doi: 10.1007/s12264-017-0200-8

Morty, R. E., and Kuebler, W. M. (2014). TRPV4: an exciting new target to promote alveolocapillary barrier function. *Am. J. Physiol. Lung Cell Mol. Physiol.* 307, 817–821. doi: 10.1152/ajplung.00254.2014

Narita, K., Sasamoto, S., Koizumi, S., Okazaki, S., Nakamura, H., Inoue, T., et al. (2015). TRPV4 regulates the integrity of the blood-cerebrospinal fluid barrier and modulates transepithelial protein transport. *FASEB J.* 29, 2247–2259. doi: 10.1096/fj.14-261396

Nilius, B., Vriens, J., Prenen, J., Droogmans, G., and Voets, T. (2004). TRPV4 calcium entry channel: a paradigm for gating diversity. *Am. J. Physiol. Cell Physiol.* 286, 195–205. doi: 10.1152/ajpcell.00365.2003

Obermeier, B., Daneman, R., and Ransohoff, R. M. (2013). Development, maintenance and disruption of the blood-brain barrier. *Nat. Med.* 19, 1584–1596. doi: 10.1038/nm.3407

Pan, J., Qu, M., Li, Y., Wang, L., Zhang, L., Wang, Y., et al. (2020). MicroRNA-126-3p/-5p overexpression attenuates blood-brain barrier disruption in a mouse model of middle cerebral artery occlusion. *Stroke* 51, 619–627. doi: 10.1161/STROKEAHA.119.027531

Radu, M., and Chernoff, J. (2013). An in vivo assay to test blood vessel permeability. *J. Vis. Exp.* 73:e50062. doi: 10.3791/50062

Ransohoff, R. M., and Engelhardt, B. (2012). The anatomical and cellular basis of immune surveillance in the central nervous system. *Nat. Rev. Immunol.* 12, 623–635. doi: 10.1038/nri3265

Ríos, M. O., Imm, R. N., Godínez, N. M. H., Cortes, A. M. B., Escalante, D. D. L., Liedtke, W., et al. (2019). TRPV4 inhibition prevents increased water diffusion and blood-retina barrier breakdown in the retina of streptozotocin-induced diabetic mice. *PLoS One* 14:e0212158. doi: 10.1371/journal.pone.0212158

Ruck, T., Bittner, S., Epping, L., Herrmann, A. M., and Meuth, S. G. (2014). Isolation of primary murine brain microvascular endothelial cells. *J. Vis. Exp* 93:e52204. doi: 10.3791/52204

Schattling, B., Steinbach, K., Thies, E., Kruse, M., Menigoz, A., Ufer, F., et al. (2012). TRPM4 cation channel mediates axonal and neuronal degeneration in experimental autoimmune encephalomyelitis and multiple sclerosis. *Nat. Med.* 18, 1805–1811. doi: 10.1038/nm.3015

Scheraga, R. G., Abraham, S., Niese, K. A., Southern, B. D., Grove, L. M., Hite, R. D., et al. (2016). TRPV4 mechanosensitive ion channel regulates lipopolysaccharide-stimulated macrophage phagocytosis. *J. Immunol.* 196, 428–436. doi: 10.4049/jimmunol.1501688

Shibasaki, K., Suzuki, M., Mizuno, A., and Tominaga, M. (2007). Effects of body temperature on neural activity in the hippocampus: regulation of resting membrane potentials by transient receptor potential vanilloid 4. *J. Neurosci.* 27, 1566–1575. doi: 10.1523/JNEUROSCI.4284-06.2007

Simpson, S., Preston, D., Schwerk, C., Schroten, H., and Blazer-Yost, B. (2019). Cytokine and inflammatory mediator effects on TRPV4 function in choroid plexus epithelial cells. *Am. J. Physiol. Cell Physiol.* 317, C881–C893. doi: 10.1152/ajpcell.00205.2019

Strotmann, R., Harteneck, C., Nunnenmacher, K., Schultz, G., and Plant, T. D. (2000). OTRPC4, a nonselective cation channel that confers sensivity to extracellular osmolarity. *Nat. Cell Biol.* 2, 695–702. doi: 10.1038/35036318

Sweeney, M. D., Sagare, A. P., and Zlokovic, B. V. (2018). Blood-brain barrier breakdown in Alzheimer's disease and other neurodegenerative disorders. *Nat. Rev. Neurol.* 14, 133–150. doi: 10.1038/nrneurol.2017.188

Thorneloe, K. S., Cheung, M., Bao, W., Alsaid, H., Lenhard, S., Jian, M., et al. (2012). An orally active TRPV4 channel blocker prevents and resolves pulmonary edema induced by heart failure. *Sci. Transl. Med.* 4:159ra148. doi: 10.1126/scitranslmed.3004276

Tietz, S., and Engelhardt, B. (2015). Brain barriers: crosstalk between complex tight junctions and adherens junctions. *J. Cell Biol.* 209, 493–506. doi: 10.1083/jcb.201412147

Tominaga, M., and Caterina, M. J. (2004). Thermosensation and pain. *J. Neurobiol.* 61, 3–12. doi: 10.1002/neu.20079

Viñuela-Berni, V., Gómez-González, B., and Quintanar-Stephano, A. (2020). Blockade of arginine vasopressin receptors prevents blood-brain barrier breakdown in experimental autoimmune encephalomyelitis. *Sci. Rep.* 10:467. doi: 10.1038/s41598-019-57134-y

Watanabe, H., Vriens, J., Prenen, J., Droogmans, G., Voets, T., and Nilius, B. (2003). Anandamide and arachidonic acid use epoxyeicosatrienoic acids to activate TRPV4 channels. *Nature* 424, 434–438. doi: 10.1038/nature01807

Weidenfeller, C., Schrot, S., Zozulya, A., and Galla, H.-J. (2005). Murine brain capillary endothelial cells exhibit improved barrier properties under the influence of hydrocortisone. *Brain Res.* 1053, 162–174. doi: 10.1016/J.BRAINRES.2005.06.049

Wissenbach, U., Bödding, M., Freichel, M., and Flockerzi, V. (2000). Trp12, a novel Trp related protein from kidney. *FEBS Lett.* 485, 127–134. doi: 10.1016/S0014-5793(00)02212-2

Zhao, H., Zhang, K., Tang, R., Meng, H., Zou, Y., Wu, P., et al. (2018). TRPV4 blockade preserves the blood-brain barrier by inhibiting stress fiber formation in a rat model of intracerebral hemorrhage. *Front. Mol. Neurosci.* 11:97. doi: 10.3389/fnmol.2018.00097

Zhao, Z., Nelson, A. R., Betsholtz, C., and Zlokovic, B. V. (2015). Establishment and dysfunction of the blood-brain barrier zhen. *Cell* 163, 1064–1078. doi: 10.1016/j.cell.2015.10.067

11

Molecular and Functional Study of Transient Receptor Potential Vanilloid 1-4 at the Rat and Human Blood–Brain Barrier Reveals Interspecies Differences

Huilong Luo[1,2], Bruno Saubamea[1], Stéphanie Chasseigneaux[1], Véronique Cochois[1], Maria Smirnova[1], Fabienne Glacial[3], Nicolas Perrière[3], Catarina Chaves[1], Salvatore Cisternino[1,4] and Xavier Declèves[1,5]*

[1] Faculté de Pharmacie, Inserm, UMRS-1144, Optimisation Thérapeutique en Neuropsychopharmacologie, Université de Paris, Paris, France, [2] Department of Chemical and Biological Engineering, University of Wisconsin-Madison, Madison, WI, United States, [3] BrainPlotting, Paris, France, [4] Service Pharmacie, Assistance Publique Hôpitaux de Paris (AP-HP), Hôpital Universitaire Necker – Enfants Malades, Paris, France, [5] Biologie du médicament et toxicologie, Assistance Publique Hôpitaux de Paris (AP-HP), Hôpital Universitaire Cochin, Paris, France

***Correspondence:**
Xavier Declèves
xavier.decleves@parisdescartes.fr*

Transient receptor potential vanilloid 1-4 (TRPV1-4) expression and functionality were investigated in brain microvessel endothelial cells (BMEC) forming the blood–brain barrier (BBB) from rat and human origins. In rat, Trpv1-4 were detected by qRT-PCR in the brain cortex, brain microvessels, and in primary cultures of brain microvessel endothelial cells [rat brain microvessel endothelial cells (rPBMEC)]. A similar *Trpv1-4* expression profile in isolated brain microvessels and rPBMEC was found with the following order: *Trpv4* > *Trpv2* > *Trpv3* > *Trpv1*. In human, TRPV1-4 were detected in the BBB cell line human cerebral microvessel endothelial cells D3 cells (hCMEC/D3) and in primary cultures of BMEC isolated from human adult and children brain resections [human brain microvascular endothelial cells (hPBMEC)], showing a similar *TRPV1-4* expression profile in both hCMEC/D3 cells and hPBMECs as follow: *TRPV2* > > *TRPV4* > *TRPV1* > *TRPV3*. Western blotting and immunofluorescence experiments confirmed that TRPV2 and TRPV4 are the most expressed TRPV isoforms in hCMEC/D3 cells with a clear staining at the plasma membrane. A fluorescent dye Fluo-4 AM ester was applied to record intracellular Ca^{2+} levels. TRPV4 functional activity was demonstrated in mediating Ca^{2+} influx under stimulation with the specific agonist GSK1016790A (ranging from 3 to 1000 nM, EC_{50} of 16.2 ± 4.5 nM), which was inhibited by the specific TRPV4 antagonist, RN1734 (30 μM). In contrast, TRPV1 was slightly activated in hCMEC/D3 cells as shown by the weak Ca^{2+} influx induced by capsaicin at a high concentration (3 μM), a highly potent and specific TRPV1 agonist. Heat-induced Ca^{2+} influx was not altered by co-treatment with a selective potent TRPV1 antagonist capsazepine (20 μM), in agreement with the low expression of *TRPV1* as assessed by qRT-PCR. Our present study reveals an interspecies difference between Rat and

Human. Functional contributions of TRPV1-4 subtype expression were not identical in rat and human tissues reflective of BBB integrity. TRPV2 was predominant in the human whereas TRPV4 had a larger role in the rat. This interspecies difference from a gene expression point of view should be taken into consideration when modulators of TRPV2 or TRPV4 are investigated in rat models of brain disorders.

Keywords: TRPV1, TRPV2, TRPV4, interspecies differences, blood–brain barrier, brain endothelial cell

INTRODUCTION

During the last decade, the transient receptor potential (TRP) channels were identified as promising pharmacological targets and some drug candidates targeting TRP have even already entered clinical trials or been approved as drugs for treating neuropathic pain, epilepsia or heart failure (Moran, 2018). Once activated possibly by heat, mechanical/shear stress, various endogenous and exogenous molecules, some TRP channels expressed at the plasma membrane increase the influx of inorganic monovalent or divalent cations (Na^+, K^+, Ca^{2+}, Mg^{2+}), triggering several downstream cell functions depending on the cell type (Rodrigues et al., 2016). Indeed, the main knowledge of TRP functions and agonists come from their expression in sensory electrically excitable cells such as neurons and their role in the nociception and pain (Mickle et al., 2015). Recently, more studies have been done and evidenced the TRP expression and their ability in modulating the functionalities of non-excitable cells such as endothelial cells using various chemical agonists and antagonists, including a requirement in vasorelaxation and vascular permeability (Kassmann et al., 2013; Grace et al., 2014; Ambrus et al., 2017). TRP channels of the vanilloid subfamily (TRPV) are divided into 6 isoforms (TRPV1-6). TRPV5 and TRPV6 are mainly expressed in intestinal and renal epithelia (Peng et al., 2018) while transient receptor potential vanilloid 1-4 (TRPV1-4) are mostly expressed in diverse cell types of the CNS, exocrine organs, skin, eye, lung, heart, and blood vessels (Steinritz et al., 2018).

Transient receptor potential vanilloid 1-4 have been evidenced in peripheral endothelial cells where they modulate the vascular tone through the release of factors that induce relaxation of smooth muscle cells (Marrelli et al., 2007), play a role in modulating endothelial permeability (Villalta and Townsley, 2013), participate in angiogenesis of peripheral vascular (Smani et al., 2018), and sense hemodynamic and chemical changes (Kohler et al., 2006). Ca^{2+} modulation has been known to be an important factor in maintaining the function of brain microvessel endothelial cells (BMEC) forming blood–brain barrier (BBB) (Brown and Davis, 2002; De Bock et al., 2013). By modulating Ca^{2+} trafficking into BMEC, a growing evidence has been achieved that TRP channels may have a critical role on the BBB properties including its permeability, angiogenesis and inflammatory responses (Berrout et al., 2012; Huang et al., 2020). However, the expression or functionality of TRPV in BBB was much less studied than in non-cerebral endothelial cells. The expression or functionality of TRPV in BMEC forming the BBB was much less studied than in non-cerebral endothelial cells although there is growing evidence that TRP channels may have a critical role at the BBB by modulating Ca^{2+} trafficking into BMEC. Dysfunctions of the BBB are increasingly recognized as a cause or a consequence in the pathophysiology of diverse brain pathologies such as stroke, neurodegenerative and psychiatric diseases (Sweeney et al., 2019; Yang et al., 2019; Kealy et al., 2020; Yu et al., 2020). A dysfunctional BBB can thus be targeted with new drug candidates, which would be a promising way for treating brain pathologies. However, pre-clinical proof of concept studies of such drug candidates are usually developed with rodent models, thus raising the question of interspecies differences regarding the BBB equipment between rodents and human. Moreover, TRPV isoforms can be specifically activated by various physical and/or chemical stimuli such as heat, osmolality, and mechanical stress (Montell, 2001). Thus, the comparative expression levels of TRPV1-4 in the BBB of rodent pharmacological models and human are meaningful in clarifying the possible involvement of each isoform in physiological and pathological BBB. A whole transcriptomic analysis revealed a relative low Trpv2 expression in murine primary BMEC (Zhang et al., 2014) and rat Trpv2 was not immunolocalized in the brain vasculature (Nedungadi et al., 2012), whereas TRPV2 was shown highly expressed in the human cerebral microvessel endothelial cells D3 cells (hCMEC/D3) human cerebral microvessel endothelial cell line (Luo et al., 2019), suggesting interspecies differences in the expression of TRPV between rat and human BMEC.

The present work aims at determining TRPV1-4 expression in primary cultured rat BMEC, rat cortex and isolated cortex microvessels, as well as in primary cultured human BMEC isolated from patient biopsies and the hCMEC/D3 human cerebral microvessel endothelial cell line. Functional activity of human TRPV1-4 channels was subsequently studied in hCMEC/D3 cells.

MATERIALS AND METHODS

Reagents and Chemicals

Cannabidiol (CBD) (1 mg/mL in methanol), tranilast (TNL), capsaicin (CAP), capsazepine (CPZ), and GSK1016790A (GSK) were all analytical grade and purchased from Sigma-Aldrich (Saint-Quentin-Fallavier, France). $CaCl_2$, $MgSO_4$, NaCl, NaH_2PO_4, $NaHCO_3$, KH_2PO_4, and KCl were purchased from Merck (Fontenay-sous-Bois, France).

RNA extraction kits were bought from Qiagen (Courtaboeuf, France). Primers, RT-PCR reagents and Lipofectamine® RNAi MAX transfection reagent were obtained from Invitrogen Life

Technologies (Cergy-Pontoise, France). The Power SYBR Green PCR Master Mix was purchased from Applied Biosystems (Applied Biosystems^{TM}, France). All other reagents and chemicals were purchased from Sigma.

Dulbecco's modified Eagle's medium (DMEM), DMEM/F12 + Glutamax, Hank's buffered salt solution (HBSS), HEPES and Penicillin/Streptomycine were from Life Technologies (Cergy-Pontoise, France). fetal bovine serum (FBS) was from GE Healthcare Life Science. Liberase DL, bovine serum albumin (BSA) (cat. # A7906), Dextran (cat. # 31390), DNase I (cat. # DN25), Puromycine and b-FGF were from Sigma-Aldrich. plasma derived bovine serum (PDBS) was from First Link (Wolverhampton, United Kingdom).

Isolation of Rat Brain Microvessels

The isolation of rat brain cortex microvessels was done according to a protocol reported previously (Chaves et al., 2020). CO_2 anesthetized animals were decapitated, rat brains were removed and immediately soaked in ice-cold HBSS containing 10 mmol/L HEPES. Brain cortices were isolated, minced and homogenized, and subsequent brain homogenates were centrifuged (2000 × *g*, 10 min), the pellets were re-suspended in 17.5% 64–76 kDa dextran (Sigma Aldrich) and centrifuged one more time (4400 × *g*, 15 min). The resulting pellets were suspended in HBSS containing 1% BSA and were firstly filtered through a 100 μm nylon mesh, and then through a 20 μm nylon mesh. The retained cerebral cortex microvessels were immediately collected and stored at −80°C before analysis (diameter size around 4–6 μ m).

Cell Culture Conditions

Human Cerebral Microvessel Endothelial Cells D3 Cells (hCMEC/D3)

The hCMEC/D3 cell line kindly given by Cochin Institute (Paris, France). were used from passages 27 to 33 and cultured with the EndoGRO complete medium (Merck), supplemented with 5% FBS,1% streptomycin-penicillin (Gibco, Carlsbad, CA, United States), and 1 ng/mL b-FGF (Sigma) under 5% CO_2 and 37°C as previously described (Luo et al., 2019). Culture flasks and plates were pre-coated with 150 μg/mL rat tail collagen type I. Assessment of intracellular calcium kinetics was carried out on confluent cultures in 24-well plates seeded at 5×10^4 cells/cm^2.

HEK-293 Cells

Human embryonic kidney HEK293 cells were cultured with DMEM (Gibco) containing 10% FBS (Thermo) and 1% streptomycin-penicillin (Gibco) under 5% CO_2 and 37°C.

Primary Cultures of Rat Brain Microvessel Endothelial Cells (rPBMEC)

Adult male Sprague-Dawley rats weighing 300–350 g were purchased from Charles River laboratory (L'arbresle, France). They were housed in groups of four per cage under standard 12:12-h light/dark conditions (light from 08:00 to 20:00 h) in a temperature- and humidity-controlled room. They had access to food and water *ad libitum*. Rats were acclimated for 7 days before experimentation. The care and treatment of animals conformed to the standards and guidelines promulgated by the European Communities Council Directive (86/609/EEC). The protocol was approved by the ethics review committee of Paris Descartes University (approval n°12-185/12-2012). Rats were deeply anesthetized by intraperitoneal administration of diazepam (5 mg/mL) and ketamine (100 mg/mL). They were perfused transcardially with Buffer 1 (HBSS, 10 mmol/L HEPES) at room temperature (RT) for 3 min. All subsequent steps were done on ice except when indicated. The cortex was dissected, cleared from adhering white matter and meninges and gently crushed in a Petri dish using a glass slide. Tissue pieces from two cortices were pooled, rinsed in Buffer 1, then centrifuged (2 min, 600 g) and resuspended in 10 mL of DMEM containing 10 mM HEPES, 0.4 WU/mL Liberase DL and 100 U/mL DNase I. Digestion was performed for 40 min at 37°C with gentle mechanical trituration with a 10 mL pipette (at 10 min), then with a P1000 pipet tip (at 20 min) and finally with a roded glass Pasteur pipette (at 30, 35, and 40 min), to obtain an homogenate with a creamy texture and almost no visible remaining piece. Digestion was stopped by adding 30 mL of DMEM + 10% FBS and the homogenate was centrifuged (5 min, 1,000 × *g*). The supernatant was discarded and the pellet was resuspended in 25 mL of Buffer 1 + 18% BSA and centrifuged (15 min, 2,000 × *g*). The compact myelin disk was eliminated and the pellet resuspended in 50 mL of Buffer 1 + 1% BSA. This suspension was filtered on a 10 μm nylon mesh (cat. # NY1004700, Millipore). Cells from the filtrate were pelleted, resuspended in DMEM + 10% FBS and counted. Cells were then seeded in 12-wells plate (1.5×10^6/well) in complete medium (DMEM/F12 + Glutamax, 20% PDBS, 10 U/mL penicillin/streptomycin, 80 μg/mL heparin, 5 ng/mL b-FGF) containing 4 μg/mL puromycin. After 3 days, medium was changed for complete medium without puromycin and cells were grown until confluency.

Primary Cultures of Human Brain Microvascular Endothelial Cells (hPBMEC)

All human samples were provided by BrainPlotting (iPEPS, Institut du Cerveau et de la Moelle épinière, Hôpital Universitaire de la Pitié-Salpêtrière, Paris, France) in partnership with Sainte-Anne Hospital, Paris (neurosurgeon Dr. Johan Pallud) and harvested during tumor scheduled resection surgery with written informed consent from the patients (authorization number CODECOH DC-2014-2229). Human brain microvessels were obtained from surgical resections of three patients: a 70-years-old female suffering from Glioblastoma, a 2-year-old child suffering from glioma and a 8-year-old child suffering from astrocytoma. Microvessels were isolated from resections of tumor, peritumoral or healthy brain tissue using an enzymatic procedure (Chaves et al., 2020) adapting methods previously published for rats (Perriere et al., 2005, 2007). Briefly, tissue samples were carefully cleaned from meninges and excess of blood; then, an enzymatic mix was used to dissociate the tissues and microvessels were isolated by retention on a 10 μM mesh. Cells were cultured in EBM-2 medium (Lonza, Basel, Switzerland) supplemented with 20% serum and growth factors (Sigma) (Perriere et al., 2005, 2007). After seeding brain capillaries in petri dishes, brain primary microvascular endothelial cells were shortly amplified and seeded (P1) on Transwell (Corning) with microporous membranes (pore size: 0.4 μm) in monoculture (CC205, CC206, and CC216) or in co-culture with the same patient's fresh primary human cultured astrocytes (CC216). Dry cell pellets were stored at −80°C before RT-qPCR experiments.

RNA Isolation, Reverse Transcription and Quantitative Real Time PCR (qPCR)

Total RNA was purified using the RNeasy Mini kit (Qiagen GmbH, Hilden, Germany). The concentration and purity of the RNA samples were determined using the NanoDrop® ND-1000 instrument (NanoDrop Technologies, United States). Reverse transcription of total RNA was achieved in a thermocycler (PTC-100 programmable thermal controller, MJ research INC, United States) using the following conditions: 25°C for 10 min, then at 42°C for 30 min and at 99°C for 5 min, as previously reported (Dauchy et al., 2009). cDNAs were stored at −80°C. Gene expression was determined by SYBR Green fluorescence detection using an ABI Prism 7900 HT Sequence Detection System (Applied Biosystems, Foster City, CA, United States) as previously reported (Luo et al., 2019). Samples were run in duplicate. Primers (**Table 1**) were designed using OLIGO 6.42 software (MedProbe, Norway). The lower the cycle threshold (Ct) value the higher the amount of mRNA, RT negative controls and no-template controls had Ct values > 40. RT negative controls and no-template controls had Ct values > 40. cDNAs from HEK293 cells were used to validate primers of human genes of interest. The relative expression of each gene of interest X as compared to the expression of the housekeeping gene encoding TATA box-binding protein (*TBP*) was calculated as $2^{-(Ct(X)-Ct(TBP))}$. Gene expression of genes having a Ct higher than 33 was not quantified.

Western Blot

Human cerebral microvessel endothelial cells D3 cells were washed twice with cold phosphate-buffered saline (PBS) on ice, then the protein lysis buffer (150 mM NaCl, 50 mM Tris–HCl pH 7.4, 0.5% Triton X100, 0.5% sodium deoxycholate), and protease inhibitor cocktail (complete®, Sigma) was added. The Bradford assay was applied to quantify the protein concentration (BSA as a standard). Total proteins were separated on a 7.5% SDS-polyacrylamide gel and transferred to polyvinylidene difluoride (PVDF) membranes (Bio-Rad), blocked for 2 h with 5% non-fat dry milk. Membranes were incubated overnight with a mouse anti-human TRPV2 primary antibody (1/250, sc-390439, Santa Cruz Biotechnology, Dallas, TX, United States), a polyclonal rabbit anti-human TRPV4 primary antibody (1/200, ab94868, Abcam) or a monoclonal mouse anti-human β-actin primary antibody (1/3000, Millipore). A secondary anti-mouse or anti-rabbit IgG conjugated to HRP (1/2000, Santa Cruz Biotechnology) was then incubated for detection using an ECL plus Western Blot Detection System (GE Healthcare, Velizy, France).

Confocal Imaging

Human cerebral microvessel endothelial cells D3 cells were cultured on a 8-well ibidi μ-Slide (1.5 polymer coverslip, tissue culture treated from CliniSciences, Nanterre, France). At 80% confluence, cells were fixed with PBS containing 3.2% paraformaldehyde and permeabilized with 0.2% Triton-X-100 (Sigma) in PBS for 10 min. After 30 min in blocking solution (0.2% Triton-X-100, 1% BSA and 10% goat serum containing PBS) at RT, cells were incubated with the rabbit anti-human TRPV2 primary antibody (1:250, Thermo Fisher Scientific, Ref: PA1-18346), rabbit anti-human TRPV4 primary antibody (1:100, ab94868, Abcam), rabbit anti-human Claudin-5 primary antibody (1:250, Santa Cruz Biotechnology) or rabbit anti human VE-Cadherin primary antibody (1:500, Enzo Life Sciences) overnight at 4°C. After washing with PBS, μ-slides were incubated for 2 h at RT with a goat anti-rabbit-555 (1:500, Santa Cruz Biotechnology) and nuclei were stained with Hoechst 33342 (1:10000, Thermo Fisher Scientific, France). Negative control cells were incubated omitting primary antibodies. Visualization of the proteins was performed using a Zeiss LSM 510 Meta confocal microscope (Oberkochen, Germany).

Intracellular Ca^{2+} Signal Measurements

Fluorescence measurement of intracellular Ca^{2+} concentration was performed as described previously (Luo et al., 2019). hCMEC/D3 cells grown to confluency in 24-well plate were loaded with 2 μM of Fluo-4-AM (λ_{ex} = 496 nm, λ_{em} = 516 nm, F14201, Thermo Fisher Scientific) for 45 min at 37°C in Hank's buffer (5.37 mM KCl, 0.44 mM KH_2PO_4, 4.2 mM $NaHCO_3$, 137.9 mM NaCl, 0.34 mM Na_2HPO_4, 1.5 mM $CaCl_2$, 0.9 mM $MgSO_4$, 5.56 mM D-Glucose at pH 7.4, all from Sigma,

TABLE 1 | Primers list for TRPVs channels and TBP applied in human and rat.

Gene	Forward primer (5′-3′)	Reverse primer (3′-5′)	Length (bp)
TBP or Tbp	TGCACAGGAGCCAAGAGTGAA	CACATCACAGCTCCCCACCA	132
Human TRPV1	ACTGCCATCATCACTGTCATCT	CTTCACAGCCAACAGGTCTACCA	83
Human TRPV2	CGTGCAGATCCCCTTCGAGA	TGGGCAACTTGTGATACAGATGG	85
Human TRPV3	TACGTGGCTGAGGGAGAG	ATCGTGGCGTGAAGTCCA	92
Human TRPV4	TCAGGGAATCACAGTTGGC	AGCTCTTCATTGATGGATTCTT	82
Rat Trpv1	CTCGCTCTCCGCCATTCTTGC	TGTGCGTGACTTATGGGAGATGT	88
Rat Trpv2	ACCACCAAAAAGTGTCCCTTCTC	CGGCCTCTTTAGGAGTCTCACC	94
Rat Trpv3	GCTCCAGCCTGTGTTGAAAAT	CCTCCCAGTCCCTTGCTAAAG	90
Rat Trpv4	CCCCCTCAGCTCTTCACGG	CCCCACCCTGTTCCACTTTTTC	114

500 μL/well). Cells were then washed and replaced with HBSS (500 μL/well). After 10 min of incubation at 37°C, fluorescence in the 24-well plates were read using a Victor® X2 fluorescent microplate reader (PerkinElmer, Villebon, France).

Fluorescence was determined with diverse activators of TRP channels. Cells were also pre-treated with TRP antagonists (capsazepine 10 and 20 μM, tranilast 50 μM, RN1734 30 μM) for 5 min before adding TRP agonists (GSK1016790A ranging from 3 to 1000 nM, capsaicin 1 and 3 μM, cannabidiol 15 μM) and the fluorescent signals were then recorded in the presence of fixed concentration of TRP antagonists. All TRP activators and antagonists were dissolved with 100% DMSO or ethanol as stock solutions and the final solvent concentration in treated cells did not exceed 1%, a solvent concentration that had no effect on Ca^{2+} entry as compared to control cells without any solvent (data not shown). Data were normalized to the control group, which is expressed as F1/F0, where F0 is the average fluorescence of the control group (no activator of TRP) and F1 is the actual fluorescence at the corresponding time for the control group (in this case the average ratio for the control group is 1 or 100%) or the treated group.

To explore heating-induced Ca^{2+} influx, hCMEC/D3 cells were plated in 24-wells plate and loaded with Fluo-4-AM. The plate was then placed in the detecting room of Victor™ X2 fluorescent microplate reader with automatically heating system. The plate was heating from RT to 50°C. The temperature and fluorescence were recorded at the same time by the Victor™ X2 in the presence or not of the specific TRPV antagonist. Data was expressed as ratio normalized to the average of fluorescence intensity at RT in each well.

Statistical Analysis

Data are expressed as mean value ± SEM (standard error of the mean). Statistical analysis was performed using ANOVA with Dunnett *a posteriori* test to compare different groups with the control. An unpaired *t*-test was applied between two groups. p value < 0.05 was considered statistically significant. To calculate the EC_{50} of the agonist (GSK1016790A), the concentration-response data were fitted to a logistic function as follows: $Y = \text{Bottom} + (\text{Top}-\text{Bottom})/(1 + 10^{(logEC50-X)})$; where X is the log of the agonist concentration. Data fitting was performed in GraphPad Prism 5.01.

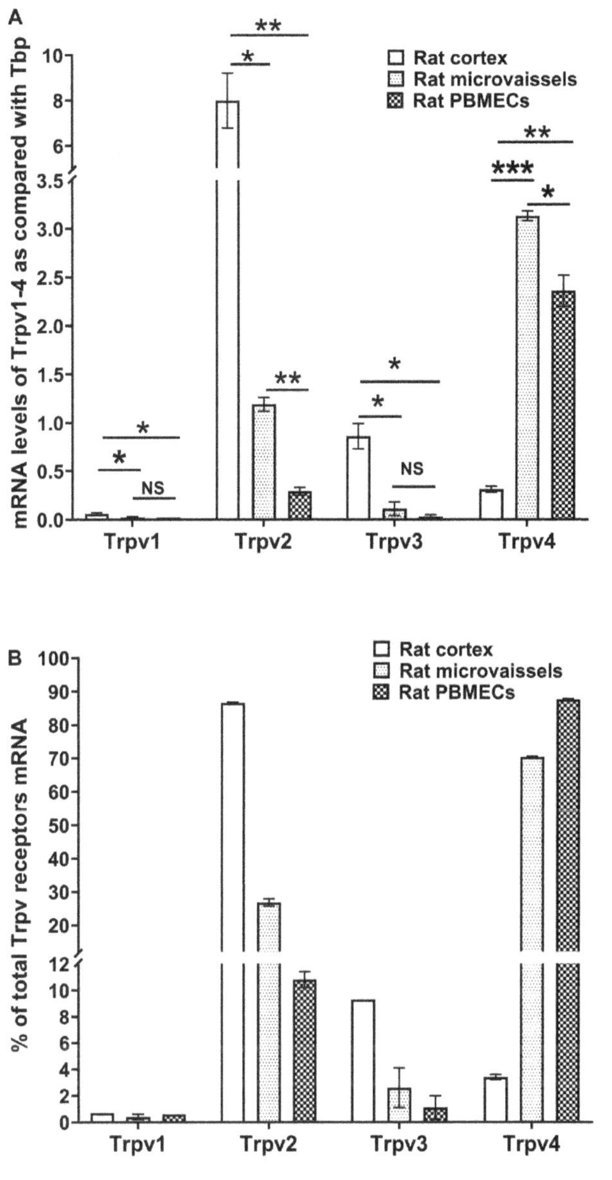

FIGURE 1 | Expression of thermo-sensitive Trpv in rat cortex, rat microvessels and BBB endothelial cells. **(A,B)** mRNA levels of *Trp1-4* were detected by qRT-PCR in rat brain cortex, rat brain isolated microvessels and primary cultures of rat brain microvessel endothelial cells (see section "Materials and Methods"). Data are expressed as ratio (mean ± SEM) of *Trpv* mRNA levels compared with those of the endogenous housekeeping gene *Tbp* in each sample from three different RNA extractions **(A)** or expressed as a percentage of total *Trpv1-4* expression set at 100% **(B)**. Inter-group comparisons were performed by ANOVA with Dunnett *a posteriori* test, NS not significant, *$p < 0.05$, **$p < 0.01$, ***$p < 0.001$.

RESULTS

Thermo-Sensitive *Trpv1-4* Gene Expression in Rat Cortex, Brain Microvessels and rPBMEC

We measured the relative expression of *Trpv1-4* by qRT-PCR in primary cultured rat brain microvessel endothelial cells (rPBMEC) (**Figure 1**). *Trpv1* mRNA levels were barely detectable in whole cortex, brain microvessels and rPBMEC (**Figure 1A**). *Trpv2* expression was much higher in the whole cortex than in both brain microvessels and rPBMEC (7.99 ± 1.21, 1.19 ± 0.07, and 0.29 ± 0.04, respectively; $p < 0.05$ rat cortex vs. microvessels, $p < 0.01$ rat cortex vs. rPBMEC) and similar results were obtained for *Trpv3* (0.86 ± 0.13, 0.11 ± 0.07, 0.03 ± 0.02, respectively; $p < 0.05$ rat cortex vs. microvessels, $p < 0.05$ rat cortex vs. rPBMEC). Among *Trpv1-4*, *Trpv4* was the most highly expressed gene in brain microvessels and rPBMEC (3.13 ± 0.05 and 2.36 ± 0.16, respectively; $p < 0.001$ rat cortex vs. microvessels, $p < 0.01$ rat cortex vs. rPBMEC) while its expression in rat cortex was far below that of *Trpv2*. Meanwhile, no significant difference was observed for the gene expression of *Trpv1* and *Trpv3* between brain microvessels and rPBMEC (**Figure 1A**), while a significant decrease of *Trpv2* and Trpv 4 gene expression was observed in rPBMEC compared with that in brain microvessels (**Figure 1A**, $p < 0.01$, $p < 0.05$ for *Trpv2* and *Trpv4*, respectively, rat microvessels vs. rPBMEC). The *Trpv1-4* gene expression profile expressed as a percentage of total *Trpv* genes expressed was similar in brain microvessels and rPBMEC with the following rank order: *Trpv4* > *Trpv2* > *Trpv3* > > *Trpv1* (**Figure 1B**). This is dramatically different from the *Trpv1-4* gene expression profile in the whole brain cortex with the following rank order: *Trpv2* > *Trpv3* > *Trpv4* > > *Trpv1*.

Thermo-Sensitive *TRPV1-4* Gene Expression in Human BMEC

We measured the relative expression of *TRPV1-4* by qRT-PCR in hCMEC/D3 cells and primary cultured human brain microvascular endothelial cells (hPBMEC) from three different brain tumor biopsies (**Figure 2A**). *TRPV1* mRNA levels were easily detected in hPBMEC of the adult patient culture CC216 and, albeit at a lower level, in hCMEC/D3 and hPBMEC from the two children cultures CC205 and CC206 (3.05 ± 0.26, 0.22 ± 0.01, 0.21 ± 0.01, and 0.76 ± 0.08, respectively, **Figure 2A**). It is noteworthy that *TRPV1* expression was increased significantly by 4.8-fold (from 3.05 ± 0.26 to 14.6 ± 2.0, $p < 0.01$) when cells were co-cultured with isolated primary astrocytes from the same patient, while no effect was found for the other 3 TRPV isoforms (**Figure 2A**). *TRPV2* was by far the most highly expressed gene in hCMEC/D3 and hPBMEC cells [*TRPV2* data for CC205 and CC206 was also shown in Luo et al. (2019)]. *TRPV4* was expressed at moderate levels in hPBMEC from the three patients (10.36 ± 2.23, 1.35 ± 0.04, and 1.79 ± 0.12) and hCMEC/D3 (1.38 ± 0.01) while *TRPV3* mRNA were barely detectable in all cells. A similar *TRPV1-4* gene expression profile expressed as a percentage of total *TRP* gene expressed was observed in hCMEC/D3 cells and hPBMEC with the following rank order: *TRPV2* > > *TRPV4* > *TRPV1* > > *TRPV3* (**Figure 2B**).

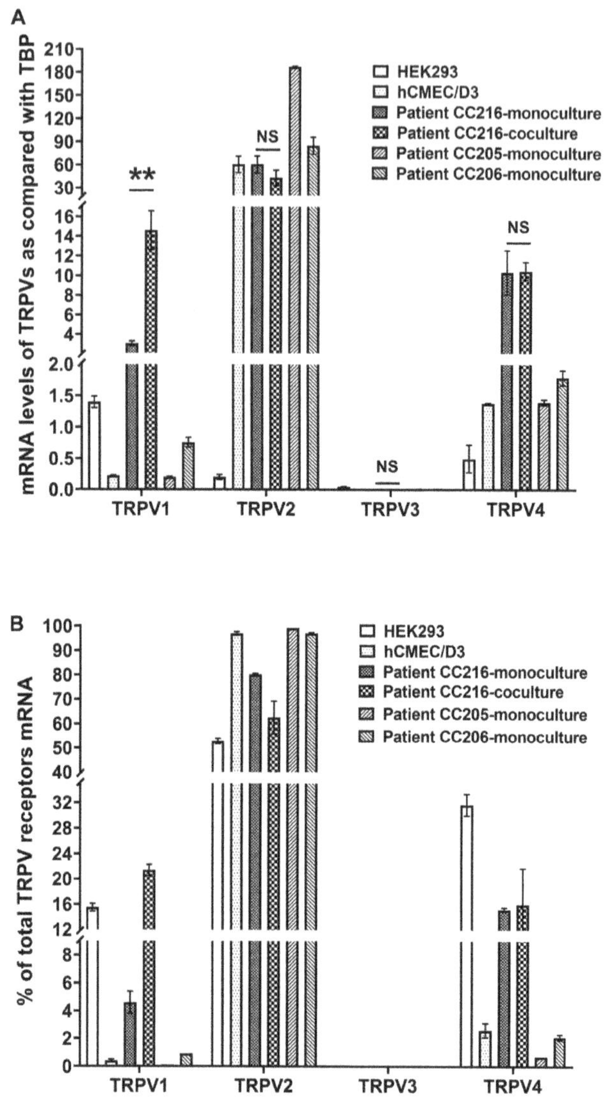

FIGURE 2 | Expression of thermo-sensitive Trpv in human BMEC. **(A,B)** mRNA levels of *TRPV1-4* were detected by qRT-PCR in primary cultures of brain microvessel endothelial cells obtained from patients (see section "Materials and Methods") and in hCMEC/D3 cells. Data are expressed as ratio (mean ± SEM) of TRPV1-4 mRNA levels compared with those of the endogenous housekeeping gene *TBP* in each sample from three different RNA extractions **(A)** or expressed as a percentage of total *TRPV1-4* expression set at 100% **(B)**. When comparing TRPV1-4 expression in human BMEC culturing alone or together with astrocytes isolated from the same patient, statistical significance was determined by an unpaired *t*-test, NS, not significant, $^{**}p < 0.01$.

Protein Expression of TRPV2 and TRPV4 in hCMEC/D3

The expression of TRPV2 and TRPV4, the two genes with the highest expression at the mRNA level in human brain endothelial cells, was then studied at the protein level. Western blot analysis showed that TRPV2 and TRPV4 proteins were expressed in hCMEC/D3 cells where they are detected in a single band at a molecular weight around 80–90 kDa, in agreement with the predicted value of TRPV2 and TRPV4 molecular weights (**Figure 3A**). This was confirmed by immunostaining and confocal microscopy which revealed a specific expression of both TRPV2 and TRPV4 at the plasma membrane of hCMEC/D3 cells as well as in intracellular compartments concentrated in the perinuclear region (**Figure 3B**). Omitting the primary antibody resulted in the absence of any detectable fluorescence signal (NEG in **Figure 3B**). The tight junction protein Claudine-5 was used as a positive control for brain endothelial cell phenotype as it was reported to be expressed in hCMEC/D3 cells (Weksler et al., 2005).

Functional Activity of TRPV in hCMEC/D3

Transient receptor potential vanilloid 1, TRPV2, and TRPV4 functional activity was then investigated in hCMEC/D3 cells.

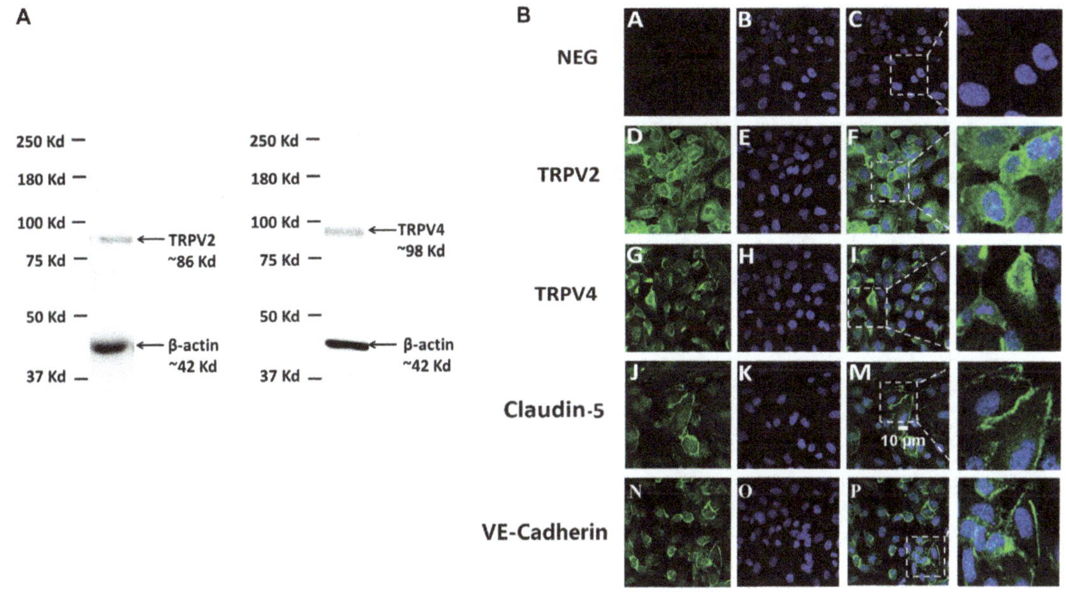

FIGURE 3 | Protein expression of TRPV2 and TRPV4 in hCMEC/D3. **(A)** Expression of TRPV2 and TRPV4 determined by Western blot of total crude proteins obtained from two different protein extractions of hCMEC/D3. β-actin served as a loading control housekeeping protein. **(B)** Confocal immunofluorescence localization of TRPV2 and TRPV4 in hCMEC/D3. TRPV2 or TRPV4 (green) and nuclei (blue) were stained in hCMEC/D3 as described in section "Materials and Methods" (second D, E, F and third G, H, I row panels). Claudin-5 (green) and nuclei (blue) were stained in hCMEC/D3 (fourth row panel J, K, M). VE-Cadherin (green) and nuclei (blue) were stained in hCMEC/D3 (fifth row panel N, O, P). Control cells (NEG) were stained omitting the primary antibodies (first row panel A, B, C).

Ionomycin, which triggers an immediate increase of the intracellular Ca^{2+} concentration, was used as a positive control (2 μM ionomycin) in all Ca^{2+} influx experiments.

The AUC of intracellular Ca^{2+} levels during 20 min were not significantly affected when cells were exposed for 20 min to 1 or 3 μM CAP, a highly specific and efficient agonist of TRPV1 (**Figures 4A,B**). By contrast, CAP, at lower concentrations than those used in our study, were high enough to fully activate human TRPV1 (Binshtok et al., 2007). In addition to compare the AUC of intracellular Ca^{2+} levels during 20 min, we further compared the intracellular Ca^{2+} levels at specific time (**Figures 4C,D**). Interestingly, a significant statistical difference between the control group and 3 μM CAP group at 7 min (p = 0.019), 11 min (p = 0.041), 12 min (p = 0.049), and 16 min (p = 0.045) were found (**Figures 4C,D**). However, no significant difference of Ca^{2+} influx at any specific times was found when cells exposed to 1 μM CAP (**Figures 4C,D**). Ca^{2+} flux levels were not significantly altered when cells exposed to CAP from 1 to 3 μM (**Figures 4C,D**). Meanwhile, a significant 3.3-fold increase of Ca^{2+} influx was observed in the positive control group treated with 2 μM ionomycin (**Figures 4A,B**, $p < 0.001$ compared with the control group). TRPV1 is a known thermo-sensitive channel (Mergler et al., 2010). Therefore, we asked whether CPZ, a well-known TRPV1 antagonist, was able to block the heat-induced increase of intracellular Ca^{2+} concentration. As shown in **Figures 4E,F**, exposing cells continuously from RT to 50°C for 40 min resulted in a significant increase in intracellular Ca^{2+} but this Ca^{2+} flux was not altered by co-treatment with CPZ (10 or 20 μM; **Figure 4E**), in agreement with the low expression of *TRPV1* assessed by qRT-PCR and the weak TRPV1 activation by CAP. Conversely, heat-induced Ca^{2+} influx could be blocked by TNL, a selective TRPV2 antagonist. Exposing the cells to CBD, a highly potent activator of TRPV2 and to a lesser extent of TRPV1, resulted in an increased Ca^{2+} influx in hCMEC/D3, an effect which was not reversed by CPZ (**Figures 4G,H**). Similar trends were demonstrated when comparing the Ca^{2+} influx at specific time (**Figures 4I,J**).

To assess TRPV4 activity in hCMEC/D3, we applied GSK1016790A (GSK), a highly selective and potent agonist of TRPV4. GSK induced a dramatic and rapid concentration-dependent increase in Ca^{2+} levels (**Figure 5A**). A maximal increase in intracellular Ca^{2+} levels (1.6-fold) was obtained with GSK ≥100 nM (**Figure 5B**). An apparent concentration-effect relationship was observed with an EC_{50} of 16.2 ± 4.5 nM (**Figure 5C**). The rise in intracellular Ca^{2+} concentration induced by 30 nM GSK1016790A was inhibited by RN1734 pretreatment (30 μM) a well-known TRPV4 antagonist (**Figures 5D,E**).

DISCUSSION

Brain microvessel endothelial cells, the main component of the BBB, are widely exposed to various stimuli from the blood and brain compartments. Among these, blood borne compounds and mechanical stress might modulate the activity of TRP channels, thus allowing Ca^{2+} entry into brain endothelial cells where Ca^{2+} concentrations need to be maintained within a certain range of concentrations through a dynamic equilibrium (Ma and Liu, 2019). Intracellular/cytosolic [Ca^{2+}] modulates

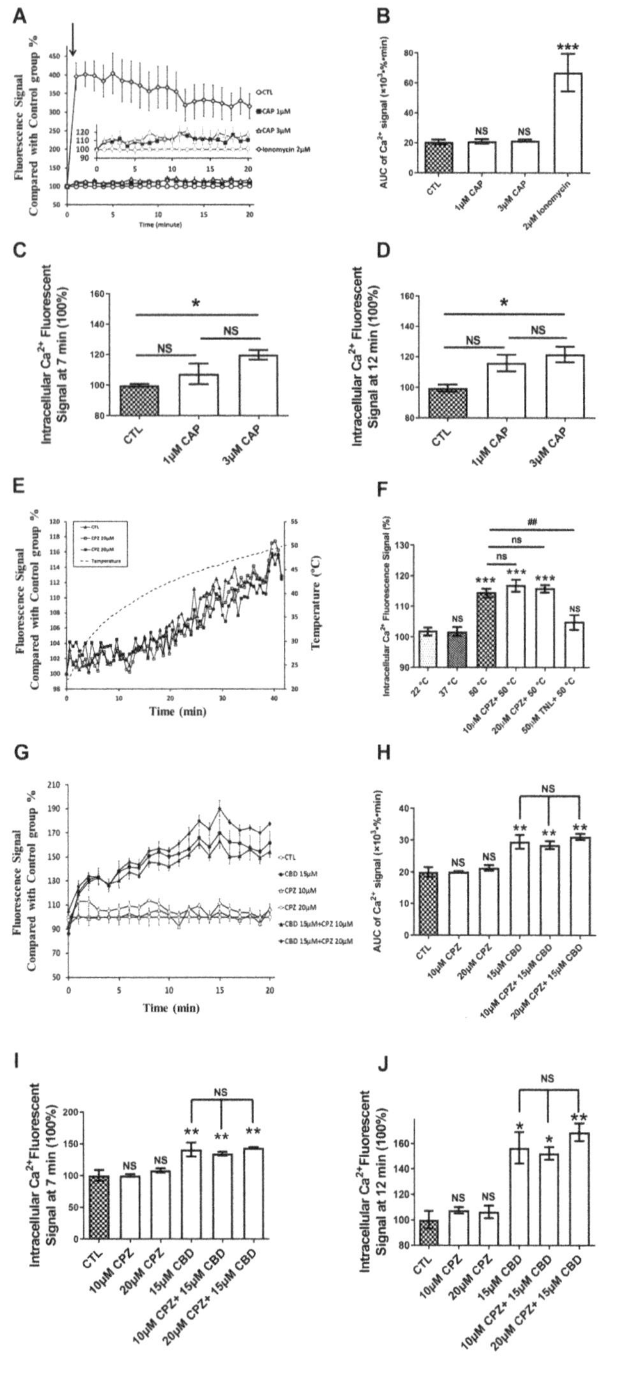

FIGURE 4 | TRPV1 is not functional in hCMEC/D3. **(A)** Representative time course of $[Ca^{2+}]_i$ in hCMEC/D3 under stimulation of TRPV1 by capsaicin (CAP). Cells were plated in 24-wells plate and loaded with Fluo-4-AM as described in section "Materials and Methods." CAP or ionomycin (as positive control of Ca^{2+} entry) was added and the fluorescence was recorded. **(B)** Change of the area under curve (AUC) over the 20 min obtained from the experiment shown in panel **(A)**. **(C)** Change in $[Ca^{2+}]_i$ at T = 7 min obtained from the experiment shown in panel **(A)**. **(D)** Change in $[Ca^{2+}]_i$ at T = 12 min obtained from the experiment shown in panel **(A)**. **(E)** Change of $[Ca^{2+}]_i$ upon heat exposure of hCMEC/D3 for 40 min from room temperature to 50°C. Cells were plated in 24-wells plate and loaded with Fluo-4-AM. The fluorescence was recorded in the presence or not of the specific TRPV1 antagonist

(Continued)

FIGURE 4 | Continued

capsazepine (CPZ; 10 or 20 μM). **(F)** Changes in $[Ca^{2+}]_i$ in hCMEC/D3 at 22, 37, or 50°C with or without CPZ or Tranilast (TNL, 50 μM) derived from panel **(E)**. **(G)** Representative time course of $[Ca^{2+}]_i$ in hCMEC/D3 stimulated by the TRPV1-2 agonist cannabidiol (CBD, 15 μM) and pre-treated or not with the TRPV1 specific antagonist CPZ. Cells were loaded with Fluo-4-AM. CBD was added and the fluorescence was recorded. When applying CPZ, cells were pre-treated with 10 or 20 μM CPZ for 5 min before incubation with 15 μM CBD and the fluorescence was recorded in the persistent presence of 10 or 20 μM CPZ. **(H)** Change of the area under curve (AUC) over the 20 min obtained from the experiment shown in panel **(G)**. **(I)** Change in $[Ca^{2+}]_i$ at T = 7 min obtained from the experiment shown in panel **(G)**. **(J)** Change in $[Ca^{2+}]_i$ at T = 12 min obtained from the experiment shown in panel **(G)**. Data are expressed as mean ± SEM and inter-group comparisons were performed by ANOVA with Dunnett *a posteriori* test. $^{*}p < 0.05$, $^{**}p < 0.01$, $^{***}p < 0.001$ compared with CTL or 22°C groups or among indicated group.

various cellular processes such as excitability, proliferation, synaptic plasticity, resistance to oxidative stress, and cell death, depending on the concentration, timing and duration of the signal (Fliniaux et al., 2018). Modifications of intracellular $[Ca^{2+}]$ can trigger the proliferation of BMEC and increase the permeability of the BBB by altering tight junction proteins (Ma and Liu, 2019). Furthermore, BBB dysfunctions observed in several brain pathologies are usually associated with increasing intracellular Ca^{2+} concentrations, suggesting that TRP-mediated Ca^{2+} signaling may play crucial roles in maintaining and regulating BBB functions (De Bock et al., 2013). Interestingly, the highly potent TRPV2 activator CBD increased Ca^{2+} entry in hCMEC/D3 cells where it induces proliferation, tubulogenesis and migration (Luo et al., 2019). Moreover, CBD has anti-inflammatory activity and is able to reduce the disruption of the BBB observed in lipopolysaccharide (LPS) (Ruiz-Valdepenas et al., 2011) and multiple sclerosis mice models (Mecha et al., 2013). CBD was demonstrated as effective in preventing disruption of an *in vitro* BBB model under hypoxic and glucose deprivation conditions (Hind et al., 2016). Altogether, these results suggest that activating TRPV2 might be a relevant strategy to positively modulate the BBB in the context of brain disorders including ischemic stroke (Calapai et al., 2020). Here, we looked at interspecies differences in the expression and activity of TRPV in rat and human BBB.

Transient receptor potential vanilloid 1-4 were first to be known for their expression in sensory neurons and their function in sensing nociception and pain (Mickle et al., 2015). However, the expression of TRPV1-4 in the brain is quite region-specific and heterogeneous (Kauer and Gibson, 2009; Cavanaugh et al., 2011; Nedungadi et al., 2012). For TRPV1, previous studies have believed that it can be widely expressed throughout the brain (Kauer and Gibson, 2009). However, a recent study applied a highly sensitive method using gene editing to modify the Trpv1 genetic locus in two lines of reporter mice, showing that TRPV1 is highly limitedly expressed in several specific brain regions, such as the caudal hypothalamus, the dorsal motor nucleus of the vagus, mesencephalic trigeminal nucleus, and parabrachial nucleus (Cavanaugh et al., 2011). Litter expression was found for the other brain regions (Cavanaugh et al., 2011). TRPV2 was found to be intensively expressed mainly in several brain

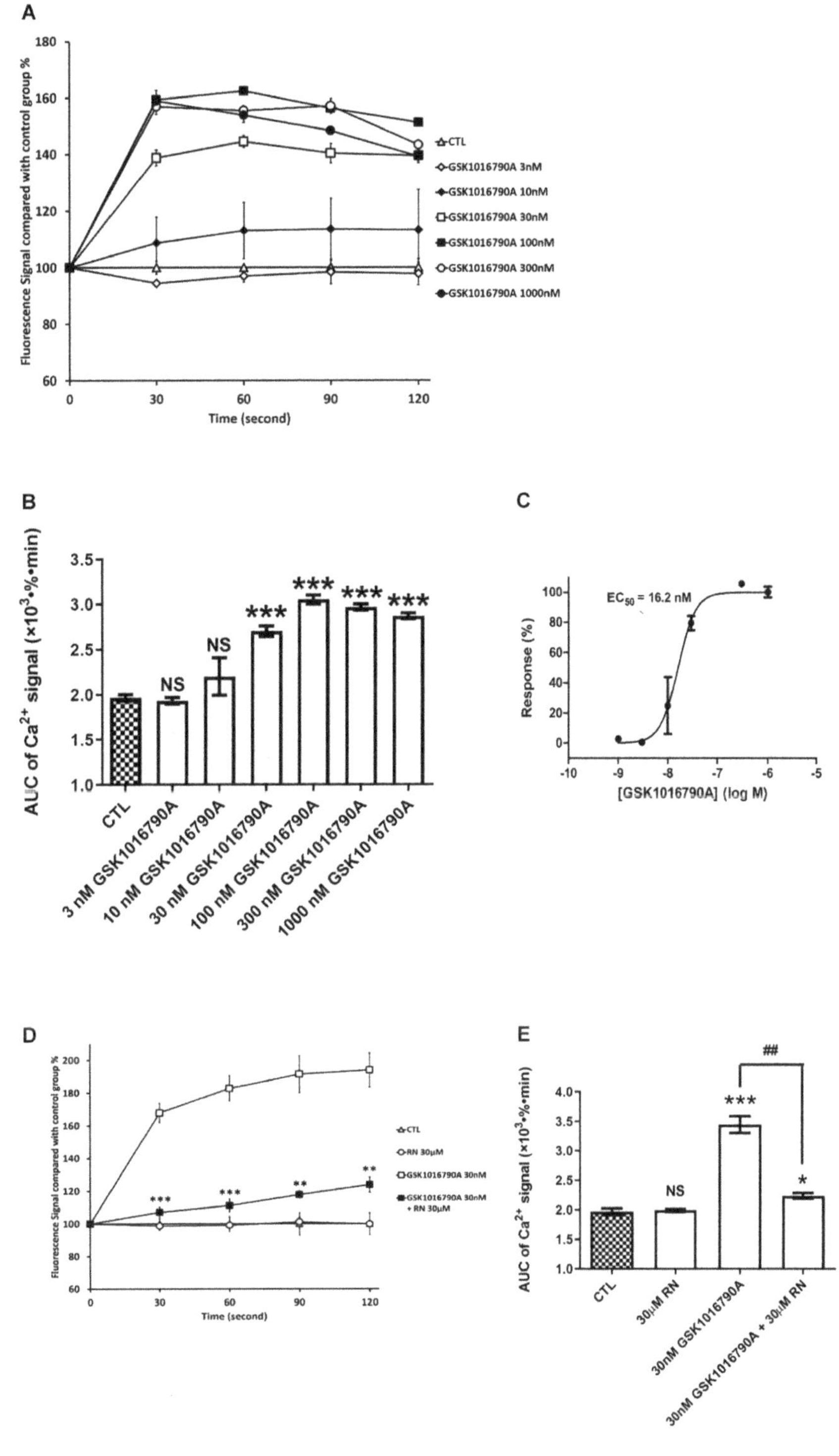

FIGURE 5 | TRPV4 is functional in hCMEC/D3. **(A)** Representative time course of $[Ca^{2+}]_i$ in hCMEC/D3 stimulated by the TRPV4 agonist GSK1016790A. Cells were plated in 24-wells plate and loaded with Fluo-4-AM as described. GSK1016790A was added and the fluorescence was recorded. **(B)** Change of the area under curve (AUC) over the 120 s obtained from the experiment shown in panel **(A)**. **(C)** Concentration-response relationship of GSK1016790A. Measurements were obtained from panel **(B)**. **(D)** Representative time course of $[Ca^{2+}]_i$ in hCMEC/D3 stimulated by GSK1016790A and pre-treated or not with the TRPV4 specific antagonist RN1734 (RN). When applying RN, cells were pre-treated with 30 μM RN for 5 min and the fluorescence was recorded in the persistent presence of 30 μM GSK1016790A. **(D)** Change of the area under curve (AUC) over the 120 s obtained from the experiment shown in panel **(C)**. Data are expressed as mean ± SEM. For panels **(B,E)**, inter-group comparisons were performed by ANOVA with Dunnett *a posteriori* test, NS, not significant, $^{*}p < 0.05$, $^{***}p < 0.001$ compared with CTL group, ##$p < 0.01$ compared with 30 nMGSK1016790A group, $n = 3$ in triplicate. For panel **(D)**, inter-group comparisons were performed by ANOVA with Dunnett *a posteriori* test, $^{*}p < 0.01$, $^{**}p < 0.01$, $^{***}p < 0.001$ compared with GSK1016790A group.

areas including: hypothalamus, the nucleus of the solitary tract, hypoglossal nucleus, and the rostral division of the ventrolateral (Nedungadi et al., 2012). TRPV3 protein expression has not been detected in the mouse brain, although TRPV3 mRNA transcripts has been detected in the brain at low levels (Luo and Hu, 2014). TRPV3 is also evidenced to be absent in the mouse bEnd.3 brain endothelial cell line and in the freshly isolated brain capillaries and primary cultured BMECs from rat (Mickle et al., 2015). This is in accordance with the whole transcriptomic analysis demonstrating the absence of Trpv3 in murine primary BMECs (Zhang et al., 2014) and by brain vascular single-cell transcriptomics study (Vanlandewijck et al., 2018). TRPV3 is most abundantly expressed in skin keratinocytes and in cells surrounding hair follicles, where it plays an essential role in cutaneous sensation. RT-PCR or q-PCR analysis showing the absence of TRPV3 in human BMECs (Golech et al., 2004; Hatano et al., 2013) and gain-of-function mutations in human TRPV3 are associated with Olmsted syndrome, which is characterized by severe palmoplantar and periorificial keratoderma (Greco et al., 2020; Zhang et al., 2020). TRPV4 has been reported to be widely expressed throughout the brain including hippocampus, hypothalamus, cerebellum, lamina terminalis and optic chiasm, as well as a special enhanced expression in the olfactory placodes (Mangos et al., 2007; Kauer and Gibson, 2009; Shibasaki et al., 2015). Unfortunately, it is still remained largely unknown which types of cells were responsible for their expression in a specific brain region (Kauer and Gibson, 2009). Our results showed significant mRNA levels of some TRPVs in human brain endothelial cells which follow this rank of expression: *TRPV2* > *TRPV4* > *TRPV1*, while *TRPV3* was barely detected. It should be noted that this rank order is based on mRNA levels and functional studies since the absolute amount of each TRPV at protein level was not investigated in this study. These observations are supported by a study showing the qualitative expression of TRPV1, 2, and 4 in human primary cultured brain endothelial cells by RT-PCR (Hatano et al., 2013). TRPV2, a thermo-sensitive TRPV channel, was by far the most highly expressed isoform in hPBMEC and hCMEC/D3 while its relative expression was much lower than that of Trpv4 in rat microvessels and rPBMEC. TRPV1 and TRPV4 were also expressed both in rPBMEC, hPBMEC and hCMEC/D3 cells, and TRPV2 was even more expressed in hPBMEC than in hCMEC/D3 cells. TRPV4 expression was further evidenced by Western blot and immunofluorescence analysis in hCMEC/D3 cells supporting previous RT-PCR and/or immunofluorescence results in human BMEC (Sullivan et al., 2012; Hatano et al., 2013). However, using specific peptides of TRPV2 and TRPV4 targeted by the primary anti-TRPV2 and antiT-RPV4 antibodies used in our study would have increased the specificity of the immunofluorescence staining. Interestingly, we detected a 4.0- and 5.8-fold higher expression of, respectively, *TRPV1* and *TRPV4* mRNA, in the brain endothelial cells derived from the adult patient (CC216) as compared with the two children (CC205 and CC206), suggesting that TRPV1 and TRPV4 expression might increase with age while that of TRPV2 might decrease. This is in agreement with the reported age-dependent expression and function of Trpvl in the rodent forebrain (Koles et al., 2013), although we cannot exclude, in our case, that these differences might result from the limited numbers of patients and/or reflect the underlying pathology or the exposure of the patients to medication. Interestingly, *TRPV* expression in hPBMEC was modulated by co-culture with astrocytes as shown by the 4.8-fold TRPV1 increase in hPBMECs co-culture with isolated primary astrocytes obtained from the same patient. In contrast, this effect was absent for *TRPV2,3,4* isoforms. Recently, Mannari et al. (2013) have reported that the astrocytic *TRPV1* could directly sense the blood-borne signals in the sensory circumventricular organs in adult mouse brains. Trpvl is regarded as a target in regulating BBB permeability (Hu et al., 2005; Beggs et al., 2010) and might be also a downstream target in the modulated BBB permeability mediated by astrocytes (Abbott, 2002; Abbott et al., 2006).

A similar expression profile was found between hPBMEC isolated from patients and the human BBB cell line hCMEC/D3, confirming previous data (Dauchy et al., 2009; Ohtsuki et al., 2013) and suggesting that hCMEC/D3 is a proper *in vitro* surrogate in exploring TRPV properties at the human BBB. *Trpv2* gene expression was 25.8-fold more expressed in brain cortex than in rPBMEC, in accordance with a more pronounced Trpv2 immunostaining in the rat brain (Nedungadi et al., 2012). Notably, we evidenced a remarkable interspecies difference regarding the expression profile of *TRPV1-4* between rPBMEC and the two human *in vitro* BBB models (hPBMEC and hCMEC/D3). Although *TRPV2* and *TRPV4* were expressed both in rat and human BMEC, *Trpv4* and *TRPV2* were the most expressed isoform in rPBMEC and hBMEC, respectively. Brown et al. (2008) have demonstrated *Trpv1-4* expression by RT-PCR in the bEnd.3 murine BBB cell line and in isolated mouse brain microvessels, showing a higher *Trpv2* expression than *Trpv4*, suggesting TRPV expression profile could be similar in murine and human BMEC. A whole transcriptomic analysis revealed a similar expression of *Trpv2* and *Trpv4* in murine primary BMEC, while *Trpvl* and *Trpv3* transcripts were undetectable (Zhang et al., 2014). Except for TRPV1-4, many other transporters and enzymes expressed at the BBB also demonstrated interspecies differences in expression and function levels (Deo et al., 2013). PET studies have demonstrated a significant interspecies differences for the expression and functionality of ABCB1 (i.e., P-gp), an important efflux transporter at the BBB (Syvanen et al., 2009). The brain-to-plasma concentration ratio of [^{11}C]GR205171, a substrate of P-gp, was almost 9-times higher in humans compared with rats (Syvanen et al., 2009; Ball et al., 2013). In fact, interspecies differences in expression and/or function levels were also verified for ABCG2 (BCRP) (Ito et al., 2011; Uchida et al., 2011; Agarwal et al., 2012), MRPs (Agarwal et al., 2012), some OATPs (Ito et al., 2011; Uchida et al., 2011) and some SLCs (Ito et al., 2011; Agarwal et al., 2012).

Our current work did not indicate whether TRPV receptors are expressed at BBB in a polarized way or not. Many receptors/transporters are localized specifically at luminal or abluminal side of the brain endothelial cells in charge of different functions (Dragoni and Turowski, 2018). Very poor data were reported regarding the subcellular localization of TRPV1-3 in brain microvessels. In the rat middle cerebral arteries, TRPV4 was found to be expressed preferentially on the abluminal membrane of endothelial cells (Marrelli et al., 2007) but the observation that a selective P2Y2 receptor agonist could induce TRPV4-mediated Ca^{2+} entry across the luminal and abluminal face of an endothelial monolayer (Guerra et al., 2018), suggests that TRPV4 could be also expressed on the luminal face of endothelial cells. Benfenati et al. (2007) confirmed that expression of TRPV4 is abundantly localized on astrocytic endfeet area abutting pial and parenchyma blood vessels. Also, TRPV2 has been shown to be prominently localized to the umbrella apical membrane of bladder epithelium cells, while TRPV4 was identified on their abluminal surfaces (Yu et al., 2011).

Transient receptor potential vanilloid-mediated modulation of the intracellular Ca^{2+} concentration was further investigated using specific agonist and antagonists. The highly potent TRPV1 agonist CAP, usually effective at nanomolar levels (Flockerzi, 2007), did not increase the AUC of intracellular Ca^{2+} during 20 min in hCMEC/D3 at a concentration of 1 or 3 μM. Further statistical tests revealed that 3 μM CAP can stimulate the Ca^{2+} influx at specific time (7, 11, and 12 min post CAP stimulation), indicating a possible weak function of TRPV1 in the BBB. This in agreement with the low gene expression of *TRPV1* in hCMEC/D3 and also with the recent observation that no functional activity with CAP up to 1 mM could be detected in human renal podocytes although these cells expressed TRPV1 (Ambrus et al., 2017). Notably, TRPV1-induced Ca^{2+} influx under CAP stimulation at specific times is not quite dose-dependently as similar Ca^{2+} influx levels were found in 1 or 3 μM CAP, from the view of either the AUC of Ca^{2+} during 20 min or the Ca^{2+} influx at any specific time, further identifying the quite lower TRPV1 expression at the membrane of hCMEC/D3 cells. In fact, the much lower expression of TRPV1 in BBB endothelial cells were also demonstrated by Golech et al. (2004) by RT-PCR and polyclonal antibodies. TRPV1 is also functional in responding to heat stimulation, however the heat-induced Ca^{2+} influx was not significantly inhibited by CPZ (10 or 20 μM), a widely used TRPV1 antagonist, suggesting that TRPV1 might not be the main functional isoform in hCMED/D3 cells. In addition, it was reported that TRPV1 could be also activated by CBD, although its agonist potency was lower than toward TRPV2 (Qin et al., 2008). Yet, no significant alteration in intracellular Ca^{2+} was observed when co-treating cells with CBD and CPZ, a TRPV1 antagonist, further suggesting the lack of TRPV1 activity or weak TRPV1 activity in hCMEC/D3 cells. However, we cannot exclude a functional activity of TRPV1 in hPBMECs since TRPV1 gene expression was much higher in those cells than in hCMEC/D3 cells, especially when they were co-cultured with astrocytes from the same patient. Moreover, CPZ is not a very potent antagonist of TRPV1 (Rigoni et al., 2003), that could only produce an insufficient/partial blocking of TRPV1. Therefore, the absence of functional activity of TRPV1 in hCMEC/D3 cells remains questionable.

The specific and potent TRPV4 agonist GSK triggered a rapid elevation of intracellular Ca^{2+} with an E_{max} at 100 nM (EC_{50} ~16.2 nM), which can be totally inhibited by the specific TRPV4 antagonist RN1734. The EC_{50} for GSK in hCMEC/D3 cells was close to that reported for stimulating Ca^{2+} influx in another study (26.9 nM) (Sullivan et al., 2012). Previous studies have identified the expression of TRPV4 in commercial human BMECs at gene and protein levels (Hatano et al., 2013). The expression and function of TRPV4 are also verified using patch-clamp electrophysiology techniques in freshly BMECs isolated from brain capillaries of C57BL/6J mouse (Harraz et al., 2018). The specific TRPV4 agonist GSK-stimulated currents was completely abolished in TRPV4-knockout mice or when co-applying the specific TRPV4 antagonist HC-067047 in murine BMECs (Harraz et al., 2018). It is also reported that TRPV4 might play a vital role in regulating the function of blood-retina barrier, similarly to BBB, via modulating Ca^{2+} homeostasis in human retinal microvascular endothelial cells (Phuong et al., 2017). Due to their diverse cellular and subcellular localizations, TRP channels could mediate Ca^{2+} influx and generate distinct cytosolic/local intracellular Ca^{2+} waves that could regulate specific subcellular downstream pathways leading to different cell responses including death or survival (Fliniaux et al., 2018). In this regard, mitochondrial expression of TRPV1-2-3 has been evidenced in human odontoblasts (Wen et al., 2017), which is consistent with the intracellular staining we observed in hCMEC/D3 cells for TRPV2 and TRPV4.

CONCLUSION

In conclusion, our present study shows that TRPV1, TRPV2 and TRPV4 are expressed in hPBMECs. Even less expressed than TRPV2, TRPV4 is functionally expressed in the human BBB. Recently, TRPV4 has been shown to be highly expressed and functional in retinal endothelial cells (Phuong et al., 2017). The authors nicely showed by different electrophysiological and Ca^{2+} imaging techniques and using an *in vitro* retinal barrier model that TRPV4 highly contributed to Ca^{2+} homeostasis and barrier function. The role of TRPV4 in BBB barrier function and physiology should be evaluated in further experiments before claiming whether or not TRPV4 could be a target to be investigated for modulating the BBB. TRPV1 is much less expressed than TRPV2 and TRPV4 in the human BBB but still shows weak or limited functionality when activated by relative high concentration of selective chemical agonist. An interspecies difference between rat and human TRPV2,4 was evidenced in the BBB using a gene expression approach which may be taken into consideration for rat to human translational pharmacological approaches targeting TRPV in the BBB. This interspecies difference between rat and human TRPV should be further confirmed from a functional point of view by using for example electrophysiological techniques like patch-clamp and measuring whole-cell currents of TRPV2 and TRPV4 between human and rat BMEC.

ETHICS STATEMENT

The studies involving human participants were reviewed and approved by French Ministry of Higher Education and Research

(CODECOH DC-2014-2229). Written informed consent to participate in this study was provided by the participants' legal guardian/next of kin. The animal study was reviewed and approved by the Ethics Review Committee of Paris Descartes University.

AUTHOR CONTRIBUTIONS

HL, BS, SCh, VC, MS, FG, and CC: experiments. HL and XD: writing - original draft preparation. BS, SCi, and XD: writing - review and editing. SCi and XD: supervision. All authors have read and agreed to the submitted version of the manuscript.

REFERENCES

Abbott, N. J. (2002). Astrocyte-endothelial interactions and blood-brain barrier permeability. *J. Anat.* 200, 629–638. doi: 10.1046/j.1469-7580.2002.00064.x

Abbott, N. J., Ronnback, L., and Hansson, E. (2006). Astrocyte-endothelial interactions at the blood-brain barrier. *Nat. Rev. Neurosci.* 7, 41–53. doi: 10.1038/nrn1824

Agarwal, S., Uchida, Y., Mittapalli, R. K., Sane, R., Terasaki, T., and Elmquist, W. F. (2012). Quantitative proteomics of transporter expression in brain capillary endothelial cells isolated from P-glycoprotein (P-gp), breast cancer resistance protein (Bcrp), and P-gp/Bcrp knockout mice. *Drug Metab. Dispos.* 40, 1164–1169. doi: 10.1124/dmd.112.044719

Ambrus, L., Kelemen, B., Szabo, T., Biro, T., and Toth, B. I. (2017). Human podocytes express functional thermosensitive TRPV channels. *Br. J. Pharmacol.* 174, 4493–4507. doi: 10.1111/bph.14052

Ball, K., Bouzom, F., Scherrmann, J. M., Walther, B., and Decleves, X. (2013). Physiologically based pharmacokinetic modelling of drug penetration across the blood-brain barrier–towards a mechanistic IVIVE-based approach. *AAPS J.* 15, 913–932. doi: 10.1208/s12248-013-9496-0

Beggs, S., Liu, X. J., Kwan, C., and Salter, M. W. (2010). Peripheral nerve injury and TRPV1-expressing primary afferent C-fibers cause opening of the blood-brain barrier. *Mol. Pain* 6:74.

Benfenati, V., Amiry-Moghaddam, M., Caprini, M., Mylonakou, M. N., Rapisarda, C., Ottersen, O. P., et al. (2007). Expression and functional characterization of transient receptor potential vanilloid-related channel 4 (TRPV4) in rat cortical astrocytes. *Neuroscience* 148, 876–892. doi: 10.1016/j.neuroscience.2007.06.039

Berrout, J., Jin, M., and O'Neil, R. G. (2012). Critical role of TRPP2 and TRPC1 channels in stretch-induced injury of blood-brain barrier endothelial cells. *Brain Res.* 1436, 1–12. doi: 10.1016/j.brainres.2011.11.044

Binshtok, A. M., Bean, B. P., and Woolf, C. J. (2007). Inhibition of nociceptors by TRPV1-mediated entry of impermeant sodium channel blockers. *Nature* 449, 607–610.

Brown, R. C., and Davis, T. P. (2002). Calcium modulation of adherens and tight junction function: a potential mechanism for blood-brain barrier disruption after stroke. *Stroke* 33, 1706–1711. doi: 10.1161/01.str.0000016405.06729.83

Brown, R. C., Wu, L., Hicks, K., and O'Neil, R. G. (2008). Regulation of blood-brain barrier permeability by transient receptor potential type C and type v calcium-permeable channels. *Microcirculation* 15, 359–371. doi: 10.1080/10739680701762656

Calapai, F., Cardia, L., Sorbara, E. E., Navarra, M., Gangemi, S., Calapai, G., et al. (2020). Cannabinoids, blood-brain barrier, and brain disposition. *Pharmaceutics* 12:265. doi: 10.3390/pharmaceutics12030265

Cavanaugh, D. J., Chesler, A. T., Jackson, A. C., Sigal, Y. M., Yamanaka, H., Grant, R., et al. (2011). Trpv1 reporter mice reveal highly restricted brain distribution and functional expression in arteriolar smooth muscle cells. *J. Neurosci.* 31, 5067–5077. doi: 10.1523/jneurosci.6451-10.2011

Chaves, C., Campanelli, F., Chapy, H., Gomez-Zepeda, D., Glacial, F., Smirnova, M., et al. (2020). An interspecies molecular and functional study of organic cation transporters at the blood-brain barrier: from rodents to humans. *Pharmaceutics* 12:308. doi: 10.3390/pharmaceutics12040308

Dauchy, S., Miller, F., Couraud, P. O., Weaver, R. J., Weksler, B., Romero, I. A., et al. (2009). Expression and transcriptional regulation of ABC transporters and cytochromes P450 in hCMEC/D3 human cerebral microvascular endothelial cells. *Biochem. Pharmacol.* 77, 897–909. doi: 10.1016/j.bcp.2008.11.001

De Bock, M., Wang, N., Decrock, E., Bol, M., Gadicherla, A. K., Culot, M., et al. (2013). Endothelial calcium dynamics, connexin channels and blood-brain barrier function. *Prog. Neurobiol.* 108, 1–20. doi: 10.1016/j.pneurobio.2013.06.001

Deo, A. K., Theil, F. P., and Nicolas, J. M. (2013). Confounding parameters in preclinical assessment of blood-brain barrier permeation: an overview with emphasis on species differences and effect of disease states. *Mol. Pharm.* 10, 1581–1595. doi: 10.1021/mp300570z

Dragoni, S., and Turowski, P. (2018). Polarised VEGFA Signalling at Vascular Blood-Neural Barriers. *Int. J. Mol. Sci.* 19:1378. doi: 10.3390/ijms19051378

Fliniaux, I., Germain, E., Farfariello, V., and Prevarskaya, N. (2018). TRPs and Ca(2+) in cell death and survival. *Cell Calc.* 69, 4–18. doi: 10.1016/j.ceca.2017.07.002

Flockerzi, V. (2007). An introduction on TRP channels. *Handb. Exper. Pharmacol.* 68, 619–647.

Golech, S. A., McCarron, R. M., Chen, Y., Bembry, J., Lenz, F., Mechoulam, R., et al. (2004). Human brain endothelium: coexpression and function of vanilloid and endocannabinoid receptors. *Brain Res. Mol. Brain Res.* 132, 87–92. doi: 10.1016/j.molbrainres.2004.08.025

Grace, M. S., Baxter, M., Dubuis, E., Birrell, M. A., and Belvisi, M. G. (2014). Transient receptor potential (TRP) channels in the airway: role in airway disease. *Br. J. Pharmacol.* 171, 2593–2607. doi: 10.1111/bph.12538

Greco, C., Leclerc-Mercier, S., Chaumon, S., Doz, F., Hadj-Rabia, S., Molina, T., et al. (2020). Use of epidermal growth factor receptor inhibitor erlotinib to treat palmoplantar keratoderma in patients with olmsted syndrome caused by TRPV3 mutations. *JAMA Dermatol.* 156, 191–195. doi: 10.1001/jamadermatol.2019.4126

Guerra, G., Lucariello, A., Perna, A., Botta, L., De Luca, A., and Moccia, F. (2018). The role of endothelial Ca(2+) signaling in neurovascular coupling: a view from the lumen. *Intern. J. Mol. Sci.* 19:938. doi: 10.3390/ijms19040938

Harraz, O. F., Longden, T. A., Hill-Eubanks, D., and Nelson, M. T. (2018). PIP2 depletion promotes TRPV4 channel activity in mouse brain capillary endothelial cells. *eLife* 7:e38689.

Hatano, N., Suzuki, H., Itoh, Y., and Muraki, K. (2013). TRPV4 partially participates in proliferation of human brain capillary endothelial cells. *Life Sci.* 92, 317–324. doi: 10.1016/j.lfs.2013.01.002

Hind, W. H., England, T. J., and O'Sullivan, S. E. (2016). Cannabidiol protects an in vitro model of the blood-brain barrier from oxygen-glucose deprivation via PPARgamma and 5-HT1A receptors. *Br. J. Pharmacol.* 173, 815–825. doi: 10.1111/bph.13368

Hu, D. E., Easton, A. S., and Fraser, P. A. (2005). TRPV1 activation results in disruption of the blood-brain barrier in the rat. *Br. J. Pharmacol.* 146, 576–584. doi: 10.1038/sj.bjp.0706350

Huang, Q., Wang, X., Lin, X., Zhang, J., You, X., and Shao, A. (2020). The role of transient receptor potential channels in blood-brain barrier dysfunction after ischemic stroke. *Biomed. Pharmacother.* 131:110647. doi: 10.1016/j.biopha.2020.110647

Ito, K., Uchida, Y., Ohtsuki, S., Aizawa, S., Kawakami, H., Katsukura, Y., et al. (2011). Quantitative membrane protein expression at the blood-brain barrier of adult and younger cynomolgus monkeys. *J. Pharm. Sci.* 100, 3939–3950. doi: 10.1002/jps.22487

Kassmann, M., Harteneck, C., Zhu, Z., Nurnberg, B., Tepel, M., and Gollasch, M. (2013). Transient receptor potential vanilloid 1 (TRPV1), TRPV4, and the kidney. *Acta Physiol.* 207, 546–564. doi: 10.1111/apha.12051

Kauer, J. A., and Gibson, H. E. (2009). Hot flash: TRPV channels in the brain. *Trends Neurosci.* 32, 215–224. doi: 10.1016/j.tins.2008.12.006

Kealy, J., Greene, C., and Campbell, M. (2020). Blood-brain barrier regulation in psychiatric disorders. *Neurosci. Lett.* 726:133664. doi: 10.1016/j.neulet.2018.06.033

Kohler, R., Heyken, W. T., Heinau, P., Schubert, R., Si, H., Kacik, M., et al. (2006). Evidence for a functional role of endothelial transient receptor potential V4 in shear stress-induced vasodilatation. *Arterioscler. Thromb. Vasc. Biol.* 26, 1495–1502. doi: 10.1161/01.atv.0000225698.36212.6a

Koles, L., Garcao, P., Zadori, Z. S., Ferreira, S. G., Pinheiro, B. S., da Silva-Santos, C. S., et al. (2013). Presynaptic TRPV1 vanilloid receptor function is age- but not CB1 cannabinoid receptor-dependent in the rodent forebrain. *Brain Res. Bull.* 97, 126–135. doi: 10.1016/j.brainresbull.2013.06.007

Luo, H., Rossi, E., Saubamea, B., Chasseigneaux, S., Cochois, V., Choublier, N., et al. (2019). Cannabidiol increases proliferation, migration, tubulogenesis, and integrity of human brain endothelial cells through TRPV2 activation. *Mol. Pharm.* 16, 1312–1326. doi: 10.1021/acs.molpharmaceut.8b01252

Luo, J., and Hu, H. (2014). Thermally activated TRPV3 channels. *Curr. Top. Membr.* 74, 325–364. doi: 10.1016/b978-0-12-800181-3.00012-9

Ma, X., and Liu, W. (2019). Calcium signaling in brain microvascular endothelial cells and its roles in the function of the blood-brain barrier. *Neuroreport* 30, 1271–1277. doi: 10.1097/wnr.0000000000001357

Mangos, S., Liu, Y., and Drummond, I. A. (2007). Dynamic expression of the osmosensory channel trpv4 in multiple developing organs in zebrafish. *Gene Expr. Patter.* 7, 480–484. doi: 10.1016/j.modgep.2006.10.011

Mannari, T., Morita, S., Furube, E., Tominaga, M., and Miyata, S. (2013). Astrocytic TRPV1 ion channels detect blood-borne signals in the sensory circumventricular organs of adult mouse brains. *Glia* 61, 957–971. doi: 10.1002/glia.22488

Marrelli, S. P., O'Neil, R. G., Brown, R. C., and Bryan, R. M. Jr. (2007). *PLA2* and TRPV4 channels regulate endothelial calcium in cerebral arteries. *Am. J. Physiol. Heart Circ. Physiol.* 292, H1390–H1397.

Mecha, M., Feliu, A., Inigo, P. M., Mestre, L., Carrillo-Salinas, F. J., and Guaza, C. (2013). Cannabidiol provides long-lasting protection against the deleterious effects of inflammation in a viral model of multiple sclerosis: a role for A2A receptors. *Neurobiol. Dis.* 59, 141–150. doi: 10.1016/j.nbd.2013.06.016

Mergler, S., Valtink, M., Coulson-Thomas, V. J., Lindemann, D., Reinach, P. S., Engelmann, K., et al. (2010). TRPV channels mediate temperature-sensing in human corneal endothelial cells. *Exp. Eye Res.* 90, 758–770. doi: 10.1016/j.exer.2010.03.010

Mickle, A. D., Shepherd, A. J., and Mohapatra, D. P. (2015). Sensory TRP channels: the key transducers of nociception and pain. *Prog. Mol. Biol. Transl. Sci.* 131, 73–118. doi: 10.1007/978-3-319-18705-1_3

Montell, C. (2001). Physiology, phylogeny, and functions of the TRP superfamily of cation channels. *Sci. STKE* 2001:re1. doi: 10.1126/stke.2001.90.re1

Moran, M. M. (2018). TRP channels as potential drug targets. *Annu. Rev. Pharmacol. Toxicol.* 58, 309–330.

Nedungadi, T. P., Dutta, M., Bathina, C. S., Caterina, M. J., and Cunningham, J. T. (2012). Expression and distribution of TRPV2 in rat brain. *Exp. Neurol.* 237, 223–237. doi: 10.1016/j.expneurol.2012.06.017

Ohtsuki, S., Ikeda, C., Uchida, Y., Sakamoto, Y., Miller, F., Glacial, F., et al. (2013). Quantitative targeted absolute proteomic analysis of transporters, receptors and junction proteins for validation of human cerebral microvascular endothelial cell line hCMEC/D3 as a human blood-brain barrier model. *Mol. Pharm.* 10, 289–296. doi: 10.1021/mp3004308

Peng, J. B., Suzuki, Y., Gyimesi, G., and Hediger, M. A. (2018). "TRPV5 and TRPV6 calcium-selective channels," in *Calcium Entry Channels in Non-Excitable Cells*, eds J. A. Kozak and J. W. Putney Jr. (Boca Raton, FL: CRC Press), 241–274. doi: 10.1201/9781315152592-13

Perriere, N., Demeuse, P., Garcia, E., Regina, A., Debray, M., Andreux, J. P., et al. (2005). Puromycin-based purification of rat brain capillary endothelial cell cultures. Effect on the expression of blood-brain barrier-specific properties. *J. Neurochem.* 93, 279–289. doi: 10.1111/j.1471-4159.2004.03020.x

Perriere, N., Yousif, S., Cazaubon, S., Chaverot, N., Bourasset, F., Cisternino, S., et al. (2007). A functional in vitro model of rat blood-brain barrier for molecular analysis of efflux transporters. *Brain Res.* 1150, 1–13. doi: 10.1016/j.brainres.2007.02.091

Phuong, T. T. T., Redmon, S. N., Yarishkin, O., Winter, J. M., Li, D. Y., and Krizaj, D. (2017). Calcium influx through TRPV4 channels modulates the adherens contacts between retinal microvascular endothelial cells. *J. Physiol.* 595, 6869–6885. doi: 10.1113/jp275052

Qin, N., Neeper, M. P., Liu, Y., Hutchinson, T. L., Lubin, M. L., and Flores, C. M. (2008). TRPV2 is activated by cannabidiol and mediates CGRP release in cultured rat dorsal root ganglion neurons. *J. Neurosci.* 28, 6231–6238. doi: 10.1523/jneurosci.0504-08.2008

Rigoni, M., Trevisani, M., Gazzieri, D., Nadaletto, R., Tognetto, M., Creminon, C., et al. (2003). Neurogenic responses mediated by vanilloid receptor-1 (TRPV1) are blocked by the high affinity antagonist, iodo-resiniferatoxin. *Br. J. Pharmacol.* 138, 977–985. doi: 10.1038/sj.bjp.0705110

Rodrigues, T., Sieglitz, F., and Bernardes, G. J. (2016). Natural product modulators of transient receptor potential (TRP) channels as potential anti-cancer agents. *Chem. Soc. Rev.* 45, 6130–6137. doi: 10.1039/c5cs00916b

Ruiz-Valdepenas, L., Martinez-Orgado, J. A., Benito, C., Millan, A., Tolon, R. M., and Romero, J. (2011). Cannabidiol reduces lipopolysaccharide-induced vascular changes and inflammation in the mouse brain: an intravital microscopy study. *J. Neuroinflamm.* 8:5. doi: 10.1186/1742-2094-8-5

Shibasaki, K., Tominaga, M., and Ishizaki, Y. (2015). Hippocampal neuronal maturation triggers post-synaptic clustering of brain temperature-sensor TRPV4. *Biochem. Biophys. Res. Commun.* 458, 168–173. doi: 10.1016/j.bbrc.2015.01.087

Smani, T., Gomez, L. J., Regodon, S., Woodard, G. E., Siegfried, G., Khatib, A. M., et al. (2018). TRP channels in angiogenesis and other endothelial functions. *Front. Physiol.* 9:1731. doi: 10.3389/fphys.2018.01731

Steinritz, D., Stenger, B., Dietrich, A., Gudermann, T., and Popp, T. (2018). TRPs in Tox: involvement of transient receptor potential-channels in chemical-induced organ toxicity-A structured review. *Cells* 7:98. doi: 10.3390/cells7080098

Sullivan, M. N., Francis, M., Pitts, N. L., Taylor, M. S., and Earley, S. (2012). Optical recording reveals novel properties of GSK1016790A-induced vanilloid transient receptor potential channel TRPV4 activity in primary human endothelial cells. *Mol. Pharmacol.* 82, 464–472. doi: 10.1124/mol.112.078584

Sweeney, M. D., Zhao, Z., Montagne, A., Nelson, A. R., and Zlokovic, B. V. (2019). Blood-brain barrier: from physiology to disease and Back. *Physiol. Rev.* 99, 21–78. doi: 10.1152/physrev.00050.2017

Syvanen, S., Lindhe, O., Palner, M., Kornum, B. R., Rahman, O., Langstrom, B., et al. (2009). Species differences in blood-brain barrier transport of three positron emission tomography radioligands with emphasis on P-glycoprotein transport. *Drug Metab. Dispos.* 37, 635–643. doi: 10.1124/dmd.108.024745

Uchida, Y., Ohtsuki, S., Katsukura, Y., Ikeda, C., Suzuki, T., Kamiie, J., et al. (2011). Quantitative targeted absolute proteomics of human blood-brain barrier transporters and receptors. *J. Neurochem.* 117, 333–345. doi: 10.1111/j.1471-4159.2011.07208.x

Vanlandewijck, M., He, L., Mae, M. A., Andrae, J., Ando, K., Del Gaudio, F., et al. (2018). A molecular atlas of cell types and zonation in the brain vasculature. *Nature* 554, 475–480. doi: 10.1038/nature25739

Villalta, P. C., and Townsley, M. I. (2013). Transient receptor potential channels and regulation of lung endothelial permeability. *Pulm. Circ.* 3, 802–815. doi: 10.1086/674765

Weksler, B. B., Subileau, E. A., Perriere, N., Charneau, P., Holloway, K., Leveque, M., et al. (2005). Blood-brain barrier-specific properties of a human adult brain endothelial cell line. *FASEB J.* 19, 1872–1874. doi: 10.1096/fj.04-3458fje

Wen, W., Que, K., Zang, C., Wen, J., Sun, G., Zhao, Z., et al. (2017). Expression and distribution of three transient receptor potential vanilloid(TRPV) channel proteins in human odontoblast-like cells. *J. Mol. Histol.* 48, 367–377. doi: 10.1007/s10735-017-9735-2

Yang, C., Hawkins, K. E., Dore, S., and Candelario-Jalil, E. (2019). Neuroinflammatory mechanisms of blood-brain barrier damage in ischemic stroke. *Am. J. Physiol. Cell Physiol.* 316, C135–C153.

Yu, W., Hill, W. G., Apodaca, G., and Zeidel, M. L. (2011). Expression and distribution of transient receptor potential (TRP) channels in bladder epithelium. *Am. J. Physiol. Ren. Physiol.* 300, F49–F59.

Yu, X., Ji, C., and Shao, A. (2020). Neurovascular unit dysfunction and neurodegenerative disorders. *Front. Neurosci.* 14:334. doi: 10.3389/fphys.2018.00334

Zhang, A., Duchatelet, S., Lakdawala, N., Tower, R. L., Diamond, C., Marathe, K., et al. (2020). Targeted inhibition of the epidermal growth factor receptor and mammalian target of rapamycin signaling pathways in olmsted syndrome. *JAMA Dermatol.* 156, 196–200. doi: 10.1001/jamadermatol.2019.4141

Zhang, Y., Chen, K., Sloan, S. A., Bennett, M. L., Scholze, A. R., O'Keeffe, S., et al. (2014). An RNA-sequencing transcriptome and splicing database of glia, neurons, and vascular cells of the cerebral cortex. *J. Neurosci.* 34, 11929–11947. doi: 10.1523/jneurosci.1860-14.2014

12

TRPC6 Attenuates Cortical Astrocytic Apoptosis and Inflammation in Cerebral Ischemic/Reperfusion Injury

Lu Liu[1†], Manli Chen[1†], Kun Lin[1], Xuwu Xiang[1], Jing Yang[1], Yueying Zheng[1], Xiaoxing Xiong[1,2] and Shengmei Zhu[1*]*

[1] *Department of Anesthesiology, The First Affiliated Hospital, Zhejiang University School of Medicine, Hangzhou, China,*
[2] *Department of Neurosurgery, Renmin Hospital of Wuhan University, Wuhan, China*

Correspondence:
Shengmei Zhu
smzhu20088@zju.edu.cn
Xiaoxing Xiong
xiaoxingxiong@whu.edu.cn

†These authors share first authorship

Transient receptor potential canonical 6 (TRPC6) channel is an important non-selective cation channel with a variety of physiological roles in the central nervous system. Evidence has shown that TRPC6 is involved in the process of experimental stroke; however, the underlying mechanisms remain unclear. In the present study, the role of astrocytic TRPC6 was investigated in an oxygen–glucose deprivation cell model and middle cerebral artery occlusion (MCAO) mouse model of stroke. HYP9 (a selective TRPC6 agonist) and SKF96365 (SKF; a TRPC antagonist) were used to clarify the exact functions of TRPC6 in astrocytes after ischemic stroke. TRPC6 was significantly downregulated during ischemia/reperfusion (IR) injury in cultured astrocytes and in cortices of MCAO mice. Application of HYP9 *in vivo* alleviated the brain infarct lesion, astrocytes population, apoptosis, and interleukin-6 (IL-6) and IL-1β release in mouse cortices after ischemia. HYP9 dose-dependently inhibited the downregulation of TRPC6 and reduced astrocytic apoptosis, cytotoxicity and inflammatory responses in IR insult, whereas SKF aggravated the damage *in vitro*. In addition, modulation of TRPC6 channel diminished IR-induced Ca^{2+} entry in astrocytes. Furthermore, decreased Ca^{2+} entry due to TRPC6 contributed to reducing nuclear factor kappa light chain enhancer of activated B cells (NF-κB) nuclear translocation and phosphorylation. Overexpression of astrocytic TRPC6 also attenuated apoptosis, cytotoxicity, inflammatory responses, and NF-κB phosphorylation in modeled ischemia in astrocytes. The results of the present study indicate that the TRPC6 channel can act as a potential target to reduce both inflammatory responses and apoptosis in astrocytes during IR injury, subsequently attenuating ischemic brain damage. In addition, we provide a novel view of stroke therapy by targeting the astrocytic TRPC6 channel.

Keywords: apoptosis, astrocytes, Ca^{2+}, inflammation, ischemic stroke, NF-κB, TRPC6

INTRODUCTION

The transient receptor potential (TRP) channels are cation-permeable membrane proteins with common structural features of six transmembrane segments. Based on the homology of amino acid sequences, the TRP superfamily can be subdivided into seven subfamilies: TRPC (canonical), TRPV (vanilloid), TRPM (melastatin), TRPA (ankyrin), TRPN (*Drosophila* NOMPC), TRPP (polycystin), and TRPML (mucolipin) (Venkatachalam and Montell, 2007). Among the channels, the TRPC channel, which is most closely related to *Drosophila* TRPs, is widely distributed in different tissues and governs the fate and functions of various cell types (Curcic et al., 2019). TRPCs are broadly expressed in brain, lung, heart, kidney, liver, spleen, and other organs in mammalian animals like human, mouse, rat, and rabbit (Montell, 2001; Venkatachalam and Montell, 2007). In terms of similarity to amino acid sequences and function, TRPC members can be further classified into four subgroups: TRPC1, TRPC2, TRPC4/5, and TRPC3/6/7 (Wang et al., 2020a).

The TRPC6 channel is emerging as an important target for the control of Ca^{2+} currents in a wide range of disorders, including immune-mediated diseases, pulmonary arterial hypertension, atherosclerosis, and central nervous system (CNS)-related diseases, such as autism spectrum disorders, glioma, depression, traumatic brain injuries, seizure, Alzheimer's disease, and ischemic stroke (Hamid and Newman, 2009; Ding et al., 2010; Du et al., 2010; Griesi-Oliveira et al., 2015; Kim and Kang, 2015; Zhang et al., 2015, 2016; Pochwat et al., 2018; Ramirez et al., 2018; Chen et al., 2019). TRPC6 is abundantly expressed in various anatomical regions of the CNS, such as the cerebellum, hippocampus, middle frontal gyrus, and cortex (Riccio et al., 2002; Du et al., 2010). As a regulator of Ca^{2+} influx, TRPC6 is involved in neuronal survival, synapse formation, neuronal nerve-growth-cone guidance, and sensory transduction (Li et al., 2005; Jia et al., 2007; Zhou et al., 2008; Quick et al., 2012). Dysfunction of the TRPC6 channel may trigger a series of downstream events and neurobiological disorders.

Ischemic stroke is a life-threatening condition caused by a vascular embolism due to cardiac events, artery-to-artery embolism, or *in-situ* small artery disease (Hankey, 2017). Several underlying mechanisms, including excitotoxicity, ionic imbalance, oxidative and nitrative stress, inflammation, and apoptosis, are involved in the pathophysiological process of cerebral ischemia (Khoshnam et al., 2017). Ca^{2+} overload has a critical role and initiates the ischemic cascade during brain ischemia/reperfusion (IR) injury. Increasing evidence indicates an important role of TRPC6 in cerebral IR injury (Liu et al., 2020). TRPC6 is identified on cortical neurons and astrocytes, and is downregulated in neurons after brain ischemic injury (Du et al., 2010; Guo et al., 2017; Qu et al., 2017; Shirakawa et al., 2017). Notably, maintaining the TRPC6 protein level in neurons improves neuronal survival and behavioral performance, thus alleviating ischemic brain damage (Du et al., 2010; Guo et al., 2017). However, the roles of the TRPC6 channel in mouse cortical astrocytes following IR injury have not been evaluated.

In the present study, the specific effects of astrocytic TRPC6 on ischemic stroke were investigated. TRPC6 protein expression in primary mouse astrocytes was downregulated following IR injury. Inhibition of TRPC6 downregulation via HYP9 or TRPC6 overexpression protected astrocytes and the brain against IR insults. These results indicate that the TRPC6 channel contributes to neuroprotection in cerebral ischemia by promoting astrocyte survival. Furthermore, this study provides therapeutic evidence for the treatment of ischemic stroke by targeting the TRPC6 channel.

MATERIALS AND METHODS

Animals

C57BL/6J male mice 8–10 weeks of age were purchased from Shanghai SLAC Laboratory Animal Co., Ltd. (Shanghai, China). All animal experiments were approved by the Animal Care Committee of the First Affiliated Hospital at Zhejiang University. Mice were housed in polypropylene cages and maintained at $25 \pm 1°C$ under 12 h light/12 h dark cycles with free access to rodent chow and water. Mice were randomly allocated to each group before any treatment. Proper anesthetic procedures were used to ensure that the mice did not suffer unnecessarily during or after the experimental procedure. A total of 82 mice were used in this study (including 10 mice that died).

In vivo Model of Focal Cerebral Ischemia

Focal cerebral ischemia was induced by middle cerebral artery occlusion (MCAO). Animals were anesthetized with 1% sodium pentobarbital (75–100 mg/kg, intraperitoneal injection); body temperature was maintained at $37 \pm 0.5°C$ during the operation using a heating pad. Transient MCAO was generally performed as previously reported (Lin et al., 2013a). Briefly, the left common carotid artery was exposed to separate the internal carotid artery (ICA) and the external carotid artery (ECA). Next, a 6-0 monofilament nylon suture (RWD Life Science Co., LTD, Shenzhen, China) with a rounded tip was inserted through the exposed left ICA and advanced into the middle cerebral artery. After 1 h of occlusion, the filament was gently withdrawn to allow reperfusion. At 24 h after reperfusion, animals were sacrificed and the brain tissues were obtained for future assays.

Intracerebroventricular Injection

Mouse intracerebroventricular injection was performed using a stereotaxic instrument (RWD Life Science Co., Ltd., Shenzhen, China) with a micro-syringe pump under anesthesia. Drugs or vehicle (5 μL in total) were slowly injected (1 μL/min) into the left ventricle at a depth of 2.5 mm below the brain surface, 1.0 mm lateral and 0.5 mm posterior to the bregma. After injection, animals were allowed to recover from anesthesia under a heating pad.

Cell Culture

As previously reported(Shen et al., 2016), primary astrocytes from cerebral cortices of 0–1-day-old post-natal C57BL/6 mice were isolated under sterile conditions. Astrocytes were grown in culture medium [Dulbecco's modified Eagle's medium (DMEM) containing 10% fetal bovine serum and 1% penicillin/streptomycin]. Dissociated cortical cells were seeded onto poly-D-lysine (PDL, 10 μg/mL; # P7405; Sigma-Aldrich St. Louis, MO, USA)-coated T-75 flasks (Costar; Corning Inc., Corning, NY, USA) at a density of three cortices per flask and incubated at 37°C with 5% CO_2 in a humidified incubator. The medium was changed every other day. After 8–10 days, confluent cultures were shaken (250 rpm at 37°C) for 12 h to reduce microglial contamination. Then, purified astrocytes were cultured in medium supplemented with 20 μM cytosine-1-β-D-arabinofuranosid (Sigma-Aldrich) for the next 2–3 days. The remaining attached cells were digested with 0.25% trypsin

(#25200056; Gibco, Grand Island, NY, USA) and then reseeded at a density of 0.03–0.05 × $10^6/cm^2$ in PDL-coated six-well plates at 37°C in an incubator with 5% CO_2. After 5–7 days when the astrocytes reached 90–95% confluence, cells were prepared for subsequent experiments. More than 95% of cells in culture were astrocytes (results not shown).

Oxygen-Glucose Deprivation and Re-oxygenation (OGD/R)

OGD/R experiments were established to mimic the *in vitro* condition of IR injury. The cultures were incubated for 1–4 h in DMEM medium without glucose in a humidified incubator chamber at 37°C with 95% N_2 and 5% CO_2. Subsequently, the astrocytes were returned to the original culture conditions and then incubated under normoxic conditions for the next 24 h.

Drugs and Experimental Groups

The TRPC6-specific agonist HYP9 (Leuner et al., 2010) (#H9791; Sigma-Aldrich), dissolved in dimethyl sulfoxide (DMSO; the final maximum DMSO concentration was <0.05%), was used to determine the role of TRCP6 in astrocytes following IR injury. To verify the optimum concentration, 0, 1, 5, 10, 15, 20, or 30 µM HYP9 was preincubated *in vitro*. SKF96365 (SKF; #ab120280; Abcam, Cambridge, MA, USA) was originally recognized as a major inhibitor of TRPC channels (Singh et al., 2010). In the present study, SKF (dissolved in deionized water) at 0, 0.05, 0.5, 5, 10, 20, 30, or 40 µM concentration was used to treat primary mouse astrocytes. The *in vitro* groups consisted of eight subgroups: (1) control group (CON + Naive); (2) control combined with vehicle (DMSO) group (CON + Vehicle); (3) control combined with HYP9 (15 µM) group (CON + HYP9); (4) control combined with SKF (30 µM) group (CON + SKF); (5) OGD/R group (OGD + Naive); (6) OGD/R combined with vehicle (DMSO) group (OGD + Vehicle); (7) OGD/R combined with HYP9 (15 µM) group (OGD + HYP9); (8) OGD/R combined with SKF (30 µM) group (OGD + SKF).

Animals were randomly assigned into eight groups before any procedure as follows: (1) sham operation group (sham + Naive) (n = 9); (2) sham operation combined with vehicle (DMSO) group (sham + Vehicle) (n = 3); (3) sham operation combined with HYP9 (5 µg) group (sham + HYP9) (n = 3); (4) sham operation combined with SKF (20 µg) group (sham + SKF) (n = 3); (5) MCAO operation group (MCAO + Naive) (n = 18); (6) MCAO operation combined with DMSO group (MCAO + Vehicle) (n = 12); (7) MCAO operation combined with HYP9 (5 µg) group (MCAO + HYP9) (n = 12); (8) MCAO operation combined with SKF (20 µg) group (MCAO + SKF) (n = 12). **Figure 1** shows the experiment paradigm.

Lentivirus Infection

Lentivirus vectors were chemically synthesized by Obio Technology (Shanghai) Corp., Ltd. To overexpress astrocytic TRPC6, we infected primary astrocytes with lentiviruses carrying FLAG-tagged full-length mCherry-WT-TRPC6 (WT-TRPC6) or mCherry-WT-TRPC6-null (Vehicle1). Besides, to knock down TRPC6 in primary astrocytes, lentiviruses

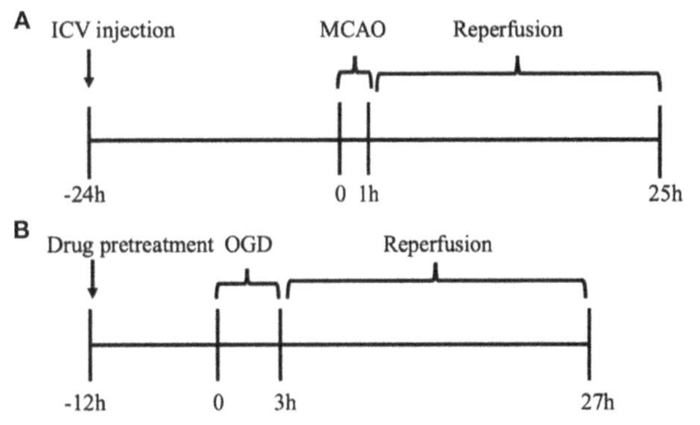

FIGURE 1 | Experiment paradigm. **(A)** *In vivo* cohort for MCAO model of ischemic stroke in mice. The drugs were administrated into left ventricles 24 h before MCAO. **(B)** *In vitro* cohort for OGD/R experiment in primary mouse astrocytes. After 12 h pre-incubation of drugs, OGD/R was developed in cultured astrocytes.

carrying mCherry-shRNA-TRPC6 (sh-TRPC6) or mCherry-shRNA-TRPC6-null (Vehicle2) were used to infect primary cortical astrocytes. Targeted sequences for TRPC6 and Vehicle2 siRNAs are: GCTTGCCAACATTGAGAAA and TTCTCCGAACGTGTCACGT, respectively. Astrocytes at 70% confluence were infected with lentiviruses according to the vendor's protocol. After 72 96 h lentiviral infection, astrocytes were used for subsequent experiments. The efficiency of infections was detected by western bolts.

TTC Staining

Animals were sacrificed at 24 h after reperfusion. The infarct volume was tested based on 2,3,5-triphenyltetrazolium chloride (TTC) staining. The brains were sectioned into 2-mm coronal slices using a brain matrix. The brain slices were incubated in 2% TTC solution staining for 20 min at 37°C and then fixed in 4% paraformaldehyde (PFA). The ischemic volume was quantified using ImageJ software (version 2.0). The infarct percentage was shown as the ratio of the ischemic area to the entire slice area.

Analysis of Cell Viability and Lactate Dehydrogenase (LDH) Release

An LDH release quantification kit (#11644793001; Sigma-Aldrich) was used to evaluate cell viability. The cell-free supernatant was obtained by centrifugation at ~250 × g for 10 min. Subsequently, the supernatant was incubated in working solutions in the dark for 1 h at room temperature (~22°C). The absorbance of the samples was measured at 490 nm using a microplate reader (SpectraMax i3x; Molecular Devices, Sunnyvale, CA, USA). To determine the cytotoxicity percentage, all groups were compared with the control groups.

Flow Cytometry

The flow cytometry measurement of astrocyte apoptosis and Ca^{2+} concentration was performed using a BD flow cytometer (BD Biosciences, San Jose, CA, USA). Astrocytes were digested with trypsin. The harvested cells were washed with phosphate-buffered saline (PBS) twice before incubating in buffer containing 5 μL of fluorescein isothiocyanate-annexin V and 5 μL of propidium iodide or 0.5 μg/ml DAPI for 15 min at room temperature in the dark. Subsequently, the cells were detected and analyzed.

The Ca^{2+} concentration was also measured using the BD flow cytometer. Cortical astrocytes were loaded with 2 μM Fluo-4 AM (#F14217; Invitrogen, Carlsbad, CA, USA) in culture medium for 1 h at 37°C in an incubator with 5% CO_2. Next, the medium was changed to Hank's balanced salt solution (#14025092; Gibco) and the astrocytes were incubated for another 30 min at 37°C. Then, the astrocytes were collected and analyzed using flow cytometry.

Western Blot

Western blot analysis was performed as previously described with slight modifications (Li et al., 2020). Samples (20–40 μg) were separated on 12% gels and transferred onto 0.45-μm polyvinylidene difluoride membranes (#IPVH00010; Millipore, Billerica, MA, USA). Membranes were blocked with 5% skim milk for 1 h and then incubated with the following primary antibodies at 4°C overnight: TRPC6 (1;1,000; #21403; SAB Biotherapeutics, Sioux Falls, SD, USA), caspase-3 (1:1,000; #ab214430; Abcam, Cambridge, MA, USA), NF-κB (1:1,000; #6956S; Cell Signaling Technology), phospho-NF-κB (1:1,000; #3033S, Cell Signaling Technology), IL-1β (1:2,000; #ab9722; Abcam), Flag (1:1000; # F1804, Sigma-Aldrich), β-actin (1:2,000; #60008-1-Ig; Proteintech, Rosemont, IL, USA). Then, the membranes were incubated for 1 h with secondary antibodies (1:8,000; #SA00001-1 and #SA00001-2; Proteintech). Protein-specific signals were visualized using the Bio-Rad ChemiDoc™ MP imaging system (Hercules, CA, USA).

Immunofluorescence

Brain tissues were cut into 20 μm slices using a cryostat (#CM1950; Leica, Wetzlar, Germany). Tissues were blocked in 5% goat serum containing 0.3% Triton X-100 for 1 h at 37°C and then incubated with the following primary antibodies overnight at 4°C: GFAP (1:400; #80788S and #3670S; Cell Signaling Technology), TRPC6 (1:100; #ab62461; Abcam). Next, the slices were washed with PBS and incubated with secondary fluorescent antibodies (1:100; #SA00013-1, SA00013-2, SA00013-3, or SA00013-4; Proteintech) for 1 h at room temperature. In addition, 4′,6-iamidino-2-phenylindole, dihydrochloride (DAPI; 1 μg/mL; #4083; Cell Signaling Technology) staining was used to visualize the nuclei. Images were acquired using a confocal laser-scanning microscope (Nikon A1 Ti, 600× magnification; Leica TCS SP8, 400× magnification).

Astrocytes plated on glass coverslips 12 mm in diameter were collected and fixed in 4% PFA for 15 min at room temperature. Subsequently, the fixed cells were permeabilized with 0.1% Triton X-100 for 15 min at room temperature followed by blocking in 10% goat serum at 37°C for 30 min. Before incubation with secondary fluorescent antibodies, the astrocytes were labeled with the following primary antibodies: GFAP (1:400; #80788S and #3670S; Cell Signaling Technology), NF-κB (1:100; #6956S; Cell Signaling Technology). Next, DAPI (1 μg/mL) was used to stain nuclei. Specific fluorescent signals were tested using a confocal microscope (Leica TCS SP8, 630× or 1,890× magnification).

Enzyme-Linked Immunosorbent Assay

The release of interleukin-6 (IL-6) and IL-1β from cortices and cultured astrocytes was quantified using enzyme-linked immunosorbent assay (IL-6, #70-EK206HS; IL-1β, #70-EK201BHS-96; MULTI SCIENCES, Hangzhou, China). The experiments were performed according to the manufacturer's instructions. The final absorbance was detected at 450 nm and the background correction was set at 570 nm on a microplate reader (SpectraMax i3x; Molecular Devices).

Statistical Analyses

Data are presented as the means ± standard error of the mean (SEM) of at least three independent analyses. SPSS ver. 25.0 software (IBM Corp., Armonk, NY, USA) and GraphPad Prism 8.0 software (GraphPad Software, San Diego, CA, USA) were used for statistical analyses. One-way analysis of variance with Tukey's test for *post-hoc* analysis were performed. P-value <0.05 was considered statistically significant.

RESULTS

TRPC6 in Mouse Cortical Astrocytes Is Downregulated After Ischemia

In several studies, TRPC6 in neurons reportedly declines after cerebral ischemia, and maintaining the expression of neuronal TRPC6 protein contributes to neuronal survival and reduced cerebral ischemic insult (Du et al., 2010; Lin et al., 2013a; Guo et al., 2017). However, the role of the astrocytic TRPC6 channel after stroke remains unclear.

Astrocytes have provided important insights into ischemic stroke (Liu and Chopp, 2016). To confirm the vital functions of the astrocytic TRPC6 channel in cerebral ischemia, we established an *in vitro* model of stroke in primary mouse astrocytes using an OGD/R experiment. Astrocytes were exposed to 1–4 h of OGD followed by 24 h reperfusion. The apoptosis rate was elevated and cell viability was decreased in astrocytes following hypoxia injury (**Figures 2A–C**). The TRPC6 protein levels in astrocytes after OGD/R were significantly downregulated (**Figures 2D,F**). Conversely, the expression of the apoptosis-specific biomarker, cleaved caspase-3, was gradually increased after stroke compared with the control groups (**Figures 2D,E**). As shown in **Figures 2A–D**, 3 h OGD and 24 h reperfusion triggered appropriate hypoxic damage in astrocytes; thus, the subsequent *in vitro* OGD/R experiments were performed under this condition.

The *in vivo* stroke model is mimicked by MCAO in mice. Immunofluorescence signals showed that astrocytic TRPC6 was downregulated in the ischemic penumbra (**Figures 2G,H**). In parallel with the *in vitro* results, the TRPC6 protein level in peri-infarct areas was decreased compared with that in contralateral cortices (**Figures 2I,K**). In addition, after ischemic stroke, the cleaved caspase-3 expression in the ipsilateral hemisphere was upregulated compared with the contralateral hemisphere (**Figures 2I,J**). Furthermore, immunofluorescence

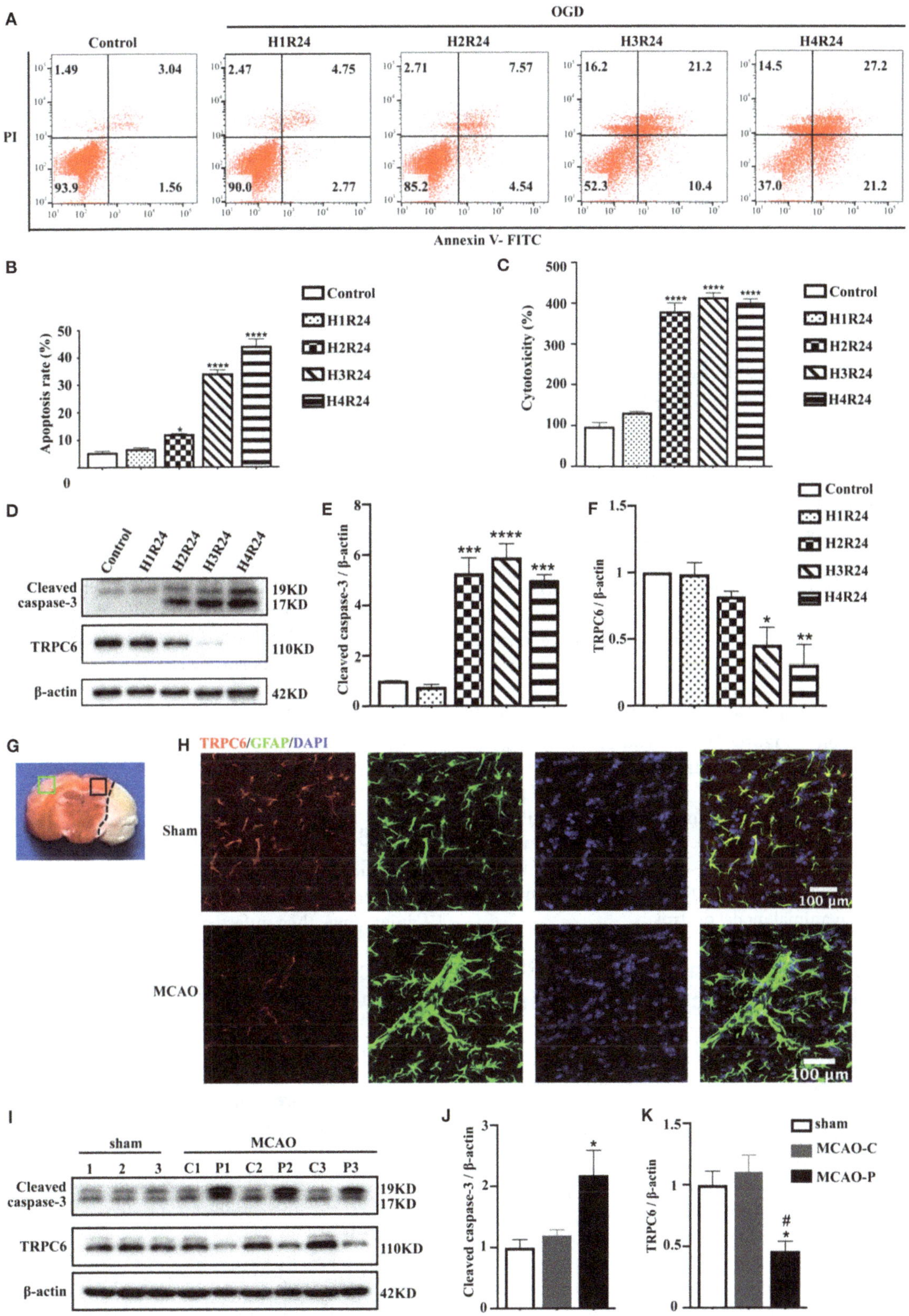

FIGURE 2 | TRPC6 in the cortical astrocytes is downregulated in ischemia. **(A)** Cultured astrocytes were exposed or not to OGD/R, and their apoptosis and death was detected by FITC/PI flow cytometry analysis. The percentage of apoptosis in scatter plots was presented as the proportion of apoptotic cells vs. total cell

(Continued)

FIGURE 2 | population (H1R24: 1 h OGD followed by 24 h reperfusion; H2R24: 2 h OGD followed by 24 h reperfusion; H3R24: 3 h OGD followed by 24 h reperfusion; H4R24: 4 h OGD followed by 24 h reperfusion). **(B)** Bar chart showed the statistical results of apoptosis rate measured by flow cytometry in each group in three independent experiments. Data were shown as mean ± SEM ($n = 3$). **(C)** LDH assay was used to measure the cytotoxicity of astrocytes in control and OGD groups. Data were shown as mean ± SEM ($n = 4$). **(D)** The protein level of TRPC6 and cleaved caspase-3 in astrocytes were tested by western blot analysis. β-actin was used as a loading control. **(E,F)** Quantifications of cleaved caspase-3 and TRPC6 protein levels shown in **(D)**. Data were shown as mean ± SEM ($n = 3$). **(G)** Brain slices with TTC staining. Green rectangle: contralateral cortex; Black rectangle: peri-infarct cortex. **(H)** Representative images of the cortex after sham or MCAO operation (peri-infarct cortex) double-stained with the TRPC6 (Red) and GFAP (Green) antibodies (Scar bar: 100 μm; 600× magnification). **(I)** Mice were exposed to sham operation or MCAO procedure ($n = 3$). The expressions of TRPC6 and cleaved caspase-3 in sham group (left hemisphere) and in contralateral (C) or peri-infarct (P) cortex were detected by western blotting. β-actin was used as a loading control. The number "1," "2," "3" represents cortices in each group were extracted form three different mice. **(J,K)** Quantifications of cleaved caspase-3 and TRPC6 protein levels shown in **(I)**. Data were shown as mean ± SEM ($n = 3$). MCAO-C, contralateral cortices in MCAO mice; MCAO-P, peri-infarct cortices in MCAO mice. $^*p < 0.05$, $^{**}p < 0.01$, $^{***}p < 0.001$, $^{****}p < 0.0001$ (all comparisons to control group or sham group). $^{\#}p < 0.05$ (comparisons to MCAO-C group).

signals showed that astrocytic TRPC6 was downregulated in the ischemic penumbra (**Figure 2H**).

These results indicate that IR injury-induced changes in TRPC6 channel protein levels may have important functions in brain ischemia.

Reducing IR-Mediated TRPC6 Downregulation With HYP9 Alleviates Ischemic Insults in the Mouse Cortex

Consequently, to determine the role of TRPC6 in an *in vivo* model of ischemic stroke, intraventricular administration of HYP9 or SKF was performed in mice. MCAO resulted in increased infarct size and pro-inflammatory cytokine release compared with the sham groups (**Figure 3**). Pretreatment with HYP9 alleviated cortical injury, reduced infarct volume (**Figures 3A,B**), astrocytic population (**Figure 3C**), cleaved caspase-3 expression (**Figures 3D,E**), and inhibited pro-inflammatory cytokine (IL-6 and IL-1β) generation after MCAO (**Figures 3G,H**). However, the effects of SKF on an animal model of stroke regarding infarction volume, astrocytic population, cleaved caspase-3 protein level, and cytokine generation were not significantly different. In conclusion, the results show that application of the TRPC6 agonist HYP9 can alleviate IR-induced cerebral injury in an animal model of stroke.

Dose-Dependent HYP9 Inhibition of TRPC6 Downregulation in Astrocytes Promotes Astrocyte Survival During IR Injury

HYP9 is a specific TRPC6 channel activator (Leuner et al., 2010). Treatment with HYP9 (0, 1, 5, 10, 15, 20, or 30 μM) was used to verify whether TRPC6 channel degradation is responsible for IR-induced astrocyte insults. Astrocytes were pre-incubated with different concentrations of HYP9 for 12 h in a CO_2 chamber and then exposed to normal or OGD/R conditions. Application of 15 μM HYP9 contributed to a significant decrease in OGD/R-induced astrocyte apoptosis and cytotoxicity (**Figures 4A–C**). Western blot results showed that HYP9 (15 μM) suppressed the downregulation of TRPC6 and decreased cleaved caspase-3 protein levels in primary mouse astrocytes in the OGD group (**Figures 4D–F**). These results indicate that maintaining the protein level of the TRPC6 channel in astrocytes with HYP9 diminishes OGD/R-induced astrocyte apoptosis and improves cell vitality.

TRPC Antagonist SKF Aggravates Astrocyte Damage Dose-Dependently in the OGD/R Experiment

Next, whether blockage of the TRPC6 channel by SKF results in increased astrocyte damage after OGD/R was investigated. Cultured astrocytes were pretreated with 0, 0.05, 0.5, 5, 10, 20, 30, or 40 μM SKF for 12 h before the OGD/R experiment. As shown in **Figures 5A,B**, the apoptosis of astrocytes was markedly increased in the OGD group supplemented with 30 or 40 μM SKF compared with the OGD group without SKF pretreatment. In addition, the effects of SKF on astrocyte cytotoxicity in the control and OGD groups were investigated using the LDH assay. Notably, IR injury-mediated astrocyte cytotoxicity was elevated after pre-incubation with 20, 30, or 40 μM SKF in OGD groups (**Figure 5C**). In addition to the increased cleaved caspase-3 expression, the OGD/R-induced degradation of TRPC6 protein was not rescued after treatment with SKF (**Figures 5D–F**). Taken together, pretreatment of cultured astrocytes with 30 or 40 μM SKF aggravates apoptosis and cytotoxicity in OGD groups.

TRPC6 Protects Astrocytes Against IR Injury in Modeled Ischemia

To further clarify the protective role of astrocytic TRPC6 during IR injury, we then infected primary cortical astrocytes with lentivirus vectors to overexpress (WT-TRPC6) or knock down (sh-TRPC6) TRPC6. The efficiency of lentiviral infections was shown in **Figure 6D**. OGD/R notably decreased the protein levels of TRPC6 compared with that in control groups in astrocytes (**Figure 6D**). Overexpression of TRPC6 strikingly reduced OGD/R-induced astrocyte apoptosis (**Figures 6A,B**), cytotoxicity (**Figure 6C**), and cleaved caspase-3 protein levels (**Figures 6D,E**). However, knocking down TRPC6 via sh-TRPC6 did not exacerbate IR injury-mediated apoptosis, cytotoxicity or cleaved caspase-3 protein levels in astrocytes (**Figure 6**). In general, TRPC6 attenuates astrocytes IR injury in modeled ischemia *in vitro*.

Maintaining the Protein Level of the TRPC6 Channel in Astrocytes Alleviates Astrocytic Inflammatory Responses

Astrocytic inflammatory response also has a critical effect on regulating the progress and prognosis of ischemic stroke (Cekanaviciute and Buckwalter, 2016; Deng et al., 2018). In

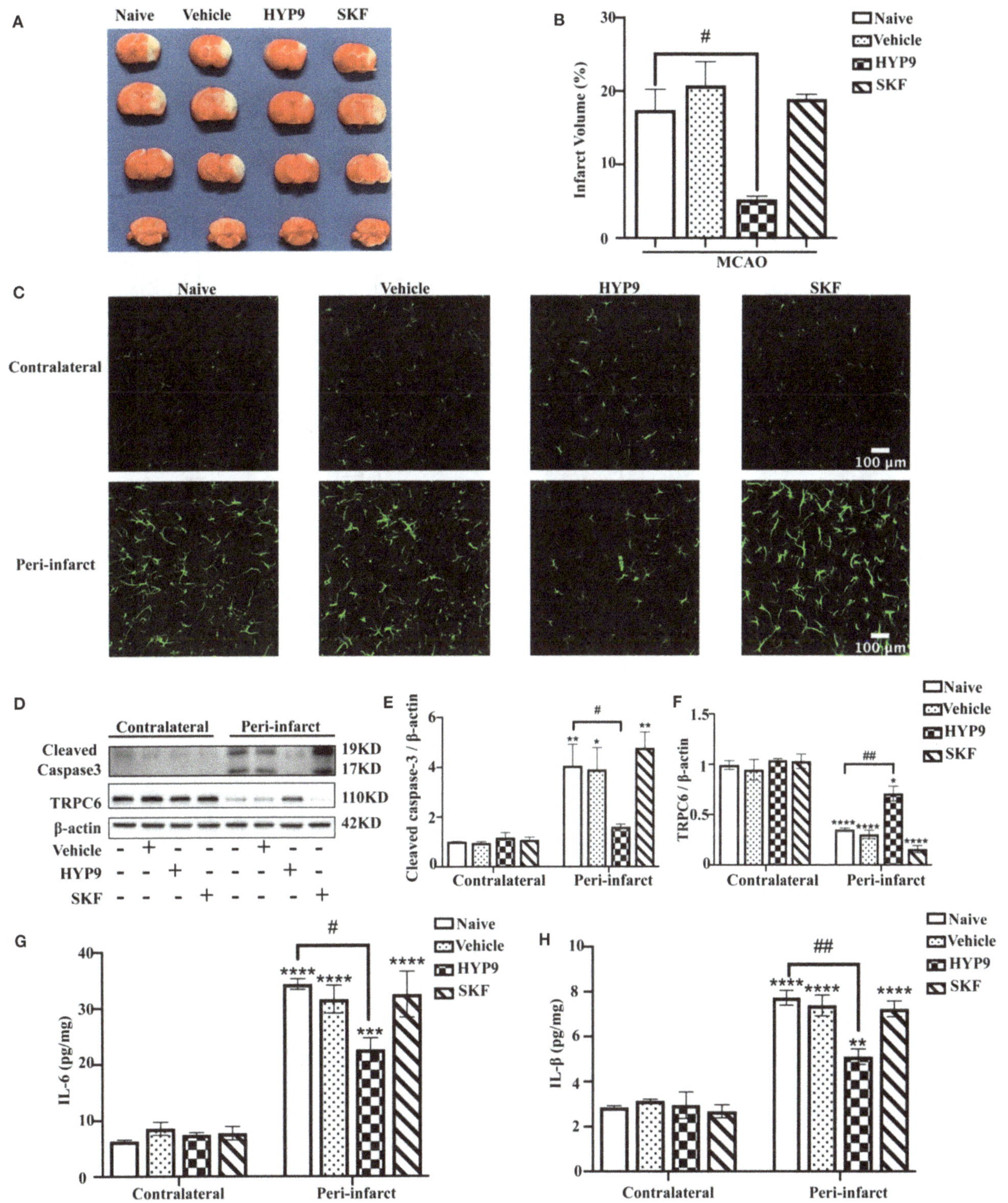

FIGURE 3 | Reducing IR-mediated TRPC6 downregulation with HYP9 alleviates ischemic damage in mice. Vehicle (DMSO), 5 μg HYP9, or 20 μg SKF were injected into left ventricles of mice 24 h before sham or MCAO operation. **(A)** TTC-stained cerebral slices indicated the infarct size in mice. **(B)** Quantification of infarct volumes after ischemia. Data were shown as mean ± SEM ($n = 3$). $^{\#}p < 0.05$ vs. MCAO + Naive group. **(C)** Representative images of astrocytes population with GFAP (green) staining in contralateral or peri-infarct cortices in MCAO mice (Scar bar: 100 μm; 400× magnification). **(D)** Western blot detecting TRPC6 and cleaved caspase-3 in mouse cortices. β-actin was used as a loading control. **(E,F)** Quantifications of cleaved caspase-3 and TRPC6 protein levels shown in **(D)**. Data were

(Continued)

FIGURE 3 | shown as mean ± SEM ($n = 3$). **(G,H)** The release of IL-6 and IL-1β was determined by ELISA assay. Data were shown as mean ± SEM ($n = 3$). *$p < 0.05$, **$p < 0.01$, ***$p < 0.001$, ****$p < 0.0001$ vs. MCAO + Naïve group in contralateral cortices; #$p < 0.05$, ##$p < 0.01$ vs. MCAO + Naive group in peri-infarct area.

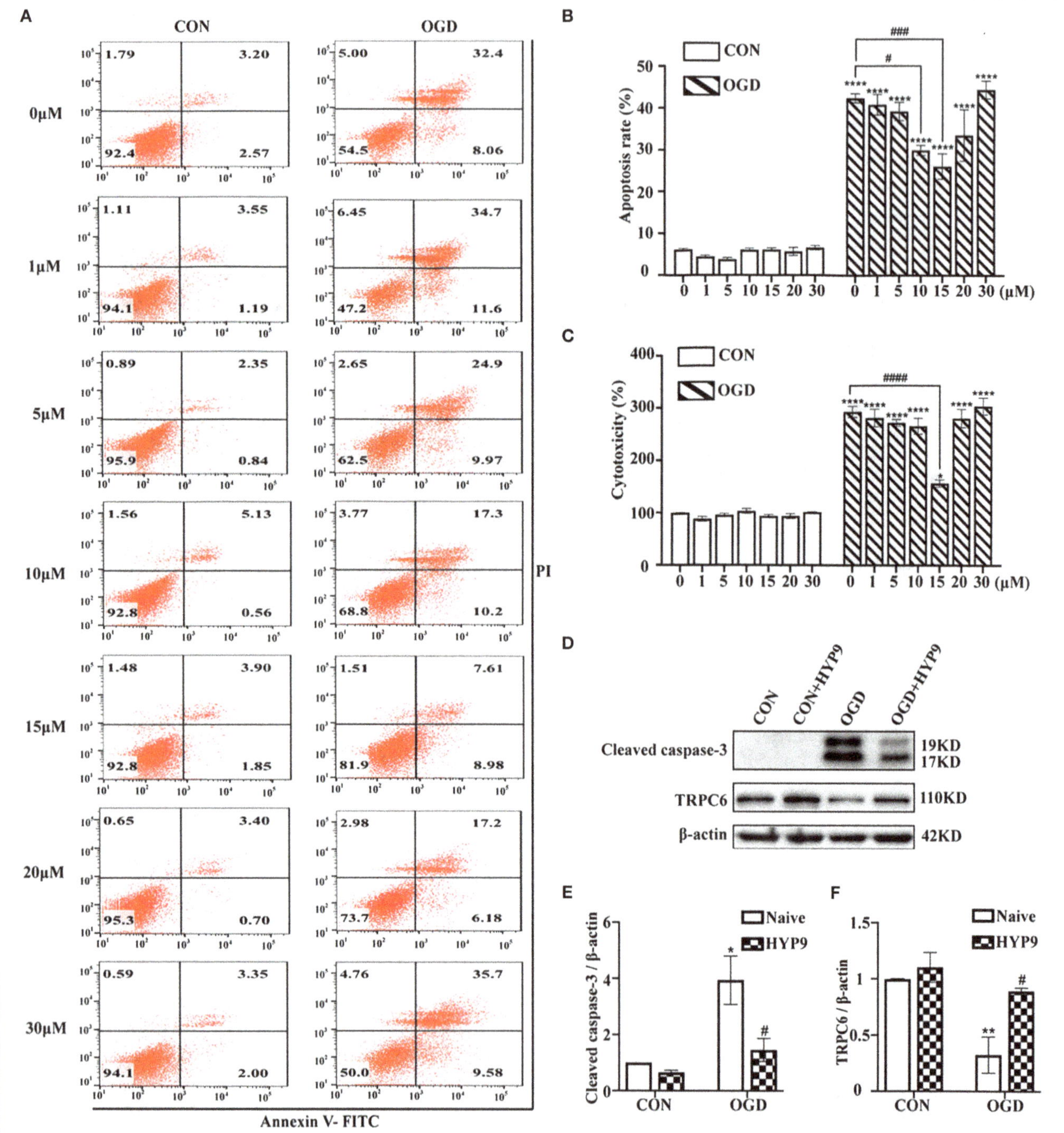

FIGURE 4 | Inhibition of TRPC6 downregulation by HYP9 protects astrocytes from ischemic damage. Astrocytes were pre-incubated with 0, 1, 5, 10, 15, 20, and 30 μM HYP9 for 12 h, and then subjected to control condition (CON) or 3 h OGD and 24 h reperfusion (OGD). **(A)** Representative scatter plots of astrocytic apoptosis measured by Annexin-V FITC/PI flow cytometry in each group. **(B)** Cell apoptosis rate was analyzed by Annexin-V FITC/PI flow cytometry, and the data were shown as mean ± SEM ($n = 4$). **(C)** Quantification of OGD/R-mediated cell cytotoxicity by LDH assay. Data were shown as mean ± SEM ($n = 4$). **(D)** Immunoblots for TRPC6 and cleaved caspase-3 of the extracts from CON or OGD-treated cortical astrocytes acquiring 15 μM HYP9 or not. β-actin was used as a loading control. **(E,F)** Quantifications of cleaved caspase-3 and TRPC6 protein levels shown in **(D)**. Data were shown as mean ± SEM ($n = 3$). *$p < 0.05$, **$p < 0.01$, ****$p < 0.0001$ vs. CON (HYP9 = 0 μM) group; #$p < 0.05$, ###$p < 0.001$, ####$p < 0.0001$ vs. OGD (HYP9 = 0 μM) group.

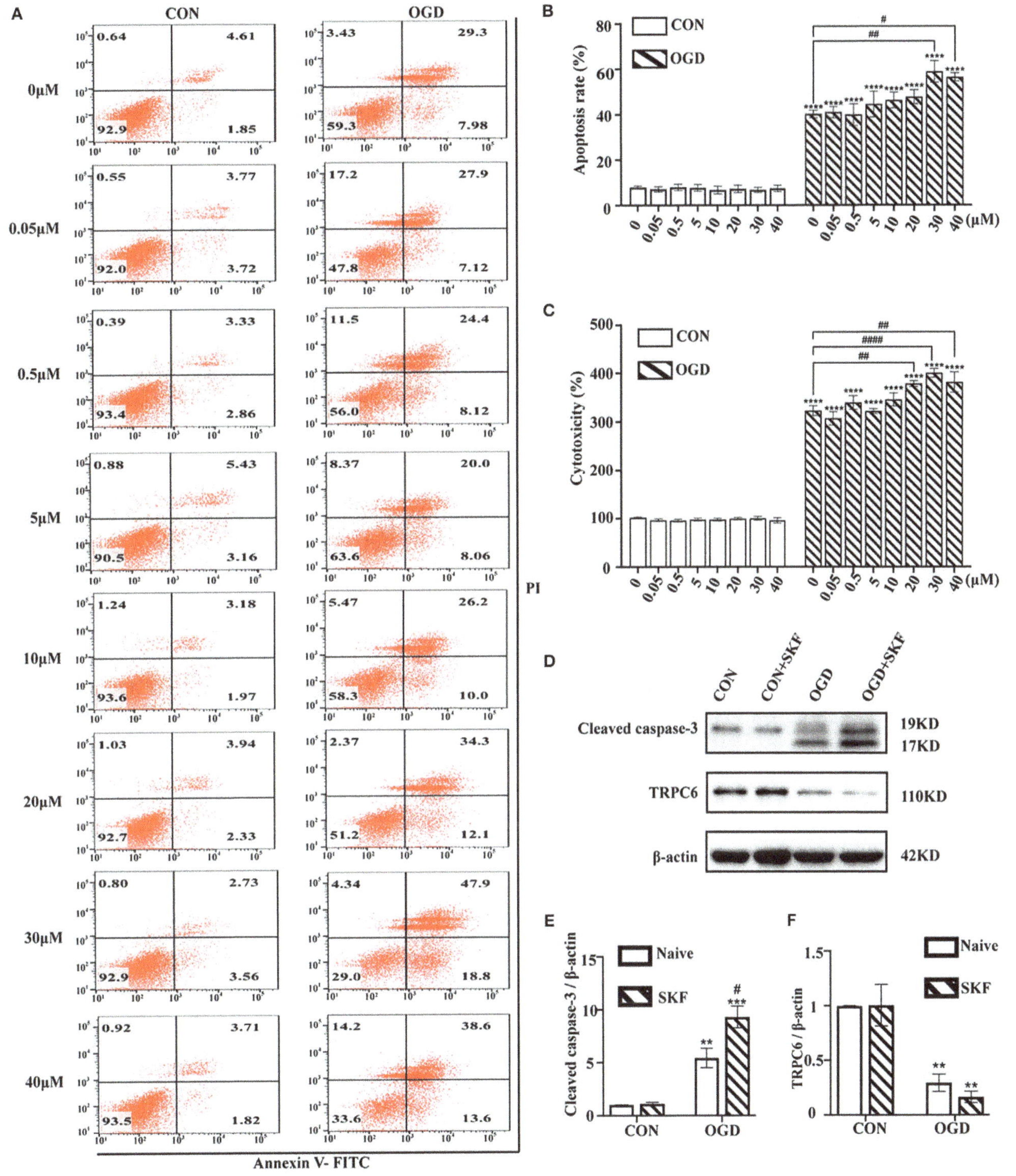

FIGURE 5 | TRPC antagonist SKF aggravates OGD/R induced astrocytes insults. Astrocytes were pre-incubated with 0, 0.05, 0.5, 5, 10, 20, 30, and 40 μM SKF for 12 h, and then subjected to control condition (CON) or 3 h OGD and 24 h reperfusion (OGD). **(A)** Representative scatter plots of astrocytic apoptosis measured by Annexin-V FITC/PI flow cytometry in each group. **(B)** Cell apoptosis rate was analyzed by Annexin-V FITC/PI flow cytometry, and the data were shown as mean ± SEM ($n = 4$). **(C)** Quantification of OGD/R-mediated cell cytotoxicity by LDH assay. Data were shown as mean ± SEM ($n = 4$). **(D)** Immunoblots for TRPC6 and cleaved caspase-3 of the extracts from CON or OGD-treated cortical astrocytes acquiring 30 μM SKF or not. β-actin was used as a loading control. **(E,F)** Quantifications of cleaved caspase-3 and TRPC6 protein levels shown in **(D)**. Data were shown as mean ± SEM ($n = 3$). $^{**}p < 0.01$, $^{***}p < 0.001$, $^{****}p < 0.0001$ vs. CON (SKF = 0 μM) group; $^{\#}p < 0.05$, $^{\#\#}p < 0.01$, $^{\#\#\#\#}p < 0.0001$ vs. OGD (SKF = 0 μM) group.

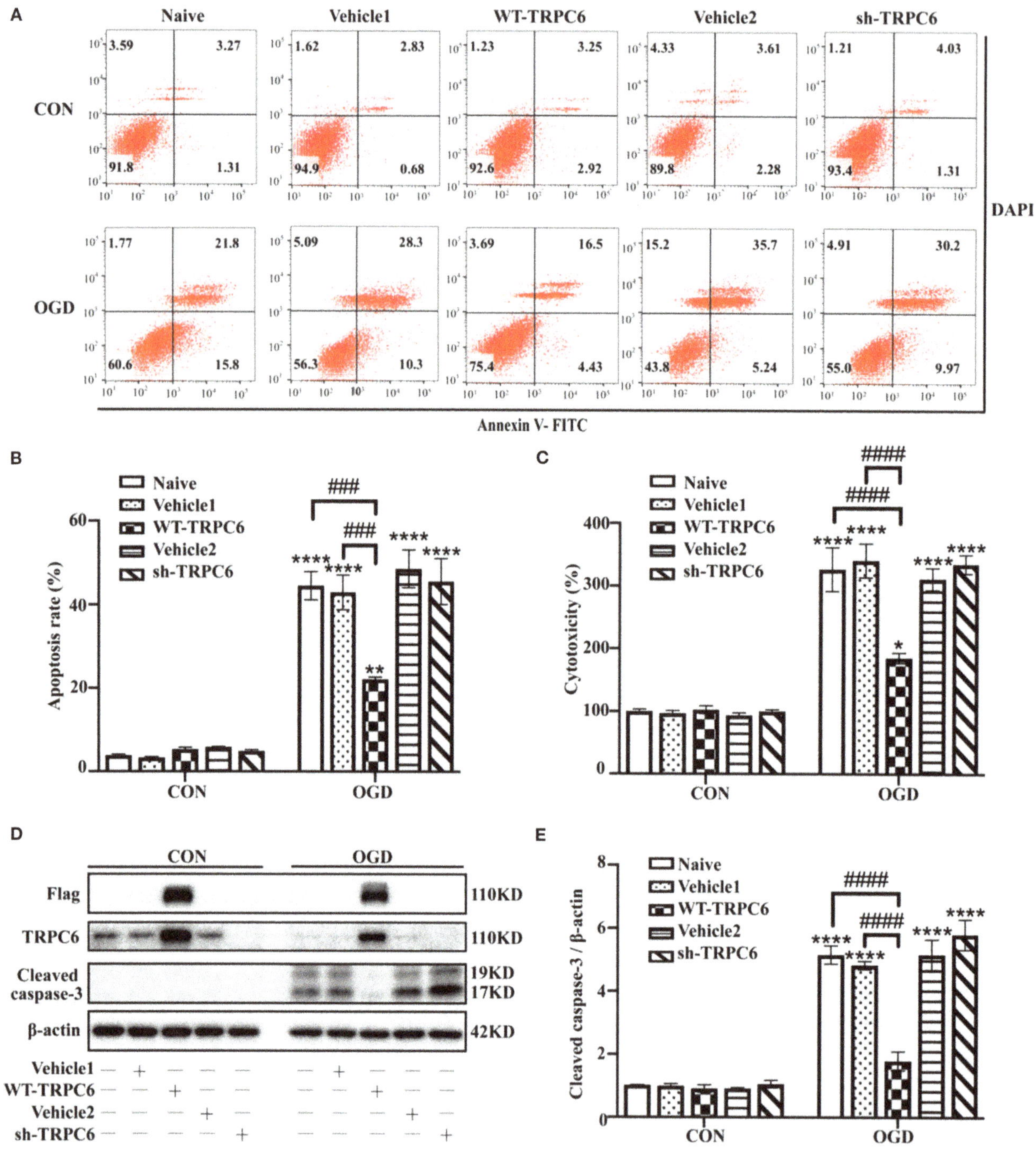

FIGURE 6 | TRPC6 protects astrocytes against IR injury in modeled ischemia. Astrocytes were infected with lentiviruses carrying mCherry-WT-TRPC6-null (Vehicle1), FLAG-tagged full-length mCherry-WT-TRPC6 (WT-TRPC6), mCherry-shRNA-TRPC6-null (Vehicle2), or mCherry-shRNA-TRPC6 (sh-TRPC6), and then exposed to control condition (CON) or 3 h OGD and 24 h reperfusion (OGD). **(A)** Representative scatter plots of astrocytic apoptosis measured by Annexin-V FITC/DAPI flow cytometry in each group. **(B)** Cell apoptosis rate was analyzed by Annexin-V FITC/DAPI flow cytometry, and the data were shown as mean ± SEM ($n = 4$). **(C)** Quantification of OGD/R-mediated cell cytotoxicity by LDH assay. Data were shown as mean ± SEM ($n = 4$). **(D)** Immunoblots for Flag, TRPC6, and cleaved caspase-3 of the extracts from control or OGD-treated cortical astrocytes acquiring Vehicle1, WT-TRPC6, Vehicle2, or sh-TRPC6 vectors. β-actin was used as a loading control. **(E)** Quantification of cleaved caspase-3 protein levels shown in **(D)**. Data were shown as mean ± SEM ($n = 3$). $^*p < 0.05$, $^{**}p < 0.01$, $^{****}p < 0.0001$ vs. CON + naive group; $^{\#\#\#}p < 0.001$, $^{\#\#\#\#}p < 0.0001$ vs. OGD + naive or OGD + Vehicle1 group.

addition to cell apoptosis and vitality, the expression of the pro-inflammatory cytokines IL-6 and IL-1β were measured to confirm the effects of HYP9 and SKF on ischemic astrocytic inflammation. The IL-6 and IL-1β protein levels were significantly increased in the OGD groups compared with the control groups. Notably, HYP9 and WT-TRPC6 reduced the elevated level of IL-6 and IL-1β in astrocytes in the OGD groups (**Figures 7A–F**).

The data show that inhibition of TRPC6 downregulation with HYP9 or WT-TRPC6 reduces inflammatory responses in astrocytes after OGD/R.

Inhibiting TRPC6 Downregulation Suppresses Intracellular Ca^{2+} Overload in Primary Astrocytes

The above reported results indicate the TRPC6 channel is closely associated with apoptosis, vitality, and inflammatory response in cultured cortical astrocytes exposed to IR damage. As a Ca^{2+} channel, TRPC6 modulates the concentration of intracellular Ca^{2+} ($[Ca^{2+}]_i$) (Wang et al., 2020a). To understand the potential mechanism of TRPC6 channel against cerebral ischemic insults in astrocytes, the effects of HYP9 and SKF on $[Ca^{2+}]_i$ in astrocytes was measured. Consistent with previous research (Li et al., 2015; Rakers and Petzold, 2017), OGD/R dramatically increased astrocytic $[Ca^{2+}]_i$ compared with control conditions (**Figures 8A,B**). Notably, application of HYP9 statistically reduced the elevated $[Ca^{2+}]_i$ in the OGD group (**Figures 8A,B**). In addition, SKF raised $[Ca^{2+}]_i$ in ischemic astrocytes (**Figures 8A,B**). These results indicate that astrocytic TRPC6 channel triggers a variety of protective cellular responses by inhibiting brain ischemia-induced Ca^{2+} overload.

TRPC6 Diminishes NF-κB Nuclear Translocation and Phosphorylation

NF-κB phosphorylation and nuclear translocation are considered vital pathways that mediate the inflammatory cascade, including cytokine generation (Kopitar-Jerala, 2015; Shih et al., 2015). Therefore, the influence of HYP9 and SKF on NF-κB nuclear translocation and phosphorylation in primary mouse astrocytes exposed to ischemic damage was investigated. Immunofluorescent signals showed the nuclear distribution of NF-κB was increased after OGD/R (**Figure 9**). Notably, the TRPC6-specific activator HYP9 attenuated IR injury-induced NF-κB nuclear translocation (**Figure 9**). Furthermore, HYP9 and WT-TRPC6 inhibited the phosphorylation of NF-κB in astrocytes subjected to OGD/R (**Figures 10A–G**). Collectively, the findings indicate that NF-κB phosphorylation and nuclear translocation may be pivotal downstream pathways that contribute to the protective effects of TRPC6 in astrocytes after stroke.

DISCUSSION

In cerebral ischemia, several clinical trials have failed due to narrow therapeutic window, adverse effects, and individual differences (Petrovic-Djergovic et al., 2016). A breakthrough in stroke therapeutic strategies is considered urgent. In the present study, significant downregulation of TRPC6 protein was observed in both cultured astrocytes and cerebral cortices after IR injury. *In vivo* results confirmed that the TRPC6 channel-specific activator HYP9 attenuated the infarct volume, astrocytes population, apoptosis, and the generation of pro-inflammatory cytokines (IL-6 and IL-1β) caused by MCAO. However, significant effects of SKF on infarct lesion or cortical IL-6 and IL-1β release in MCAO mice were not observed. In addition, HYP9 was shown to attenuate apoptosis rate, improve cell vitality, and reduce the generation of IL-6 and IL-1β in cultured astrocytes subjected to OGD/R. Furthermore, the TRPC channel antagonist SKF aggravated astrocytic apoptosis and cytotoxicity in OGD groups. In addition, inhibition of the TRPC6 channel downregulation with HYP9 suppressed the increase in $[Ca^{2+}]_i$ in ischemic astrocytes. The IR-mediated increased NF-κB phosphorylation and nuclear translocation were inhibited by HYP9 pretreatment in primary mouse astrocytes. In parallel, overexpression of TRPC6 also decreased IR injury-induced astrocytic apoptosis, cytotoxicity, inflammatory responses and NF-κB phosphorylation in modeled ischemia *in vitro*.

Previously, neuron-specific-related mechanisms are primarily considered in the pathogenesis of brain ischemia. As knowledge increased, astrocytes and other CNS cells are shown to be closely involved in ischemic stroke (Pekny et al., 2016; Werner et al., 2020). Astrocytes interact with neurons and participate in structural support, neuronal metabolism, synaptogenesis, synaptic transmission, axonal remodeling, and neurogenesis (Halassa and Haydon, 2010; Liu and Chopp, 2016). IR injury-activated astrocytes initiate the CNS inflammatory response, which in turn exacerbates brain insults during ischemic stroke (Cekanaviciute and Buckwalter, 2016). Thus, maintaining the normal function of astrocytes likely promotes post-ischemic neurological recovery. Therapeutic targeting of astrocytes is expected to be a future area of research regarding treatment and prognosis of brain ischemia (Neuhaus et al., 2017).

Evidence shows that TRPC6 is a crucial regulator of inflammatory cascades, especially in pulmonary inflammation (Chen et al., 2020; Ortiz-Muñoz et al., 2020). TRPC6 contributes to platelet activation, leukocyte transendothelial migration, lung vascular barrier disruption, and airway inflammation (Tauseef et al., 2012; Weber et al., 2015; Chen et al., 2020; Ortiz-Muñoz et al., 2020). In addition, activation of the TRPC6 channel promotes apoptosis in neonatal glomerular mesangial cells and renal tubular epithelial cells under different injury conditions (Soni and Adebiyi, 2016; Hou et al., 2018). TRPC6 inhibits N-methyl-D-aspartate (NMDA)-mediated Ca^{2+} elevation and reduces neuronal ischemic excitotoxity (Li et al., 2012). Furthermore, inhibition of TRPC6 degradation in neurons through cAMP-response element binding protein (CREB) pathway alleviates ischemic cerebral insults (Du et al., 2010). (-)-Epigallocatechin-3-gallate, resveratrol, and neuroprotectin D1 contribute to neuroprotective effect on brain IR damage through TRPC6/CREB pathways (Lin et al., 2013b; Yao et al., 2013, 2014). In particular, Hyperforin, a selective TRPC6 agonist, alleviates cerebral IR injury by suppressing the degradation of TRPC6 and increasing phosphorylated CREB in Ca^{2+}/calmodulin-dependent kinase IV (CaMKIV) signaling pathway (Lin et al., 2013a). Collectively, these

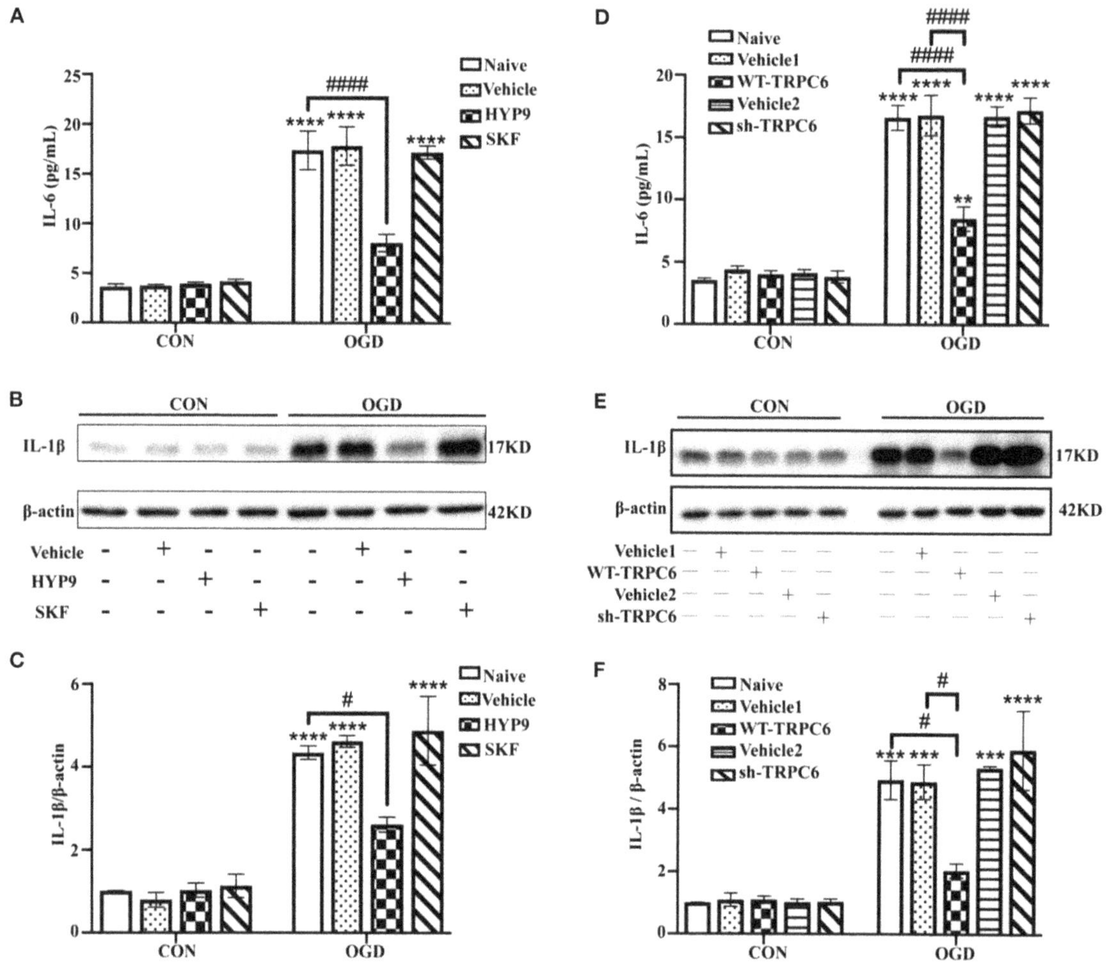

FIGURE 7 | Maintaining the protein level of TRPC6 attenuates astrocytic inflammatory responses. Astrocytes were pre-incubated with DMSO (as vehicle, the final DMSO concentration was 0.025%), 15 μM HYP9 or 30 μM SKF for 12 h, and then exposed to control condition (CON) or 3 h OGD and 24 h reperfusion (OGD). **(A)** The protein level of IL-6 was determined by ELISA assay. Data were shown as mean ± SEM ($n = 4$). **(B)** The expression of pro-inflammatory cytokine IL-1β in cortical astrocytes was measured using western blotting. β-actin was used as a loading control. **(C)** Quantification of IL-1β protein levels shown in **(B)**. Data were shown as mean ± SEM ($n = 3$). Astrocytes were infected with lentiviruses carrying Vehicle1, WT-TRPC6, Vehicle2, or sh-TRPC6, and then exposed to control condition (CON) or 3 h OGD and 24 h reperfusion (OGD). **(D)** The protein level of IL-6 was determined by ELISA assay. Data were shown as mean ± SEM ($n = 4$). **(E)** The expression of pro-inflammatory cytokine IL-1β in cortical astrocytes was measured using western blotting. β-actin was used as a loading control. **(F)** Quantification of IL-1β protein levels shown in **(E)**. Data were shown as mean ± SEM ($n = 3$). $^{**}p < 0.01$, $^{***}p < 0.001$, $^{****}p < 0.0001$ vs. CON + Naive group; $^{\#}p < 0.05$, $^{\#\#\#\#}p < 0.0001$ vs. OGD + Naive or OGD + Vehicle1 group.

evidences suggest the vital role of TRPC6/CREB pathway in ischemic stroke. Studies have shown that TRPC6 channel is expressed in microglia and involved in microglial activation and neuroinflammatory response in different diseases including hypertension, epilepsy, Alzheimer's disease, infectious diseases and neuropathic pain (Toth et al., 2013; Lee et al., 2014; Liu et al., 2017; Shinjyo et al., 2020; Wang et al., 2020b). However, the relevance of the TRPC6 channel in IR injury-induced astrocytic apoptosis and inflammation remains unclear. In addition, other downstream mechanisms beyond TRCP6/CREB pathways are worth exploring.

Hyperforin, a main compound of St. John's wort, can activate the TRPC6 channel and induce changes in $[Ca^{2+}]_i$ currents (Leuner et al., 2007); however, hyperforin is chemically unstable when subjected to oxygen and light. HYP9 is a stable synthetic phloroglucinol derivative of hyperforin that maintains the biological function of hyperforin in activating the TRPC6 channel (Leuner et al., 2010). Consequently, HYP9 was used in the present study to explore its function in the TRPC6 channel and the associated downstream cellular mechanisms in ischemic stroke. Inflammatory responses and apoptosis in ischemic astrocytes were inhibited by maintaining the protein level of the TRPC6 channel *via* HYP9. Overexpression of TRPC6 also reduced IR injury-induced astrocytic apoptosis, cytotoxicity, and inflammatory responses in experimental stroke *in vitro*. Meanwhile, SKF is a TRPC channel blocker (Song et al., 2014; Jing et al., 2016). SKF also affects other channels belonging to the TRPC channel subfamily. Evidence shows that TRPC1, TRPC3,

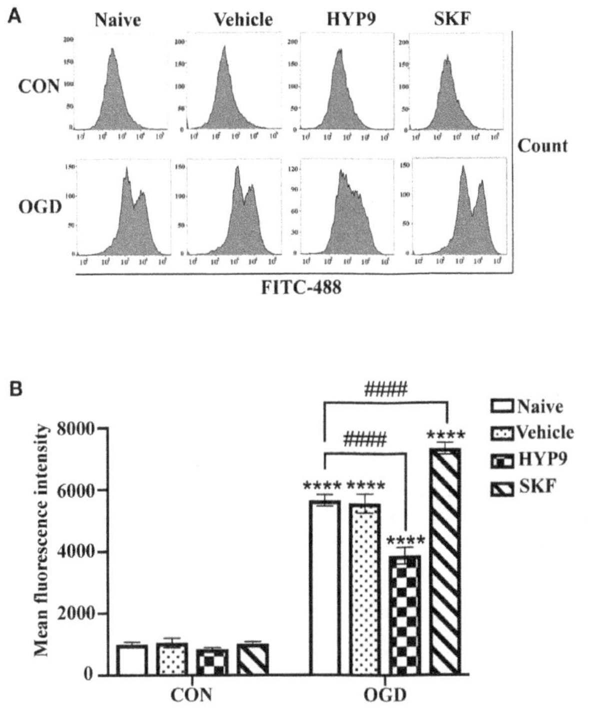

FIGURE 8 | TRPC6-specific agonists HYP9 suppresses intracellular Ca^{2+} overload in primary astrocytes. Astrocytes were pre-incubated with Vehicle (DMSO, the final concentration was 0.025%), 15 μM HYP9 or 30 μM SKF for 12 h, and then exposed to control condition (CON) or 3 h OGD and 24 h reperfusion (OGD). **(A)** Representative charts of average fluorescence intensity. The level of intracellular Ca^{2+} in astrocytes was measured by Ca^{2+} fluorescence probe Fluo-4 AM through FITC-488 flow cytometry. **(B)** Quantification of Ca^{2+} concentration in astrocytes by flow cytometry. Data were shown as mean ± SEM ($n = 4$). $^{****}p < 0.0001$ vs. CON + Naive group; $^{\#\#\#\#}p < 0.0001$ vs. OGD + Naive group.

and TRPC7 are involved in cerebral ischemic stroke (Chen et al., 2017; Xu et al., 2018). In the present study, SKF aggravated astrocyte injury after ischemia *in vitro*. However, significant changes in infarct volume, cleaved caspase-3 expression, and cytokine release were not observed in the MCAO model after SKF application. The inconsistent results between cell and animal models of stroke may be due to the complex effects of SKF on cortical non-astrocytic cells. Noticeably, knocking down TRPC6 via sh-TRPC6 shown no significant effects on apoptosis, cytotoxicity, and inflammatory responses in primary astrocytes after OGD/R. Since TRPC6 is strikingly downregulated in astrocytes exposed to IR insults, knocking down of TRPC6 did not significantly aggravate astrocytic damage in OGD group. The dissimilar effects of SKF and sh-TRPC6 on ischemic astrocytes might be related to the side-effect of SKF on other TRPCs (TRPC3/7). Overall, further *in vivo* studies using astrocytic TRPC6-, siRNA-, or shRNA-targeted transgenic mice are needed to fully clarify the role of the astrocytic TRPC6 channel in stroke.

Activation of the cerebral inflammatory cascade has important roles in acute brain IR insults. The inflammatory response induced by IR injury directly affect the progress of cerebral ischemia (Petrovic-Djergovic et al., 2016; Ramiro et al., 2018). Notably, astrocytes regulate the neuroinflammatory response by affecting the generation and release of diverse cytokines in ischemic stroke (Sofroniew, 2014). Astrocytes generate several pro-inflammatory cytokines and chemokines, including IL-6, IL-1β, tumor necrosis factor-α (TNF-α), C-C motif chemokine ligand (CCL)-2, CCL-5, CCL-7, C-X-C motif chemokine ligand (CXCL)-10, and vasoactive endothelial growth factor (John et al., 2005; Hamby et al., 2012; Sofroniew, 2015). Astrocyte-derived IL-6 and IL-1β are essential for secondary inflammatory damage in brain ischemia (John et al., 2005; Diaz-Cañestro et al., 2019). The pro-inflammatory nuclear transcription factor NF-κB belongs to the detrimental astrocytic signaling pathways (Colombo and Farina, 2016). NF-κB is involved in astrocyte inflammation and apoptosis (Su et al., 2019; Bai et al., 2020). Compelling evidence has shown that inhibition of NF-κB nuclear translocation or phosphorylation alleviates IR-mediated cytokine production and brain inflammation (Colombo and Farina, 2016; Liu et al., 2019; Xie et al., 2019; Bai et al., 2020). NF-κB activation is tightly modulated by various typical upstream signaling molecules, which include toll-like receptors, TNF receptors, IL-1 receptors, CAMKII, and stromal interaction molecule or Orai-mediated Ca^{2+} signals (Verstrepen et al., 2008; Berry et al., 2018; Pires et al., 2018; Ye et al., 2019).

A crucial relationship exists between Ca^{2+} and NF-κB signaling pathways (Wei et al., 2019). As a vital second messenger, Ca^{2+} governs a variety of functions causing cellular pathological and physiological changes. Modulation of the Ca^{2+} current has attracted interest as a promising medical strategy for ischemic stroke (Kalogeris et al., 2016; Secondo et al., 2018). The TRPC6 channel, a Ca^{2+} permeable cation channel, has been associated with Ca^{2+} entry and brain ischemic pathogenesis (Liu et al., 2020). In the present study, TRPC6 was dramatically downregulated during IR injury. The TRPC6-specific agonist HYP9 rescued TRPC6 degradation in primary cultured astrocytes and reduced $[Ca^{2+}]_i$. Consistently, the TRPC channel antagonist SKF contributed to increased $[Ca^{2+}]_i$. How a Ca^{2+} entry activator reduces and a Ca^{2+} channel blocker increases the Ca^{2+} influx in primary astrocytes is notable. TRPC6 has been shown to block the NMDA receptor (NMDAR)-triggered $[Ca^{2+}]_i$ increase and neurotoxicity in neurons after brain IR damage (Li et al., 2012). Overexpression of TRPC6 inhibits $[Ca^{2+}]_i$ overload, prevents neuronal death, lessen infarct size, and improves behavior performance after ischemia. Similarly, another research team suggests that the TRPC6 channel selectively suppresses the NMDAR-mediated current in hippocampal neurons, which is increased *via* TRPC6 knockdown or interference with SKF (Shen et al., 2013). In another study, SKF increases intracellular Ca^{2+} by promoting the reverse mode of the Na^+/Ca^{2+} exchanger (Song et al., 2014). Thus, we hypothesized that the underlying mechanism of TRPC6-induced $[Ca^{2+}]_i$ decrease in astrocytes after ischemic insults may be associated with the complex interaction between the TRPC6 channel and other ion exchangers.

Although the present study showed a protective role of the TRPC6 channel in astrocytes after ischemia, various questions remain unanswered. The effects of the astrocytic TRPC6

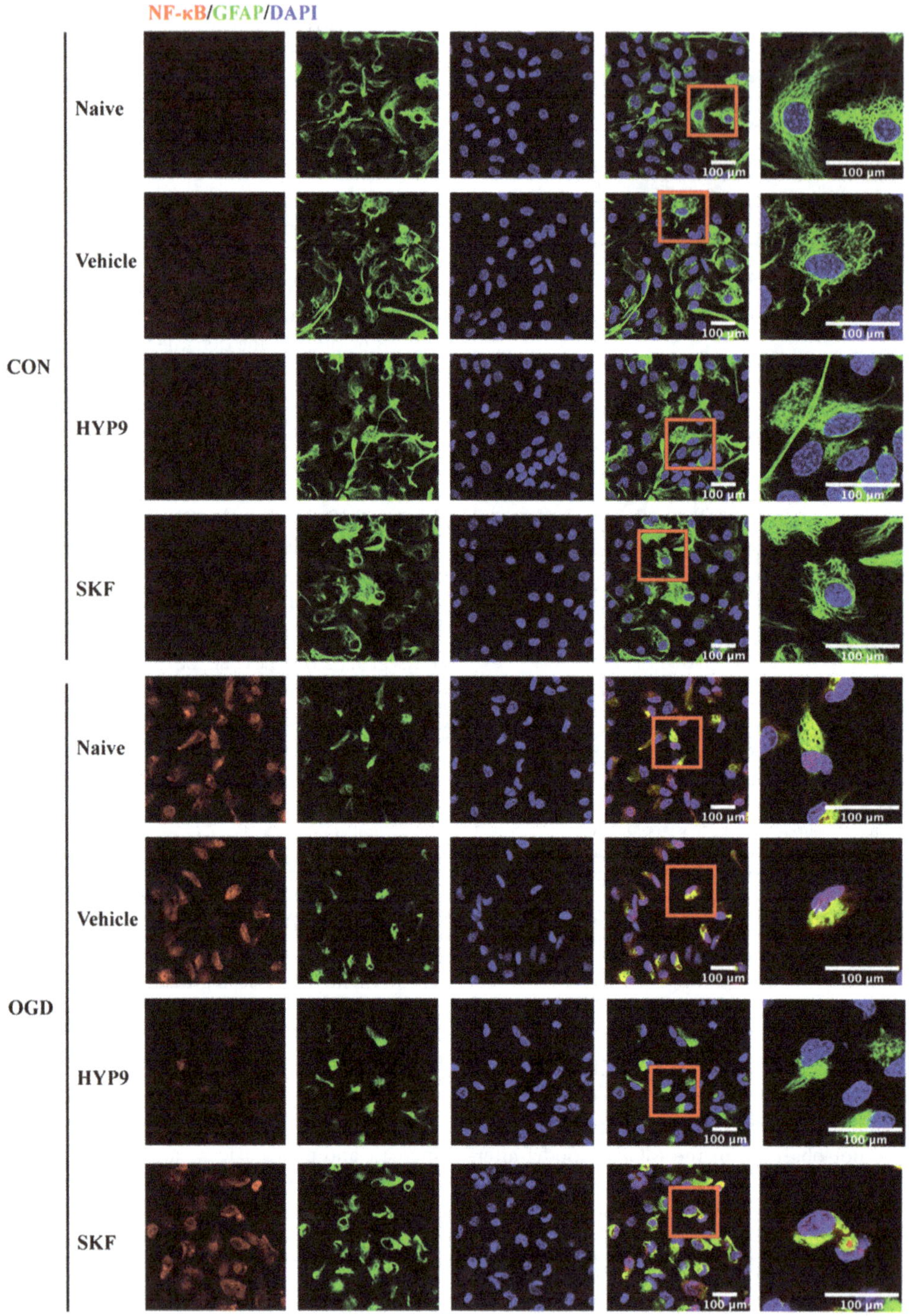

FIGURE 9 | TRPC6 diminishes NF-κB nuclear translocation in astrocytes after ishcemia. Astrocytes were pre-incubated with Vehicle (DMSO, the final concentration is 0.025%), 15 μM HYP9 or 30 μM SKF for 12 h, and then expose to control condition (CON) or 3 h OGD and 24 h reperfusion (OGD). Representative images of cortical astrocytes after OGD/R double-stained with the NF-κB (red) and GFAP (green) antibodies (Scar bar: 100 μm; 630× or 1,890× magnification).

channel on ischemic neurons will be addressed in our future work. Furthermore, the underlying mechanisms of TRPC6-triggered astrocytic Ca^{2+} changes in ischemic stroke warrant further investigations.

CONCLUSION

The results of the present study indicate that HYP9 reduces the infarct size, apoptosis, and pro-inflammatory cytokine release in

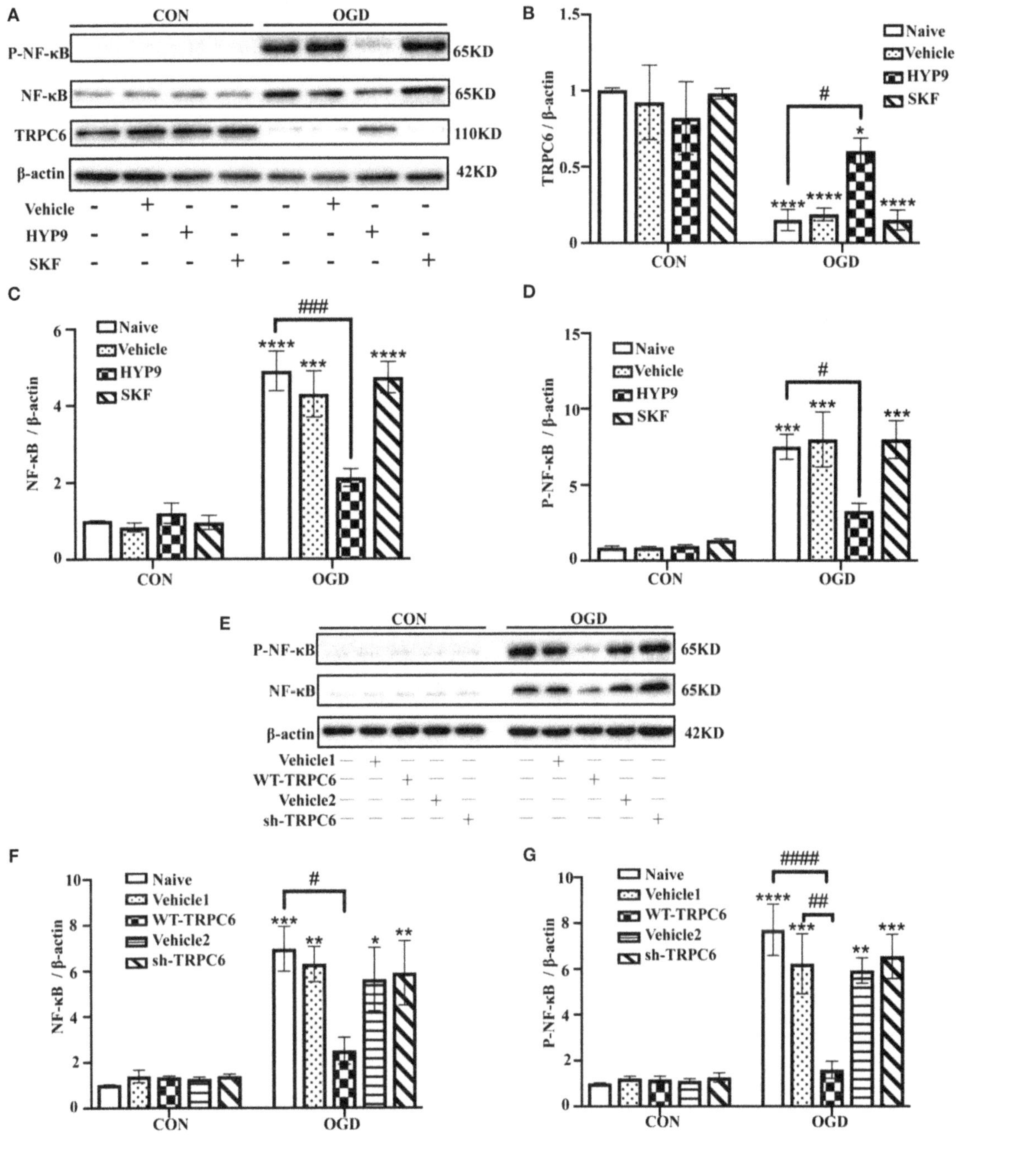

FIGURE 10 | TRPC6 diminishes OGD/R-induced NF-κB phosphorylation in astrocytes. Astrocytes were pre-incubated with Vehicle (DMSO, the final concentration is 0.025%), 15 μM HYP9 or 30 μM SKF for 12 h, and then expose to control condition (CON) or 3 h OGD and 24 h reperfusion (OGD). **(A)** Immunoblots for TRPC6, NF-κB, and phosphorylated-NF-κB (P-NF-κB) of the extracts from cortical astrocytes. β-actin was used as a loading control. **(B–D)** Quantification of TRPC6, NF-κB, and P-NF-κB protein levels shown in **(A)**. Data were shown as mean ± SEM ($n = 3$). Astrocytes were infected with lentiviruses carrying Vehicle1, WT-TRPC6, Vehicle2, or sh-TRPC6, and then exposed to control condition (CON) or 3 h OGD and 24 h reperfusion (OGD). **(E)** Immunoblots for NF-κB and P-NF-κB of the extracts from cortical astrocytes. β-actin was used as a loading control. **(F,G)** Quantification of NF-κB, and P-NF-κB protein levels shown in **(E)**. Data were shown as mean ± SEM ($n = 3$). $^{*}p < 0.05$, $^{**}p < 0.01$, $^{***}p < 0.001$, $^{****}p < 0.0001$ vs. CON + Naive group; $^{\#}p < 0.05$, $^{\#\#}p < 0.01$, $^{\#\#\#}p < 0.001$, $^{\#\#\#\#}p < 0.0001$ vs. OGD + Naive or OGD + Vehicle1 group.

a mouse model of ischemic stroke. Inhibition of TRPC6 channel downregulation *via* HYP9 or TRPC6 overexpression alleviates apoptosis and inflammatory response in astrocytes exposed to ischemic damage. Furthermore, the protective role of TRPC6 in stroke is associated with Ca^{2+}/NF-κB-dependent pathways. The results of this study indicate that the astrocytic TRPC6 channel and TRPC6 agonist HYP9 might be a novel therapeutic approach to prevent ischemic stroke induced by brain injury.

ETHICS STATEMENT

The animal study was reviewed and approved by Animal Care Committee of the First Affiliated Hospital at Zhejiang University.

AUTHOR CONTRIBUTIONS

LL wrote the manuscript. LL, MC, and KL finished the experiment. SZ and XXio designed the general idea. All authors edited the drafts of the manuscript.

REFERENCES

Bai, X., Zhang, Y. L., and Liu, L. N. (2020). Inhibition of TRIM8 restrains ischaemia-reperfusion-mediated cerebral injury by regulation of NF-κB activation associated inflammation and apoptosis. *Exp. Cell Res.* 388:111818. doi: 10.1016/j.yexcr.2020.111818

Berry, C. T., May, M. J., and Freedman, B. D. (2018). STIM- and Orai-mediated calcium entry controls NF-κB activity and function in lymphocytes. *Cell Calcium* 74, 131–143. doi: 10.1016/j.ceca.2018.07.003

Cekanaviciute, E., and Buckwalter, M. S. (2016). Astrocytes: integrative regulators of neuroinflammation in stroke and other neurological diseases. *Neurotherapeutics* 13, 685–701. doi: 10.1007/s13311-016-0477-8

Chen, Q., Zhou, Y., Zhou, L., Fu, Z., Yang, C., Zhao, L., et al. (2020). TRPC6-dependent Ca(2+) signaling mediates airway inflammation in response to oxidative stress via ERK pathway. *Cell Death Dis.* 11:170. doi: 10.1038/s41419-020-2360-0

Chen, X., Lu, M., He, X., Ma, L., Birnbaumer, L., and Liao, Y. (2017). TRPC3/6/7 knockdown protects the brain from cerebral ischemia injury via astrocyte apoptosis inhibition and effects on NF-κB translocation. *Mol. Neurobiol.* 54, 7555–7566. doi: 10.1007/s12035-016-0227-2

Chen, X., Taylor-Nguyen, N. N., Riley, A. M., Herring, B. P., White, F. A., and Obukhov, A. G. (2019). The TRPC6 inhibitor, larixyl acetate, is effective in protecting against traumatic brain injury-induced systemic endothelial dysfunction. *J. Neuroinflamm.* 16:21. doi: 10.1186/s12974-019-1407-6

Colombo, E., and Farina, C. (2016). Astrocytes: key regulators of neuroinflammation. *Trends Immunol.* 37, 608–620. doi: 10.1016/j.it.2016.06.006

Curcic, S., Tiapko, O., and Groschner, K. (2019). Photopharmacology and opto-chemogenetics of TRPC channels-some therapeutic visions. *Pharmacol. Ther.* 200, 13–26. doi: 10.1016/j.pharmthera.2019.04.003

Deng, Y. L., Ma, Y. L., Zhang, Z. L., Zhang, L. X., Guo, H., Qin, P., et al. (2018). Astrocytic N-Myc downstream-regulated gene-2 is involved in nuclear transcription factor κB-mediated inflammation induced by global cerebral ischemia. *Anesthesiology* 128, 574–586. doi: 10.1097/aln.0000000000002044

Diaz-Cañestro, C., Reiner, M. F., Bonetti, N. R., Liberale, L., Merlini, M., Wüst, P., et al. (2019). AP-1 (activated protein-1) transcription factor JunD regulates ischemia/reperfusion brain damage via IL-1β (interleukin-1β). *Stroke* 50, 469–477. doi: 10.1161/strokeaha.118.023739

Ding, X., He, Z., Zhou, K., Cheng, J., Yao, H., Lu, D., et al. (2010). Essential role of TRPC6 channels in G2/M phase transition and development of human glioma. *J. Natl. Cancer Inst.* 102, 1052–1068. doi: 10.1093/jnci/djq217

Du, W., Huang, J., Yao, H., Zhou, K., Duan, B., and Wang, Y. (2010). Inhibition of TRPC6 degradation suppresses ischemic brain damage in rats. *J. Clin. Invest.* 120, 3480–3492. doi: 10.1172/jci43165

Griesi-Oliveira, K., Acab, A., Gupta, A. R., Sunaga, D. Y., Chailangkarn, T., Nicol, X., et al. (2015). Modeling non-syndromic autism and the impact of TRPC6 disruption in human neurons. *Mol. Psychiatry* 20, 1350–1365. doi: 10.1038/mp.2014.141

Guo, C., Ma, Y., Ma, S., Mu, F., Deng, J., Duan, J., et al. (2017). The role of TRPC6 in the neuroprotection of calycosin against cerebral ischemic injury. *Sci. Rep.* 7:3039. doi: 10.1038/s41598-017-03404-6

Halassa, M. M., and Haydon, P. G. (2010). Integrated brain circuits: astrocytic networks modulate neuronal activity and behavior. *Annu. Rev. Physiol.* 72, 335–355. doi: 10.1146/annurev-physiol-021909-135843

Hamby, M. E., Coppola, G., Ao, Y., Geschwind, D. H., Khakh, B. S., and Sofroniew, M. V. (2012). Inflammatory mediators alter the astrocyte transcriptome and calcium signaling elicited by multiple G-protein-coupled receptors. *J. Neurosci.* 32, 14489–14510. doi: 10.1523/jneurosci.1256-12.2012

Hamid, R., and Newman, J. H. (2009). Evidence for inflammatory signaling in idiopathic pulmonary artery hypertension: TRPC6 and nuclear factor-kappaB. *Circulation* 119, 2297–2298. doi: 10.1161/circulationaha.109.855197

Hankey, G. J. (2017). Stroke. *Lancet* 389, 641–654. doi: 10.1016/s0140-6736(16) 30962-x

Hou, X., Xiao, H., Zhang, Y., Zeng, X., Huang, M., Chen, X., et al. (2018). Transient receptor potential channel 6 knockdown prevents apoptosis of renal tubular epithelial cells upon oxidative stress via autophagy activation. *Cell Death Dis.* 9:1015. doi: 10.1038/s41419-018-1052-5

Jia, Y., Zhou, J., Tai, Y., and Wang, Y. (2007). TRPC channels promote cerebellar granule neuron survival. *Nat. Neurosci.* 10, 559–567. doi: 10.1038/nn1870

Jing, Z., Sui, X., Yao, J., Xie, J., Jiang, L., Zhou, Y., et al. (2016). SKF-96365 activates cytoprotective autophagy to delay apoptosis in colorectal cancer cells through inhibition of the calcium/CaMKIIγ/AKT-mediated pathway. *Cancer Lett.* 372, 226–238. doi: 10.1016/j.canlet.2016.01.006

John, G. R., Lee, S. C., Song, X., Rivieccio, M., and Brosnan, C. F. (2005). IL-1-regulated responses in astrocytes: relevance to injury and recovery. *Glia* 49, 161–176. doi: 10.1002/glia.20109

Kalogeris, T., Baines, C. P., Krenz, M., and Korthuis, R. J. (2016). Ischemia/reperfusion. *Compr. Physiol.* 7, 113–170. doi: 10.1002/cphy.c160006

Khoshnam, S. E., Winlow, W., Farzaneh, M., Farbood, Y., and Moghaddam, H. F. (2017). Pathogenic mechanisms following ischemic stroke. *Neurol. Sci.* 38, 1167–1186. doi: 10.1007/s10072-017-2938-1

Kim, Y. J., and Kang, T. C. (2015). The role of TRPC6 in seizure susceptibility and seizure-related neuronal damage in the rat dentate gyrus. *Neuroscience* 307, 215–230. doi: 10.1016/j.neuroscience.2015.08.054

Kopitar-Jerala, N. (2015). Innate immune response in brain, NF-kappaB signaling and cystatins. *Front. Mol. Neurosci.* 8:73. doi: 10.3389/fnmol.2015.00073

Lee, S. K., Kim, J. E., Kim, Y. J., Kim, M. J., and Kang, T. C. (2014). Hyperforin attenuates microglia activation and inhibits p65-Ser276 NFκB phosphorylation in the rat piriform cortex following status epilepticus. *Neurosci. Res.* 85, 39–50. doi: 10.1016/j.neures.2014.05.006

Leuner, K., Heiser, J. H., Derksen, S., Mladenov, M. I., Fehske, C. J., Schubert, R., et al. (2010). Simple 2,4-diacylphloroglucinols as classic transient receptor potential-6 activators–identification of a novel pharmacophore. *Mol. Pharmacol.* 77, 368–377. doi: 10.1124/mol.109.057513

Leuner, K., Kazanski, V., Müller, M., Essin, K., Henke, B., Gollasch, M., et al. (2007). Hyperforin–a key constituent of St. John's wort specifically activates TRPC6 channels. *FASEB J.* 21, 4101–4111. doi: 10.1096/fj.07-8110com

Li, H., Huang, J., Du, W., Jia, C., Yao, H., and Wang, Y. (2012). TRPC6 inhibited NMDA receptor activities and protected neurons from ischemic excitotoxicity. *J. Neurochem.* 123, 1010–1018. doi: 10.1111/jnc.12045

Li, H., Xie, Y., Zhang, N., Yu, Y., Zhang, Q., and Ding, S. (2015). Disruption of IP3R2-mediated Ca^{2+} signaling pathway in astrocytes ameliorates neuronal death and brain damage while reducing behavioral deficits after focal ischemic stroke. *Cell Calcium* 58, 565–576. doi: 10.1016/j.ceca.2015.09.004

Li, Q., Cao, Y., Dang, C., Han, B., Han, R., Ma, H., et al. (2020). Inhibition of double-strand DNA-sensing cGAS ameliorates brain injury after ischemic stroke. *EMBO Mol. Med.* 12:e11002. doi: 10.15252/emmm.201911002

Li, Y., Jia, Y. C., Cui, K., Li, N., Zheng, Z. Y., Wang, Y. Z., et al. (2005). Essential role of TRPC channels in the guidance of nerve growth cones by brain-derived neurotrophic factor. *Nature* 434, 894–898. doi: 10.1038/nature03477

Lin, Y., Chen, F., Zhang, J., Wang, T., Wei, X., Wu, J., et al. (2013b). Neuroprotective effect of resveratrol on ischemia/reperfusion injury in rats through TRPC6/CREB pathways. *J. Mol. Neurosci.* 50, 504–513. doi: 10.1007/s12031-013-9977-8

Lin, Y., Zhang, J. C., Fu, J., Chen, F., Wang, J., Wu, Z. L., et al. (2013a). Hyperforin attenuates brain damage induced by transient middle cerebral artery occlusion

(MCAO) in rats via inhibition of TRPC6 channels degradation. *J. Cereb. Blood Flow Metab.* 33, 253–262. doi: 10.1038/jcbfm.2012.164

Liu, H., Wu, X., Luo, J., Wang, X., Guo, H., Feng, D., et al. (2019). Pterostilbene attenuates astrocytic inflammation and neuronal oxidative injury after ischemia-reperfusion by inhibiting NF-κB phosphorylation. *Front. Immunol.* 10:2408. doi: 10.3389/fimmu.2019.02408

Liu, L., Gu, L., Chen, M., Zheng, Y., Xiong, X., and Zhu, S. (2020). Novel targets for stroke therapy: special focus on TRPC channels and TRPC6. *Front. Aging Neurosci.* 12:70. doi: 10.3389/fnagi.2020.00070

Liu, N., Zhuang, Y., Zhou, Z., Zhao, J., Chen, Q., and Zheng, J. (2017). NF-κB dependent up-regulation of TRPC6 by Aβ in BV-2 microglia cells increases COX-2 expression and contributes to hippocampus neuron damage. *Neurosci. Lett.* 651, 1–8. doi: 10.1016/j.neulet.2017.04.056

Liu, Z., and Chopp, M. (2016). Astrocytes, therapeutic targets for neuroprotection and neurorestoration in ischemic stroke. *Prog. Neurobiol.* 144, 103–120. doi: 10.1016/j.pneurobio.2015.09.008

Montell, C. (2001). Physiology, phylogeny, and functions of the TRP superfamily of cation channels. *Sci. STKE* 2001:re1. doi: 10.1126/stke.2001.90.re1

Neuhaus, A. A., Couch, Y., Hadley, G., and Buchan, A. M. (2017). Neuroprotection in stroke: the importance of collaboration and reproducibility. *Brain* 140, 2079–2092. doi: 10.1093/brain/awx126

Ortiz-Muñoz, G., Yu, M. A., Lefrançais, E., Mallavia, B., Valet, C., Tian, J. J., et al. (2020). Cystic fibrosis transmembrane conductance regulator dysfunction in platelets drives lung hyperinflammation. *J. Clin. Invest.* 130, 2041–2053. doi: 10.1172/jci129635

Pekny, M., Pekna, M., Messing, A., Steinhäuser, C., Lee, J. M., Parpura, V., et al. (2016). Astrocytes: a central element in neurological diseases. *Acta Neuropathol.* 131, 323–345. doi: 10.1007/s00401-015-1513-1

Petrovic-Djergovic, D., Goonewardena, S. N., and Pinsky, D. J. (2016). Inflammatory disequilibrium in stroke. *Circ. Res.* 119, 142–158. doi: 10.1161/circresaha.116.308022

Pires, B. R. B., Silva, R., Ferreira, G. M., and Abdelhay, E. (2018). NF-kappaB: two sides of the same coin. *Genes (Basel)* 9:24. doi: 10.3390/genes9010024

Pochwat, B., Szewczyk, B., Kotarska, K., Rafało-Ulińska, A., Siwiec, M., Sowa, J. E., et al. (2018). Hyperforin potentiates antidepressant-like activity of lanicemine in mice. *Front. Mol. Neurosci.* 11:456. doi: 10.3389/fnmol.2018.00456

Qu, Z., Wang, Y., Li, X., Wu, L., and Wang, Y. (2017). TRPC6 expression in neurons is differentially regulated by NR2A- and NR2B-containing NMDA receptors. *J. Neurochem.* 143, 282–293. doi: 10.1111/jnc.14215

Quick, K., Zhao, J., Eijkelkamp, N., Linley, J. E., Rugiero, F., Cox, J. J., et al. (2012). TRPC3 and TRPC6 are essential for normal mechanotransduction in subsets of sensory neurons and cochlear hair cells. *Open Biol.* 2:120068. doi: 10.1098/rsob.120068

Rakers, C., and Petzold, G. C. (2017). Astrocytic calcium release mediates peri-infarct depolarizations in a rodent stroke model. *J. Clin. Invest.* 127, 511–516. doi: 10.1172/jci89354

Ramirez, G. A., Coletto, L. A., Sciorati, C., Bozzolo, E. P., Manunta, P., Rovere-Querini, P., et al. (2018). Ion channels and transporters in inflammation: special focus on TRP channels and TRPC6. *Cells* 7:70. doi: 10.3390/cells7070070

Ramiro, L., Simats, A., García-Berrocoso, T., and Montaner, J. (2018). Inflammatory molecules might become both biomarkers and therapeutic targets for stroke management. *Ther. Adv. Neurol. Disord.* 11:1756286418789340. doi: 10.1177/17562864187 89340

Riccio, A., Medhurst, A. D., Mattei, C., Kelsell, R. E., Calver, A. R., Randall, A. D., et al. (2002). mRNA distribution analysis of human TRPC family in CNS and peripheral tissues. *Brain Res. Mol. Brain Res.* 109, 95–104. doi: 10.1016/s0169-328x(02)00527-2

Secondo, A., Bagetta, G., and Amantea, D. (2018). On the role of store-operated calcium entry in acute and chronic neurodegenerative diseases. *Front. Mol. Neurosci.* 11:87. doi: 10.3389/fnmol.2018.00087

Shen, H., Pan, J., Pan, L., and Zhang, N. (2013). TRPC6 inhibited NMDA current in cultured hippocampal neurons. *Neuromol. Med.* 15, 389–395. doi: 10.1007/s12017-013-8226-1

Shen, Y., Qin, H., Chen, J., Mou, L., He, Y., Yan, Y., et al. (2016). Postnatal activation of TLR4 in astrocytes promotes excitatory synaptogenesis in hippocampal neurons. *J. Cell Biol.* 215, 719–734. doi: 10.1083/jcb.201605046

Shih, R. H., Wang, C. Y., and Yang, C. M. (2015). NF-kappaB signaling pathways in neurological inflammation: a mini review. *Front. Mol. Neurosci.* 8:77. doi: 10.3389/fnmol.2015.00077

Shinjyo, N., Nakayama, H., Li, L., Ishimaru, K., Hikosaka, K., Suzuki, N., et al. (2020). Hypericum perforatum extract and hyperforin inhibit the growth of neurotropic parasite *Toxoplasma gondii* and infection-induced inflammatory responses of glial cells *in vitro*. *J. Ethnopharmacol.* doi: 10.1016/j.jep.2020.113525. [Epub ahead of print].

Shirakawa, H., Katsumoto, R., Iida, S., Miyake, T., Higuchi, T., Nagashima, T., et al. (2017). Sphingosine-1-phosphate induces Ca(2+) signaling and CXCL1 release via TRPC6 channel in astrocytes. *Glia* 65, 1005–1016. doi: 10.1002/glia.23141

Singh, A., Hildebrand, M. E., Garcia, E., and Snutch, T. P. (2010). The transient receptor potential channel antagonist SKF96365 is a potent blocker of low-voltage-activated T-type calcium channels. *Br. J. Pharmacol.* 160, 1464–1475. doi: 10.1111/j.1476-5381.2010.00786.x

Sofroniew, M. V. (2014). Multiple roles for astrocytes as effectors of cytokines and inflammatory mediators. *Neuroscientist.* 20, 160–172. doi: 10.1177/1073858413504466

Sofroniew, M. V. (2015). Astrocyte barriers to neurotoxic inflammation. *Nat. Rev. Neurosci.* 16, 249–263. doi: 10.1038/nrn3898

Song, M., Chen, D., and Yu, S. P. (2014). The TRPC channel blocker SKF 96365 inhibits glioblastoma cell growth by enhancing reverse mode of the Na(+)/Ca(2+) exchanger and increasing intracellular Ca(2+). *Br. J. Pharmacol.* 171, 3432–3447. doi: 10.1111/bph.12691

Soni, H., and Adebiyi, A. (2016). TRPC6 channel activation promotes neonatal glomerular mesangial cell apoptosis via calcineurin/NFAT and FasL/Fas signaling pathways. *Sci Rep.* 6:29041. doi: 10.1038/srep29041

Su, Y., Zong, S., Wei, C., Song, F., Feng, H., Qin, A., et al. (2019). Salidroside promotes rat spinal cord injury recovery by inhibiting inflammatory cytokine expression and NF-κB and MAPK signaling pathways. *J. Cell Physiol.* 234, 14259–14269. doi: 10.1002/jcp.28124

Tauseef, M., Knezevic, N., Chava, K. R., Smith, M., Sukriti, S., Gianaris, N., et al. (2012). TLR4 activation of TRPC6-dependent calcium signaling mediates endotoxin-induced lung vascular permeability and inflammation. *J. Exp. Med.* 209, 1953–1968. doi: 10.1084/jem.20111355

Toth, P., Tucsek, Z., Sosnowska, D., Gautam, T., Mitschelen, M., Tarantini, S., et al. (2013). Age-related autoregulatory dysfunction and cerebromicrovascular injury in mice with angiotensin II-induced hypertension. *J. Cereb. Blood Flow Metab.* 33, 1732–1742. doi: 10.1038/jcbfm.2013.143

Venkatachalam, K., and Montell, C. (2007). TRP channels. *Annu. Rev. Biochem.* 76, 387–417. doi: 10.1146/annurev.biochem.75.103004.142819

Verstrepen, L., Bekaert, T., Chau, T. L., Tavernier, J., Chariot, A., and Beyaert, R. (2008). TLR-4, IL-1R and TNF-R signaling to NF-kappaB: variations on a common theme. *Cell Mol. Life Sci.* 65, 2964–2978. doi: 10.1007/s00018-008-8064-8

Wang, H., Cheng, X., Tian, J., Xiao, Y., Tian, T., Xu, F., et al. (2020a). TRPC channels: structure, function, regulation and recent advances in small molecular probes. *Pharmacol. Ther.* 209:107497. doi: 10.1016/j.pharmthera.2020.107497

Wang, J., Zhao, M., Jia, P., Liu, F. F., Chen, K., Meng, F. Y., et al. (2020b). The analgesic action of larixyl acetate, a potent TRPC6 inhibitor, in rat neuropathic pain model induced by spared nerve injury. *J. Neuroinflamm.* 17:118. doi: 10.1186/s12974-020-01767-8

Weber, E. W., Han, F., Tauseef, M., Birnbaumer, L., Mehta, D., and Muller, W. A. (2015). TRPC6 is the endothelial calcium channel that regulates leukocyte transendothelial migration during the inflammatory response. *J. Exp. Med.* 212, 1883–1899. doi: 10.1084/jem.20150353

Wei, T., Wang, Y., Xu, W., Liu, Y., Chen, H., and Yu, Z. (2019). KCa3.1 deficiency attenuates neuroinflammation by regulating an astrocyte phenotype switch involving the PI3K/AKT/GSK3β pathway. *Neurobiol. Dis.* 132:104588. doi: 10.1016/j.nbd.2019.104588

Werner, Y., Mass, E., Ashok Kumar, P., Ulas, T., Händler, K., Horne, A., et al. (2020). Cxcr4 distinguishes HSC-derived monocytes from microglia and reveals monocyte immune responses to experimental stroke. *Nat. Neurosci.* 23, 351–362. doi: 10.1038/s41593-020-0585-y

Xie, W., Zhu, T., Dong, X., Nan, F., Meng, X., Zhou, P., et al. (2019). HMGB1-triggered inflammation inhibition of notoginseng leaf triterpenes against cerebral ischemia and reperfusion injury via MAPK and NF-κB signaling pathways. *Biomolecules* 9:512. doi: 10.3390/biom9100512

Xu, N., Meng, H., Liu, T., Feng, Y., Qi, Y., and Wang, H. (2018). TRPC1 deficiency exacerbates cerebral ischemia/reperfusion-induced neurological injury by potentiating Nox4-derived reactive oxygen species generation. *Cell Physiol. Biochem.* 51, 1723–1738. doi: 10.1159/000495676

Yao, C., Zhang, J., Chen, F., and Lin, Y. (2013). Neuroprotectin D1 attenuates brain damage induced by transient middle cerebral artery occlusion in rats through TRPC6/CREB pathways. *Mol. Med. Rep.* 8, 543–550. doi: 10.3892/mmr.2013.1543

Yao, C., Zhang, J., Liu, G., Chen, F., and Lin, Y. (2014). Neuroprotection by (-)-epigallocatechin-3-gallate in a rat model of stroke is mediated through inhibition of endoplasmic reticulum stress. *Mol. Med. Rep.* 9, 69–76. doi: 10.3892/mmr.2013.1778

Ye, J., Das, S., Roy, A., Wei, W., Huang, H., Lorenz-Guertin, J. M., et al. (2019). Ischemic injury-induced CaMKIIδ and CaMKIIγ confer neuroprotection through the NF-κB signaling pathway. *Mol. Neurobiol.* 56, 2123–2136. doi: 10.1007/s12035-018-1198-2

Zhang, H., Sun, S., Wu, L., Pchitskaya, E., Zakharova, O., Fon Tacer, K., et al. (2016). Store-operated calcium channel complex in postsynaptic spines: a new therapeutic target for Alzheimer's disease treatment. *J. Neurosci.* 36, 11837–11850. doi: 10.1523/jneurosci.1188-16.2016

Zhang, Y., Qin, W., Zhang, L., Wu, X., Du, N., Hu, Y., et al. (2015). MicroRNA-26a prevents endothelial cell apoptosis by directly targeting TRPC6 in the setting of atherosclerosis. *Sci. Rep.* 5:9401. doi: 10.1038/srep09401

Zhou, J., Du, W., Zhou, K., Tai, Y., Yao, H., Jia, Y., et al. (2008). Critical role of TRPC6 channels in the formation of excitatory synapses. *Nat. Neurosci.* 11, 741–743. doi: 10.1038/nn.2127

13

Functional Importance of Transient Receptor Potential (TRP) Channels in Neurological Disorders

Kihwan Lee[1†], Youn Yi Jo[2†], Gehoon Chung[3], Jung Hoon Jung[4], Yong Ho Kim[1] and Chul-Kyu Park[1*]*

[1] Gachon Pain Center and Department of Physiology, Gachon University College of Medicine, Incheon, South Korea, [2] Department of Anesthesiology and Pain Medicine, Gil Medical Center, Gachon University, Incheon, South Korea, [3] Department of Oral Physiology and Program in Neurobiology, School of Dentistry, Seoul National University, Seoul, South Korea, [4] Program in Neurosciences and Mental Health, The Hospital for Sick Children, Toronto, ON, Canada

***Correspondence:**
Yong Ho Kim
euro16@gachon.ac.kr
Chul-Kyu Park
pck0708@gachon.ac.kr

† These authors have contributed equally to this work

Transient receptor potential (TRP) channels are transmembrane protein complexes that play important roles in the physiology and pathophysiology of both the central nervous system (CNS) and the peripheral nerve system (PNS). TRP channels function as non-selective cation channels that are activated by several chemical, mechanical, and thermal stimuli as well as by pH, osmolarity, and several endogenous or exogenous ligands, second messengers, and signaling molecules. On the pathophysiological side, these channels have been shown to play essential roles in the reproductive system, kidney, pancreas, lung, bone, intestine, as well as in neuropathic pain in both the CNS and PNS. In this context, TRP channels have been implicated in several neurological disorders, including Alzheimer's disease, Parkinson's disease, Huntington's disease, amyotrophic lateral sclerosis, and epilepsy. Herein, we focus on the latest involvement of TRP channels, with a special emphasis on the recently identified functional roles of TRP channels in neurological disorders related to the disruption in calcium ion homeostasis.

Keywords: TRP channels, neurological disorders, calcium homeostasis, Alzheimer's disease, Parkinson's disease, Huntington's disease, amyotrophic lateral sclerosis, epilepsy

INTRODUCTION

TRP Channel Subfamily

Transient receptor potential (TRP) channels are classified into 28 members that function as a group of unique non-selective cation channels in mammals. TRP channels are conserved in yeast, invertebrates, and vertebrates and share a common three-dimensional structure with six transmembrane helical segments (S1–S6), two variable and intracellular amino (-NH_2) and a carboxy (-COOH) terminal cytosolic domain, and the channel pore formed by S5 and S6, which allow transport of various ions including sodium (Na^+), potassium (K^+), calcium (Ca^{2+}), and magnesium ions (Mg^{2+}). Based on significant sequence homology and a common structure, TRP channels are divided into six subfamilies: TRPC (canonical), TRPM (melastatin), TRPV (vanilloid), TRPA (ankyrin), TRPP (polycystin), and TRPML (mucolipin). TRP subfamilies are divided into Group 1 (TRPC, TRPM, TRPV, and TRPA) and Group 2 (TRPP and TRPML) according to differences in their sequence and topology. Subfamilies of TRP channels are divided into groups and subtypes as represented in the phylogenetic tree in **Supplementary Figure 1**.

Transient receptor potential channels are ubiquitously expressed in many cell types (especially neurons and non-neuronal cells in the central nervous system, CNS) and tissues, including brain, kidney, pancreas, lung, bone, intestine, reproductive system as well as dorsal root ganglia (DRG) neurons in the peripheral nervous system (PNS). In addition, TRP channels are primarily expressed in plasma membranes that play critical roles in stimulus perception (i.e., thermosensation, mechanosensation, and chemosensation) and ion homeostasis (Nishida et al., 2006; Nilius and Owsianik, 2011).

Initially, TRP channels were shown to regulate cellular Ca^{2+} influx through the so-called store-operated channels (Nilius, 2004; Ramsey et al., 2006; Yazgan and Naziroglu, 2017). Several studies have shown that TRP channels regulate neuronal excitability, intracellular Ca^{2+} and Mg^{2+} homeostasis, as well as cell proliferation and differentiation (Nilius, 2004).

In addition to their physiological functions, TRP channels are known to contribute to various pathophysiological roles in neurological disorders of the CNS (Nilius, 2007; Colsoul et al., 2013; Takada et al., 2013).

Neurological Disorders

Neurodegenerative diseases, such as Alzheimer's disease (AD), Parkinson's disease (PD), Huntington's disease (HD), and amyotrophic lateral sclerosis (ALS) and epilepsy, collectively known as "neurological disorders," have distinct pathologies and represent a significant medical burden in the modern world.

Alzheimer's disease is the most common neurodegenerative disease in the world and is characterized by the accumulation of beta-amyloid (Aβ) plaques from amyloid precursor protein (APP) and hyperphosphorylated tau protein (Iqbal et al., 2010; Murphy and Levine, 2010). PD is also a common brain disorder, primarily characterized by a resting tremor, postural instability, rigidity, and bradykinesia caused by dopaminergic (DA) neuronal loss in the substantia nigra (SN) pars compacta (SNpc) (Michel et al., 2013; Kalia and Lang, 2015). HD is an inherited neurodegenerative disorder that causes cognitive deficits, emotional imbalance, and uncontrolled excessive motor movements caused by a CAG trinucleotide repeat expansion within the Huntingtin gene that leads to the synthesis of polyglutamine tracts (Kremer et al., 1994). ALS, also known as Lou Gehrig's disease, is another fatal type of neurodegenerative motor disease characterized by the deterioration of motor neurons in the motor cortex, brainstem, and spinal cord that leads to impairments in voluntary movement (Guatteo et al., 2007). Finally, epilepsy is a neurological disorder characterized by recurrent epileptic seizures, abnormal brain activity, and unusual behavior.

Over the past few decades, enormous efforts have been made to unveil the pathogenesis of neurological disorders. For example, endoplasmic reticulum (ER) stress, also known as oxidative stress, which is caused by misfolded proteins and abnormal Ca^{2+} homeostasis, neuroinflammation, and mitochondrial dysfunction have been shown to lead to neuronal cell death. Most notably, Ca^{2+} regulation, which is involved in normal physiological functions such as neuronal survival, proliferation, differentiation, gene transcription, and exocytosis at synapses, has been shown to be dysregulated in various neurological disorders (Bojarski et al., 2008; Bezprozvanny, 2009; Grosskreutz et al., 2010; Surmeier et al., 2010; Wu et al., 2011; Nikoletopoulou and Tavernarakis, 2012).

Interestingly, several studies have reported a correlation between intracellular Ca^{2+} concentrations ($[Ca^{2+}]_i$) and other pathogenic mechanisms, including the imbalance between antioxidant function and reactive oxygen species (ROS) production (Gorlach et al., 2015) as well as mitochondrial dysfunction (Contreras et al., 2010; Pivovarova and Andrews, 2010).

In fact, exposure of neuronal cells to Aβ peptides, induces an elevation of $[Ca^{2+}]_i$ that leads to cell death as observed in *in vitro* experiments (Adhya and Sharma, 2019). Aggregation of α-synuclein, which is associated with the pathology of PD, can also induce neuronal cell death via the disruption of cellular Ca^{2+} homeostasis (Fonfria et al., 2005; Danzer et al., 2007). Furthermore, the polyglutamine-expanded huntingtin protein and mutant superoxide dismutase-1 (SOD1), which are implicated in the pathogenesis of HD and ALS, respectively, also disrupt cellular Ca^{2+} homeostasis (Giacomello et al., 2013; Barrett et al., 2014). The disruption of intracellular Ca^{2+} concentration in epilepsy induces ROS production, apoptosis, and caspase activation through mitochondrial oxidative stress (Yilmaz et al., 2011; Naziroglu and Ovey, 2015). Therefore, alleviating disturbances in Ca^{2+} homeostasis may represent a potential therapeutic target for the treatment of neurological disorders (Nilius, 2007; Colsoul et al., 2013; Takada et al., 2013).

TRP CHANNELS IN NEUROLOGICAL DISORDERS

TRP Channels in AD

Importantly, a strong correlation between the pathological hallmarks of AD (Aβ accumulation and neurofibrillary tangles) and perturbed cellular Ca^{2+} homeostasis have been reported in AD patients as well as in animal and cell culture models of AD (Mattson and Chan, 2001). To date, TRPC1, TRPC3, TRPC6, TRPM2, TRPM7, TRPV1, TRPV4, TRPA1, and TRPML1 have been shown to be involved in AD (**Figure 1A**). TRPC1 is a member of the most prevalent TRPC channels in the brain and is linked to the store-operated Ca^{2+} channel-mediated Ca^{2+} entry (SOCE) channels. Interestingly, SOCE was reduced by downregulation of TRPC1 in astrocytes in APP knockout (KO) mice (Linde et al., 2011). Additionally, the alteration of the brain-derived neurotrophic factor-tropomyosin receptor kinase B-TRPC3 (BDNF-TrkB-TRPC3) signaling pathway led to hyperphosphorylation of tau protein caused by increased $[Ca^{2+}]_i$ levels in AD (Elliott and Ginzburg, 2006). Moreover, it has been reported that TRPC1 and TRPC3 are associated with caveolin-1, which is the main component of the plasma membrane caveolae that interacts with APP (Ikezu et al., 1998). Several studies have reported that TRPC6 in neurons promotes neuronal survival (Jia et al., 2007), synaptogenesis, and learning and memory (Zhou J. et al., 2008). Furthermore, in pharmacological studies using hyperforin, one of the

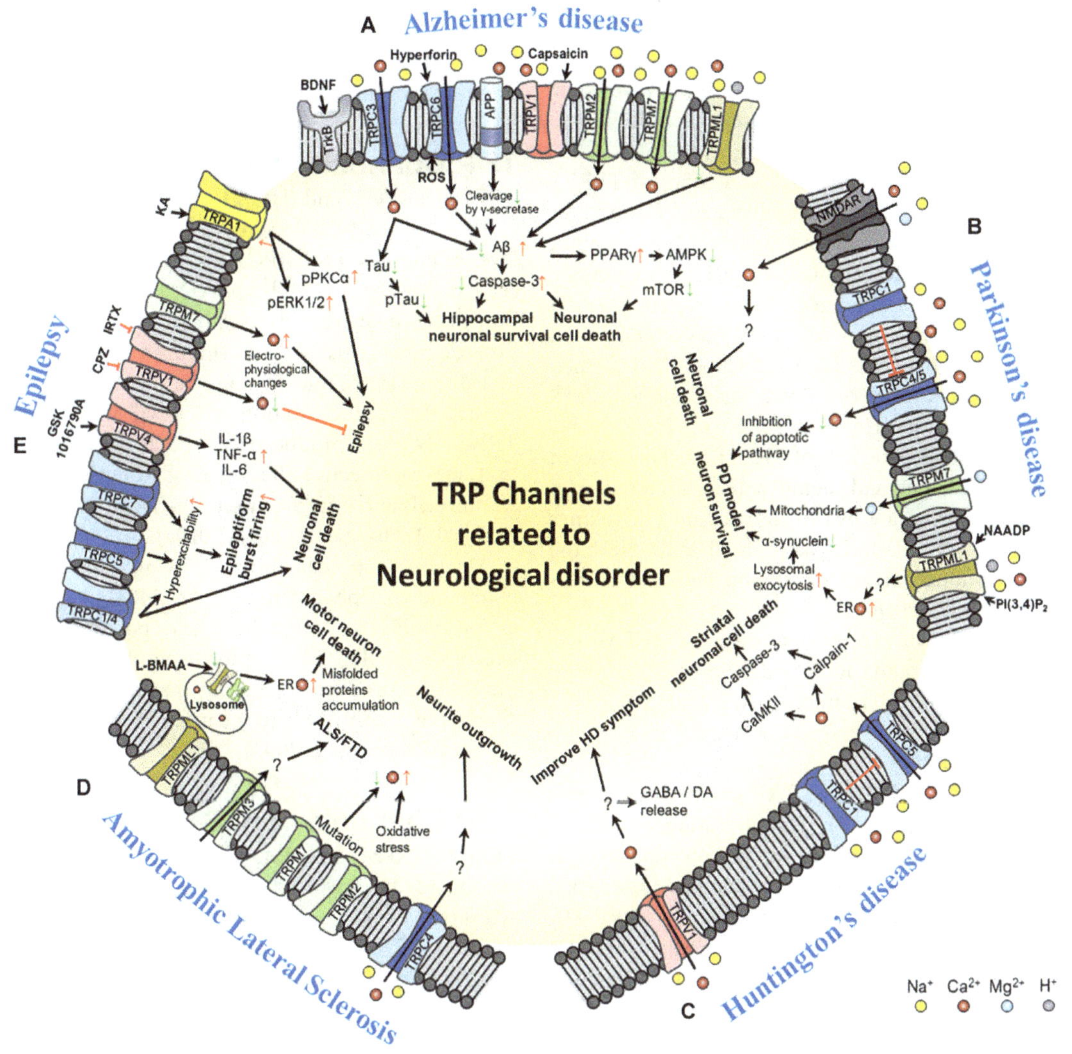

FIGURE 1 | Schematic of the molecular mechanism of TRP channel-mediated pathogenesis of neurological disorders: **(A)** Alzheimer's disease, **(B)** Parkinson's disease, **(C)** Huntington's disease, **(D)** Amyotrophic lateral sclerosis, and **(E)** epilepsy. In the figure, red arrows represent increase or up-regulation; green arrows, decrease or down-regulation; red thick bar, inhibition of the signaling pathway; and black arrows, activation of the signaling pathway. Ion channels involved in each of the neurological disorders and their transporting ions, channel agonists, and antagonists are also shown in the figure. *Abbreviations*: BDNF, brain-derived neurotrophic factor; ROS, reactive oxygen species; Aβ, beta-amyloid; PPAR, peroxisome proliferator-activated receptor gamma; AMPK, 5′ adenosine monophosphate-activated protein kinase; mTOR, mechanistic target of rapamycin; NMDAR, N-methyl-D-aspartate receptor; NAADP, Nicotinic acid adenine dinucleotide phosphate; $PI(3,4)P_2$, phosphatidylinositol (3,4)-bisphosphate; PD, Parkinson's disease; ER, endoplasmic reticulum; GABA, gamma-aminobutyric acid; DA, dopamine; ALS/FTD, amyotrophic lateral sclerosis patients with frontotemporal dementia; L-BMAA, L-beta-methylamino-L-alanine; IL, interleukin; TNF-α, tumor necrosis factor alpha; CPZ, capsazepine; IRTX, 5′-Iodoresiniferatoxin; KA, kainic acid; pPKCα, phospho-protein kinase C alpha; pERK1/2, phospho-extracellular signal-regulated kinase 1/2.

main natural compounds of the medicinal plant Saint John's wort that acts as an antidepressant drug (Zanoli, 2004) and TRPC6 activator (Tu et al., 2010), or tetrahydrohyperforin, a stable semisynthetic compound derived from hyperforin (Rozio et al., 2005), TRPC6 was shown to play a potential role in AD through the reduction of Aβ accumulation due to increased cerebrovascular P-glycoprotein (Brenn et al., 2014) and increased adult hippocampal neurogenesis and long-term spatial memory (Abbott et al., 2013), respectively. In contrast, AD-linked presenilin (PS)-2 mutants influenced TRPC6-mediated neurotoxic Ca^{2+} entry (Lessard et al., 2005), whereas TRPC6 was shown to be neuroprotective against AD through interaction with the cleavage of APP (Wang et al., 2015). In fact, a recent study observed that hyperforin induced activation of TRPC6, reduced Aβ levels, and improved mild cognitive impairment in AD models and that TRPC6 mRNA levels in the blood cells were reduced in AD patients (Lu et al., 2018).

While APP/PS1 transgenic (Tg) mice were observed to have age-dependent spatial memory deficits through TRPM2 channel activation by toxic oligomeric Aβ, genetic elimination of TRPM2 in APP/PS1 Tg mice ameliorated the synaptic loss and spatial memory deficits (Ostapchenko et al., 2015). It has been suggested that the TRPM2 channel may be a possible therapeutic agent of neuronal toxicity and memory impairment in AD. In contrast, TRPM7, which is another TRPM channel, plays an important role in not only inducing anoxic neuronal cell death by disrupting Ca^{2+} and Mg^{2+} homeostasis but also increasing susceptibility to degenerative processes (Aarts et al., 2003).

In recent studies of TRPV channels, the activity of TRPV1 was reported to reduce oxidative/nitrosative stress (Hofrichter et al., 2013; Jayant et al., 2016), rescue Aβ-induced degradation of hippocampal neurons (Balleza-Tapia et al., 2018), and increase levels of presynaptic synapsin I and postsynaptic density 93 (PSD93). In contrast, increased TRPV4 expression has been observed in the brain of aged rats (Lee and Choe, 2014), which is known to increase neuronal cell death via increased Ca^{2+} influx and ROS production (Hong et al., 2016). In APP/PS1 Tg/TRPA1 KO mice, the genetic loss of TRPA1 has been shown to exacerbate spatial learning and memory deficits, increase Aβ deposition, promote the release of pro-inflammatory cytokines such as interleukin (IL)-1β, IL-4, IL-6, and IL-10, and inhibit the activities of transcriptional factors NF-κB and nuclear factor of activated T cells (Lee et al., 2016).

Lastly, it has been shown that overexpression of TRPML1 is sufficient to rescue memory and cognitive deficits by diminishing neuronal apoptosis in APP/PS1 Tg mice (Zhang et al., 2017).

TRP Channels in PD

TRPC1, TRPC3, TRPM2, TRPM7, and TRPV1 have been shown to be involved in PD (**Figure 1B**). The activation of TRPC1 channels has been reported to induce neuroprotection against apoptosis in SH-SY5Y neuroblastoma cells (Bollimuntha et al., 2006), as well as to regulate SOCE channels and reduce DA neuronal cell death in the SN of TRPC1 KO mice (Selvaraj et al., 2009, 2012). Consistent with these reports, decreased levels of TRPC1 have been detected in brain lysates from the SNpc of PD patients (Sun et al., 2017). In contrast to TRPC1 levels, TRPC3 levels are not altered in SNpc DA neurons in PD patients (Sun et al., 2017) although their levels are increased by the compensatory effect of decreased TRPC1 in 1-methyl-4-phenyl-1,2,3,6-tetrahyrdropyridine (MPTP)-induced PD-like conditions (Selvaraj et al., 2009). Constitutively active TRPC3 channels are known to express and regulate firing intensity and pattern in GABAergic neurons of the SN pars reticulata (SNpr) (Zhou F. W. et al., 2008). Therefore, this channel may also be involved in different brain subregions or pathophysiological mechanisms of PD.

Additionally, 1-methyl-4-phenylpyridinium ion (MPP^+)-induced oxidative stress has been shown to increase intracellular Ca^{2+} influx via TRPM2 channel activity and promote DA neuronal cell death in the SNpc (Sun et al., 2018). Importantly, TRPM7 channels regulate Mg^{2+} homeostasis in cells, and increased concentrations of Mg^{2+} significantly inhibit MPP + -induced neurotoxicity by reducing the number of DA neurons and ameliorating the length of DA neurites (Hashimoto et al., 2008; Paravicini et al., 2012).

The activation of TRPV1 has also been shown to induce cell death in DA neurons, increase Ca^{2+} influx, and mediate mitochondrial disruption (Kim et al., 2005; Nam et al., 2015).

Furthermore, activation of TRPML1 evokes global ER Ca^{2+} release and Ca^{2+} influx (Kilpatrick et al., 2016) and results in upregulated lysosomal exocytosis, thus preventing α-synuclein accumulation in DA neurons (Tsunemi et al., 2019).

TRP Channels in HD

TRPC1, TRPC5, and TRPV1 have been shown to be involved in HD (**Figure 1C**). Recently, it was shown that the expression level of endogenous TRPC1 was decreased in Q111 HD striatal cells compared to wild-type (Q7) cells (Hong et al., 2015). Furthermore, increased glutathionylation of TRPC5, activated by oxidants, leads to Ca^{2+}-induced apoptosis of the striatal neurons in HD Tg mice (Hong et al., 2015). However, knockdown by siTRPC5 and inhibition of TRPC5 with ML204, a selective TRPC4 blocker produced by the Molecular Libraries Probe, produces a protective effect against oxidative stress in Q111 HD striatal cells and improves motor behavior in HD Tg mice (Miller et al., 2011; Hong et al., 2015, 2020a).

Moreover, it has been shown that administration of N-arachidonoylphenolamine (AM404), an inhibitor of endocannabinoid reuptake, has potential antihyperkinetic effects via the TRPV1 receptor using the 3-nitropropionic acid-induced HD model, suggesting that the activity of the TRPV1 channel may contribute to the motor dysfunction in HD patients (Lastres-Becker et al., 2003).

TRP Channels in ALS

TRPC4, TRPM2, TRPM3, TRPM7, and TRPML1 have been shown to be involved in ALS (**Figure 1D**). The clinical symptoms of ALS overlap with those of Parkinsonism dementia complex (PDC), a neurodegenerative disorder characterized by symptoms of PD and dementia (Garruto, 2006; Hermosura and Garruto, 2007). While the pathogenesis of ALS/PDC is not fully understood, it is thought to be caused by two potential scenarios: (i) low levels of Ca^{2+} and Mg^{2+}, which cause excess ROS production and cell death, and (ii) excess exposure to putative neurotoxin β-methylamino-L-alanine (L-BMAA), derived from the cycad plant, which causes an increase of $[Ca^{2+}]_i$ (Brownson et al., 2002).

A previous study demonstrated that the expression of TRPC4 is increased by nerve growth factor and dibutyryl-cAMP treatment in cultured DRG neurons. Conversely, inhibition of TRPC4 using a selective siRNA approach reduces neurite outgrowth in cultured DRG neurons (Wu et al., 2008). In ALS, reactive astrocytes accelerate nerve growth factor production (Pehar et al., 2004). In addition, a recent study demonstrated that ALS-resistant motor neurons from mutant SOD1 ALS models upregulate axonal outgrowth and dendritic branching (Osking et al., 2019). Taken together, these findings suggest that TRPC4 regulates DRG differentiation and plays a pivotal role in ALS.

In contrast, mutations in both $TRPM2^{P1018L}$ and $TRPM7^{T1482I}$ have been found in Guamanian ALS/PDC patients. Importantly, the $TRPM2^{P1018L}$ variant was shown to attenuate oxidative stress-induced Ca^{2+} influx through inactivation of the channel (Hermosura et al., 2008). In contrast, the $TRPM7^{T1482I}$ variant promotes an imbalance in Ca^{2+} and Mg^{2+} homeostasis

(Hermosura and Garruto, 2007). TRPM3, which is in the same group as TRPM2, has also been considered as a possible candidate gene involved in the pathogenesis of ALS with frontotemporal dementia (Lee et al., 2003).

TRPML1 was expressed in cell lysosomes or in the endosomal membrane and in the main Ca^{2+}-releasing channel used as a regulator of lysosomal storage via phosphatidylinositol 3,5-biphosphate ($PI(3,5)P_2$) (Cheng et al., 2010; Li et al., 2013). In addition, TRPML1 also regulates the maintenance of lysosome homeostasis and accumulation of autophagy (Cheng et al., 2010; Curcio-Morelli et al., 2010; Morgan et al., 2011). Interestingly, $PI(3,5)P_2$ levels are significantly impaired in some forms of ALS (Chow et al., 2009; Osmanovic et al., 2017). Moreover, in an experimental model of ALS/PDC, the expression of TRPML1 was shown to be reduced through autophagy leading to the loss of motor neurons. Additionally, with an L-BMAA-induced ALS mouse model, it was discovered that TRPML1 is downregulated, and autophagy is impaired in primary motor neurons, which leads to ER stress and neuronal cell death (Tedeschi et al., 2019).

TRP Channels in Epilepsy

TRPC1, TRPC3-7, TRPM2, TRPM7, TRPV1, TRPV4, and TRPA1 have been shown to be involved in epilepsy (**Figure 1E**). As mentioned above, TRPC channels are not only known to play an important role in neuronal outgrowth and survival during brain development but are also believed to play a pivotal role in various epileptogenic processes. For example, the expression of TRPC1 is increased in cortical lesions of epilepsy patients and regulated by the mediation of astrocyte-induced epilepsy (Zang et al., 2015). Using a pilocarpine (muscarinic agonist)-induced status epilepticus (PISE) model, studies have shown that the genetic elimination of TRPC3 reduces the susceptibility of seizures to pilocarpine, while enhancing the expression of TRPC3 induces hyperexcitability and increases susceptibility to epileptiform activity in the cortex (Zhou and Roper, 2014; Phelan et al., 2017). In contrast, the expression of TRPC6 has been shown to be down-regulated in chronic epileptic rats, whereas the genetic ablation by siTRPC6 increases seizure susceptibility and seizure-induced neuronal damage in the dentate gyrus but not in CA1 and CA3 neurons of the hippocampus (Kim and Kang, 2015). In addition, in other members of the TRPC family, the genetic deletion of TRPC1/4 reduces seizure-induced neuronal cell death. Furthermore, TRPC5 KO mice exhibit significantly reduced seizures as well as minimal seizure-induced neuronal cell death in the CA1 and CA3 areas of the hippocampus (Phelan et al., 2013). Conversely, the TRPC7 channel plays an important role in spontaneous epileptiform bursting in the CA3, the reduction of which is correlated with a reduction in PISE in TRPC7 KO mice (Phelan et al., 2014).

The TRPM family is also involved in the pathogenesis of epilepsy. For example, TRPM2 channels are co-expressed with the EF-hand domain-containing protein 1 gene, which is related to an increased susceptibility to juvenile myoclonic epilepsy, and are regulated in the hippocampal neurons (Katano et al., 2012). Moreover, TRPM7 has been shown to be activated during epilepsy (Aarts and Tymianski, 2005). Importantly, genetic ablation of TRPM7 blocks the activation of a cation current, which is produced by oxygen-glucose deprivation (I_{OGD}), and prevents ROS-mediated I_{OGD} activation (Aarts et al., 2003).

Although the TRPV1 channel is believed to play an essential role in the development of neurogenic pain and inflammation in the sensory neurons (Caterina and Julius, 2001; Julius and Basbaum, 2001), it is also expressed in other brain regions, including the cerebral cortex, hippocampus, cerebellum, thalamus, hypothalamus, striatum, midbrain, and amygdala (Cristino et al., 2006). Furthermore, increased expression of TRPV1 has been found in the hippocampus of rats and the dentate gyrus of mice with temporal lobe epilepsy as well as in the cortex of patients with temporal lobe epilepsy (Bhaskaran and Smith, 2010; Sun et al., 2013; Saffarzadeh et al., 2015). In fact, a recent study suggested that the activation of the TRPV1 channel may play a key role in the development of epilepsy (Naziroglu and Ovey, 2015). Using capsazepine, 5′-iodoresiniferatoxin, and resolvins, the authors showed that inhibition of the TRPV1 channel induced protective effects against epilepsy and epilepsy-induced Ca^{2+} entry in the hippocampal and DRG neurons (Naziroglu and Ovey, 2015).

Activation of TRPV3 by eugenol was shown to suppress epileptiform field potentials and decrease the amplitude of field postsynaptic potentials evoked in CA1 neurons of the hippocampus and the third layer of the neocortex (Muller et al., 2006). Another study using the PISE model of epilepsy found that activation of TRPV4 by the specific agonist GSK1016790A increased pro-inflammatory cytokines (TNF-α, IL-1β, and IL-6), while the inhibition of TRPV4 by HC-067047, a selective TRPV4 antagonist, significantly increased cell survival post status epilepticus (Wang et al., 2019).

Using a kainic acid-induced seizure model, TRPA1 was found to be upregulated while TRPV4 was not, which is contradictory to the earlier findings concerning TRPV4 (Hunt et al., 2012; Wang et al., 2019).

CONCLUSION AND FUTURE PERSPECTIVES

In this review, we described the functional importance of TRP channels in the regulation of Ca^{2+} and oxidative stress responses as well as their contributions to neurological disorders, including AD, PD, HD, ALS, and epilepsy.

Overall, in addition to playing a broad range of physiological roles throughout the CNS and PNS, TRP channels also contribute to pathophysiology across a wide range of diseases and disorders through abnormalities in Ca^{2+} homeostasis. In the CNS, TRP channels are expressed in several brain regions (including the spinal cord) and have been shown to be key regulatory proteins involved in lipid metabolism, glucose homeostasis (Liu et al., 2009; Zhu et al., 2011), and the pathobiology of aforementioned neurological disorders.

Apart from their important role in neurological disorders of the CNS, TRP channels are also expressed in the neurons of the DRG, trigeminal ganglion, and sympathetic ganglion, and contribute to both normal and pathological sensory processing in the PNS (Lee et al., 2019). For example, TRP channels are known to be involved in diabetic peripheral neuropathy, chemotherapy-induced peripheral neuropathy, and autonomic neuropathy.

In light of the physiological and pathophysiological functions of TRP channels in both the CNS and PNS, we believe that they represent potential therapeutic targets for treating neurological disorders of the CNS as well as neuropathic pain in the PNS.

AUTHOR CONTRIBUTIONS

KL, YYJ, YHK, and C-KP contributed to the conception and design. KL and YYJ drafted the manuscript. KL, GC, JHJ, YHK, and C-KP revised the manuscript. All authors contributed to the article and approved the submitted version.

SUPPLEMENTARY MATERIAL

Supplementary Figure 1 | Summary of TRP subfamilies-mediated studies related to neurological disorders [modified from Nilius (2007), Hong et al. (2020b), Thapak et al. (2020)]. Different colors are used in the table for better classification and the gray boxes in the "Related Disease" column represent the roles of specific TRP subfamilies in each neurological disorders as reported in the published literature. *Abbreviations*: AD, Alzheimer's disease; ALS, amyotrophic lateral sclerosis; AMG, amygdala; APP, amyloid precursor protein; BBB, blood-brain barrier; BG, basal ganglia; Bs, brainstem; CB, cerebellum; CC, corpus callosum; Cd, caudate; Cg, cingulate gyrus; CNS, central nervous system; CTX, cortex; DA, dopamine; DG, dentate gyrus; DRG, dorsal root ganglion; ER, endoplasmic reticulum; FB, forebrain; fCTX, frontal cortex; GABA, gamma-aminobutyric acid; GP, globus pallidus; HD, Huntington's disease; HPC, hippocampus; HT, hypothalamus; IC, inferior colliculus; JME, juvenile myoclonic epilepsy; KA, kainic acid; LS, lateral septum; MB, midbrain; mFBb, medial forebrain bundle; mPFC, medial prefrontal cortex; mTOR, mechanistic target of rapamycin; n.d., not determined; OB, olfactory bulb; PD, Parkinson's disease; PISE, pilocarpine-induced status epilepticus; PNS, peripheral nervous system; Pm, putamen; PS1, presenilin 1; RCh, retrochiasmatic area; SC, spinal cord; Sep, septum; SN, substantia nigra; SNpc, substantia nigra pars compacta; SNpr, substantia nigra pars reticulata; SOCE, store-operated calcium entry; Str, striatum; TH, thalamus; vS, ventral subiculum.

REFERENCES

Aarts, M., Iihara, K., Wei, W. L., Xiong, Z. G., Arundine, M., Cerwinski, W., et al. (2003). A key role for TRPM7 channels in anoxic neuronal death. *Cell* 115, 863–877. doi: 10.1016/s0092-8674(03)01017-1

Aarts, M. M., and Tymianski, M. (2005). TRsPMs and neuronal cell death. *Pflugers Arch.* 451, 243–249.

Abbott, A. C., Calderon Toledo, C., Aranguiz, F. C., Inestrosa, N. C., and Varela-Nallar, L. (2013). Tetrahydrohyperforin increases adult hippocampal neurogenesis in wild-type and APPswe/PS1DeltaE9 mice. *J. Alzheimers Dis.* 34, 873–885. doi: 10.3233/jad-121714

Adhya, P., and Sharma, S. S. (2019). Redox TRPs in diabetes and diabetic complications: mechanisms and pharmacological modulation. *Pharmacol. Res.* 146:104271. doi: 10.1016/j.phrs.2019.104271

Balleza-Tapia, H., Crux, S., Andrade-Talavera, Y., Dolz-Gaiton, P., Papadia, D., Chen, G., et al. (2018). TrpV1 receptor activation rescues neuronal function and network gamma oscillations from Abeta-induced impairment in mouse hippocampus in vitro. *Elife* 7:e37703.

Barrett, E. F., Barrett, J. N., and David, G. (2014). Dysfunctional mitochondrial Ca(2+) handling in mutant SOD1 mouse models of fALS: integration of findings from motor neuron somata and motor terminals. *Front. Cell. Neurosci.* 8:184.

Bezprozvanny, I. (2009). Calcium signaling and neurodegenerative diseases. *Trends Mol. Med.* 15, 89–100. doi: 10.1016/j.molmed.2009.01.001

Bhaskaran, M. D., and Smith, B. N. (2010). Effects of TRPV1 activation on synaptic excitation in the dentate gyrus of a mouse model of temporal lobe epilepsy. *Exp. Neurol.* 223, 529–536. doi: 10.1016/j.expneurol.2010.01.021

Bojarski, L., Herms, J., and Kuznicki, J. (2008). Calcium dysregulation in Alzheimer's disease. *Neurochem. Int.* 52, 621–633.

Bollimuntha, S., Ebadi, M., and Singh, B. B. (2006). TRPC1 protects human SH-SY5Y cells against salsolinol-induced cytotoxicity by inhibiting apoptosis. *Brain Res.* 1099, 141–149. doi: 10.1016/j.brainres.2006.04.104

Brenn, A., Grube, M., Jedlitschky, G., Fischer, A., Strohmeier, B., Eiden, M., et al. (2014). St. John's Wort reduces beta-amyloid accumulation in a double transgenic Alzheimer's disease mouse model-role of P-glycoprotein. *Brain Pathol.* 24, 18–24. doi: 10.1111/bpa.12069

Brownson, D. M., Mabry, T. J., and Leslie, S. W. (2002). The cycad neurotoxic amino acid, beta-N-methylamino-L-alanine (BMAA), elevates intracellular calcium levels in dissociated rat brain cells. *J. Ethnopharmacol.* 82, 159–167. doi: 10.1016/s0378-8741(02)00170-8

Caterina, M. J., and Julius, D. (2001). The vanilloid receptor: a molecular gateway to the pain pathway. *Annu. Rev. Neurosci.* 24, 487–517. doi: 10.1146/annurev.neuro.24.1.487

Cheng, X., Shen, D., Samie, M., and Xu, H. (2010). Mucolipins: intracellular TRPML1-3 channels. *FEBS Lett.* 584, 2013–2021. doi: 10.1016/j.febslet.2009.12.056

Chow, C. Y., Landers, J. E., Bergren, S. K., Sapp, P. C., Grant, A. E., Jones, J. M., et al. (2009). Deleterious variants of FIG4, a phosphoinositide phosphatase, in patients with ALS. *Am. J. Hum. Genet.* 84, 85–88. doi: 10.1016/j.ajhg.2008.12.010

Colsoul, B., Nilius, B., and Vennekens, R. (2013). Transient receptor potential (TRP) cation channels in diabetes. *Curr. Top. Med. Chem.* 13, 258–269. doi: 10.2174/1568026611313030004

Contreras, L., Drago, I., Zampese, E., and Pozzan, T. (2010). Mitochondria: the calcium connection. *Biochim. Biophys. Acta* 1797, 607–618. doi: 10.1016/j.bbabio.2010.05.005

Cristino, L., De Petrocellis, L., Pryce, G., Baker, D., Guglielmotti, V., and Di Marzo, V. (2006). Immunohistochemical localization of cannabinoid type 1 and vanilloid transient receptor potential vanilloid type 1 receptors in the mouse brain. *Neuroscience* 139, 1405–1415. doi: 10.1016/j.neuroscience.2006.02.074

Curcio-Morelli, C., Charles, F. A., Micsenyi, M. C., Cao, Y., Venugopal, B., Browning, M. F., et al. (2010). Macroautophagy is defective in mucolipin-1-deficient mouse neurons. *Neurobiol. Dis.* 40, 370–377. doi: 10.1016/j.nbd.2010.06.010

Danzer, K. M., Haasen, D., Karow, A. R., Moussaud, S., Habeck, M., Giese, A., et al. (2007). Different species of alpha-synuclein oligomers induce calcium influx and seeding. *J. Neurosci.* 27, 9220–9232.

Elliott, E., and Ginzburg, I. (2006). The role of neurotrophins and insulin on tau pathology in Alzheimer's disease. *Rev. Neurosci.* 17, 635–642.

Fonfria, E., Marshall, I. C., Boyfield, I., Skaper, S. D., Hughes, J. P., Owen, D. E., et al. (2005). Amyloid beta-peptide(1-42) and hydrogen peroxide-induced toxicity are mediated by TRPM2 in rat primary striatal cultures. *J. Neurochem.* 95, 715–723. doi: 10.1111/j.1471-4159.2005.03396.x

Garruto, R. M. (2006). A commentary on neuronal degeneration and cell death in Guam ALS and PD: an evolutionary process of understanding. *Curr. Alzheimer Res.* 3, 397–401. doi: 10.2174/156720506778249425

Giacomello, M., Oliveros, J. C., Naranjo, J. R., and Carafoli, E. (2013). Neuronal Ca(2+) dyshomeostasis in Huntington disease. *Prion* 7, 76–84. doi: 10.4161/pri.23581

Gorlach, A., Bertram, K., Hudecova, S., and Krizanova, O. (2015). Calcium and ROS: a mutual interplay. *Redox Biol.* 6, 260–271. doi: 10.1016/j.redox.2015.08.010

Grosskreutz, J., Van Den Bosch, L., and Keller, B. U. (2010). Calcium dysregulation in amyotrophic lateral sclerosis. *Cell Calcium* 47, 165–174. doi: 10.1016/j.ceca.2009.12.002

Guatteo, E., Carunchio, I., Pieri, M., Albo, F., Canu, N., Mercuri, N. B., et al. (2007). Altered calcium homeostasis in motor neurons following AMPA receptor but not voltage-dependent calcium channels' activation in a genetic model of amyotrophic lateral sclerosis. *Neurobiol. Dis.* 28, 90–100. doi: 10.1016/j.nbd.2007.07.002

Hashimoto, T., Nishi, K., Nagasao, J., Tsuji, S., and Oyanagi, K. (2008). Magnesium exerts both preventive and ameliorating effects in an in vitro rat Parkinson disease model involving 1-methyl-4-phenylpyridinium (MPP+) toxicity in dopaminergic neurons. *Brain Res.* 1197, 143–151. doi: 10.1016/j.brainres.2007.12.033

Hermosura, M. C., Cui, A. M., Go, R. C., Davenport, B., Shetler, C. M., Heizer, J. W., et al. (2008). Altered functional properties of a TRPM2 variant in Guamanian ALS and PD. *Proc. Natl. Acad. Sci. U.S.A.* 105, 18029–18034. doi: 10.1073/pnas.0808218105

Hermosura, M. C., and Garruto, R. M. (2007). TRPM7 and TRPM2-Candidate susceptibility genes for Western Pacific ALS and PD? *Biochim. Biophys. Acta* 1772, 822–835. doi: 10.1016/j.bbadis.2007.02.008

Hofrichter, J., Krohn, M., Schumacher, T., Lange, C., Feistel, B., Walbroel, B., et al. (2013). Reduced Alzheimer's disease pathology by St. John's Wort treatment is independent of hyperforin and facilitated by ABCC1 and microglia activation in mice. *Curr. Alzheimer Res.* 10, 1057–1069. doi: 10.2174/15672050113106660171

Hong, C., Choi, S. H., Kwak, M., Jeong, B., Ko, J., Park, H. J., et al. (2020a). TRPC5 channel instability induced by depalmitoylation protects striatal neurons against oxidative stress in Huntington's disease. *Biochim. Biophys. Acta Mol. Cell Res.* 1867:118620. doi: 10.1016/j.bbamcr.2019.118620

Hong, C., Jeong, B., Park, H. J., Chung, J. Y., Lee, J. E., Kim, J., et al. (2020b). TRP channels as emerging therapeutic targets for neurodegenerative diseases. *Front. Physiol.* 11:238. doi: 10.3389/fphys.2020.00238

Hong, C., Seo, H., Kwak, M., Jeon, J., Jang, J., Jeong, E. M., et al. (2015). Increased TRPC5 glutathionylation contributes to striatal neuron loss in Huntington's disease. *Brain* 138, 3030–3047. doi: 10.1093/brain/awv188

Hong, Z., Tian, Y., Yuan, Y., Qi, M., Li, Y., Du, Y., et al. (2016). Enhanced oxidative stress is responsible for TRPV4-induced neurotoxicity. *Front. Cell. Neurosci.* 10:232. doi: 10.3389/fncel.2016.00232

Hunt, R. F., Hortopan, G. A., Gillespie, A., and Baraban, S. C. (2012). A novel zebrafish model of hyperthermia-induced seizures reveals a role for TRPV4 channels and NMDA-type glutamate receptors. *Exp. Neurol.* 237, 199–206. doi: 10.1016/j.expneurol.2012.06.013

Ikezu, T., Trapp, B. D., Song, K. S., Schlegel, A., Lisanti, M. P., and Okamoto, T. (1998). Caveolae, plasma membrane microdomains for alpha-secretase-mediated processing of the amyloid precursor protein. *J. Biol. Chem.* 273, 10485–10495. doi: 10.1074/jbc.273.17.10485

Iqbal, K., Liu, F., Gong, C. X., and Grundke-Iqbal, I. (2010). Tau in Alzheimer disease and related tauopathies. *Curr. Alzheimer Res.* 7, 656–664. doi: 10.2174/156720510793611592

Jayant, S., Sharma, B. M., and Sharma, B. (2016). Protective effect of transient receptor potential vanilloid subtype 1 (TRPV1) modulator, against behavioral, biochemical and structural damage in experimental models of Alzheimer's disease. *Brain Res.* 1642, 397–408. doi: 10.1016/j.brainres.2016.04.022

Jia, Y., Zhou, J., Tai, Y., and Wang, Y. (2007). TRPC channels promote cerebellar granule neuron survival. *Nat. Neurosci.* 10, 559–567. doi: 10.1038/nn1870

Julius, D., and Basbaum, A. I. (2001). Molecular mechanisms of nociception. *Nature* 413, 203–210. doi: 10.1038/35093019

Kalia, L. V., and Lang, A. E. (2015). Parkinson's disease. *Lancet* 386, 896–912.

Katano, M., Numata, T., Aguan, K., Hara, Y., Kiyonaka, S., Yamamoto, S., et al. (2012). The juvenile myoclonic epilepsy-related protein EFHC1 interacts with the redox-sensitive TRPM2 channel linked to cell death. *Cell Calcium* 51, 179–185. doi: 10.1016/j.ceca.2011.12.011

Kilpatrick, B. S., Yates, E., Grimm, C., Schapira, A. H., and Patel, S. (2016). Endo-lysosomal TRP mucolipin-1 channels trigger global ER Ca2+ release and Ca2+ influx. *J. Cell Sci.* 129, 3859–3867. doi: 10.1242/jcs.190322

Kim, S. R., Lee, D. Y., Chung, E. S., Oh, U. T., Kim, S. U., and Jin, B. K. (2005). Transient receptor potential vanilloid subtype 1 mediates cell death of mesencephalic dopaminergic neurons in vivo and in vitro. *J. Neurosci.* 25, 662–671. doi: 10.1523/jneurosci.4166-04.2005

Kim, Y. J., and Kang, T. C. (2015). The role of TRPC6 in seizure susceptibility and seizure-related neuronal damage in the rat dentate gyrus. *Neuroscience* 307, 215–230. doi: 10.1016/j.neuroscience.2015.08.054

Kremer, B., Goldberg, P., Andrew, S. E., Theilmann, J., Telenius, H., Zeisler, J., et al. (1994). A worldwide study of the Huntington's disease mutation. The sensitivity and specificity of measuring CAG repeats. *N. Engl. J. Med.* 330, 1401–1406. doi: 10.1056/nejm199405193302001

Lastres-Becker, I., De Miguel, R., De Petrocellis, L., Makriyannis, A., Di Marzo, V., and Fernandez-Ruiz, J. (2003). Compounds acting at the endocannabinoid and/or endovanilloid systems reduce hyperkinesia in a rat model of Huntington's disease. *J. Neurochem.* 84, 1097–1109. doi: 10.1046/j.1471-4159.2003.01595.x

Lee, J. C., and Choe, S. Y. (2014). Age-related changes in the distribution of transient receptor potential vanilloid 4 channel (TRPV4) in the central nervous system of rats. *J. Mol. Histol.* 45, 497–505. doi: 10.1007/s10735-014-9578-z

Lee, K., Lee, B. M., Park, C. K., Kim, Y. H., and Chung, G. (2019). Ion channels involved in tooth pain. *Int. J. Mol. Sci.* 20:2266. doi: 10.3390/ijms20092266

Lee, K. I., Lee, H. T., Lin, H. C., Tsay, H. J., Tsai, F. C., Shyue, S. K., et al. (2016). Role of transient receptor potential ankyrin 1 channels in Alzheimer's disease. *J. Neuroinflammation* 13:92.

Lee, N., Chen, J., Sun, L., Wu, S., Gray, K. R., Rich, A., et al. (2003). Expression and characterization of human transient receptor potential melastatin 3 (hTRPM3). *J. Biol. Chem.* 278, 20890–20897. doi: 10.1074/jbc.m211232200

Lessard, C. B., Lussier, M. P., Cayouette, S., Bourque, G., and Boulay, G. (2005). The overexpression of presenilin2 and Alzheimer's-disease-linked presenilin2 variants influences TRPC6-enhanced Ca2+ entry into HEK293 cells. *Cell. Signal.* 17, 437–445. doi: 10.1016/j.cellsig.2004.09.005

Li, X., Garrity, A. G., and Xu, H. (2013). Regulation of membrane trafficking by signalling on endosomal and lysosomal membranes. *J. Physiol.* 591, 4389–4401. doi: 10.1113/jphysiol.2013.258301

Linde, C. I., Baryshnikov, S. G., Mazzocco-Spezzia, A., and Golovina, V. A. (2011). Dysregulation of Ca2+ signaling in astrocytes from mice lacking amyloid precursor protein. *Am. J. Physiol. Cell Physiol.* 300, C1502–C1512.

Liu, H., Dear, A. E., Knudsen, L. B., and Simpson, R. W. (2009). A long-acting glucagon-like peptide-1 analogue attenuates induction of plasminogen activator inhibitor type-1 and vascular adhesion molecules. *J. Endocrinol.* 201, 59–66. doi: 10.1677/joe-08-0468

Lu, R., Wang, J., Tao, R., Wang, J., Zhu, T., Guo, W., et al. (2018). Reduced TRPC6 mRNA levels in the blood cells of patients with Alzheimer's disease and mild cognitive impairment. *Mol. Psychiatry* 23, 767–776. doi: 10.1038/mp.2017.136

Mattson, M. P., and Chan, S. L. (2001). Dysregulation of cellular calcium homeostasis in Alzheimer's disease: bad genes and bad habits. *J. Mol. Neurosci.* 17, 205–224. doi: 10.1385/jmn:17:2:205

Michel, P. P., Toulorge, D., Guerreiro, S., and Hirsch, E. C. (2013). Specific needs of dopamine neurons for stimulation in order to survive: implication for Parkinson disease. *FASEB J.* 27, 3414–3423. doi: 10.1096/fj.12-220418

Miller, M., Shi, J., Zhu, Y., Kustov, M., Tian, J. B., Stevens, A., et al. (2011). Identification of ML204, a novel potent antagonist that selectively modulates native TRPC4/C5 ion channels. *J. Biol. Chem.* 286, 33436–33446. doi: 10.1074/jbc.m111.274167

Morgan, A. J., Platt, F. M., Lloyd-Evans, E., and Galione, A. (2011). Molecular mechanisms of endolysosomal Ca2+ signalling in health and disease. *Biochem. J.* 439, 349–374. doi: 10.1042/bj20110949

Muller, M., Pape, H. C., Speckmann, E. J., and Gorji, A. (2006). Effect of eugenol on spreading depression and epileptiform discharges in rat neocortical and hippocampal tissues. *Neuroscience* 140, 743–751. doi: 10.1016/j.neuroscience.2006.02.036

Murphy, M. P., and Levine, H. III (2010). Alzheimer's disease and the amyloid-beta peptide. *J. Alzheimers Dis.* 19, 311–323.

Nam, J. H., Park, E. S., Won, S. Y., Lee, Y. A., Kim, K. I., Jeong, J. Y., et al. (2015). TRPV1 on astrocytes rescues nigral dopamine neurons in Parkinson's disease via CNTF. *Brain* 138, 3610–3622. doi: 10.1093/brain/awv297

Naziroglu, M., and Ovey, I. S. (2015). Involvement of apoptosis and calcium accumulation through TRPV1 channels in neurobiology of epilepsy. *Neuroscience* 293, 55–66. doi: 10.1016/j.neuroscience.2015.02.041

Nikoletopoulou, V., and Tavernarakis, N. (2012). Calcium homeostasis in aging neurons. *Front. Genet.* 3:200. doi: 10.3389/fgene.2012.00200

Nilius, B. (2004). Store-operated Ca2+ entry channels: still elusive! *Sci. STKE* 2004:e36.

Nilius, B. (2007). TRP channels in disease. *Biochim. Biophys. Acta* 1772, 805–812.

Nilius, B., and Owsianik, G. (2011). The transient receptor potential family of ion channels. *Genome Biol.* 12:218. doi: 10.1186/gb-2011-12-3-218

Nishida, M., Hara, Y., Yoshida, T., Inoue, R., and Mori, Y. (2006). TRP channels: molecular diversity and physiological function. *Microcirculation* 13, 535–550. doi: 10.1080/10739680600885111

Osking, Z., Ayers, J. I., Hildebrandt, R., Skruber, K., Brown, H., Ryu, D., et al. (2019). ALS-Linked SOD1 mutants enhance neurite outgrowth and branching in adult motor neurons. *iScience* 19, 448–449. doi: 10.1016/j.isci.2019.08.004

Osmanovic, A., Rangnau, I., Kosfeld, A., Abdulla, S., Janssen, C., Auber, B., et al. (2017). FIG4 variants in central European patients with amyotrophic lateral sclerosis: a whole-exome and targeted sequencing study. *Eur. J. Hum. Genet.* 25, 324–331. doi: 10.1038/ejhg.2016.186

Ostapchenko, V. G., Chen, M., Guzman, M. S., Xie, Y. F., Lavine, N., Fan, J., et al. (2015). The transient receptor potential melastatin 2 (TRPM2) channel contributes to beta-amyloid oligomer-related neurotoxicity and memory impairment. *J. Neurosci.* 35, 15157–15169. doi: 10.1523/jneurosci.4081-14.2015

Paravicini, T. M., Chubanov, V., and Gudermann, T. (2012). TRPM7: a unique channel involved in magnesium homeostasis. *Int. J. Biochem. Cell Biol.* 44, 1381–1384. doi: 10.1016/j.biocel.2012.05.010

Pehar, M., Cassina, P., Vargas, M. R., Castellanos, R., Viera, L., Beckman, J. S., et al. (2004). Astrocytic production of nerve growth factor in motor neuron apoptosis: implications for amyotrophic lateral sclerosis. *J. Neurochem.* 89, 464–473. doi: 10.1111/j.1471-4159.2004.02357.x

Phelan, K. D., Shwe, U. T., Abramowitz, J., Birnbaumer, L., and Zheng, F. (2014). Critical role of canonical transient receptor potential channel 7 in initiation of seizures. *Proc. Natl. Acad. Sci. U.S.A.* 111, 11533–11538. doi: 10.1073/pnas.1411442111

Phelan, K. D., Shwe, U. T., Abramowitz, J., Wu, H., Rhee, S. W., Howell, M. D., et al. (2013). Canonical transient receptor channel 5 (TRPC5) and TRPC1/4 contribute to seizure and excitotoxicity by distinct cellular mechanisms. *Mol. Pharmacol.* 83, 429–438. doi: 10.1124/mol.112.082271

Phelan, K. D., Shwe, U. T., Cozart, M. A., Wu, H., Mock, M. M., Abramowitz, J., et al. (2017). TRPC3 channels play a critical role in the theta component of pilocarpine-induced status epilepticus in mice. *Epilepsia* 58, 247–254. doi: 10.1111/epi.13648

Pivovarova, N. B., and Andrews, S. B. (2010). Calcium-dependent mitochondrial function and dysfunction in neurons. *FEBS J.* 277, 3622–3636. doi: 10.1111/j.1742-4658.2010.07754.x

Ramsey, I. S., Delling, M., and Clapham, D. E. (2006). An introduction to TRP channels. *Annu. Rev. Physiol.* 68, 619–647.

Rozio, M., Fracasso, C., Riva, A., Morazzoni, P., and Caccia, S. (2005). High-performance liquid chromatography measurement of hyperforin and its reduced derivatives in rodent plasma. *J. Chromatogr. B Analyt. Technol. Biomed. Life Sci.* 816, 21–27. doi: 10.1016/j.jchromb.2004.10.015

Saffarzadeh, F., Eslamizade, M. J., Ghadiri, T., Modarres Mousavi, S. M., Hadjighassem, M., and Gorji, A. (2015). Effects of TRPV1 on the hippocampal synaptic plasticity in the epileptic rat brain. *Synapse* 69, 375–383. doi: 10.1002/syn.21825

Selvaraj, S., Sun, Y., Watt, J. A., Wang, S., Lei, S., Birnbaumer, L., et al. (2012). Neurotoxin-induced ER stress in mouse dopaminergic neurons involves downregulation of TRPC1 and inhibition of AKT/mTOR signaling. *J. Clin. Invest.* 122, 1354–1367. doi: 10.1172/jci61332

Selvaraj, S., Watt, J. A., and Singh, B. B. (2009). TRPC1 inhibits apoptotic cell degeneration induced by dopaminergic neurotoxin MPTP/MPP(+). *Cell Calcium* 46, 209–218. doi: 10.1016/j.ceca.2009.07.008

Sun, F. J., Guo, W., Zheng, D. H., Zhang, C. Q., Li, S., Liu, S. Y., et al. (2013). Increased expression of TRPV1 in the cortex and hippocampus from patients with mesial temporal lobe epilepsy. *J. Mol. Neurosci.* 49, 182–193. doi: 10.1007/s12031-012-9878-2

Sun, Y., Sukumaran, P., Selvaraj, S., Cilz, N. I., Schaar, A., Lei, S., et al. (2018). TRPM2 promotes neurotoxin MPP(+)/MPTP-induced cell death. *Mol. Neurobiol.* 55, 409–420. doi: 10.1007/s12035-016-0338-9

Sun, Y., Zhang, H., Selvaraj, S., Sukumaran, P., Lei, S., Birnbaumer, L., et al. (2017). Inhibition of L-type Ca(2+) channels by TRPC1-STIM1 complex is essential for the protection of dopaminergic neurons. *J. Neurosci.* 37, 3364–3377. doi: 10.1523/jneurosci.3010-16.2017

Surmeier, D. J., Guzman, J. N., and Sanchez-Padilla, J. (2010). Calcium, cellular aging, and selective neuronal vulnerability in Parkinson's disease. *Cell Calcium* 47, 175–182. doi: 10.1016/j.ceca.2009.12.003

Takada, Y., Numata, T., and Mori, Y. (2013). Targeting TRPs in neurodegenerative disorders. *Curr. Top. Med. Chem.* 13, 322–334. doi: 10.2174/1568026611313030009

Tedeschi, V., Petrozziello, T., Sisalli, M. J., Boscia, F., Canzoniero, L. M. T., and Secondo, A. (2019). The activation of Mucolipin TRP channel 1 (TRPML1) protects motor neurons from L-BMAA neurotoxicity by promoting autophagic clearance. *Sci. Rep.* 9:10743.

Thapak, P., Vaidya, B., Joshi, H. C., Singh, J. N., and Sharma, S. S. (2020). Therapeutic potential of pharmacological agents targeting TRP channels in CNS disorders. *Pharmacol. Res.* 159:105026. doi: 10.1016/j.phrs.2020.105026

Tsunemi, T., Perez-Rosello, T., Ishiguro, Y., Yoroisaka, A., Jeon, S., Hamada, K., et al. (2019). Increased lysosomal exocytosis induced by lysosomal Ca(2+) channel agonists protects human dopaminergic neurons from alpha-synuclein toxicity. *J. Neurosci.* 39, 5760–5772. doi: 10.1523/jneurosci.3085-18.2019

Tu, P., Gibon, J., and Bouron, A. (2010). The TRPC6 channel activator hyperforin induces the release of zinc and calcium from mitochondria. *J. Neurochem.* 112, 204–213. doi: 10.1111/j.1471-4159.2009.06446.x

Wang, J., Lu, R., Yang, J., Li, H., He, Z., Jing, N., et al. (2015). TRPC6 specifically interacts with APP to inhibit its cleavage by gamma-secretase and reduce Abeta production. *Nat. Commun.* 6:8876.

Wang, Z., Zhou, L., An, D., Xu, W., Wu, C., Sha, S., et al. (2019). TRPV4-induced inflammatory response is involved in neuronal death in pilocarpine model of temporal lobe epilepsy in mice. *Cell Death Dis.* 10:491.

Wu, D., Huang, W., Richardson, P. M., Priestley, J. V., and Liu, M. (2008). TRPC4 in rat dorsal root ganglion neurons is increased after nerve injury and is necessary for neurite outgrowth. *J. Biol. Chem.* 283, 416–426. doi: 10.1074/jbc.m703177200

Wu, J., Shih, H. P., Vigont, V., Hrdlicka, L., Diggins, L., Singh, C., et al. (2011). Neuronal store-operated calcium entry pathway as a novel therapeutic target for Huntington's disease treatment. *Chem. Biol.* 18, 777–793. doi: 10.1016/j.chembiol.2011.04.012

Yazgan, Y., and Naziroglu, M. (2017). Ovariectomy-induced mitochondrial oxidative stress, apoptosis, and calcium ion influx through TRPA1, TRPM2, and TRPV1 are prevented by 17beta-estradiol, tamoxifen, and raloxifene in the hippocampus and dorsal root ganglion of rats. *Mol. Neurobiol.* 54, 7620–7638. doi: 10.1007/s12035-016-0232-5

Yilmaz, M., Naziroglu, M., Kutluhan, S., Yilmaz, N., Yurekli, V. A., and Vural, H. (2011). Topiramate modulates hippocampus NMDA receptors via brain Ca(2+) homeostasis in pentylentetrazol-induced epilepsy of rats. *J. Recept. Signal Transduct. Res.* 31, 173–179. doi: 10.3109/10799893.2011.555914

Zang, Z., Li, S., Zhang, W., Chen, X., Zheng, D., Shu, H., et al. (2015). Expression patterns of TRPC1 in cortical lesions from patients with focal cortical dysplasia. *J. Mol. Neurosci.* 57, 265–272. doi: 10.1007/s12031-015-0615-5

Zanoli, P. (2004). Role of hyperforin in the pharmacological activities of St. John's Wort. *CNS Drug Rev.* 10, 203–218. doi: 10.1111/j.1527-3458.2004.tb00022.x

Zhang, L., Fang, Y., Cheng, X., Lian, Y., Xu, H., Zeng, Z., et al. (2017). TRPML1 participates in the progression of Alzheimer's disease by regulating the PPARgamma/AMPK/Mtor signalling pathway. *Cell. Physiol. Biochem.* 43, 2446–2456. doi: 10.1159/000484449

Zhou, F. W., Matta, S. G., and Zhou, F. M. (2008). Constitutively active TRPC3 channels regulate basal ganglia output neurons. *J. Neurosci.* 28, 473–482. doi: 10.1523/jneurosci.3978-07.2008

Zhou, F. W., and Roper, S. N. (2014). TRPC3 mediates hyperexcitability and epileptiform activity in immature cortex and experimental cortical dysplasia. *J. Neurophysiol.* 111, 1227–1237. doi: 10.1152/jn.00607.2013

Zhou, J., Du, W., Zhou, K., Tai, Y., Yao, H., Jia, Y., et al. (2008). Critical role of TRPC6 channels in the formation of excitatory synapses. *Nat. Neurosci.* 11, 741–743. doi: 10.1038/nn.2127

Zhu, Z., Luo, Z., Ma, S., and Liu, D. (2011). TRP channels and their implications in metabolic diseases. *Pflugers Arch.* 461, 211–223. doi: 10.1007/s00424-010-0902-5

14

Contribution of TRPC Channels in Neuronal Excitotoxicity Associated with Neurodegenerative Disease and Ischemic Stroke

Jaepyo Jeon[1], Fan Bu[2], Guanghua Sun[2], Jin-Bin Tian[1], Shun-Ming Ting[2], Jun Li[2], Jaroslaw Aronowski[2], Lutz Birnbaumer[3,4,5], Marc Freichel[6,7] and Michael X. Zhu[1]*

[1] Department of Integrative Biology and Pharmacology, McGovern Medical School, The University of Texas Health Science Center at Houston, Houston, TX, United States, [2] Department of Neurology, McGovern Medical School, The University of Texas Health Science Center at Houston, Houston, TX, United States, [3] Institute for Biomedical Research (BIOMED UCA-CONICET), Buenos Aires, Argentina, [4] School of Medical Sciences, Catholic University of Argentina (UCA), Buenos Aires, Argentina, [5] Neurobiology Laboratory, National Institute of Environmental Health Sciences, Durham, NC, United States, [6] Department of Pharmacology, Heidelberg University, Heidelberg, Germany, [7] DZHK (German Centre for Cardiovascular Research), partner site Heidelberg/Mannheim, Heidelberg, Germany

***Correspondence:**
Michael X. Zhu
Michael.X.Zhu@uth.tmc.edu

The seven canonical members of transient receptor potential (TRPC) proteins form cation channels that evoke membrane depolarization and intracellular calcium concentration ($[Ca^{2+}]_i$) rise, which are not only important for regulating cell function but their deregulation can also lead to cell damage. Recent studies have implicated complex roles of TRPC channels in neurodegenerative diseases including ischemic stroke. Brain ischemia reduces oxygen and glucose supply to neurons, i.e., Oxygen and Glucose Deprivation (OGD), resulting in $[Ca^{2+}]_i$ elevation, ion dyshomeostasis, and excitotoxicity, which are also common in many forms of neurodegenerative diseases. Although ionotropic glutamate receptors, e.g., *N*-methyl-D-aspartate receptors, are well established to play roles in excitotoxicity, the contribution of metabotropic glutamate receptors and their downstream effectors, i.e., TRPC channels, should not be neglected. Here, we summarize the current findings about contributions of TRPC channels in neurodegenerative diseases, with a focus on OGD-induced neuronal death and rodent models of cerebral ischemia/reperfusion. TRPC channels play both detrimental and protective roles to neurodegeneration depending on the TRPC subtype and specific pathological conditions involved. When illustrated the mechanisms by which TRPC channels are involved in neuronal survival or death seem differ greatly, implicating diverse and complex regulation. We provide our own data showing that TRPC1/C4/C5, especially TRPC4, may be generally detrimental in OGD and cerebral ischemia/reperfusion. We propose that although TRPC channels significantly contribute to ischemic neuronal death, detailed mechanisms and specific roles of TRPC subtypes in brain injury at different stages of ischemia/reperfusion and in different brain regions need to be carefully and systematically investigated.

Keywords: neurological disease, TRPC4 knockout, calcium, neuroprotection, neurodegeneration, neuronal death

INTRODUCTION

Stroke occurs when a part of the brain is deprived of oxygen and glucose. Each year, about 795,000 Americans suffer a new or recurrent stroke, making it the No. 5 cause of death and a leading cause of disability in the United States (Virani et al., 2020). In 70–80% of the cases, the precipitating cause of stroke is a blood clot that blocks the supply of oxygenated blood to a region of the brain, a situation termed ischemic stroke (Woodruff et al., 2011). The damage to neurons during ischemia is caused by a reduction of oxygen and glucose supply, i.e., oxygen and glucose deprivation (OGD) (Ying et al., 1997; Lipton, 1999).

Cell death after cerebral ischemia may result from a number of events, including acidosis, inflammation, generation of arachidonic acid, elevation in intracellular calcium concentrations ($[Ca^{2+}]_i$), loss of cellular ion homeostasis, free radical-mediated toxicity, energy failure, infiltration of leukocytes, cytokine-mediated cytotoxicity and glutamate-induced excitotoxicity (Woodruff et al., 2011). Particularly, excessive extracellular glutamate can elicit multiple neurotoxic effects. Initially, energy depletion-induced depolarization of the neuronal membrane leads to the influx of Ca^{2+} through voltage-gated Ca^{2+} channels (VGCCs), which triggers Ca^{2+}-dependent glutamate release from axonal terminals of excitatory neurons (Bonde et al., 2005). In the past, much of the focus on glutamate-induced excitotoxicity had been on ionotropic glutamate receptors (iGluRs), mainly NMDA (*N*-methyl-D-aspartate) receptors and AMPA (a-amino-3-hydroxy-5-methyl-4-isoxazolepropionic acid) receptors, but more recently, metabotropic glutamate receptors (mGluRs) have also been recognized to play a crucial role in excitotoxicity (Hilton et al., 2006).

The mGluR family consists of three groups, group I-III, and 8 subtypes, mGluR1-8, of which the group I mGluRs, i.e., mGluR1 and mGluR5, are coupled to $G_{q/11}$-phospholipase C (PLC) pathway and the rest are all linked to $G_{i/o}$ proteins (Swanson et al., 2005). On one hand, the activation of $G_{q/11}$-PLC pathway by glutamate through stimulation of mGluR1/5 is to enhance neuronal excitability via a number of mechanisms, such as the suppression of K^+ channels caused by the breakdown of phosphatidylinositol 4,5-bisphosphate (PIP_2), a phospholipid that supports the activity of many K^+ channels (Hille et al., 2015), and the production of inositol 1,4,5-trisphosphate (IP_3), a second messenger that acts at the IP_3 receptors to mobilize Ca^{2+} from the endoplasmic reticulum (ER) Ca^{2+} stores (Berridge, 2009). On the other hand, the activation of $G_{i/o}$-coupled group II and group III mGluRs are generally thought to inhibit neuronal excitation through, among others, activation of G protein-gated inwardly rectifying K^+ (GIRK) channels and inhibition of VGCCs (Logothetis et al., 2015). Therefore, the excessive extracellular glutamate associated with OGD may lead to both excitatory and inhibitory effects through mGluRs depending on the abundance and types of the mGluRs and downstream signaling pathways involved.

A major class of Ca^{2+}-permeable non-selective cation channels activated downstream from mGluRs is the Transient Receptor Potential Canonical (TRPC) channels. The TRPC channel family consists of 7 members, TRPC1-7, in which TRPC2 is a pseudogene in humans (Montell et al., 2002). These channels are typically activated downstream from receptors linked to PLC signaling, with $G_{q/11}$-PLCβ pathway being the most common. Thus, glutamate activation of $G_{q/11}$-coupled mGluR1/5 is likely linked to TRPC channel activation, leading to consequent membrane depolarization and $[Ca^{2+}]_i$ elevation. Ironically, despite the widespread expression of TRPCs in brain neurons (Riccio et al., 2002) and their much-longer lasting activities in response to $G_{q/11}$-PLCβ signaling than iGluRs (Hartmann et al., 2008; Riccio et al., 2009), not much is known about the contributions of TRPC channels in excitotoxicity to neurons except for a few examples. It was shown that in the pilocarpine-induced epilepsy model, the epileptiform burst firing in lateral septal and hippocampal neurons involves the activation of TRPC channels downstream from mGluRs, which is critical for the glutamate excitotoxicity (Phelan et al., 2012, 2013; Zheng and Phelan, 2014). In brain injury induced by focal cerebral ischemia, the roles of TRPC channels can be rather complex. For instance, while TRPC1 and TRPC4 mediate glutamate-induced neuronal death, TRPC6 may exert a protective role against ischemic neuronal death (Du et al., 2010).

Here, we explore the current evidence on contributions of TRPC channels in ischemic neuronal death, taking into account that these channels are activated downstream from mGluRs and likely work in concert with VGCCs and iGluRs to induce neuronal excitation and produce $[Ca^{2+}]_i$ signals, and such activities can have a pivotal impact on glutamate excitotoxicity. Because excitotoxicity occurs commonly in many types of neurodegenerative diseases, including Alzheimer's disease, epilepsy, Huntington's disease, and Parkinson's disease, we also discuss the involvement of TRPC channels in these diseases in attempt to shed some lights on the mechanistic insights of TRPC regulation of excitotoxicity. Finally, we present some of our own data demonstrating the specific role of TRPC4/C5 channels in ischemic cell death and neuroprotective potential of targeting these channels using small molecular probes.

THE BASIS OF EXCITOTOXIC NEURONAL DEATH IN ISCHEMIC STROKE

Cerebral ischemic stroke is caused by interruption of blood supply through the middle cerebral artery (MCA). The MCA has large surface branches to supply blood into its territory that encompasses almost the entire boundary of the cortex and white matter of the hemisphere, including the major lobes (frontal, parietal, temporal, and occipital) and insula cortex (Brust, 2013). Occlusion of the MCA (MCAO) is the most frequently encountered stroke signs and symptoms, which may produce paralysis on the left or right side of the body, vision loss, and speech impairment (Rathore et al., 2002). The neurological deficits in ischemic stroke resulted from the deprivation of glucose and oxygen supply, or OGD, which leads to brain tissue damages. When the MCAO is prolonged, neurons lose glucose-dependent ATP generation, which in turn disrupts electrogenic pumps, e.g., plasma membrane Ca^{2+} ATPase (PMCA) and Na^+/K^+ ATPase.

The failure of the ATPases subsequently results in $[Ca^{2+}]_i$ increase and membrane depolarization, which causes glutamate release, as well as an elevation of extracellular K^+ concentration. These also alter the ionic composition of the cytoplasm, with increases in Na^+, Ca^{2+}, and Cl^- and a decrease in K^+ levels, leading to an osmolarity change and more commonly hyperosmolarity (Tanaka et al., 1997; Tanaka et al., 1999; Brisson and Andrew, 2012). Consequently, the inflow of water into the neuron in response to the osmolality change causes cell swelling and disruption of the membrane structure, which constitutes one of the multiple causes of neuronal death (Toyoda et al., 2020).

In addition to ionic imbalance caused by the failure of ATPases, excessive extracellular accumulation of glutamate also leads to toxic increases in $[Ca^{2+}]_i$, which activate multiple signaling pathways and ultimately lead to cell death (Durukan and Tatlisumak, 2007; Doyle et al., 2008). For many years, NMDA and AMPA receptors have been considered the pivotal targets of excitotoxicity associated with ischemic stroke. The activation of postsynaptic NMDA and AMPA receptors by synaptic glutamate causes membrane depolarization and Ca^{2+} influx, which definitely accounts for excitotoxicity. However, this is not the only way by which glutamate can elicit excitotoxicity. The abundant presence of mGluRs in both pre- and postsynaptic membranes, as well as extrasynaptic membranes, suggests that these metabotropic receptors are also activated under conditions of excessive glutamate release and accumulation both inside and outside the synapse. At least for mGluR1 and mGluR5, the activation will increase excitability through $[Ca^{2+}]_i$ elevation first by causing ER Ca^{2+} release. This will be followed by store- and/or receptor-operated Ca^{2+} entry, and in the case of coupling to TRPC channels, the activation of these mGluRs will also lead to membrane depolarization, given the non-selective nature of these channels, and the subsequent Ca^{2+} influx through both TRPC channels and VGCCs. Although permeable to both Na^+ and Ca^{2+} as the NMDA and AMPA receptors, the conductance and activation kinetics of TRPC channels are vastly different from that of the iGluRs, typically being slower and longer lasting than the iGluRs as has been demonstrated during synaptic transmission (Hartmann et al., 2008; Riccio et al., 2009; Pressler and Regehr, 2013; Reiner and Levitz, 2018). Thus, in addition to iGluRs, the mGluR-TRPC coupling represents another main mechanism by which glutamate can induce excitotoxicity through $[Ca^{2+}]_i$ elevation and membrane depolarization, along with the consequent ionic imbalance, osmolarity changes and Ca^{2+} signaling (Toyoda et al., 2020), resulting in spatiotemporally distinct signaling effects that work in concert with those generated by iGluRs to induce cell demise.

Importantly, in spite of the promising results in reducing ischemic damage of brain tissues in animal models and the tremendous efforts made, antagonists of NMDA and AMPA receptors have not been effective in terms of neuroprotection against brain injury associated with ischemic stroke in clinical trials. Therefore, it would be beneficial to gain a better understanding of ischemic stroke pathology of the brain by exploring additional pathways, which will help identify new therapeutic candidates and approaches. Based on the current literature and our own experimental findings, we propose that TRPC channels play a critical part in neurological damage associated with ischemic stroke and should be evaluated as viable therapeutic targets for neuroprotection (**Figure 1**).

THE ROLES OF TRPC CHANNELS IN CELL DEATH

The seven mammalian TRPC members are divided into 4 subgroups (TRPC1, TRPC2, TRPC3/6/7, and TRPC4/5). Among them, TRPC1, C3, C4, C5, and C6 are highly expressed in neurons at various brain regions, with distinct distributions and functions; for example, TRPC3 is highly expressed in cerebellar Purkinje neurons and involved in motor coordination, TRPC4 and TRPC5 are highly expressed in cerebral cortex, hippocampus and amygdala and functionally implicated in anxiety and fear learning (Clapham, 2003; Venkatachalam and Montell, 2007; Hartmann et al., 2008; Riccio et al., 2009; Riccio et al., 2014). In general, the TRPC channels in neurons are activated downstream from stimulation of $G_{q/11}$-coupled receptors, including mGluR1/5 (Kim et al., 2003; El-Hassar et al., 2011; Phelan et al., 2012), M1 muscarinic receptors (Yan et al., 2009; Tai et al., 2011), 5-HT2 serotonin receptor (Munsch et al., 2003; Sohn et al., 2011; Gao et al., 2017), H1 histamine receptor (Tabarean, 2012), kisspeptin receptor (Zhang et al., 2008), cholecystokinin (CCK) type 1 and type 2 receptors (Riccio et al., 2009; Wang et al., 2011), and thyrotropin-releasing hormone (TRH) receptors (Zhang et al., 2015). In addition, receptor tyrosine kinases, such as TrkB receptor through stimulation by brain-derived neurotrophic factor (BDNF) (Amaral and Pozzo-Miller, 2007; Li et al., 2010) and leptin receptor by leptin (Qiu et al., 2010), are also linked to TRPC channel activation in neurons through activation of PLCγ's. However, there are some exceptions. For instance, in olfactory bulb granule cells, the TRPC1/C4 heteromeric channels are dependent on NMDA receptors, instead of mGluRs, for activation that causes long lasting depolarization and sustained Ca^{2+} influx (Storch et al., 2012); the activation of TRPC-like channels in thalamic paraventricular nucleus neurons requires not only the $G_{q/11}$-coupled thyrotropin-releasing hormone receptors but also $G_{i/o}$-coupled cannabinoid receptors CB1 and CB2 (Zhang et al., 2015). This latter observation is very interesting in light of the recent findings that receptor-operated activation of TRPC4-containing channels requires coincident stimulation of $G_{i/o}$ protein signaling and PLC activities (Thakur et al., 2016, 2020; Jeon et al., 2020). In addition, some TRPC channels are also reported to be activated by nitric oxide, reactive oxygen species (ROS), thioredoxin, and Ca^{2+} store depletion (Yoshida et al., 2006; Xu et al., 2008; Ogawa et al., 2016). For more comprehensive discussions on activation mechanisms of TRPC channels, readers are referred to our recent review article (Wang et al., 2020).

All TRPC proteins form Ca^{2+}-permeable non-selective cation channels, which are tetramers composed of either identical (homotetramers) or different (heterotetramers) TRPC subunits.

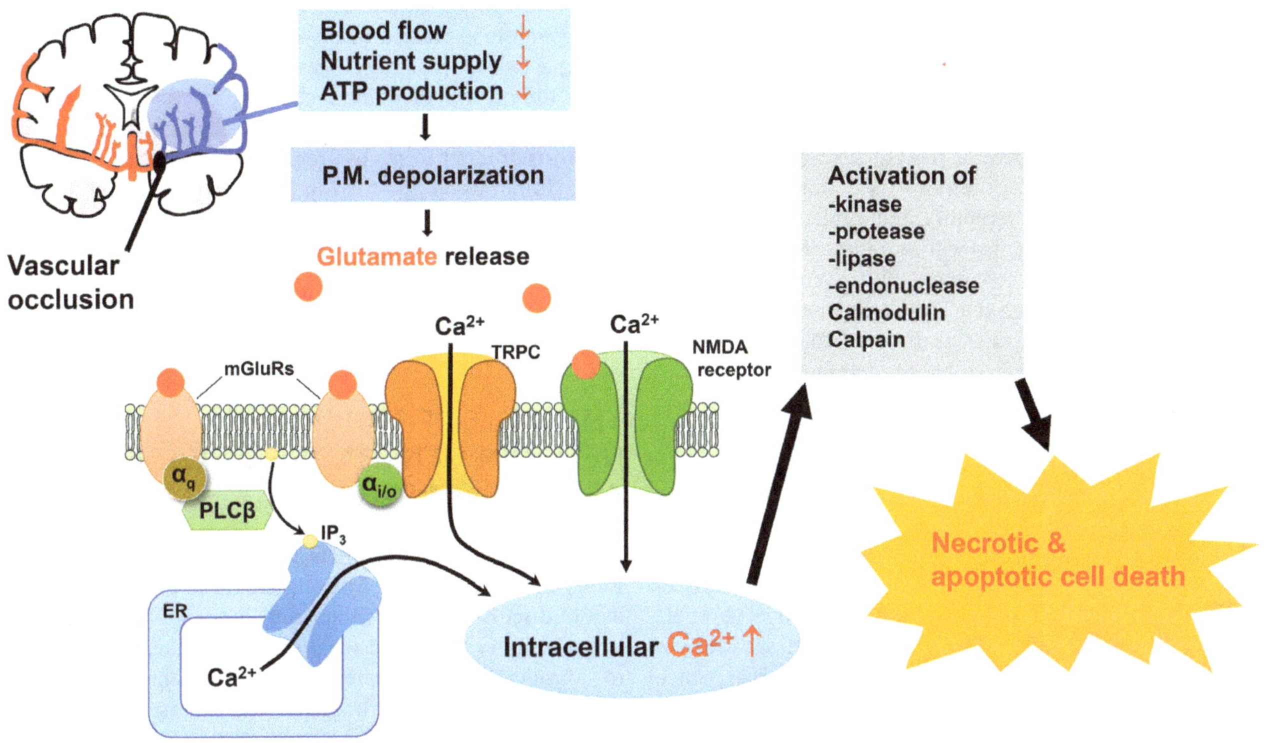

FIGURE 1 | Possible mechanisms for the involvement of TRPC channels in excitotoxic neuronal death in ischemic stroke. Oxygen and glucose deprivation due to the blockade of blood flow to brain areas in ischemic stroke causes excess accumulation of extracellular glutamate. The subsequent activation of NMDA receptors and mGluRs causes elevation of intracellular Ca^{2+} levels through Ca^{2+} influx from extracellular space and Ca^{2+} release from the ER, respectively. TRPC channels are activated downstream from mGluRs, causing more sustained Ca^{2+} elevation by mediating additional Ca^{2+} influx. TRPC4 and TRPC5 channels are also activated downstream from mGluR subtypes that couple to PTX-sensitive $G_{i/o}$ proteins, further expanding the repertoire of receptors that convey glutamate stimulation to Ca^{2+} signaling. Moreover, membrane depolarization resulting from activation of NMDA receptors and TRPC channels leads to excitation which also triggers additional Ca^{2+} influx through voltage-gated Ca^{2+} channels. The rise in intracellular Ca^{2+} due to these mechanisms causes activity changes of a plethora of enzymes, ion channels and transcription factors, as well as mitochondria, which when dysregulated induce cell death via either necrosis or apoptosis. ER, endoplasmic reticulum; IP_3, inositol 1,4,5-trisphosphate; mGluRs, metabotropic glutamate receptors; NMDA, *N*-methyl-D-aspartate; P.M., plasma membrane; PTX, pertussis toxin.

Among the seven TRPC isoforms, TRPC1 has been the most frequently studied in the context of heteromeric channels (Storch et al., 2012), especially in the forms of TRPC1/C4 and TRPC1/C4/C5 heteromers (Phelan et al., 2012; Storch et al., 2012; Broker-Lai et al., 2017). However, TRPC1/C3 heteromers also form, at least in cortical astrocytes where they regulate astrogliosis in response to traumatic brain injury (Belkacemi et al., 2017). As is the case of TRPC1/C4 and TRPC1/C5 channels where TRPC1 reduced the channel conductance (Strubing et al., 2001), TRPC1 also serves to dampen the Ca^{2+} signal and the astrogliosis-promoting effect of TRPC3 (Belkacemi et al., 2017).

The activation of TRPC channels causes Na^{+} and Ca^{2+} influxes into the cell, leading to membrane depolarization and $[Ca^{2+}]_i$ elevation. Both effects are important for TRPC channels to carry out their physiological functions. However, under conditions when these effects were not properly controlled, they can also contribute to pathology, reminiscent of iGluRs and other channels that damage cells through disrupting the membrane potential and/or causing Ca^{2+} overload. Due to differences in the biophysical properties, mechanisms of regulation, cell-type specific expression and subcellular distributions, the amplitudes, durations and subcellular locations of the depolarization and Ca^{2+} signals brought about by the activation of TRPC channels are likely very different from that by other channels. Furthermore, besides membrane depolarization and Ca^{2+} signals, TRPC channels also exert their effects on cell survival through other mechanisms, such as direct physical interactions with proteins involved in the cell death pathways (see later). Thus, the TRPC channels can have unique contributions to cell damage in difference diseases and different experimental models.

At least for TRPC4, a self-propagating positive-feedback mechanism has been proposed that allows persistent and prolonged channel activation (Thakur et al., 2020). In lateral septal neurons, this results in typically a depolarization plateau reaching to about −5 mV that lasts for about 1 s even when the stimulus, an agonist of mGluR1/5, is given for only 30 ms (Tian et al., 2014a). The all-or-none feature of the depolarization plateau is also consistent with the positive feedback mechanism. It was shown that this mechanism involves complex interactions among several intracellular messengers and protein partners, e.g., Ca^{2+}, H^{+}, and PLCδ1 (Thakur et al., 2020), the specific ranges of Ca^{2+} and PIP_2 concentrations as well as the optimal membrane potentials required for channel activation (Thakur et al., 2016). The functional coupling with PLCδ1 is probably a major reason for the self-propagating activation of the TRPC4 channel, as the PLC isozyme is targeted by its own products, Ca^{2+} and H^+ (Thakur et al., 2020). PLC catalyzes the hydrolysis of PIP_2, producing diacylglycerol (DAG), IP_3 and H^+ (Huang et al., 2010). Subsequently, IP_3 releases Ca^{2+} from the ER store through activation of IP_3 receptors and depletion of the ER Ca^{2+} store is often accompanied with store-operated Ca^{2+} entry from the extracellular space (Putney, 2017). When coupled to TRPC4, Ca^{2+} influx through the TRPC4 channel also provides an additional source for greater and more prolonged $[Ca^{2+}]_i$ increase, and the Ca^{2+} then feeds back to reinforce the activities of both PLCδ1 and TRPC4. In excitable cells, VGCCs also strongly impact native TRPC4 activation by bringing additional Ca^{2+}, and perhaps also a part of the voltage sensitivity even though the TRPC channels are intrinsically voltage sensitive on their own (Gordienko and Zholos, 2004; Tian et al., 2014a). In addition, PIP_2, which is continuously replenished upon hydrolysis through the actions of phosphatidylinositol 4 kinases and phosphatidylinositol-4-phosphate 5-kinases (Myeong et al., 2018), serves as both the membrane anchor and substrate of PLCδ1, as well as the source of DAG, IP_3 and H^+, which are all implicated in TRPC4 activation one way or the other (Storch et al., 2017; Thakur et al., 2020). However, at high concentrations, PIP_2 also exerts a tonic block on TRPC4 activation (Otsuguro et al., 2008; Thakur et al., 2016), and similarly, high cytosolic Ca^{2+} concentrations also suppress the channel activity (Thakur et al., 2016, 2020). Moreover, the optimal membrane potentials for TRPC4 activation, especially native TRPC4-containing channels, have been observed at −40 to −60 mV, and are influenced by $[Ca^{2+}]_i$ (Gordienko and Zholos, 2004). Therefore, an intricate balance is created through complex interactions among Ca^{2+}, PIP_2, DAG, H^+, and membrane voltage to support the coupled activities of PLCδ1 and TRPC4, leading to sustained channel activity that lasts much longer than the time of exposure to the triggering stimuli. Notably, for TRPC4, the triggering stimuli include coincident activations of $G_{i/o}$ proteins and PLC signaling through either $G_{q/11}$-PLCβ or receptor tyrosine kinase-PLCγ pathways (Jeon et al., 2020). For other TRPC channels, $G_{i/o}$ proteins may not be involved and the depolarization amplitude and duration may not be as strong and as long, respectively, as that of TRPC4. However, the dual (both stimulatory and inhibitory) regulation by PIP_2 and Ca^{2+}, and the sensitivity to DAG are common among the TRPCs (Wang et al., 2020), although whether or not they exhibit a specific dependence on a specific PLC isozyme, as in the case of PLCδ1 for TRPC4 (Thakur et al., 2016), remains to be elucidated. It is possible that other TRPC channels also exhibit self-propagating activation like TRPC4, but with different kinetics, amplitudes, and durations.

At the cellular level, the most direct evidence of TRPC channel contribution to cell death comes from cytotoxic effect of (−)-englerin A, a guaiane sesquiterpenoid found in the bark of *Phyllanthus engleri*, on renal carcinoma cells (Akbulut et al., 2015; Carson et al., 2015) and triple-negative breast cancer (TNBC) cell lines (Grant et al., 2019) that express high levels of TRPC4 and/or TRPC1. It was found that englerin A exerts its cytotoxic effect through activation of TRPC4 and TRPC1/C4 channels endogenously expressed in the cancer cells. Intuitively, the cell killing action of englerin A was attributed to TRPC4-mediated Ca^{2+} influx and then intracellular Ca^{2+} overload, as Ca^{2+} overload by TRPC channels has indeed been reported to regulate apoptosis or other forms of programmed cell death in some cell types (Kondratskyi et al., 2015; Maher et al., 2018; Elzamzamy et al., 2020). However, a later study suggested that the cytotoxicity effect might largely result from the excessive Na^+ influx (Ludlow et al., 2017). It would appear that both the Na^+ and Ca^{2+} influxes mediated by TRPC channels are potentially harmful to the cell, if not properly controlled.

THE ROLE OF TRPCs IN NEURODEGENERATIVE DISEASES ASIDE FROM STROKE

Pathologically, excess glutamate accumulation is relevant to brain injury in many forms of neurodegenerative diseases. Therefore, before discussing the possible contributions of TRPC channels to brain injury associated with ischemic stroke, it is worthwhile to consider the involvement of TRPC channels in neuronal cell death in other neurodegenerative diseases, as they likely share some common mechanisms of excitotoxicity with ischemic stroke in damaging brain neurons. TRPC channels have been reported to play roles in a number of neurological disorders. Depending on the type of disease and the specific TRPC subtype, the activation of TRPC channels is not always detrimental to the neuron. Some TRPCs may actually be neuroprotective in certain neurodegenerative diseases.

A likely consequence of pathological accumulation of excess glutamate is coincident stimulation of both $G_{q/11}$- and $G_{i/o}$-coupled mGluRs. This provides conditions for strong and prolonged self-propagating activation of TRPC4 and TRPC5 channels, leading to membrane potential disruption and Ca^{2+} overload. Indeed, TRPC1/C4 and TRPC5 channels have been implicated in seizure-induced neuronal death in mouse lateral septum and hippocampus, respectively, in the pilocarpine-induced model of epilepsy (Phelan et al., 2012). Inhibiting TRPC5 also protected neurons in pyriform cortex, amygdala, and hippocampus from death in kainate-treated rats with prolonged seizures (Park et al., 2019) and in hippocampal CA3 neurons in a tramatic brain injury model (Park et al., 2020). In these models, TRPC5 was thought to be activated by oxidation which first triggered a rise in cytosolic Zn^{2+} levels and then opening of TRPC5 channels to mediate Ca^{2+} influx, leading to neuronal cell death (Park et al., 2019). In the Huntington's disease model, activation of TRPC5 through glutathionylation has also been shown to cause the loss of striatal neurons (Hong et al., 2015), and this effect can be mitigated through destabilizing the presence of TRPC5 on plasma membrane via depalmitoylation (Hong et al., 2020).

On the other hand, TRPC4-containing channels are not always associated with neuronal cell injury. TRPC1/C4 heteromeric channels have been reported to exert a protective role in neuronal cell death induced by subarachnoid hemorrhage

(Wang et al., 2016). This was suggested to occur through Ca^{2+} activation of calcineurin which suppresses NMDA receptor activity through dephosphorylation. Likewise, TRPC1 has been found to be neuroprotective in animal models of Parkinson's disease and Alzheimer's disease. In dopaminergic neurons of substantia nigra, TRPC1 inhibits L-type VGCCs by facilitating the interaction of STIM1 with Cav1.3 in response to ER Ca^{2+} store depletion and thereby dampening the neurotoxin-induced VGCC function that causes neuronal death (Sun et al., 2017). In addition, through store-operated Ca^{2+} entry, TRPC1 protects the dopaminergic neurons from neurotoxin-induced ER stress and the decrease of AKT/mTOR signaling (Selvaraj et al., 2012). Conversely, dopaminergic neurons respond to neurotoxin with decreased store-operated Ca^{2+} entry via attenuation of TRPC1 transcription, which is regulated by NF-κB (Sukumaran et al., 2018). Furthermore, the inhibition of TRPC1-mediated Ca^{2+} entry by neurotoxin is facilitated by sigma 1 receptor, an ER membrane protein acting as a chaperone to regulate Ca^{2+} release and other functions, which ultimately leads to the loss of dopaminergic neurons (Sun et al., 2020). In the mouse model of Alzheimer's disease, the deletion of *trpc1* gene was found to aggravate amyloid-β (Aβ)-induced learning and memory deficits and TRPC1 was shown to interact with Aβ precursor protein (APP) at the transmembrane region, resulting in reduced Aβ levels in hippocampal neurons and attenuation of apoptosis (Li et al., 2018). By contrast, the upregulated TRPC1 expression seen in SK-N-SH human neuroblastoma cells expressing a polyglutamine Huntingtin mutant was found to support a store-operated non-selective cation current and this activity contributed to glutamate-induced apoptosis of primary cultured striatal medium spiny neurons prepared from YAC128 mice that mimic neurodegeneration of Huntington's disease (Wu et al., 2011). Indeed, eliminating TRPC1 in YAC128 mice improved motor performance and rescued neuronal spines from progressive loss (Wu et al., 2018). Therefore, TRPC1 may be either detrimental or beneficial to brain neurons depending on the models and neuronal cell types.

TRPC3 has been speculated to play a part in ischemic injury of the cerebellum owning to it higher expression in this than in other brain regions (Cederholm et al., 2019). However, this regional specific effect of TRPC3 was found to change in aging monkeys and transgenic mice overexpressing human α-synuclein, where TRPC3 was found to become enriched in the mitochondria of striatal neurons and contribute to the disruption of mitochondrial membrane potential and cell apoptosis commonly seen in Parkinson's disease (Chen M. et al., 2017). Thus far, TRPC3 represents the only TRPC isoform that has been localized to mitochondria, in addition to its common plasma membrane localization, and involved in Ca^{2+} uptake into the organelle (Feng et al., 2013). Thus, the link of TRPC3 expression and function in mitochondria to α-synuclein upregulation implicates a role of TRPC3 in the pathogenesis of Parkinson's disease (Chen M. et al., 2017). In a rodent model of pilocarpine-induced status epilepticus, while the expression of TRPC3 was found to be increased, that of TRPC6 was decreased in CA1 and CA3 pyramidal neurons and dentate granule cells. It was reported that either inhibiting TRPC3 or enhancing TRPC6 function and/or expression protected neurons from seizure-induced injury (Kim et al., 2013). These findings support the detrimental effect of TRPC3 hyperactivation on brain neurons, but implicate that TRPC6 may exert an opposite effect.

Indeed, although closely related to TRPC3, TRPC6 has mainly been shown to be protective against neurodegeneration. For example, a system wide reduction of TRPC6 expression was found in patients with Alzheimer's disease and mild cognitive impairment, including blood cells, which negatively correlated with the cognitive performance (Lu et al., 2018; Chen et al., 2019). Moreover, neurons differentiated from induced pluripotent stem cells (iPSCs) derived from peripheral blood of sporadic Alzheimer's disease patients also exhibit decreased TRPC6 expression, as well as elevated Aβ and phosphorylated tau levels, hallmarks of Alzheimer's disease (Tao et al., 2020). Mechanistically, TRPC6 has been proposed to physically interact with APP via its second transmembrane segment, through which it inhibits the cleavage of APP by γ-secretase, leading to reduced Aβ production (Wang et al., 2015). That increasing TRPC6 expression or using a membrane penetrating peptide representing TRPC6's second transmembrane segment effectively lowered the levels of Aβ and phosphorylated tau in iPSC neurons derived from sporadic Alzheimer's disease patients supports a role of TRPC6 in suppressing the disease pathogenesis (Tao et al., 2020).

In a separate study, TRPC6 was found to form a complex with Orai2 that is regulated by STIM2 to conduct store-operated Ca^{2+} influx in dendritic mushroom spines of hippocampal neurons (Zhang et al., 2016). When this is impaired, the mushroom spines become unstable and disrupted, leading to memory loss. The beneficial effect of TRPC6 to Alzheimer's disease was demonstrated by showing that stimulating TRPC6 or the store-operated Ca^{2+} entry improved hippocampal long-term potentiation of the APP-presenilin 1 mutant mice, an experimental model of Alzheimer's disease (Zhang et al., 2016; Popugaeva et al., 2019). However, in a different model, where the expression of a familial Alzheimer's disease (FAD) presenilin 1 mutation bearing the deletion of the 9th exon (PSEN1ΔE9) in hippocampal neurons caused mushroom spine loss through enhancing, instead of suppressing, TRPC6-mediated store-operated Ca^{2+} entry, inhibiting such activity then becomes beneficial (Chernyuk et al., 2019). Therefore, depending on the nature of dysregulation, TRPC6 can be either beneficial or detrimental to neurons, highlighting the importance of maintaining the proper Ca^{2+} homeostasis. Previously, an inhibitory effect of presenilin 2 and its Alzheimer's-disease-linked variants on receptor-operated TRPC6 function has been demonstrated in heterologous expression systems, suggesting functional interaction between presenilins and TRPC6 (Lessard et al., 2005). In status epilepticus, TRPC6 serves to protect granule neurons of dentate gyrus from degeneration through activation of ERK1/2 and the subsequent phosphorylation of dynamin-related proteins 1 (DRP1) at Ser-616 (Ko and Kang, 2017) and an increase in the expression of a mitochondrial protease, Lon protease-1 (Kim et al., 2019). In the absence of TRPC6, the hypo-phosphorylation of DRP1 and reduction in Lon protease-1 then lead to mitochondrial elongation and dysfunction, which increase the vulnerability of granule cells to seizure-induced death (Kim and Kang, 2015).

Taken together, the above findings suggest that TRPC channels exert differential effects on neurodegeneration in isoform and disease specific fashions. Although $[Ca^{2+}]_i$ dysregulation and membrane depolarization may be the common effects of TRPC channel activation, other mechanisms, including protein–protein interactions that involve specific regions of particular TRPC subtypes with certain disease-related protein partners and unique signaling pathways pertaining to the regulation of specific TRPC channels, are also involved. These diverse mechanisms underlie the differential outcomes resulting from TRPC channel function, ranging from neuroprotection to neurodegeneration. Therefore, it cannot be generalized that the extended activation of TRPC channels always leads to cell death, despite the high risk of Ca^{2+} overload.

THE ROLE OF TRPCs IN ISCHEMIC BRAIN INJURY

Brain injury after focal ischemic insult has been linked to the reduction of oxygen and nutrient (glucose) supply to the affected brain region (Lipton, 1999; Lo et al., 2003). Both *in vivo* MCAO model and the *in vitro* OGD model are commonly used to evaluate the involvement and mechanisms of TRPC channels in neuronal cell death associated with ischemic stroke. Like with the other neurodegenerative diseases discussed above, these studies revealed complex roles of different TRPC channels in ischemic brain injury.

For TRPC1, both the MCAO model and OGD assay suggested that TRPC1 plays a protective role against neuronal injuries caused by cerebral ischemia/reperfusion through suppression of ROS generation (Xu et al., 2018). TRPC1 expression was shown to be downregulated not only in brain tissues of mice subject to 90 min MCAO followed by 24 h reperfusion, but also in the cultured murine hippocampal cell line, HT22, that was exposed to an OGD culture for 4 h and then placed in the reoxygenated normal medium for 6–24 h. It was demonstrated that the amplitude of store-operated Ca^{2+} entry in the hippocampal cells was positively corrected with the expression TRPC1, but negatively correlated with the NADPH oxidase activity, and unrelated to the expression of STIM1 and Orai1 as well as mitochondrial ROS generation. However, no evidence was provided to suggest a direct inhibitory effect of Ca^{2+} on NADPH oxidase activity. Rather, TRPC1 inhibited NADPH oxidase-mediated ROS production through physically interacting with a catalytic component of the oxidase, Nox4, which facilitated Nox4 degradation along with cytoplasmic retention of the cytosolic subunits of the NADPH oxidase complex, p47phox and p67phox (Xu et al., 2018). This protective role of TRPC1 is opposite from the results of an earlier work, which showed that SKF96365 prevented cortical neuron death induced by 1.5 h OGD and 24 h reoxygenation (Wang et al., 2016). Since SKF96365 is a non-specific drug that inhibits all TRPC channels, and all forms of store- and receptor-operated Ca^{2+} entry, it did not inform which specific channel type was responsible for the protective effect.

On the other hand, the TRPC3/6/7 triple knockout mice were reported to be resistant to brain injury induced by MCAO followed by reperfusion (Chen X. et al., 2017). Here, the detrimental role of TRPC3/6/7 channels was attributed at least in part to astrocytes, in which these channels contributed to the enhanced NF-κB phosphorylation, reduced AKT phosphorylation and increased cell apoptosis following OGD and reoxygenation treatment (Chen X. et al., 2017). How this function of TRPC3/6/7, which promotes the death of astrocytes, is related or coordinated with astrogliosis, an abnormal proliferation of brain astrocytes observed after stroke and shown to be positively regulated by TRPC3 (Shirakawa et al., 2010; Munakata et al., 2013; Belkacemi et al., 2017), is an interesting question that needs to be addressed in future studies.

Although TRPC6 expression in mouse cortical neurons has been reported to be increased following brain ischemia/reperfusion *in vivo* and OGD/reoxygenation *in vitro*, and this increase contributed to neuronal injury in an NMDA receptor-dependent manner (Chen J. et al., 2017), nearly all other studies argue for a protective role of TRPC6 in neurological damage associated with ischemic stroke. The neuroprotective role of TRPC6 was suggested to occur through activation of cAMP response element-binding protein (CREB) signaling, which is disrupted following cerebral ischemia due to degradation of TRPC6 proteins in neurons by proteolytic cleavage mediated by calpain, non-lysosomal cysteine proteases activated as a result of $[Ca^{2+}]_i$ rise from NMDA receptor activation by elevated extracellular glutamate (Du et al., 2010). It was found that attenuating the calpain-mediated TRPC6 degradation could underlie the neuroprotective effects of several natural compounds, such as resveratrol, neuroprotectin D1, and (–)-epigallocatechin-3-gallate (the main ingredient of green tea), and calycosin (Lin et al., 2013a; Yao et al., 2013, 2014; Guo et al., 2017). That these protective effects were obliviated by inhibiting mitogen-activated protein kinase kinase (MEK) and/or calmodulin kinases suggests that these kinases mediate CREB activation downstream from TRPC6 (Lin et al., 2013b; Yao et al., 2013). On the other hand, increasing TRPC6 expression or its function through overexpression or treatment with hyperforin also inhibited NMDA receptor function and suppressed calpain activity (Li et al., 2012; Lin et al., 2013b), indicative of reciprocal regulations between TRPC6 and NMDA receptors/calpain. Once suggested as a TRPC6 agonist (Leuner et al., 2007), hyperforin was found to increase TRPC6 expression in mouse hippocampus following ischemia/reperfusion (Lin et al., 2013b). Hyperforin was also reported not to change TRPC6 channel activity, but acts independently of TRPC6 as a protonophore, which may explain its anti-depressive effects (Sell et al., 2014). Furthermore, the calpain cleavage of TRPC6 has also been reported to be activated by interleukin 17 (IL-17) (Zhang et al., 2014), a T-cell derived pro-inflammatory cytokine shown to contribute to ischemic brain injury (Gelderblom et al., 2012), suggesting an immune-neural interaction that exacerbates ischemic neurological damage through downregulating TRPC6.

In contrast to the rich information on TRPC6, little is known about the roles of TRPC4 and TRPC5 in brain injury associated with ischemic stroke. In one study, it was reported that TRPC4 protein expression was increased in rat striatal and hippocampal neurons at 12 h to 3 days after MCAO (Gao et al., 2004). Other studies speculating a detrimental function of TRPC5 in neurological deficits following stroke had based on the activation of TRPC5 by oxidation, without experimentation in the stroke model (Ishii et al., 2011; Park et al., 2019, 2020). In a very recent study, TRPC5 was found to directly interact with phospholipid scramblase 1 (PLSCR1) on the plasma membrane to facilitate externalization of phosphatidylserine (PS) and apoptosis of cortical neurons in response to cerebral ischemia/reperfusion (Guo et al., 2020). The same protein complex likely also includes TRPC1 and TRPC4. While the examination of cerebral slices of animals subject to ischemia/reperfusion revealed reduced PS externalization and apoptosis in TRPC5 knockout mice, whether these translate into protection against cerebral infarction and/or behavioral neurological impairments remains to be elucidated (Guo et al., 2020). On the other hand, overexpression of TRPC5 in spinal cord via adeno-associated viruses attenuated spinal cord ischemia/reperfusion injury in rats (Shen et al., 2020). This could result from the angiogenic function of TRPC5 which dampens the injury induced inflammation. Indeed, TRPC5 has been reported to promote endothelial cell sprouting, angiogenesis, and blood perfusion in ischemic tissues through activation of nuclear factor of activated T cell (NFAT) isoform c3 and angiopoietin-1 (Zhu et al., 2019). Therefore, the effect of TRPC4/C5 on ischemic brain injury may be very complex, including both positive and negative regulations that either exacerbate or prevent neuronal cell death.

TRPC4 IN ISCHEMIC BRAIN INJURY – OUR OWN STUDY

The above analysis indicates that despite the common mechanisms that link G protein and PLC pathways to TRPC channel activation and the likelihood that these channels participate in excitotoxicity triggered by excessive extracellular accumulation of glutamate through mGluRs, it is not easy to predict whether a specific TRPC channel type is detrimental or beneficial to brain neurons under conditions of cerebral ischemia/reperfusion. Depending on the TRPC isoforms, cell types involved, and mechanisms of actions, the TRPC channel may be neuroprotective or destructive.

To define the overall contributions of TRPC channels in brain damage associated with cerebral ischemia, we first compared neurological scores and brain infarction volumes of wild type and quadruple TRPC1, C4, C5, C6 knockout (QuadKO) mice subject to 40 min of MCAO using the standard intraluminal suture (thread) method, followed by 24 h reperfusion. In this method, a monofilament nylon surgical suture with a heat-rounded tip is inserted from an opening at external carotid artery and advanced through internal carotid artery until it reaches the middle cerebral artery to block the blood flow there. After the desired time period of occlusion, the filament was withdrawn to allow resupply of the blood to the blocked brain area (Alkayed et al., 1998; Sun et al., 2019). Since TRPC2 is mainly expressed in the vomeronasal system (Liman et al., 1999), TRPC3 mainly present in the cerebellum (Hartmann et al., 2008), and TRPC7 mostly found in peripheral tissues (Okada et al., 1999), we consider TRPC1, C4, C5, and C6 as the main cerebral TRPC subtypes expressed in areas typically affected in the MCAO model. As described above, both TRPC1 and C6 have been suggested to play protective roles against ischemic brain injury, but the function of TRPC4 and C5 remains unclear. Therefore, the QuadKO mice provide a good model to learn if TRPC channels generally serve a protective or detrimental role in cerebral ischemia. We found that on average, TRPC-QuadKO mice had better neurological scores (**Figure 2A**) and smaller brain infarct areas (shown by staining with 2,3,5-triphenyltetrazolium chloride, TTC) than the wild type mice (**Figures 2B,C**), suggesting that overall, TRPC channels contribute to causing damage of the brain in response to cerebral ischemia/reperfusion. Given that TRPC1 and TRPC6 may play some neuroprotective function during ischemia/reperfusion, it is plausible that the detrimental actions are mainly mediated by TRPC4 and/or TRPC5, and these two TRPC isoforms may dominate the cortical neuronal responses to ischemic insults. This interpretation is consistent with the finding that TRPC4/C5 expression is more abundant than other TRPC isoforms in several major areas of rat brain, including the prefrontal cortex (Fowler et al., 2007). Clearly, the distinct contributions of different TRPC isoforms in brain injury at different stages of cerebral ischemia/reperfusion warrant more detailed investigation.

Given that among the major brain TRPC isoforms, only TRPC4 has not been evaluated for its role in ischemic stroke, we then set out to compare brain damages caused by cerebral ischemia/reperfusion in wild type and TRPC4 knockout mice. Here, we performed transient focal middle cerebral artery/common carotid artery occlusion (MCA/CCAO) on the animals for 30, 90, and 120 min, followed by 24 h reperfusion. The MCA/CCAO is surgically performed using craniotomy to directly occlude distal MCA with a thin stainless wire (Aronowski et al., 1994; Zhao et al., 2015). This type of method was reported to produce reversible infarction and confined focal cerebral ischemia at distal MCA territory (Braeuninger and Kleinschnitz, 2009; Tavafoghi et al., 2016). We found that the infarct areas were markedly smaller in brains of *Trpc4*$^{-/-}$ mice than wild type animals, especially with shorter time of ischemia, i.e., 30 and 90 min (**Figures 2D,E**). Specifically, with the 30 min ischemia followed by 24 h reperfusion, whereas the infarctions were readily visible in wild type brains, they were hardly detectable in *Trpc4*$^{-/-}$ specimens. However, with a longer time (120 min) ischemia, the protective effect of TRPC4 knockout diminished (**Figures 2D,E**). These data indicate that TRPC4-containing channels contribute positively to ischemic brain damage, particularly during the early time period of the ischemia.

Next and to attribute underlying mechanisms more directly to TRPC4 function in neurons, we used cortical neuron cultures prepared from newborn wild type, *Trpc1*$^{-/-}$, *Trpc4*$^{-/-}$ and TRPC QuadKO mice to examine the effect of OGD-reoxygenation on cultured neurons *in vitro* (Ying et al., 1997). As illustrated in **Figure 3A**, cells were cultured for 16–18 days *in vitro* (DIV). On the day of the experiment, the culture medium was replaced with either a deoxygenated bicarbonate buffer without glucose (OGD) or an oxygenated bicarbonate

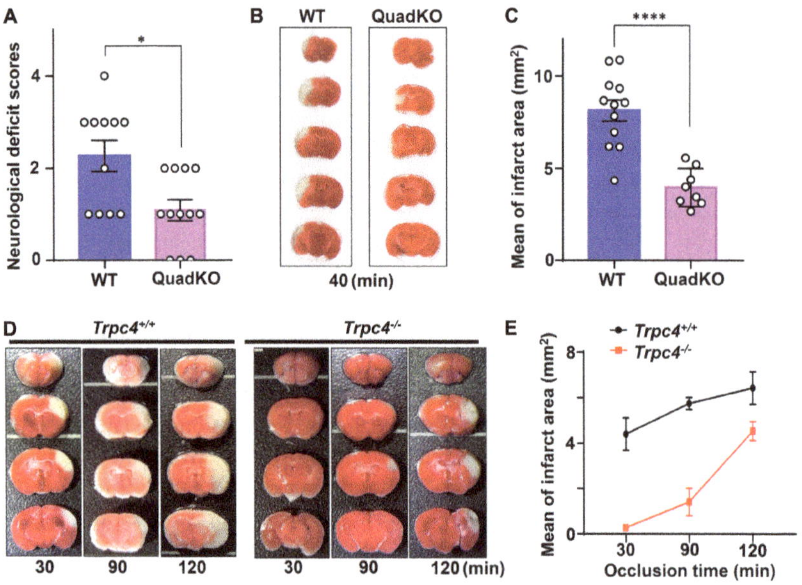

FIGURE 2 | Transient receptor potential canonical (TRPC) deficiency attenuates cerebral ischemic damage. **(A–C)** TRPC1, C4, C5, C6 quadruple knockout (QuadKO) and wild type control mice were subjected to reversible MCAO for 40 min using intraluminal suture method, followed by 22–24 h reperfusion. After assessing neurological deficits as described (Li et al., 2011) **(A)**, the animals were sacrificed and brain sections stained with TTC for quantification of infarct areas **(B,C)**. **(A)** Neurological scores of animals subjected to ischemia/reperfusion. Data represent means ± SEM for $n = 11$ (wild type) and 12 (QuadKO) mice. $^{*}P < 0.05$ by Mann–Whitney test. **(B)** Representative photographs of TTC-stained brain sections demarcating infarction. **(C)** Infarct areas at rostrocaudal plains were determined from morphometric analyses of TTC-stained brain sections. Data represent means ± SEM for $n = 12$ (wild type) and 8 (QuadKO) mice. $^{****}P < 0.0001$ by unpaired *t*-test. **(D,E)** *Trpc4*$^{-/-}$ and wild type control mice were subjected to reversible 30, 90, and 120 min MCA/CCAO, followed by 24 h reperfusion. **(D)** Representative photographs of TTC-stained brain sections. **(E)** Infarct areas at rostrocaudal plains were determined from morphometric analyses of TTC-stained brain sections. Data are presented as means ± range for $n = 2$ mice for each time point.

buffer with glucose (Control), and the cultures were maintained in a 37°C hypoxic incubator for 2 h with the oxygen level kept at 1% atmosphere. After the treatment, the neurons were either immediately evaluated for cell death by staining with propidium iodide (PI) or returned to the normal culture medium and maintained in the regular incubator at the normal oxygen level for 24 h before the PI staining. All cells were also stained with DAPI (4′,6-diamidino-2-phenylindole) to label the nuclei (**Figure 3B**). A comparison of the ratios of PI-positive/DAPI-positive labels, which represent percental cell death, revealed that wild type neurons were more vulnerable than the TRPC knockout neurons to the 2 h exposure of the bicarbonate buffer no matter if the buffer was oxygenated or not (**Figure 3C**). The reason for this is unclear, but could be related to the differences in the developmental status between the wild type and TRPC knockout cortical neurons cultured *in vitro*. Indeed, TRPCs play roles in several different aspects of neuronal development (Greka et al., 2003; Jeon et al., 2013; Tian et al., 2014b) and some of these could influence the sensitivity of the neurons to nutrient deprivation, given that the bicarbonate buffer does not contain serum and amino acids. This protective effect of TRPC depletion on neuronal survival in the serum and amino acid-deprived but glucose-containing buffer requires further investigation. Despite this, while the 2-h OGD treatment (without reoxygenation) did not immediately increase cell death further in wild type cortical neurons, it did so in all TRPC knockout neurons (**Figure 3C**), suggesting that OGD may interfere with the protective effect of TRPC knockout on cultured cortical neurons subject to serum and amino acid deprivation.

With the 24 h reoxygenation and nutrient replenishment (herein referred to as refeeding), cell death nearly doubled in wild type neurons that had been treated with OGD but not those exposed to the control buffer. The response to refeeding, however, was quite different between the three different TRPC knockout lines. The control buffer-treat QuadKO neurons displayed a marked increase in cell death after 24 h refeeding, but OGD-treated ones virtually did not change. However, while the *Trpc1*$^{-/-}$ neurons did not show any increase in death after refeeding regardless of the oxygen and glucose status during the starvation, the *Trpc4*$^{-/-}$ neurons exhibited a marked refeeding-dependent increase in cell death only when OGD treatment was applied (**Figure 3C**). These results, although difficult to interpret without more extensive investigations, underscore the complex and diverse roles different TRPC channels play in neuronal cell responses to nutrient shortage, OGD, and the subsequent replenishment of all nutrients, including oxygen.

To avoid the complications with the cultured neurons and the developmental effects of the TRPC knockout, we also performed OGD experiments using brain slices following a previous protocol (Taylor et al., 1999; Tasca et al., 2015). As illustrated in **Figure 4A**, the cerebral slices from wild type mice were recovered in artificial cerebrospinal fluid (aCSF) bubbled with 95% O_2 and 5% CO_2 at 35°C for 1–2 h after cutting. Then they were transferred to a modified aCSF omitting glucose

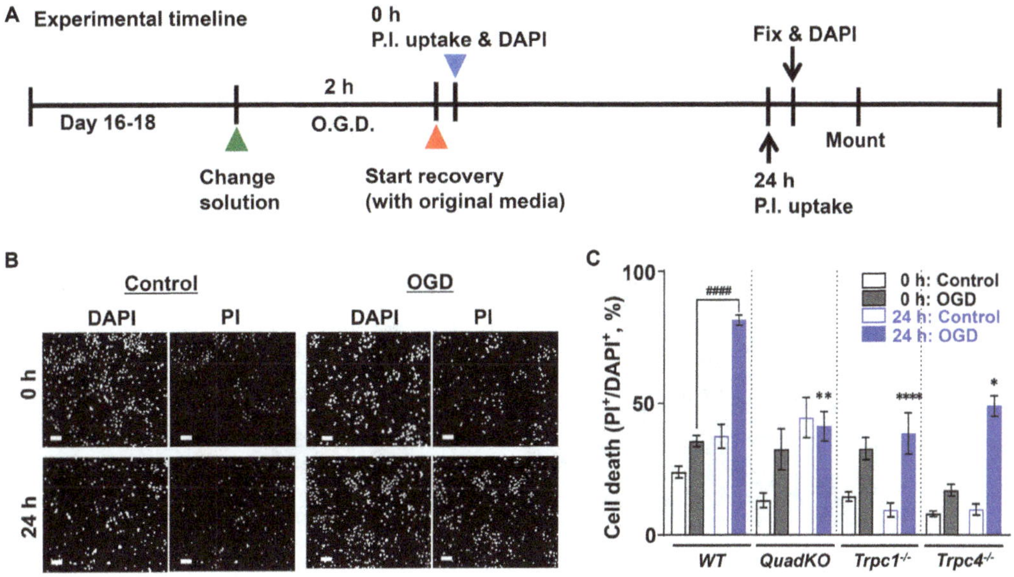

FIGURE 3 | Oxygen and glucose deprivation (OGD)-induced cell death of cultured cortical neurons from wild type, *Trpc1*$^{-/-}$, *Trpc4*$^{-/-}$, and *Trpc1/c4/c5/c6*$^{-/-}$ mice. **(A)** Schematic of the experimental timeline. Primary cultures of cortical neurons (16–18 DIV) from WT, *Trpc1*$^{-/-}$, *Trpc4*$^{-/-}$, and *Trpc1/c4/c5/c6*$^{-/-}$ (QuadKO) mice were treated without or with OGD for 2 h and then allowed to grow in normal medium for 0 or 24 h. **(B)** Representative images of DAPI staining (Bocksch et al., 2010) and PI uptake of cultured cortical neurons from wild type (WT) mice grown under control conditions or subjected to OGD for 2 h. Cells were stained either immediately after the treatment (0 h) or returned to normal culture conditions for 24 h before staining (24 h). Scale bars, 50 μm. **(C)** Summary data of PI-positive cells, normalized to the total cell number determined by DAPI staining. Data represent means ± SEM of $n = 20$ to 30 fields of views for each condition pooled from 4 coverslips of neurons from two separately prepared primary cultures. $^{\#\#\#\#}P < 0.0001$, $^{*}P < 0.05$, $^{**}P < 0.01$, $^{****}P < 0.0001$ vs. WT 24 h: OGD by one-way ANOVA.

and bubbled with N_2 (OGD) and maintained for 30 min at the same temperature. Control slices were treated with fresh oxygenated aCSF in parallel. After that, all slices were returned to fresh oxygenated aCSF and incubated for another 3 h. PI and Hoechst were added at 40 and 10 min, respectively, before the end of the incubation to label dead cells and nuclei of all cells. This was followed by fixation with 4% paraformaldehyde (12 h at 4°C) and mounting. In order to examine to what extent inhibiting TRPC4/C5 channels can protect against OGD-induced neuronal death and the possible therapeutic windows of targeting these channels, we also applied TRPC4/C5 antagonists, ML204 (Miller et al., 2011) and compounds 9 and 13 (cpd 9, cpd 13, analogs of M084) (Zhu et al., 2015), either at the beginning or the end of the OGD treatment. As shown in **Figures 4B,C**, after 30 min OGD and 3 h reoxygenation, the number and intensity of PI labeling in the cortex area were dramatically increased as compared to the control. Including the TRPC4/C5 antagonists either during or post OGD significantly decreased the damage. Since the TRPC4/C5 antagonists inhibit both TRPC4 or TRPC5 homomeric channels and TRPC1/C4 and TRPC1/C5 heteromeric channels, these data support the general idea that targeting TRPC1/C4/C5 channels can be beneficial to stroke therapy including post ischemic protection. Clearly, additional studies are needed to illustrate the details on how these TRPC channels contribute to neurological damage in response to ischemia and reperfusion and the appropriate intervention strategies that bring the most benefit with minimal detrimental effects.

DISCUSSION

Recent studies have demonstrated that TRPC channels play complex and even opposing functions in neuronal cell survival and death. Depending on the different TRPC subtypes, brain locations and cell types, as well as the specific pathological conditions, TRPC channels can be either detrimental or beneficial to neurons. However, the general theme is that for nearly every neurodegenerative disease, TRPC channels play crucial roles, and these include ischemic stroke and other conditions that cause brain injury. Because of the diverse mechanisms that have been revealed so far, it is also clear that no generalized mechanism should be used to explain or predict how a specific TRPC channel contributes to brain injury. Even for TRPC6, although most studies have indicated a pro-survival role, the molecular and cellular mechanisms elucidated from various studies have been very different, ranging from a direct interaction of the channel with a specific disease-causing protein (Wang et al., 2015), regulation of mitochondrial fission (Ko and Kang, 2017), to CREB-dependent transcription (Du et al., 2010) and suppression of NMDA receptor and calpain function (Li et al., 2012; Lin et al., 2013b). Therefore, future studies should focus not only on unique mechanism(s) that underlies the regulation of a specific TRPC channel in a particular form of neuronal injury, but also make attempts to reconcile the mechanism with existing knowledge and identify a common theme(s), if possible, that would enrich the mechanistic understanding of how the TRPC channel contributes to disease pathogenesis.

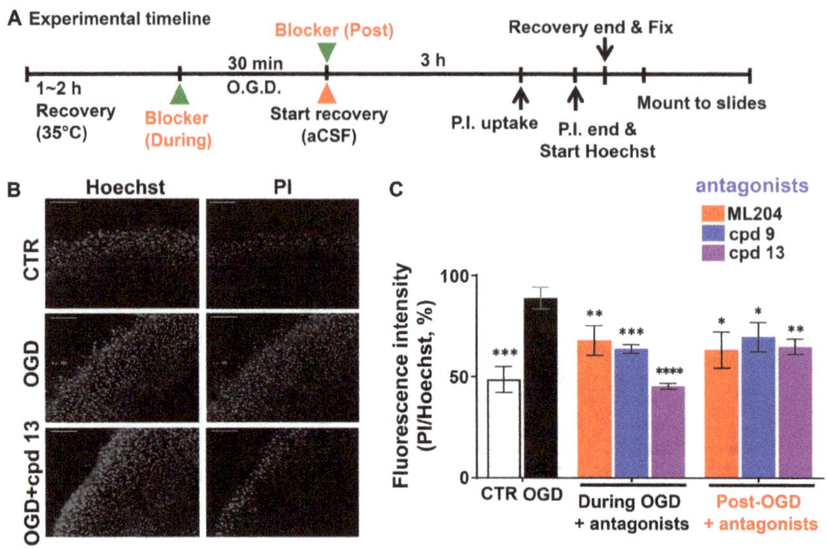

FIGURE 4 | Oxygen and glucose deprivation -induced neuronal death in the cerebral cortex of mouse brain slices. TRPC4/C5 blockers rescued OGD-induced neuronal death in the cerebral cortex of brain slices. **(A)** Schematic of the experimental timeline. **(B)** Representative images of Hoechst staining (left panels) and PI uptake (right panels) of acute brain slices (P15) from wild type (WT) mice without (CTR) or with OGD for 30 min in the absence or presence of TRPC4/C5 blocker, compound 13 (cpd 13). After the treatment, the slices were recovered for 3 h and stained with PI and Hoechst at 40 and 10 min, respectively, before the end of the 3 hr incubation. Scale bars, 100 μm. **(C)** Summary data of PI/Hoechst fluorescence ratios (random unit, but the same settings used for all conditions). TRPC4/C5 blockers, ML204 (at 50 μM), cpd 9, and cpd 13 (at 30 μM) prevented the OGD-induced cell death to varying degrees no matter if they were added during or after (post) the OGD treatment. Data represent means ± SEM of $n = 8$ to 15 fields of view of independently treated slices. *$P < 0.05$, **$P < 0.01$, ***$P < 0.001$, ****$P < 0.0001$ vs. OGD without antagonist by Student *t*-test.

Particularly for brain damage associated with ischemic stroke, the roles of TRPC channels at different stages of the ischemia/reperfusion and in different brain areas are far from clear. The acute deprivation of oxygen and glucose, as well as other nutrient supplies, certainly exerts a tremendous stress on neurons, causing many changes in signal transduction and intracellular and extracellular messengers that are linked to TRPC channels through either functional or physical coupling or both. These can be factors that directly activate the channel, such as DAG or ROS, or transmitters that work through G protein-coupled receptors, like glutamate, as well as neurotrophic factors that stimulate tyrosine kinases, e.g., BDNF. The combination of some of these factors may even bring synergistic effect, making some otherwise insignificant molecules into important contributors to TRPC channel activation that either induces neuronal death or protects them from the damages caused by other signals. Importantly, changes that occur in the ischemic stage do not just revert back to their original states after reperfusion or oxygenation. The restoration of nutrient supply and blood circulation also causes inflammation and oxidation, leading to stress responses that may evoke TRPC activation as well. Thus, a TRPC subtype may be involved in either the ischemic or reperfusion stage, or both stages, of the ischemia/reperfusion injury but with different outcomes. Furthermore, while irreversible damages can occur immediately at the ischemic core during OGD through necrosis, neurons in the neighboring regions (ischemic penumbra) more often display delayed cell death or apoptosis (Rami and Kogel, 2008). It is not known how different TRPC isoforms are involved in the different forms of cell death pathways, and therefore, it remains to be elucidated whether and how each of them plays a part in different stages and different brain regions (core *vs.* penumbra) in neurological damages associated with ischemia/reperfusion. These, together with the diverse mechanisms that have been reported for TRPC channel activation under pathological conditions, argue for the need of more careful and systematic examinations of TRPC channels in ischemic brain damage.

In practice, a stroke therapy is more useful in post-stroke than during or pre-stroke application since in most cases, the need for treatment is only realized after the stroke has occurred. Therefore, a better understanding of mechanisms that contribute to neuronal death during reperfusion and/or in ischemic penumbra instead of the core area, or any intervention that would facilitate the recovery of damaged neurons, if possible, from the death pathway will be desirable for therapeutic development. However, despite all the studies that have been discussed above, nothing is available on whether any TRPC channel would be a good target of post-stroke neuroprotection. Our *in vitro* experiment (**Figure 4**) suggests that it might be possible for the TRPC4/C5 inhibitors to have such a function, even though it might not be a complete protection. It may be common that targeting a single pathway or molecule post-stroke or post-OGD will not completely protect all neurons from ischemic injury, since even if the targeting is effective and represents the most critical one, irreversible damages that have occurred during ischemia will unlikely be rescued. Recently, the TRPC channel field has experienced an explosion of newly identified small molecular probes that can act as either selective agonists or antagonists of specific TRPC channel subtypes (Wang et al., 2020). This gives an opportunity to test whether selectively enhancing or suppressing the function of a specific TRPC subtype at different time points post MCAO will exacerbate or inhibit brain damage and neurological deficits. Of course, these experiments will need to be followed by cell type specific manipulation of TRPC channel function or expression and other approaches in order to gain mechanistic insights on how the channel contributes to the delayed neuronal death.

Mechanistically, even though Ca^{2+} signal is an obvious downstream event of TRPC channel activation, there can be many different kinds of consequences which may or may not be related to the Ca^{2+} signal. The downstream targets of Ca^{2+} also remain largely undefined, although both CaMKII and calcineurin have been implicated. Ca^{2+}-dependent kinases could also include those that phosphorylate NMDA receptor NR2B subunits, e.g., DAPK1, which is known to play a role in stroke (Nair et al., 2013). TRPC channels can mediate DAPK1 activation through calcineurin or calmodulin (Shamloo et al., 2005; Nair et al., 2013). Also, as has been illustrated for TRPC6, calpain is another possible candidate of Ca^{2+} regulation and it is known to play a role in NMDA receptor-mediated cell death (Lankiewicz et al., 2000; Simpkins et al., 2003). Therefore, specific inhibitors of the above Ca^{2+}-regulated enzymes, calpain, CaMKII, calcineurin, and DAPK1 may be used to dissect their roles.

In summary, although TRPC channels appear to be ideally suited for integrating mGluR signaling to contribute to excitotoxicity to neurons under conditions of ischemic stroke, critical data demonstrating their involvement in neuronal damage or protection are only beginning to emerge. The pathological significance and roles of TRPC channels in ischemia/reperfusion remain to be fully elucidated. More detailed studies on regulatory mechanisms of TRPC channels will also shed lights on their functional significance in stroke pathology and future drug development.

METHODS

Animals

All animal procedures were carried out in accordance with the NIH guidelines for the Care and Use of Laboratory Animals and approved by the Animal Welfare Committee of the University of Texas Health Science Center at Houston. TRPC1 KO (*Trpc1*$^{-/-}$) and quadruple TRPC1, C4, C5, C6 KO (QuadKO) mice (129/SvEv and C57BL/6J mixed background) were created and maintained as described (Dietrich et al., 2007; Formoso et al., 2020); TRPC4 KO (*Trpc4*$^{-/-}$) in C57BL/6 background were generated and maintained as previously described (Freichel et al., 2001).

Mouse Ischemic Models

Focal ischemia (intraluminal suture) model of MCAO was carried out for 40 min followed by reperfusion as previously described (Sun et al., 2019). Animals were male QuadKO mice (8–9 weeks, ~25 g) and age-matched wild type controls (C57BL/6J). In the MCA\CCAO model, unilateral occlusion of the left middle cerebral artery (MCA) and the left common carotid artery (CCA) was made as previously described (Aronowski et al., 1994; Zhao et al., 2015) using male wild type C57BL/6J and TRPC4 KO mice (8 weeks old). The occlusion times were 30, 90, and 120 min followed by reperfusion. With this method, the infarction is limited to the cortical tissue.

Oxygen and Glucose Deprivation (OGD) Models

Primary cultures of cortical neurons were established using postnatal day 0 mouse pups (M/F) according to the description (Facci and Skaper, 2012). Cortical tissues from wild type (C57BL/6J), TRPC1 KO, TRPC4 KO, and QuadKO pups were triturated in a papain dissociation solution (Worthington) supplemented with DNase (200 units/ml) and incubated for 1 h in 37°C CO_2 incubator. After stopping the reaction by adding ovomucoid (10 mg/ml), DNase (200 units/ml), and 10% fetal bovine serum in Earle's balanced salt solution, cells were plated at 2×10^5 per well in 500 μl of neurobasal medium supplemented with B27 (Invitrogen) and Glutamax (invitrogen) on poly-D-lysine (Sigma)-coated 12-mm round coverslips in 24-well culture plates. Another 500 μl of medium with arabinofuranosyl cytidine (1 μM final) was then added, and 20–30% of the medium was exchanged every other day until the cells were used for experiments (usually 16–18 days). For OGD, the medium was replaced with the deoxygenated glucose-free bicarbonate solution and the plate transferred to an anaerobic incubator containing 5% CO_2 and 94% N_2 (1% O_2) atmosphere for 2 h. After OGD, the cells were rinsed with oxygenated glucose (20 mM)-containing bicarbonate solution, fed with the original neurobasal medium, and cultured for 0 or 24 h at 37°C, 5% CO_2 (Ying et al., 1997).

Acute brain slices were prepared from wild type and TRPC4 KO mice (M, P15) as previously described (Tian et al., 2014a). Coronal slices (350 μm) were incubated in normal artificial cerebrospinal fluid (aCSF) consisting of (in mM): 125 NaCl, 26 $NaHCO_3$, 1 $MgSO_4$, 2.5 KCl, 1.25 NaH_2PO_4, 2 $CaCl_2$, and 10 glucose, bubbled with 95% O_2/5% CO_2 at 35°C for at least 90 min before experiments. To induce OGD, slices were transferred to 15 ml conical tubes containing aCSF without glucose, which were bubbled with N_2/CO_2 at 35°C for 30 min. After the OGD treatment, the slices were returned to the glucose containing aCSF bubbled with 95% O_2/5% CO_2 at 35°C for 3 h.

ETHICS STATEMENT

The animal study was reviewed and approved by Animal Welfare Committee of University of Texas Health Science Center at Houston.

AUTHOR CONTRIBUTIONS

JJ prepared illustrations and wrote the manuscript. MZ wrote the manuscript. All authors proofread and approved the manuscript.

ACKNOWLEDGMENTS

We thank Prof. Veit Flockerzi (Saarland University, Germany) for the TRPC4 knockout mice.

REFERENCES

Akbulut, Y., Gaunt, H. J., Muraki, K., Ludlow, M. J., Amer, M. S., Bruns, A., et al. (2015). (−)-Englerin A is a potent and selective activator of TRPC4 and TRPC5 calcium channels. *Angew. Chem. Int. Ed. Engl.* 54, 3787–3791. doi: 10.1002/anie.201411511

Alkayed, N. J., Harukuni, I., Kimes, A. S., London, E. D., Traystman, R. J., and Hurn, P. D. (1998). Gender-linked brain injury in experimental stroke. *Stroke* 29, 159–165. doi: 10.1161/01.str.29.1.159

Amaral, M. D., and Pozzo-Miller, L. (2007). TRPC3 channels are necessary for brain-derived neurotrophic factor to activate a nonselective cationic current and to induce dendritic spine formation. *J. Neurosci.* 27, 5179–5189. doi: 10.1523/JNEUROSCI.5499-06.2007

Aronowski, J., Ostrow, P., Samways, E., Strong, R., Zivin, J. A., and Grotta, J. C. (1994). Graded bioassay for demonstration of brain rescue from experimental acute ischemia in rats. *Stroke* 25, 2235–2240. doi: 10.1161/01.str.25.11.2235

Belkacemi, T., Niermann, A., Hofmann, L., Wissenbach, U., Birnbaumer, L., Leidinger, P., et al. (2017). TRPC1- and TRPC3-dependent Ca(2+) signaling in mouse cortical astrocytes affects injury-evoked astrogliosis in vivo. *Glia* 65, 1535–1549. doi: 10.1002/glia.23180

Berridge, M. J. (2009). Inositol trisphosphate and calcium signalling mechanisms. *Biochim. Biophys. Acta* 1793, 933–940. doi: 10.1016/j.bbamcr.2008.10.005

Bocksch, W., Pomar, F., Dziarmaga, M., Tresukosol, D., Ismail, O., Janek, B., et al. (2010). Clinical safety and efficacy of a novel thin-strut cobalt-chromium coronary stent system: results of the real world coroflex blue registry. *Catheter. Cardiovasc. Interv* 75, 78–85. doi: 10.1002/ccd.22208

Bonde, C., Noraberg, J., Noer, H., and Zimmer, J. (2005). Ionotropic glutamate receptors and glutamate transporters are involved in necrotic neuronal cell death induced by oxygen-glucose deprivation of hippocampal slice cultures. *Neuroscience* 136, 779–794. doi: 10.1016/j.neuroscience.2005.07.020

Braeuninger, S., and Kleinschnitz, C. (2009). Rodent models of focal cerebral ischemia: procedural pitfalls and translational problems. *Exp. Transl. Stroke Med.* 1:8. doi: 10.1186/2040-7378-1-8

Brisson, C. D., and Andrew, R. D. (2012). A neuronal population in hypothalamus that dramatically resists acute ischemic injury compared to neocortex. *J. Neurophysiol.* 108, 419–430. doi: 10.1152/jn.00090.2012

Broker-Lai, J., Kollewe, A., Schindeldecker, B., Pohle, J., Nguyen Chi, V., Mathar, I., et al. (2017). Heteromeric channels formed by TRPC1, TRPC4 and TRPC5 define hippocampal synaptic transmission and working memory. *EMBO J.* 36, 2770–2789. doi: 10.15252/embj.201696369

Brust, J. C. M. (2013). *Principles of Neural Science*, 5th Edn. New York: McGraw-Hill, 1550–1554.

Carson, C., Raman, P., Tullai, J., Xu, L., Henault, M., Thomas, E., et al. (2015). Englerin a agonizes the TRPC4/C5 cation channels to inhibit tumor cell line proliferation. *PLoS One* 10:e0127498. doi: 10.1371/journal.pone.0127498

Cederholm, J. M. E., Kim, Y., von Jonquieres, G., and Housley, G. D. (2019). Human brain region-specific alternative splicing of TRPC3, the type 3 canonical transient receptor potential non-selective cation channel. *Cerebellum* 18, 536–543. doi: 10.1007/s12311-019-01026-4

Chen, J., Li, Z., Hatcher, J. T., Chen, Q. H., Chen, L., Wurster, R. D., et al. (2017). Deletion of TRPC6 attenuates NMDA receptor-mediated Ca(2+) entry and Ca(2+)-induced neurotoxicity following cerebral ischemia and oxygen-glucose deprivation. *Front. Neurosci.* 11:138. doi: 10.3389/fnins.2017.00138

Chen, J. M., Li, Q. W., Liu, J. S., Jiang, G. X., Liu, J. R., Chen, S. D., et al. (2019). TRPC6 mRNA levels in peripheral leucocytes of patients with Alzheimer's disease and mild cognitive impairment: a case-control study. *Prog. Neuropsychopharmacol. Biol. Psychiatry* 92, 279–284. doi: 10.1016/j.pnpbp.2019.01.009

Chen, M., Liu, J., Lu, Y., Duan, C., Lu, L., Gao, G., et al. (2017). Age-dependent alpha-synuclein accumulation is correlated with elevation of mitochondrial TRPC3 in the brains of monkeys and mice. *J. Neural Transm.* 124, 441–453. doi: 10.1007/s00702-016-1654-y

Chen, X., Lu, M., He, X., Ma, L., Birnbaumer, L., and Liao, Y. (2017). TRPC3/6/7 knockdown protects the brain from cerebral ischemia injury via astrocyte apoptosis inhibition and effects on NF-small ka, CyrillicB translocation. *Mol. Neurobiol.* 54, 7555–7566. doi: 10.1007/s12035-016-0227-2

Chernyuk, D., Zernov, N., Kabirova, M., Bezprozvanny, I., and Popugaeva, E. (2019). Antagonist of neuronal store-operated calcium entry exerts beneficial effects in neurons expressing PSEN1DeltaE9 mutant linked to familial Alzheimer disease. *Neuroscience* 410, 118–127. doi: 10.1016/j.neuroscience.2019.04.043

Clapham, D. E. (2003). TRP channels as cellular sensors. *Nature* 426, 517–524. doi: 10.1038/nature02196

Dietrich, A., Kalwa, H., Storch, U., Mederos y Schnitzler, M., Salanova, B., Pinkenburg, O., et al. (2007). Pressure-induced and store-operated cation influx in vascular smooth muscle cells is independent of TRPC1. *Pflugers Arch.* 455, 465–477. doi: 10.1007/s00424-007-0314-3

Doyle, K. P., Simon, R. P., and Stenzel-Poore, M. P. (2008). Mechanisms of ischemic brain damage. *Neuropharmacology* 55, 310–318. doi: 10.1016/j.neuropharm.2008.01.005

Du, W., Huang, J., Yao, H., Zhou, K., Duan, B., and Wang, Y. (2010). Inhibition of TRPC6 degradation suppresses ischemic brain damage in rats. *J. Clin. Invest.* 120, 3480–3492. doi: 10.1172/JCI43165

Durukan, A., and Tatlisumak, T. (2007). Acute ischemic stroke: overview of major experimental rodent models, pathophysiology, and therapy of focal cerebral ischemia. *Pharmacol. Biochem. Behav.* 87, 179–197. doi: 10.1016/j.pbb.2007.04.015

El-Hassar, L., Hagenston, A. M., D'Angelo, L. B., and Yeckel, M. F. (2011). Metabotropic glutamate receptors regulate hippocampal CA1 pyramidal neuron excitability via Ca(2)(+) wave-dependent activation of SK and TRPC channels. *J. Physiol.* 589(Pt 13), 3211–3229. doi: 10.1113/jphysiol.2011.209783

Elzamzamy, O. M., Penner, R., and Hazlehurst, L. A. (2020). The role of TRPC1 in modulating cancer progression. *Cells* 9:388. doi: 10.3390/cells9020388

Facci, L., and Skaper, S. D. (2012). Culture of rodent cortical and hippocampal neurons. *Methods Mol. Biol.* 846, 49–56. doi: 10.1007/978-1-61779-536-7_5

Feng, S., Li, H., Tai, Y., Huang, J., Su, Y., Abramowitz, J., et al. (2013). Canonical transient receptor potential 3 channels regulate mitochondrial calcium uptake. *Proc. Natl. Acad. Sci. U.S.A.* 110, 11011–11016. doi: 10.1073/pnas.1309531110

Formoso, K., Susperreguy, S., Freichel, M., and Birnbaumer, L. (2020). RNA-seq analysis reveals TRPC genes to impact an unexpected number of metabolic and regulatory pathways. *Sci. Rep.* 10:7227. doi: 10.1038/s41598-020-61177-x

Fowler, M. A., Sidiropoulou, K., Ozkan, E. D., Phillips, C. W., and Cooper, D. C. (2007). Corticolimbic expression of TRPC4 and TRPC5 channels in the rodent brain. *PLoS One* 2:e573. doi: 10.1371/journal.pone.0000573

Freichel, M., Suh, S. H., Pfeifer, A., Schweig, U., Trost, C., Weissgerber, P., et al. (2001). Lack of an endothelial store-operated Ca2+ current impairs agonist-dependent vasorelaxation in TRP4−/− mice. *Nat. Cell Biol.* 3, 121–127. doi: 10.1038/35055019

Gao, Y., Yao, T., Deng, Z., Sohn, J. W., Sun, J., Huang, Y., et al. (2017). TrpC5 mediates acute leptin and serotonin effects via pomc neurons. *Cell. Rep.* 18, 583–592. doi: 10.1016/j.celrep.2016.12.072

Gao, Y. Q., Gao, H., Zhou, Z. Y., Lu, S. D., and Sun, F. Y. (2004). [Expression of transient receptor potential channel 4 in striatum and hippocampus of rats is increased after focal cerebral ischemia]. *Sheng Li Xue Bao* 56, 153–157.

Gelderblom, M., Weymar, A., Bernreuther, C., Velden, J., Arunachalam, P., Steinbach, K., et al. (2012). Neutralization of the IL-17 axis diminishes neutrophil invasion and protects from ischemic stroke. *Blood* 120, 3793–3802. doi: 10.1182/blood-2012-02-412726

Gordienko, D. V., and Zholos, A. V. (2004). Regulation of muscarinic cationic current in myocytes from guinea-pig ileum by intracellular Ca2+ release: a central role of inositol 1,4,5-trisphosphate receptors. *Cell Calcium* 36, 367–386. doi: 10.1016/j.ceca.2004.02.021

Grant, C. V., Carver, C. M., Hastings, S. D., Ramachandran, K., Muniswamy, M., Risinger, A. L., et al. (2019). Triple-negative breast cancer cell line sensitivity to englerin A identifies a new, targetable subtype. *Breast Cancer Res. Treat.* 177, 345–355. doi: 10.1007/s10549-019-05324-7

Greka, A., Navarro, B., Oancea, E., Duggan, A., and Clapham, D. E. (2003). TRPC5 is a regulator of hippocampal neurite length and growth cone morphology. *Nat. Neurosci.* 6, 837–845. doi: 10.1038/nn1092

Guo, C., Ma, Y., Ma, S., Mu, F., Deng, J., Duan, J., et al. (2017). The role of TRPC6 in the neuroprotection of calycosin against cerebral ischemic injury. *Sci. Rep.* 7:3039. doi: 10.1038/s41598-017-03404-6

Guo, J., Li, J., Xia, L., Wang, Y., Zhu, J., Du, J., et al. (2020). Transient receptor potential canonical 5-scramblase signaling complex mediates neuronal phosphatidylserine externalization and apoptosis. *Cells* 9:547. doi: 10.3390/cells9030547

Hartmann, J., Dragicevic, E., Adelsberger, H., Henning, H. A., Sumser, M., Abramowitz, J., et al. (2008). TRPC3 channels are required for synaptic transmission and motor coordination. *Neuron* 59, 392–398. doi: 10.1016/j.neuron.2008.06.009

Hille, B., Dickson, E. J., Kruse, M., Vivas, O., and Suh, B. C. (2015). Phosphoinositides regulate ion channels. *Biochim. Biophys. Acta* 1851, 844–856. doi: 10.1016/j.bbalip.2014.09.010

Hilton, G. D., Nunez, J. L., Bambrick, L., Thompson, S. M., and McCarthy, M. M. (2006). Glutamate-mediated excitotoxicity in neonatal hippocampal neurons is mediated by mGluR-induced release of Ca++ from intracellular stores and is prevented by estradiol. *Eur. J. Neurosci.* 24, 3008–3016. doi: 10.1111/j.1460-9568.2006.05189.x

Hong, C., Choi, S. H., Kwak, M., Jeong, B., Ko, J., Park, H. J., et al. (2020). TRPC5 channel instability induced by depalmitoylation protects striatal neurons against oxidative stress in Huntington's disease. *Biochim. Biophys. Acta Mol. Cell Res.* 1867:118620. doi: 10.1016/j.bbamcr.2019.118620

Hong, C., Seo, H., Kwak, M., Jeon, J., Jang, J., Jeong, E. M., et al. (2015). Increased TRPC5 glutathionylation contributes to striatal neuron loss in Huntington's disease. *Brain* 138(Pt 10), 3030–3047. doi: 10.1093/brain/awv188

Huang, J., Liu, C. H., Hughes, S. A., Postma, M., Schwiening, C. J., and Hardie, R. C. (2010). Activation of TRP channels by protons and phosphoinositide depletion in Drosophila photoreceptors. *Curr. Biol.* 20, 189–197. doi: 10.1016/j.cub.2009.12.019

Ishii, M., Iizuka, R., Kiuchi, Y., Mori, Y., and Shimizu, S. (2011). Neuroprotection by lomerizine, a prophylactic drug for migraine, against hydrogen peroxide-induced hippocampal neurotoxicity. *Mol. Cell. Biochem.* 358, 1–11. doi: 10.1007/s11010-011-0913-3

Jeon, J., Tian, J. B., and Zhu, M. X. (2020). TRPC4 as a coincident detector of Gi/o and Gq/11 signaling: mechanisms and pathophysiological implications. *Curr. Opin. Physiol.* 17, 34–41. doi: 10.1016/j.cophys.2020.06.008

Jeon, J. P., Roh, S. E., Wie, J., Kim, J., Kim, H., Lee, K. P., et al. (2013). Activation of TRPC4beta by Galphai subunit increases Ca2+ selectivity and controls neurite morphogenesis in cultured hippocampal neuron. *Cell Calcium* 54, 307–319. doi: 10.1016/j.ceca.2013.07.006

Kim, D. S., Ryu, H. J., Kim, J. E., and Kang, T. C. (2013). The reverse roles of transient receptor potential canonical channel-3 and -6 in neuronal death following pilocarpine-induced status epilepticus. *Cell. Mol. Neurobiol.* 33, 99–109. doi: 10.1007/s10571-012-9875-6

Kim, J. E., Park, H., Choi, S. H., Kong, M. J., and Kang, T. C. (2019). TRPC6-Mediated ERK1/2 activation increases dentate granule cell resistance to status epilepticus via regulating lon protease-1 expression and mitochondrial dynamics. *Cells* 8:1376. doi: 10.3390/cells8111376

Kim, S. J., Kim, Y. S., Yuan, J. P., Petralia, R. S., Worley, P. F., and Linden, D. J. (2003). Activation of the TRPC1 cation channel by metabotropic glutamate receptor mGluR1. *Nature* 426, 285–291. doi: 10.1038/nature02162

Kim, Y. J., and Kang, T. C. (2015). The role of TRPC6 in seizure susceptibility and seizure-related neuronal damage in the rat dentate gyrus. *Neuroscience* 307, 215–230. doi: 10.1016/j.neuroscience.2015.08.054

Ko, A. R., and Kang, T. C. (2017). TRPC6-mediated ERK1/2 phosphorylation prevents dentate granule cell degeneration via inhibiting mitochondrial elongation. *Neuropharmacology* 121, 120–129. doi: 10.1016/j.neuropharm.2017.05.004

Kondratskyi, A., Kondratska, K., Skryma, R., and Prevarskaya, N. (2015). Ion channels in the regulation of apoptosis. *Biochim. Biophys. Acta* 1848(10 Pt B), 2532–2546. doi: 10.1016/j.bbamem.2014.10.030

Lankiewicz, S., Marc Luetjens, C., Truc Bui, N., Krohn, A. J., Poppe, M., Cole, G. M., et al. (2000). Activation of calpain I converts excitotoxic neuron death into a caspase-independent cell death. *J. Biol. Chem.* 275, 17064–17071. doi: 10.1074/jbc.275.22.17064

Lessard, C. B., Lussier, M. P., Cayouette, S., Bourque, G., and Boulay, G. (2005). The overexpression of presenilin2 and Alzheimer's-disease-linked presenilin2 variants influences TRPC6-enhanced Ca2+ entry into HEK293 cells. *Cell. Signal.* 17, 437–445. doi: 10.1016/j.cellsig.2004.09.005

Leuner, K., Kazanski, V., Müller, M., Essin, K., Henke, B., Gollasch, M., et al. (2007). Hyperforin—a key constituent of St. John's wort specifically activates TRPC6 channels. *FASEB J.* 21, 4101–4111. doi: 10.1096/fj.07-8110com

Li, H., Huang, J., Du, W., Jia, C., Yao, H., and Wang, Y. (2012). TRPC6 inhibited NMDA receptor activities and protected neurons from ischemic excitotoxicity. *J. Neurochem.* 123, 1010–1018. doi: 10.1111/jnc.12045

Li, J., Siegel, M., Yuan, M., Zeng, Z., Finnucan, L., Persky, R., et al. (2011). Estrogen enhances neurogenesis and behavioral recovery after stroke. *J. Cereb. Blood Flow Metab.* 31, 413–425. doi: 10.1038/jcbfm.2010.181

Li, M., Liu, E., Zhou, Q., Li, S., Wang, X., Liu, Y., et al. (2018). TRPC1 null exacerbates memory deficit and apoptosis induced by Amyloid-beta. *J. Alzheimers. Dis.* 63, 761–772. doi: 10.3233/JAD-180077

Li, Y., Calfa, G., Inoue, T., Amaral, M. D., and Pozzo-Miller, L. (2010). Activity-dependent release of endogenous BDNF from mossy fibers evokes a TRPC3 current and Ca2+ elevations in CA3 pyramidal neurons. *J. Neurophysiol.* 103, 2846–2856. doi: 10.1152/jn.01140.2009

Liman, E. R., Corey, D. P., and Dulac, C. (1999). TRP2: a candidate transduction channel for mammalian pheromone sensory signaling. *Proc. Natl. Acad. Sci. U.S.A.* 96, 5791–5796. doi: 10.1073/pnas.96.10.5791

Lin, Y., Chen, F., Zhang, J., Wang, T., Wei, X., Wu, J., et al. (2013a). Neuroprotective effect of resveratrol on ischemia/reperfusion injury in rats through TRPC6/CREB pathways. *J. Mol. Neurosci.* 50, 504–513. doi: 10.1007/s12031-013-9977-8

Lin, Y., Zhang, J. C., Fu, J., Chen, F., Wang, J., Wu, Z. L., et al. (2013b). Hyperforin attenuates brain damage induced by transient middle cerebral artery occlusion (MCAO) in rats via inhibition of TRPC6 channels degradation. *J. Cereb. Blood Flow Metab.* 33, 253–262. doi: 10.1038/jcbfm.2012.164

Lipton, P. (1999). Ischemic cell death in brain neurons. *Physiol. Rev.* 79, 1431–1568. doi: 10.1152/physrev.1999.79.4.1431

Lo, E. H., Dalkara, T., and Moskowitz, M. A. (2003). Mechanisms, challenges and opportunities in stroke. *Nat. Rev. Neurosci.* 4, 399–415. doi: 10.1038/nrn1106

Logothetis, D. E., Mahajan, R., Adney, S. K., Ha, J., Kawano, T., Meng, X. Y., et al. (2015). Unifying mechanism of controlling Kir3 channel activity by G proteins and phosphoinositides. *Int. Rev. Neurobiol.* 123, 1–26. doi: 10.1016/bs.irn.2015.05.013

Lu, R., Wang, J., Tao, R., Wang, J., Zhu, T., Guo, W., et al. (2018). Reduced TRPC6 mRNA levels in the blood cells of patients with Alzheimer's disease and mild cognitive impairment. *Mol. Psychiatry* 23, 767–776. doi: 10.1038/mp.2017.136

Ludlow, M. J., Gaunt, H. J., Rubaiy, H. N., Musialowski, K. E., Blythe, N. M., Vasudev, N. S., et al. (2017). (−)-Englerin A-evoked cytotoxicity is mediated by Na+ influx and counteracted by Na+/K+-ATPase. *J. Biol. Chem.* 292, 723–731. doi: 10.1074/jbc.M116.755678

Maher, P., van Leyen, K., Dey, P. N., Honrath, B., Dolga, A., and Methner, A. (2018). The role of Ca(2+) in cell death caused by oxidative glutamate toxicity and ferroptosis. *Cell Calcium* 70, 47–55. doi: 10.1016/j.ceca.2017.05.007

Miller, M., Shi, J., Zhu, Y., Kustov, M., Tian, J. B., Stevens, A., et al. (2011). Identification of ML204, a novel potent antagonist that selectively modulates native TRPC4/C5 ion channels. *J. Biol. Chem.* 286, 33436–33446. doi: 10.1074/jbc.M111.274167

Montell, C., Birnbaumer, L., Flockerzi, V., Bindels, R. J., Bruford, E. A., Caterina, M. J., et al. (2002). A unified nomenclature for the superfamily of TRP cation channels. *Mol. Cell.* 9, 229–231. doi: 10.1016/s1097-2765(02)00448-3

Munakata, M., Shirakawa, H., Nagayasu, K., Miyanohara, J., Miyake, T., Nakagawa, T., et al. (2013). Transient receptor potential canonical 3 inhibitor Pyr3 improves outcomes and attenuates astrogliosis after intracerebral hemorrhage in mice. *Stroke* 44, 1981–1987. doi: 10.1161/STROKEAHA.113.679332

Munsch, T., Freichel, M., Flockerzi, V., and Pape, H. C. (2003). Contribution of transient receptor potential channels to the control of GABA release from dendrites. *Proc. Natl. Acad. Sci. U.S.A.* 100, 16065–16070. doi: 10.1073/pnas.2535311100

Myeong, J., Ko, J., Kwak, M., Kim, J., Woo, J., Ha, K., et al. (2018). Dual action of the Galphaq-PLCbeta-PI(4,5)P2 pathway on TRPC1/4 and TRPC1/5 heterotetramers. *Sci. Rep.* 8:12117. doi: 10.1038/s41598-018-30625-0

Nair, S., Hagberg, H., Krishnamurthy, R., Thornton, C., and Mallard, C. (2013). Death associated protein kinases: molecular structure and brain injury. *Int. J. Mol. Sci.* 14, 13858–13872. doi: 10.3390/ijms140713858

Ogawa, N., Kurokawa, T., and Mori, Y. (2016). Sensing of redox status by TRP channels. *Cell Calcium* 60, 115–122. doi: 10.1016/j.ceca.2016.02.009

Okada, T., Inoue, R., Yamazaki, K., Maeda, A., Kurosaki, T., Yamakuni, T., et al. (1999). Molecular and functional characterization of a novel mouse transient receptor potential protein homologue TRP7. Ca(2+)-permeable cation channel that is constitutively activated and enhanced by stimulation of G protein-coupled receptor. *J. Biol. Chem.* 274, 27359–27370. doi: 10.1074/jbc.274.39.27359

Otsuguro, K., Tang, J., Tang, Y., Xiao, R., Freichel, M., Tsvilovskyy, V., et al. (2008). Isoform-specific inhibition of TRPC4 channel by phosphatidylinositol 4,5-bisphosphate. *J. Biol. Chem.* 283, 10026–10036. doi: 10.1074/jbc.M707306200

Park, M. K., Choi, B. Y., Kho, A. R., Lee, S. H., Hong, D. K., Jeong, J. H., et al. (2020). Effects of transient receptor potential cation 5 (TRPC5) inhibitor, NU6027, on hippocampal neuronal death after traumatic brain injury. *Int. J. Mol. Sci.* 21:8256. doi: 10.3390/ijms21218256

Park, S. E., Song, J. H., Hong, C., Kim, D. E., Sul, J. W., Kim, T. Y., et al. (2019). Contribution of zinc-dependent delayed calcium influx via TRPC5 in oxidative neuronal death and its prevention by novel TRPC antagonist. *Mol. Neurobiol.* 56, 2822–2835. doi: 10.1007/s12035-018-1258-1257

Phelan, K. D., Mock, M. M., Kretz, O., Shwe, U. T., Kozhemyakin, M., Greenfield, L. J., et al. (2012). Heteromeric canonical transient receptor potential 1 and 4 channels play a critical role in epileptiform burst firing and seizure-induced neurodegeneration. *Mol. Pharmacol.* 81, 384–392. doi: 10.1124/mol.111.075341

Phelan, K. D., Shwe, U. T., Abramowitz, J., Wu, H., Rhee, S. W., Howell, M. D., et al. (2013). Canonical transient receptor channel 5 (TRPC5) and TRPC1/4 contribute to seizure and excitotoxicity by distinct cellular mechanisms. *Mol. Pharmacol.* 83, 429–438. doi: 10.1124/mol.112.082271

Popugaeva, E., Chernyuk, D., Zhang, H., Postnikova, T. Y., Pats, K., Fedorova, E., et al. (2019). Derivatives of piperazines as potential therapeutic agents for Alzheimer's disease. *Mol. Pharmacol.* 95, 337–348. doi: 10.1124/mol.118.114348

Pressler, R. T., and Regehr, W. G. (2013). Metabotropic glutamate receptors drive global persistent inhibition in the visual thalamus. *J. Neurosci.* 33, 2494–2506. doi: 10.1523/JNEUROSCI.3458-12.2013

Putney, J. W. (2017). Store-operated calcium entry: an historical overview. *Adv. Exp. Med. Biol.* 981, 205–214. doi: 10.1007/978-3-319-55858-5_9

Qiu, J., Fang, Y., Ronnekleiv, O. K., and Kelly, M. J. (2010). Leptin excites proopiomelanocortin neurons via activation of TRPC channels. *J. Neurosci.* 30, 1560–1565. doi: 10.1523/JNEUROSCI.4816-09.2010

Rami, A., and Kogel, D. (2008). Apoptosis meets autophagy-like cell death in the ischemic penumbra: two sides of the same coin? *Autophagy* 4, 422–426. doi: 10.4161/auto.5778

Rathore, S. S., Hinn, A. R., Cooper, L. S., Tyroler, H. A., and Rosamond, W. D. (2002). Characterization of incident stroke signs and symptoms: findings from the atherosclerosis risk in communities study. *Stroke* 33, 2718–2721. doi: 10.1161/01.str.0000035286.87503.31

Reiner, A., and Levitz, J. (2018). Glutamatergic signaling in the central nervous system: ionotropic and metabotropic receptors in concert. *Neuron* 98, 1080–1098. doi: 10.1016/j.neuron.2018.05.018

Riccio, A., Li, Y., Moon, J., Kim, K. S., Smith, K. S., Rudolph, U., et al. (2009). Essential role for TRPC5 in amygdala function and fear-related behavior. *Cell* 137, 761–772. doi: 10.1016/j.cell.2009.03.039

Riccio, A., Li, Y., Tsvetkov, E., Gapon, S., Yao, G. L., Smith, K. S., et al. (2014). Decreased anxiety-like behavior and Galphaq/11-dependent responses in the amygdala of mice lacking TRPC4 channels. *J. Neurosci.* 34, 3653–3667. doi: 10.1523/JNEUROSCI.2274-13.2014

Riccio, A., Medhurst, A. D., Mattei, C., Kelsell, R. E., Calver, A. R., Randall, A. D., et al. (2002). mRNA distribution analysis of human TRPC family in CNS and peripheral tissues. *Brain Res. Mol. Brain Res.* 109, 95–104. doi: 10.1016/s0169-328x(02)00527-2

Sell, T. S., Belkacemi, T., Flockerzi, V., and Beck, A. (2014). Protonophore properties of hyperforin are essential for its pharmacological activity. *Sci. Rep.* 4:7500. doi: 10.1038/srep07500

Selvaraj, S., Sun, Y., Watt, J. A., Wang, S., Lei, S., Birnbaumer, L., et al. (2012). Neurotoxin-induced ER stress in mouse dopaminergic neurons involves downregulation of TRPC1 and inhibition of AKT/mTOR signaling. *J. Clin. Invest.* 122, 1354–1367. doi: 10.1172/JCI61332

Shamloo, M., Soriano, L., Wieloch, T., Nikolich, K., Urfer, R., and Oksenberg, D. (2005). Death-associated protein kinase is activated by dephosphorylation in response to cerebral ischemia. *J. Biol. Chem.* 280, 42290–42299. doi: 10.1074/jbc.M505804200

Shen, N., Wang, L., Wu, Y., Liu, Y., Pei, H., and Xiang, H. (2020). Adeno-associated virus packaged TRPC5 gene therapy alleviated spinal cord ischemic reperfusion injury in rats. *Neuroreport* 31, 29–36. doi: 10.1097/WNR.0000000000001359

Shirakawa, H., Sakimoto, S., Nakao, K., Sugishita, A., Konno, M., Iida, S., et al. (2010). Transient receptor potential canonical 3 (TRPC3) mediates thrombin-induced astrocyte activation and upregulates its own expression in cortical astrocytes. *J. Neurosci.* 30, 13116–13129. doi: 10.1523/JNEUROSCI.1890-10.2010

Simpkins, K. L., Guttmann, R. P., Dong, Y., Chen, Z., Sokol, S., Neumar, R. W., et al. (2003). Selective activation induced cleavage of the NR2B subunit by calpain. *J. Neurosci.* 23, 11322–11331.

Sohn, J. W., Xu, Y., Jones, J. E., Wickman, K., Williams, K. W., and Elmquist, J. K. (2011). Serotonin 2C receptor activates a distinct population of arcuate pro-opiomelanocortin neurons via TRPC channels. *Neuron* 71, 488–497. doi: 10.1016/j.neuron.2011.06.012

Storch, U., Forst, A. L., Pardatscher, F., Erdogmus, S., Philipp, M., Gregoritza, M., et al. (2017). Dynamic NHERF interaction with TRPC4/5 proteins is required for channel gating by diacylglycerol. *Proc. Natl. Acad. Sci. U.S.A.* 114, E37–E46. doi: 10.1073/pnas.1612263114

Storch, U., Forst, A. L., Philipp, M., Gudermann, T., and Mederos y Schnitzler, M. (2012). Transient receptor potential channel 1 (TRPC1) reduces calcium permeability in heteromeric channel complexes. *J. Biol. Chem.* 287, 3530–3540. doi: 10.1074/jbc.M111.283218

Strubing, C., Krapivinsky, G., Krapivinsky, L., and Clapham, D. E. (2001). TRPC1 and TRPC5 form a novel cation channel in mammalian brain. *Neuron* 29, 645–655. doi: 10.1016/s0896-6273(01)00240-9

Sukumaran, P., Sun, Y., Antonson, N., and Singh, B. B. (2018). Dopaminergic neurotoxins induce cell death by attenuating NF-kappaB-mediated regulation of TRPC1 expression and autophagy. *FASEB J.* 32, 1640–1652. doi: 10.1096/fj.201700662RR

Sun, P., Bu, F., Min, J. W., Munshi, Y., Howe, M. D., Liu, L., et al. (2019). Inhibition of calcium/calmodulin-dependent protein kinase kinase (CaMKK) exacerbates impairment of endothelial cell and blood-brain barrier after stroke. *Eur. J. Neurosci.* 49, 27–39. doi: 10.1111/ejn.14223

Sun, Y., Sukumaran, P., and Singh, B. B. (2020). Sigma1 receptor inhibits TRPC1-mediated Ca(2+) entry that promotes dopaminergic cell death. *Cell Mol. Neurobiol.* [Epub ahead of print]. doi: 10.1007/s10571-020-00892-5

Sun, Y., Zhang, H., Selvaraj, S., Sukumaran, P., Lei, S., Birnbaumer, L., et al. (2017). Inhibition of L-Type Ca(2+) Channels by TRPC1-STIM1 Complex Is Essential for the Protection of Dopaminergic Neurons. *J. Neurosci.* 37, 3364–3377. doi: 10.1523/JNEUROSCI.3010-16.2017

Swanson, C. J., Bures, M., Johnson, M. P., Linden, A. M., Monn, J. A., and Schoepp, D. D. (2005). Metabotropic glutamate receptors as novel targets for anxiety and stress disorders. *Nat. Rev. Drug Discov.* 4, 131–144. doi: 10.1038/nrd1630

Tabarean, I. V. (2012). Persistent histamine excitation of glutamatergic preoptic neurons. *PLoS One* 7:e47700. doi: 10.1371/journal.pone.0047700

Tai, C., Hines, D. J., Choi, H. B., and MacVicar, B. A. (2011). Plasma membrane insertion of TRPC5 channels contributes to the cholinergic plateau potential in hippocampal CA1 pyramidal neurons. *Hippocampus* 21, 958–967. doi: 10.1002/hipo.20807

Tanaka, E., Yamamoto, S., Inokuchi, H., Isagai, T., and Higashi, H. (1999). Membrane dysfunction induced by in vitro ischemia in rat hippocampal CA1 pyramidal neurons. *J. Neurophysiol.* 81, 1872–1880. doi: 10.1152/jn.1999.81.4.1872

Tanaka, E., Yamamoto, S., Kudo, Y., Mihara, S., and Higashi, H. (1997). Mechanisms underlying the rapid depolarization produced by deprivation of oxygen and glucose in rat hippocampal CA1 neurons in vitro. *J. Neurophysiol.* 78, 891–902. doi: 10.1152/jn.1997.78.2.891

Tao, R., Lu, R., Wang, J., Zeng, S., Zhang, T., Guo, W., et al. (2020). Probing the therapeutic potential of TRPC6 for Alzheimer's disease in live neurons from patient-specific iPSCs. *J. Mol. Cell. Biol.* [Epub ahead of print]. doi: 10.1093/jmcb/mjaa027

Tasca, C. I., Dal-Cim, T., and Cimarosti, H. (2015). In vitro oxygen-glucose deprivation to study ischemic cell death. *Methods Mol. Biol.* 1254, 197–210. doi: 10.1007/978-1-4939-2152-2_15

Tavafoghi, M., Brodusch, N., Gauvin, R., and Cerruti, M. (2016). Hydroxyapatite formation on graphene oxide modified with amino acids: arginine versus glutamic acid. *J. R. Soc. Interface* 13:20150986. doi: 10.1098/rsif.2015.0986

Taylor, C. P., Weber, M. L., Gaughan, C. L., Lehning, E. J., and LoPachin, R. M. (1999). Oxygen/glucose deprivation in hippocampal slices: altered intraneuronal elemental composition predicts structural and functional damage. *J. Neurosci.* 19, 619–629.

Thakur, D. P., Tian, J. B., Jeon, J., Xiong, J., Huang, Y., Flockerzi, V., et al. (2016). Critical roles of Gi/o proteins and phospholipase C-delta1 in the activation of receptor-operated TRPC4 channels. *Proc. Natl. Acad. Sci. U.S.A.* 113, 1092–1097. doi: 10.1073/pnas.1522294113

Thakur, D. P., Wang, Q., Jeon, J., Tian, J. B., and Zhu, M. X. (2020). Intracellular acidification facilitates receptor-operated TRPC4 activation through PLCdelta1 in a Ca(2+) -dependent manner. *J. Physiol.* 598, 2651–2667. doi: 10.1113/JP279658

Tian, J., Thakur, D. P., Lu, Y., Zhu, Y., Freichel, M., Flockerzi, V., et al. (2014a). Dual depolarization responses generated within the same lateral septal neurons by TRPC4-containing channels. *Pflugers. Arch.* 466, 1301–1316. doi: 10.1007/s00424-013-1362-5

Tian, J., Thakur, D. P., and Zhu, M. X. (2014b). TRPC channels. *Handb. Ion Chann.* 27, 411–426.

Toyoda, H., Kawano, T., Sato, H., and Kato, T. (2020). Cellular mechanisms underlying the rapid depolarization caused by oxygen and glucose deprivation in layer III pyramidal cells of the somatosensory cortex. *Neurosci. Res.* [Epub ahead of print]. doi: 10.1016/j.neures.2020.03.003

Venkatachalam, K., and Montell, C. (2007). TRP channels. *Annu. Rev. Biochem.* 76, 387–417. doi: 10.1146/annurev.biochem.75.103004.142819

Virani, S. S., Alonso, A., Benjamin, E. J., Bittencourt, M. S., Callaway, C. W., Carson, A. P., et al. (2020). Heart disease and stroke statistics-2020 update: a report from the american heart association. *Circulation* 141, e139–e596. doi: 10.1161/CIR.0000000000000757

Wang, H., Cheng, X., Tian, J., Xiao, Y., Tian, T., Xu, F., et al. (2020). TRPC channels: structure, function, regulation and recent advances in small molecular probes. *Pharmacol. Ther.* 209:107497. doi: 10.1016/j.pharmthera.2020.107497

Wang, J., Lu, R., Yang, J., Li, H., He, Z., Jing, N., et al. (2015). TRPC6 specifically interacts with APP to inhibit its cleavage by gamma-secretase and reduce Abeta production. *Nat. Commun.* 6:8876. doi: 10.1038/ncomms9876

Wang, S., Zhang, A. P., Kurada, L., Matsui, T., and Lei, S. (2011). Cholecystokinin facilitates neuronal excitability in the entorhinal cortex via activation of TRPC-like channels. *J. Neurophysiol.* 106, 1515–1524. doi: 10.1152/jn.00025.2011

Wang, Z., Wang, Y., Tian, X., Shen, H., Dou, Y., Li, H., et al. (2016). Transient receptor potential channel 1/4 reduces subarachnoid hemorrhage-induced early brain injury in rats via calcineurin-mediated NMDAR and NFAT dephosphorylation. *Sci. Rep.* 6:33577. doi: 10.1038/srep33577

Woodruff, T. M., Thundyil, J., Tang, S. C., Sobey, C. G., Taylor, S. M., and Arumugam, T. V. (2011). Pathophysiology, treatment, and animal and cellular models of human ischemic stroke. *Mol. Neurodegener.* 6:11. doi: 10.1186/1750-1326-6-11

Wu, J., Ryskamp, D., Birnbaumer, L., and Bezprozvanny, I. (2018). Inhibition of TRPC1-dependent store-operated calcium entry improves synaptic stability and motor performance in a mouse model of Huntington's disease. *J. Huntingtons. Dis.* 7, 35–50. doi: 10.3233/JHD-170266

Wu, J., Shih, H. P., Vigont, V., Hrdlicka, L., Diggins, L., Singh, C., et al. (2011). Neuronal store-operated calcium entry pathway as a novel therapeutic target for Huntington's disease treatment. *Chem. Biol.* 18, 777–793. doi: 10.1016/j.chembiol.2011.04.012

Xu, N., Meng, H., Liu, T., Feng, Y., Qi, Y., and Wang, H. (2018). TRPC1 deficiency exacerbates cerebral ischemia/reperfusion-induced neurological injury by potentiating Nox4-derived reactive oxygen species generation. *Cell Physiol. Biochem.* 51, 1723–1738. doi: 10.1159/000495676

Xu, S. Z., Sukumar, P., Zeng, F., Li, J., Jairaman, A., English, A., et al. (2008). TRPC channel activation by extracellular thioredoxin. *Nature* 451, 69–72. doi: 10.1038/nature06414

Yan, H. D., Villalobos, C., and Andrade, R. (2009). TRPC channels mediate a muscarinic receptor-induced afterdepolarization in cerebral cortex. *J. Neurosci.* 29, 10038–10046. doi: 10.1523/JNEUROSCI.1042-09.2009

Yao, C., Zhang, J., Chen, F., and Lin, Y. (2013). Neuroprotectin D1 attenuates brain damage induced by transient middle cerebral artery occlusion in rats through TRPC6/CREB pathways. *Mol. Med. Rep.* 8, 543–550. doi: 10.3892/mmr.2013.1543

Yao, C., Zhang, J., Liu, G., Chen, F., and Lin, Y. (2014). Neuroprotection by (−)-epigallocatechin-3-gallate in a rat model of stroke is mediated through inhibition of endoplasmic reticulum stress. *Mol. Med. Rep.* 9, 69–76. doi: 10.3892/mmr.2013.1778

Ying, H. S., Weishaupt, J. H., Grabb, M., Canzoniero, L. M., Sensi, S. L., Sheline, C. T., et al. (1997). Sublethal oxygen-glucose deprivation alters hippocampal neuronal AMPA receptor expression and vulnerability to kainate-induced death. *J. Neurosci.* 17, 9536–9544.

Yoshida, T., Inoue, R., Morii, T., Takahashi, N., Yamamoto, S., Hara, Y., et al. (2006). Nitric oxide activates TRP channels by cysteine S-nitrosylation. *Nat. Chem. Biol.* 2, 596–607. doi: 10.1038/nchembio821

Zhang, C., Roepke, T. A., Kelly, M. J., and Ronnekleiv, O. K. (2008). Kisspeptin depolarizes gonadotropin-releasing hormone neurons through activation of TRPC-like cationic channels. *J. Neurosci.* 28, 4423–4434. doi: 10.1523/JNEUROSCI.5352-07.2008

Zhang, H., Sun, S., Wu, L., Pchitskaya, E., Zakharova, O., Fon Tacer, K., et al. (2016). Store-operated calcium channel complex in postsynaptic spines: a new therapeutic target for Alzheimer's disease treatment. *J. Neurosci.* 36, 11837–11850. doi: 10.1523/JNEUROSCI.1188-16.2016

Zhang, J., Mao, X., Zhou, T., Cheng, X., and Lin, Y. (2014). IL-17A contributes to brain ischemia reperfusion injury through calpain-TRPC6 pathway in mice. *Neuroscience* 274, 419–428. doi: 10.1016/j.neuroscience.2014.06.001

Zhang, L., Kolaj, M., and Renaud, L. P. (2015). Intracellular postsynaptic cannabinoid receptors link thyrotropin-releasing hormone receptors to TRPC-like channels in thalamic paraventricular nucleus neurons. *Neuroscience* 311, 81–91. doi: 10.1016/j.neuroscience.2015.10.015

Zhao, X., Wang, H., Sun, G., Zhang, J., Edwards, N. J., and Aronowski, J. (2015). Neuronal interleukin- 4 as a modulator of microglial pathways and ischemic brain damage. *J. Neurosci.* 35, 11281–11291. doi: 10.1523/JNEUROSCI.1685-15.2015

Zheng, F., and Phelan, K. D. (2014). The role of canonical transient receptor potential channels in seizure and excitotoxicity. *Cells* 3, 288–303. doi: 10.3390/cells3020288

Zhu, Y., Gao, M., Zhou, T., Xie, M., Mao, A., Feng, L., et al. (2019). The TRPC5 channel regulates angiogenesis and promotes recovery from ischemic injury in mice. *J. Biol. Chem.* 294, 28–37. doi: 10.1074/jbc.RA118.005392

Zhu, Y., Lu, Y., Qu, C., Miller, M., Tian, J., Thakur, D. P., et al. (2015). Identification and optimization of 2-aminobenzimidazole derivatives as novel inhibitors of TRPC4 and TRPC5 channels. *Br. J. Pharmacol.* 172, 3495–3509. doi: 10.1111/bph.13140

15

Novel Targets for Stroke Therapy: Special Focus on TRPC Channels and TRPC6

Lu Liu[1], Lijuan Gu[2], Manli Chen[1], Yueying Zheng[1], Xiaoxing Xiong[1,2] and Shengmei Zhu[1]**

[1] Department of Anesthesiology, The First Affiliated Hospital, College of Medicine, Zhejiang University, Hangzhou, China,
[2] Central Laboratory, Renmin Hospital of Wuhan University, Wuhan, China

***Correspondence:**
Shengmei Zhu
smzhu20088@zju.edu.cn
Xiaoxing Xiong
xiaoxingxiong@whu.edu.cn

Stroke remains a leading cause of death, disability, and medical care burden worldwide. However, transformation from laboratory findings toward effective pharmacological interventions for clinical stroke has been unsatisfactory. Novel evidence has been gained on the underlying mechanisms and therapeutic potential related to the transient receptor potential (TRP) channels in several disorders. The TRP superfamily consists of a diverse group of Ca^{2+} permeable non-selective cation channels. In particular, the members of TRP subfamilies, TRP canonical (TRPC) channels and TRPC6, have been found in different cell types in the whole body and have high levels of expression in the central nervous system (CNS). Notably, the TRPCs and TRPC6 channel have been implicated in neurite outgrowth and neuronal survival during normal development and in a range of CNS pathological conditions. Recent studies have shown that suppression of TRPC6 channel degradation prevents ischemic neuronal cell death in experimental stroke. Accumulating evidence supports the important functions of TRPC6 in brain ischemia. We have highlighted some crucial advancement that points toward an important involvement of TRPCs and TRPC6 in ischemic stroke. This review will make an overview of the TRP and TRPC channels due to their roles as targets for clinical trials and CNS disorders. Besides, the primary goal is to discuss and update the critical role of TRPC6 channels in stroke and provide a promising target for stroke prevention and therapy.

Keywords: TRP ion channels, TRPCs, TRPC6 channel, neuronal survival, ischemic stroke

INTRODUCTION

Ischemic stroke is induced by the obstruction of an artery or multiple arteries leading to the brain. Focal impairment or occlusion of blood circulation to the brain impairs the normal function of neurons. The mechanisms underlying ischemic stroke are complex, and include excitotoxicity, oxidative and nitrosative stress, Ca^{2+} overload, inflammation, and apoptosis (Szydlowska and Tymianski, 2010; Khoshnam et al., 2017). Among these mechanisms, intracellular Ca^{2+} overload remains a vital role in neuronal injury associated with ischemic stroke (Choi, 1995). Glutamate receptors, such as *N*-methyl-D-aspartate receptor (NMDAR), are thought to be major pathways for intracellular Ca^{2+} influx in the central nervous system (CNS) after cerebral ischemia-reperfusion (IR) injury. Excessive NMDARs activation and the following Ca^{2+} influx through NMDARs are crucial steps required for initiating ischemic cell death (Szydlowska and Tymianski, 2010; Lai et al., 2011).To date, pre-clinical studies have provided substantial evidences for the neuroprotective effect of NMDAR antagonists in experimental ischemic stroke (Ginsberg, 2008). However, for several decades, clinical trials of NMDAR antagonists have all ended up with failure to show beneficial effects due to their narrow therapeutic windows and adverse effects (Wu and Tymianski, 2018). Thus, effective therapeutic interventions for ischemic stroke are urgently required.

Despite the pivotal functions of NMDARs, non-glutamate mechanisms have drawn attention as promising Ca^{2+} influx pathways involved in brain ischemia. In this respect, researchers shifted focus toward the transient receptor potential (TRP) channels (Szydlowska and Tymianski, 2010). TRPs are non-selective cationic channels which have key functions in different disorders (Moran, 2018). The TRP canonical (TRPC) subfamily was proved to be extensively distributed in CNS and have important functions in neuronal development (Tai et al., 2009). Understanding of these channels may drive the researchers to make a significant breakthrough in CNS diseases therapy. Recently, growing evidence indicates that TRPC6 channel has been involved in Ca^{2+} homeostasis and shown to participate in the molecular pathophysiology of ischemic stroke. TRPC6 was reported to have an critical role in neuroprotection in both *in vitro* and *in vivo* models of ischemic stroke (Du et al., 2010). In this review, we present a general description of the current understanding of TRPs and TRPC subfamily, with an emphasis on their involvement in clinical trials and CNS dysfunctions. Furthermore, this review concentrates on evidence-based advancements of TRPC6 in CNS disorders and cerebral ischemia. The primary aim is to clarify the relationship between TRPC6 and ischemic stroke and discuss future perspectives.

THE TRP ION CHANNEL FAMILY

The TRP channels comprise a big family of cation channels that are involved in various physiological and pathological processes. TRPs were first discovered in *Drosophila* in 1960s as a conditional phototransduction mutant (Minke, 1977; Montell et al., 1985). TRPs are commonly distributed in different cell types and tissues, and possess many vital functions in ion homeostasis, sensory transduction, inflammatory responses, innate and adaptive immune responses, and cell survival (Clapham, 2003; Nilius et al., 2007; Ramirez et al., 2018). The channel subunits consist of six transmembrane domains (TDs) that assemble as cation-permeable tetramers (Clapham et al., 2001). However, TRP channels have relatively low selectivity for the transport of cations, such as Na^{+} and Ca^{2+}, into the cytoplasm.

The TRPs are divided into seven subfamilies, TRPC (canonical), TRPV (vanilloid), TRPM (melastatin), TRPP (polycystin), TRPML (mucolipin), TRPA (ankyrin), and TRPN (NO-mechano-potential), based on amino acid homology (Nilius et al., 2007). These channels can receive multiple types of intracellular and extracellular information, which in turn can induce a series of different responses. Dysfunctions of these proteins are related to many disorders (Kaneko and Szallasi, 2014); e.g., progressive kidney diseases (TRPC5 and TRPC6) (Winn et al., 2005; Zhou et al., 2017), pulmonary edema (TRPC6) (Weissmann et al., 2012), stroke (TRPC6) (Du et al., 2010), myocardial IR injury (TRPC3/6/7) (He et al., 2017), Huntington's disease (HD) (TRPC5) (Hong et al., 2015), pruritus (TRPV1,TRPA1) (Moran, 2018), lower urinary tract disorders (TRPV4), pain (TRPV1, TRPA1, TRPM8, and TRPM3), and type 2 diabetes (TRPM5) (Voets et al., 2019), idiopathic rhinitis (TRPA1 and TRPV1) (Van Gerven et al., 2017), irritable bowel syndrome (TRPV1) (Wouters et al., 2016), and genetic diseases (TRPA1, TRPC6, TRPV3/4, TRPM1/4/6, TRPML1, TRPP2) (Moran, 2018).

There have been a number of clinical trials of compounds that regulate TRPV1, TRPV3, TRPV4, TRPA1, and TRPM8 (Moran, 2018). The vanilloid receptor, TRPV1, is identified as an important detector of pain, including heat hyperalgesia, postherpetic neuralgia, and osteoarthritic pain (Moran, 2018). Small molecule antagonists and agonists targeting TRPV1, such as NEO6860, V116517, and capsaicin, have attracted attention in research on multiple pain pathways and have been shown to have clinical potential for use in sustained pain relief (Szallasi et al., 2006; Arendt-Nielsen et al., 2016; Brown et al., 2017; Blair, 2018). However, safety issues, such as impaired noxious heat sensation and hyperthermia, require special consideration. Although several recent clinical trials suggested no increase in body temperature in humans (Arendt-Nielsen et al., 2016; Brown et al., 2017), most TRPV1 antagonists examined previously showed on-target adverse effects (Lee et al., 2017; Manitpisitkul et al., 2018), thus limiting their clinical acceptance. The balance between drug efficacy and side effects in clinical trials remains to be explored. TRPV3 is sensitive to warm temperatures (>33°C) and is predominantly found in skin keratinocytes (Xu et al., 2002; Moqrich et al., 2005). The TRPV3 antagonist, GRC 15300, has successfully finished a phase 1 clinical trial and appears to have potential for pain treatment (Pharmaceuticals, 2018). TRPV3 is also an emerging target for itch and skin diseases in animal models; further studies are required to confirm its utility in treatment of clinical skin diseases. TRPV4 was originally characterized in 2000 as an osmosensor that responds to extracellular osmolarity (Liedtke et al., 2000; Strotmann et al., 2000). TRPV4 performs essential roles in various diseases by regulating Ca^{2+} influx. A clinical trial of TRPV4 blockers and their promising roles in the treatment of dyspnea and pulmonary edema in heart failure and acute decompensated heart failure cases is currently finished in phase 1 stage (GlaxoSmithKline, 2019). Similarly, another single-center study designed to estimate the effects of GSK2798745, a novel TRPV4 inhibitor, on pulmonary gas exchange and pulmonary function in participants with heart failure has already completed a phase 2 clinical trial (GlaxoSmithKline, 2018). TRPA1 has been regarded as a gatekeeper of chronic inflammatory diseases (Bautista et al., 2013). A phase 2a clinical study yielded data indicating that the TRPA1 antagonist, GRC 17536, alleviates pain with no other drug-related side effects in patients with painful diabetic neuropathy, which supports the promising therapeutic efficacy of TRPA1 blockade in pain management (Pharmaceuticals, 2014).

PF-05105679 is a TRPM8 antagonist that was shown to reverse cold pain sensation in the cold presser test in humans (Andrews et al., 2015; Gosset et al., 2017). Importantly, blockade of TRPM8 by PF-05105679 showed no effects on core body temperature.

Overall, TRPs have good potential as therapeutic targets for various diseases. Further efforts are still required to explore the specific and detailed functions of TRPs in different disorders.

THE TRPC SUBFAMILY AND THEIR ROLES IN CNS

The mammalian C-type TRP channels (TRPC proteins) are most closely related to *Drosophila* TRPs. In terms of amino acid similarity, TRPCs can be classified into four subsets: TRPC1, TRPC2, TRPC3/6/7, and TRPC4/5 (Clapham et al., 2001). At a molecular level, all TRPCs consist of a pore–loop motif, three to four NH_2-terminal ankyrin repeat domains (ARDs), and a COOH-terminal TRP domain (Venkatachalam and Montell, 2007). The ARD is a common protein–protein interaction module, typically consisting of 33 amino acid residues, which forms a canonical helix-loop-helix fold followed by a β-hairpin loop (Islam et al., 2018). ARDs perform crucial roles in various cellular processes, including thetranscription, signal transduction, inflammatory responses, cell development, and cell cycle (Islam et al., 2018). Confocal Förster resonance energy transfer (FRET) measurements revealed that the first ARD in TRPC5 is crucial for homomultimerization (Schindl et al., 2008). ADRs are also closely involved in TRPC4 tetramer assembly (Lepage et al., 2009). In addition, ARDs in TRPC3 in skeletal muscle could mediate TRPC3/1 heteromerization, thus regulating resting cytosolic Ca^{2+} levels (Woo et al., 2014). The novel membrane RING-H2 protein, RNF24, binds with the ARDs of TRPC6 in the Golgi apparatus and results in intracellular retention of TRPC6 without affecting channel activity (Lussier et al., 2008). Thus, ARDs of TRPCs likely participate in their channel heteromerization and trafficking. The TRP domain is a highly conserved sequence of 25 amino acids containing a proline-rich motif and an invariant sequence called the TRP box (Glu-Trp-Lys-Phe-Ala-Arg) (Montell, 2001). A previous study indicated that the TRP domain in TRPC3 is an essential element in regulating the cell response to erythropoietin (Hirschler-Laszkiewicz et al., 2011). The pore region of TRPCs, situated between the fifth and sixth TDs, is associated with an intracellular gate and an extracellular selectivity filter. The conserved LFW motif is a key feature of the TRPC pore loop, which has a pivotal role in hydrophobic interactions and in sustaining the appropriate structure of the ion pore (Li J. et al., 2019).

Transient receptor potential canonical channels are non-selective cation channels with different Ca^{2+} and Na^+ permeability ratios. TRPCs activation is involved in changes in $[Ca^{2+}]_i$, which governs diverse complex and crucial cellular functions. Evidence suggests that all TRPCs can be commonly activated by phospholipase C (PLC) within numerous stimulation, like inflammatory and IR injury, subsequently mediating Ca^{2+} entry into the cell (Weissmann et al., 2012; Wu et al., 2015). TRPCs are closely connected to PLC activity controlled by modulation of the endogenous agonists diacylglycerols (DAGs) and phosphoinositides. TRPCs were originally identified in sensory nerve endings followed by axons and dendrites of central neurons in the CNS. There have been shown that TRPCs are involved in nerve-growth-cone guidance, neuronal survival, synapse formation, synaptic transmission, and sensory transduction (Li et al., 2005; Jia et al., 2007; Zhou et al., 2008; Quick et al., 2012; Hartmann and Konnerth, 2015). Notably, TPRCs are responsible for inflammation, IR injury, and excitotoxicity (Ramirez et al., 2018).

Alzheimer's disease (AD) is driven by the cerebral deposition of amyloid-β protein (Aβ), the primary element of the senile plaques seen in the pathological brains. Loss of TRPC1 aggravates memory deficits and cell apoptosis induced by Aβ (Li et al., 2018). It is widely recognized that Aβ generation is closely related to amyloid precursor protein cleavage by γ-secretase. Wang et al. (2015) demonstrated that TRPC6 regulates γ-secretase of amyloid precursor protein. Importantly, a recent clinical case-control research revealed that the TRPC6 mRNA level in peripheral leukocytes is markedly reduced in patients with AD, which provides new insight for clinical diagnosis of AD (Chen et al., 2019). In addition, piperazine, a novel TRPC6 agonist, was shown to decrease long-term potentiation in the 5xFAD mouse, suggesting that piperazine may have potential for AD therapy (Popugaeva et al., 2019). Heteromultimeric channels of TRPC1/4/5 subunits regulate flexible relearning and working memory in mice (Broker-Lai et al., 2017). A study in TRPC5 transgenic mice identified an essential role of TRPC5, activated by G protein-coupled neuronal receptors, in the modulation of innate fear. This result provided strong evidence that TRPC5 channels may be a potential target for the alleviation of fear behavior (Riccio et al., 2009). Previous study has shown that TRPC1 aggravates hippocampal neuronal cell death (Narayanan et al., 2008). A subsequent research suggested that the TRPC1 mediates store-operated Ca^{2+} influx in neurons with mutant Huntingtin protein, suggesting a novel treatment for HD (Wu et al., 2011). Inhibition of TRPC1 is a potentially useful neuroprotective and therapeutic strategy against HD (Wu et al., 2018). In addition, generation of endogenous TRPC5 is increased in both transgenic mice and patients with HD. Knockdown or blockage of TRPC5 promotes neuronal survival and improved neurodegeneration in HD (Hong et al., 2015). The novel TRPC4/5 blocker, M084, was reported to show rapid antidepressant and anxiolytic-like effects in male C57BL/6 mice (Yang et al., 2015). Furthermore, TRPC channels have gained focus on the treatment of ischemic stroke. Decreased TRPC1 expression was shown in ischemic brain tissues. Overexpression of TRPC1 inhibits cerebral I/R injury, whereas TRPC1 knockout has the opposite effects. The underlying mechanism refers to the generation of reactive oxygen species via nicotinamide adenine dinucleotide phosphate (NADPH) oxidase family 4-containing-NADPH oxidase (Xu et al., 2018). Additionally, TRPC6 also holds important roles in stroke therapy, which will be discussed in further detail below.

Taken together, the observations outlined above indicating the importance of TRPCs in CNS disorders suggest that agents targeting TRPCs have great potential for clinical use. While

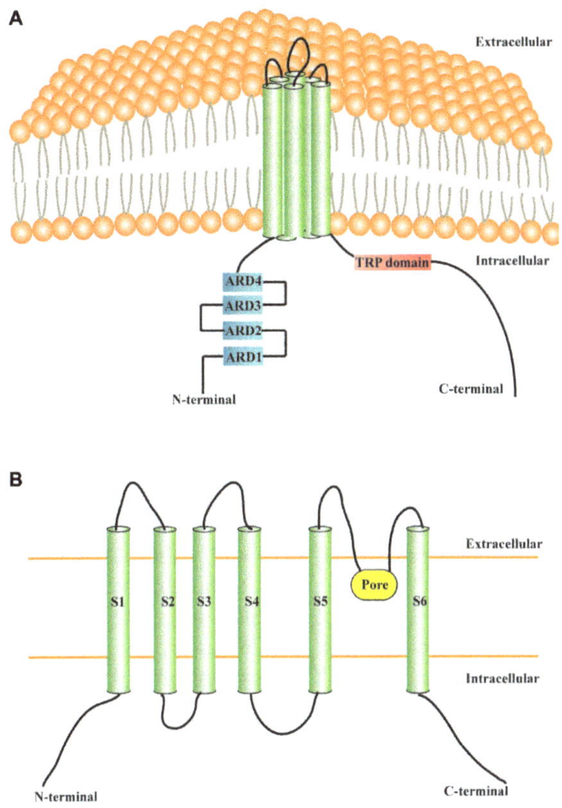

FIGURE 1 | Structural features of TRPC6 channel. **(A)** Transmembrane protein TRPC6 contains six TDs, four NH_2-terminal ARDs, and a COOH-terminal TRP domain. **(B)** S1–S6 are TDs. The pore region of TRPC6, situated between the S5 and S6, allows the passage of cations. TRP: transient receptor potential; TRPC6: transient receptor potential canonical channel 6; TD: transmembrane domain; ARD: ankyrin repeat domain; S1–S6: S1–S6 are the abbreviations of the first to sixth transmembrane domains.

highly selective and specific agonists and antagonists of TRPCs are needed for future study to deeply explore their roles in the treatment of CNS diseases. Even though there is limited evidence, specific channel characters of TRPC channels make them possible to be novel targets for brain ischemia. Therefore, further research efforts are required to find the possible mechanisms underlying the roles of TRPCs in CNS diseases and particularly in ischemic stroke.

STRUCTURE AND CHARACTERISTICS OF TRPC6

The TRPC6 channel protein is composed of six TDs, intracellular NH_2-ARDs, and the COOH-terminal TRPC6 domain (**Figure 1**). TRPC6 has a molecular weight of approximately 110 kDa and consists of 930 and 931 amino acid residues in mice and humans, respectively. The intracellular cytoplasmic domain and TD are indispensable for TRPC6 assembly (Tang et al., 2018). The TRPC6 channel is permeable to several cations, including Ca^{2+}, Na^+, K^+, Cs^+, and Ba^{2+} (Hofmann et al., 1999; Estacion et al., 2006). The relative ion permeability ratio (P_{Ca}/P_{Na}) of TRPC6 is about 5 (Hofmann et al., 1999; Owsianik et al., 2006). Particularly, TRPC6 governs the function and fate of Ca^{2+} homeostasis in various cells and tissues. TRPC6 channel activation in neurons usually occurs in parallel with cytosolic entry of Ca^{2+} ions and the elevation of intracellular Ca^{2+} (Jia et al., 2007; Bouron et al., 2016). TRPC6 is widely expressed in different anatomical regions of the CNS, and is also highly distributed in placenta, lung, pancreas, adipose, heart, kidney, muscle, and other tissues (Riccio et al., 2002). TRPC6 can be activated by DAG, store-depletion, Hyperforin (*St. John's wort* extract), or H_2O_2 (Bouron et al., 2016). DAG is a second messenger that acts as a regulator of key signaling molecules, cellular membrane constituents, and fatty acid metabolism (Massart and Zierath, 2019). It is widely accepted that activation of TRPC6 channels by DAG promotes various cellular responses, although the precise underlying mechanisms remain to be elucidated. By contrast, several studies have indicated that TRPC6 channels could also be store-operated (Yu et al., 2003; El Boustany et al., 2008). Hyperforin has been shown to specifically activate TRPC6 channels, which is mainly responsible for the antidepressant effect of *St. John's wort* (Yang et al., 2018). There is also a close relation between TRPC6 and reactive oxygen species. H_2O_2 was reported to directly activate TRPC6 channels in different cell types (Bouron et al., 2016).

THE BIOLOGICAL FUNCTION OF TRPC6 IN CNS

In the postnatal rat cerebellum, TRPC6 is identified on Purkinje cell bodies, on interneurons in the molecular layer and mature granule cells in the internal granule cell layer, and is required for postnatal cerebellar neuron development (Huang et al., 2007). In cultured cerebellar granule cells, brain-derived neurotrophic factor (BDNF) induces Ca^{2+} elevation and nerve growth-cone extension through TRPC3/6 channels (Li et al., 2005). Besides, TRPC3 and TRPC6 contribute to BDNF-induced cerebellar granule neuron survival (Jia et al., 2007). siRNAs against TRPC3 and TRPC6 reduce BDNF-mediated intracellular Ca^{2+} elevation, neuroprotection, and cAMP-response element binding protein (CREB) activation in cerebellar granule neurons. By contrast, upregulation of TRPC3 or TRPC6 was shown to suppress neuronal apoptosis and promote the transcription of CREB-dependent reporter gene. Additionally, Ca^{2+} influx-dependent TRPC6 channel function is involved in hippocampal neuron dendritic growth via the Ca^{2+}/calmodulin-dependent kinase IV (CaMKIV) and CREB pathway (Tai et al., 2008). In particular, the CaMKIV-CREB pathway seems to be a vital downstream molecular mechanism of TRPC6 function in the CNS. Another study showed that TRPC6 is predominantly presented in excitatory synapses and plays important roles in promoting synapse and dendritic spine formation, spatial memory, and learning through the CaMKIV-CREB pathway (Zhou et al., 2008). As an important intracellular second messenger, Ca^{2+} contributes to neuronal development and survival. The interaction between TRPC3/6 channels and the Na^+/Ca^{2+} exchanger could regulate Ca^{2+} influx in neuronal cells, suggesting that TRPC3/6 may govern the fate of neurons by modulating Ca^{2+} influx (Louhivuori et al., 2010). TRPC6 also acts as a negative regulator that suppresses NMDA-induced Ca^{2+} currents in hippocampal neurons (Shen et al., 2013). Interestingly, NMDAR was shown to regulate transcription and degradation of TRPC6 in neurons in a bidirectional manner through NR2A or NR2B activation (Qu et al., 2017). Hyperforin, a specific agonist of TRPC6, regulates dendritic spine morphology in the hippocampus via TRPC6 activation and increasing intracellular Ca^{2+} transients (Leuner et al., 2013). However, the underlying signaling cascade has not yet been clarified. The same research team also reported the involvement of phosphatidylinositide 3-kinase (PI3K)/protein kinase B (PKB), Ras/mitogen-activated protein kinase/extracellular signal-regulated kinases (Ras/MAPK/ERK), and CaMKIV-CREB pathways (Heiser et al., 2013). Moreover, hyperforin also raises the number of excitatory synapses, dendritic spine density, and dendritic length in experimentally depressed rats by rescuing the decline of TRPC6 expression (Liu et al., 2015). High-throughput sequencing based on TRPC6 in autism spectrum disorder (ASD) patients and controls revealed the presence of more non-synonymous mutations in ASD individuals, suggesting that TRPC6 may carry out as a potential predisposing factor for ASD (Griesi-Oliveira et al., 2015). Furthermore, TRPC3 and TRPC6 could promote normal sensory mechanotransduction in touch and hearing neurons, and therefore knocking out both TRPC3 and TRPC6 resulted in deficits in sensory conduction (Quick et al., 2012). TRPC6 and TRPC7 channels also function in phototransduction in murine retinal ganglion cells (Jiang et al., 2018).

In general, TRPC6 channels are extensively expressed in the CNS and have various crucial functions. Therefore, agents targeting TRPC6 may have potential for the cure of brain disorders.

TRPC6 AND ISCHEMIC STROKE

During the process of ischemic stroke, increasing evidences support that TRPC6 seems to be a protective pathway. In comparison with TRPC1/3/4/5, TRPC6 is significantly degraded in neurons following exposure to ischemia, resulting in ischemic neuronal death. The maintenance of TRPC6 expression via CREB-dependent mechanisms has a neuroprotective effect, and has potential as a protective strategy against ischemic stroke (Du et al., 2010). In addition, TRPC6 suppresses NMDAR-induced Ca^{2+} elevation and neuronal excitotoxicity, and protects neurons from ischemic brain injury (Li et al., 2012). Resveratrol, neuroprotectin D1, and the main compound of green tea, (−)-epigallocatechin-3-gallate, inhibit calpain-mediated TRPC6 proteolysis and activate MEK/ERK or CaMKIV-dependent CREB pathways, therefore improving neurological status in experimental stroke (Lin et al., 2013a; Yao et al., 2013, 2014). Particularly, the TRPC6 activator, hyperforin, also contributes to neuroprotection after ischemic stroke by blocking TRPC6 degradation accompanied by elevation of phosphorylated CREB in CaMKIV and Ras/MEK/ERK-dependent mechanisms (Lin et al., 2013b). Furthermore, calycosin increases neuronal TRPC6 and phosphorylated CREB expression in response to brain ischemic damage (Guo et al., 2017). We believe that the TRPC6-CaMKIV-CREB pathway may be an important mechanism of ischemic stroke (**Figure 2**). There is increasing research interest in stem cell therapy for ischemic stroke. Animal researches have indicated that bone marrow-derived stromal cells (BMSCs) improve outcomes in stroke, although the regulatory mechanisms have yet to be clarified (Yang et al., 2014). Surprisingly, TRPC6 channels have been shown to participate in the neuroprotective effect of BMSCs and oxiracetam combination therapies in acute brain IR damage (Wang et al., 2019). Furthermore, overexpression of TRPC6 in BMSCs improves neuronal functions in rats after ischemic stroke, which is associated with BDNF/CREB pathway (Li W. et al., 2019). The inflammatory response plays a critical role in the pathophysiology of ischemic stroke. The proinflammatory cytokine, interleukin (IL)-17A, was shown to be linked with brain IR injury (Gelderblom et al., 2012). Another study suggested that TRPC6 may act downstream of IL-17A, and indicated that IL-17A could promote degradation of TRPC6, thus exacerbating cerebral IR injury (Zhang et al., 2014). Taken together, the evidences outlined above indicate that TRPC6 has a positive function in neuroprotection and that TRPC6 expression is reduced during ischemic stroke. However, it should be noted that TRPC6 may also have harmful effects on neurons following cerebral IR injury. In contrast to previous studies, TRPC6 expression was proved to be increased in wild-type mice neurons after ischemic stroke. Increased TRPC6 levels or overexpression of TRPC6 exacerbated IR injury-induced infarct volume, Ca^{2+} elevation, and neuronal death (Chen J. et al., 2017). Deletion of TRPC3/6/7 was shown to decrease activation of the proapoptotic factor and nuclear factor (NF)-κB, attenuate NF-κB nuclear translocation, and enhance activation of PKB, finally leading to resistance against cerebral IR injury (Chen X. et al., 2017). The causes for these discrepancies among studies remain unclear; however, they might have been due to species differences, distinct animal ischemic stroke models, dissimilar experimental environments, and researchers. Therefore, more studies are required to clarify the specific function of the TRPC6 channel in ischemic stroke.

The evidence discussed here indicates that compounds targeting TRPC6 may have clinical potential as novel agents for prevention and treatment of ischemic stroke. It should be noted that interventions for most of the experiments mentioned above are performed under intracerebroventricular injection or *in vitro* cell condition. However, taking into consideration that TRPC6 is broadly distributed in human tissues (Riccio et al., 2002), both agonists and antagonists of TRPC6 might bring some systematic adverse effects. Besides, hyperforin had been shown to induce TRPC6-dependent Na^+ currents and entry and subsequently decrease the Na^+ gradients across the membrane thus may inhibit the neuronal amine uptake (Leuner et al., 2007; Wang et al., 2020). Furthermore, hyperforin could also function as a protonophore and generate H^+ currents in a TRPC6-independent way in several cells (cortical microglial cells, chromaffin cells, lipid bilayers, and HEK-293 cells), and thereby suppress the neurotransmitter uptake through sodium-proton exchangers (Sell et al., 2014). Thus, many factors should be

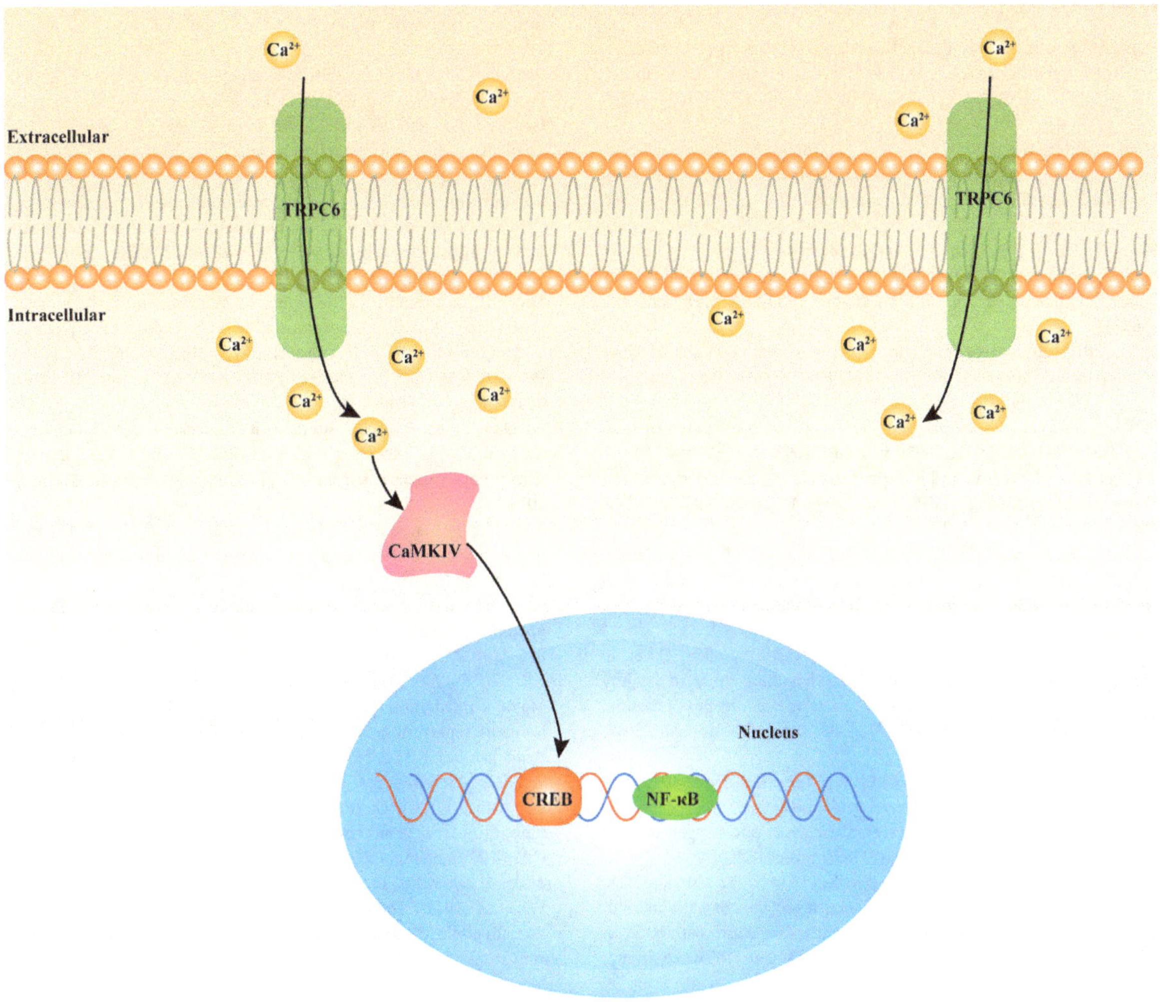

FIGURE 2 | Underlying signaling cascade of TRPC6 in ischemic stroke. TRPC6/Ca^{2+}/CAMKIV/CREB pathway is closely involved in the pathophysiological mechanism of cerebral IR injury. TRPC6: transient receptor potential canonical channel 6; Ca^{2+}: calcium; CAMKIV: Ca^{2+}/calmodulin-dependent kinase IV; CREB: cAMP-response element binding protein; NF-κB: nuclear factor (NF)-κB.

thoroughly considered before studies are conducted to explore the effect TRPC6 on ischemic stroke.

CONCLUSION AND PERSPECTIVE

Due to its high prevalence adjuvant and novel treatments for ischemic stroke are all under active investigation; e.g., digital therapeutics, microRNA-based therapeutics, cell therapy, and exosome therapy (Sun et al., 2018; Venkat et al., 2018a,b; Bayraktutan, 2019; Choi et al., 2019). Despite advances in therapy, stroke remains a major health issue. The studies discussed in this review suggest that investigation of the TRPC and TRPC6 channels may hold promise for the development of novel directions in ischemic stroke therapies. We have emphasized some important clues regarding the involved mechanisms of TRPC6 in physiology and pathophysiology of cerebral ischemia. More data and solid evidence of TRPCs and TRPC6 in stroke therapy are urgently needed to bridge the gap between current pre-clinical medical researches and clinical practice. Further studies are required to support the speculations regarding the promising therapeutic roles of TRPCs and TRPC6 in ischemic stroke, and to determine the mechanisms underlying these roles.

AUTHOR CONTRIBUTIONS

LL wrote this manuscript. SZ and XX designed the general idea. All authors edited the drafts of the manuscript.

REFERENCES

Andrews, M. D., Af Forselles, K., Beaumont, K., Galan, S. R., Glossop, P. A., Grenie, M., et al. (2015). Discovery of a selective TRPM8 antagonist with clinical efficacy in cold-related pain. *ACS Med. Chem. Lett.* 6, 419–424. doi: 10.1021/ml500479v

Arendt-Nielsen, L., Harris, S., Whiteside, G. T., Hummel, M., Knappenberger, T., O'Keefe, S., et al. (2016). A randomized, double-blind, positive-controlled, 3-way cross-over human experimental pain study of a TRPV1 antagonist (V116517) in healthy volunteers and comparison with preclinical profile. *Pain* 157, 2057–2067. doi: 10.1097/j.pain.0000000000000610

Bautista, D. M., Pellegrino, M., and Tsunozaki, M. (2013). TRPA1: a gatekeeper for inflammation. *Annu. Rev. Physiol.* 75, 181–200. doi: 10.1146/annurev-physiol-030212-183811

Bayraktutan, U. (2019). Endothelial progenitor cells: potential novel therapeutics for ischaemic stroke. *Pharmacol. Res.* 144, 181–191. doi: 10.1016/j.phrs.2019.04.017

Blair, H. A. (2018). Capsaicin 8% dermal patch: a review in peripheral neuropathic pain. *Drugs* 78, 1489–1500. doi: 10.1007/s40265-018-0982-7

Bouron, A., Chauvet, S., Dryer, S., and Rosado, J. A. (2016). Second messenger-operated calcium entry through TRPC6. *Adv. Exp. Med. Biol.* 898, 201–249. doi: 10.1007/978-3-319-26974-0_10

Broker-Lai, J., Kollewe, A., Schindeldecker, B., Pohle, J., Nguyen Chi, V., Mathar, I., et al. (2017). Heteromeric channels formed by TRPC1, TRPC4 and TRPC5 define hippocampal synaptic transmission and working memory. *EMBO J.* 36, 2770–2789. doi: 10.15252/embj.201696369

Brown, W., Leff, R. L., Griffin, A., Hossack, S., Aubray, R., Walker, P., et al. (2017). Safety, pharmacokinetics, and Pharmacodynamics study in healthy subjects of oral NEO6860, a modality selective transient receptor potential vanilloid subtype 1 antagonist. *J. Pain* 18, 726–738. doi: 10.1016/j.jpain.2017.01.009

Chen, J., Li, Z., Hatcher, J. T., Chen, Q. H., Chen, L., Wurster, R. D., et al. (2017). Deletion of TRPC6 attenuates NMDA receptor-mediated Ca^{2+} Entry and Ca^{2+}-induced neurotoxicity following cerebral ischemia and oxygen-glucose deprivation. *Front. Neurosci.* 11:138. doi: 10.3389/fnins.2017.00138

Chen, J. M., Li, Q. W., Liu, J. S., Jiang, G. X., Liu, J. R., Chen, S. D., et al. (2019). TRPC6 mRNA levels in peripheral leucocytes of patients with Alzheimer's disease and mild cognitive impairment: a case-control study. *Prog. Neuropsychopharmacol. Biol. Psychiatry* 92, 279–284. doi: 10.1016/j.pnpbp.2019.01.009

Chen, X., Lu, M., He, X., Ma, L., Birnbaumer, L., and Liao, Y. (2017). TRPC3/6/7 knockdown protects the brain from cerebral ischemia injury via astrocyte apoptosis inhibition and effects on NF-small ka. CyrillicB Translocation. *Mol. Neurobiol.* 54, 7555–7566. doi: 10.1007/s12035-016-0227-2

Choi, D. W. (1995). Calcium: still center-stage in hypoxic-ischemic neuronal death. *Trends Neurosci.* 18, 58–60. doi: 10.1016/0166-2236(95)80018-w

Choi, M. J., Kim, H., Nah, H. W., and Kang, D. W. (2019). Digital therapeutics: emerging new therapy for neurologic deficits after stroke. *J. Stroke* 21, 242–258. doi: 10.5853/jos.2019.01963

Clapham, D. E. (2003). TRP channels as cellular sensors. *Nature* 426, 517–524. doi: 10.1038/nature02196

Clapham, D. E., Runnels, L. W., and Strubing, C. (2001). The TRP ion channel family. *Nat. Rev. Neurosci.* 2, 387–396. doi: 10.1038/35077544

Du, W., Huang, J., Yao, H., Zhou, K., Duan, B., and Wang, Y. (2010). Inhibition of TRPC6 degradation suppresses ischemic brain damage in rats. *J. Clin. Investig.* 120, 3480–3492. doi: 10.1172/jci43165

El Boustany, C., Bidaux, G., Enfissi, A., Delcourt, P., Prevarskaya, N., and Capiod, T. (2008). Capacitative calcium entry and transient receptor potential canonical 6 expression control human hepatoma cell proliferation. *Hepatology* 47, 2068–2077. doi: 10.1002/hep.22263

Estacion, M., Sinkins, W. G., Jones, S. W., Applegate, M. A., and Schilling, W. P. (2006). Human TRPC6 expressed in HEK 293 cells forms non-selective cation channels with limited Ca^{2+} permeability. *J. Physiol.* 572, 359–377. doi: 10.1113/jphysiol.2005.103143

Gelderblom, M., Weymar, A., Bernreuther, C., Velden, J., Arunachalam, P., Steinbach, K., et al. (2012). Neutralization of the IL-17 axis diminishes neutrophil invasion and protects from ischemic stroke. *Blood* 120, 3793–3802. doi: 10.1182/blood-2012-02-412726

Ginsberg, M. D. (2008). Neuroprotection for ischemic stroke: past, present and future. *Neuropharmacology* 55, 363–389. doi: 10.1016/j.neuropharm.2007.12.007

GlaxoSmithKline (2018). A Study to Evaluate the Effect of the Transient Receptor Potential Vanilloid 4 (TRPV4) Channel Blocker, GSK2798745, on Pulmonary Gas Transfer and Respiration in Patients With Congestive Heart Failure. Available online at: https://clinicaltrials.gov/ct2/show/NCT02497937 (accessed October 25, 2019).

GlaxoSmithKline (2019). *A Method Validation Study for Evaluation of Novel Treatments Limiting Pulmonary Oedema in Cardiac Failure.* Available online at: https://clinicaltrials.gov/ct2/show/NCT02135861?term=trpv4&rank=2 (accessed October 25, 2019).

Gosset, J. R., Beaumont, K., Matsuura, T., Winchester, W., Attkins, N., Glatt, S., et al. (2017). A cross-species translational pharmacokinetic-pharmacodynamic evaluation of core body temperature reduction by the TRPM8 blocker PF-05105679. *Eur. J. Pharm.* 109S, S161–S167. doi: 10.1016/j.ejps.2017.06.009

Griesi-Oliveira, K., Acab, A., Gupta, A. R., Sunaga, D. Y., Chailangkarn, T., Nicol, X., et al. (2015). Modeling non-syndromic autism and the impact of TRPC6 disruption in human neurons. *Mol. Psychiatry* 20, 1350–1365. doi: 10.1038/mp.2014.141

Guo, C., Ma, Y., Ma, S., Mu, F., Deng, J., Duan, J., et al. (2017). The role of TRPC6 in the neuroprotection of calycosin against cerebral ischemic injury. *Sci. Rep.* 7:3039. doi: 10.1038/s41598-017-03404-6

Hartmann, J., and Konnerth, A. (2015). TRPC3-dependent synaptic transmission in central mammalian neurons. *J. Mol. Med.* 93, 983–989. doi: 10.1007/s00109-015-1298-7

He, X., Li, S., Liu, B., Susperreguy, S., Formoso, K., Yao, J., et al. (2017). Major contribution of the 3/6/7 class of TRPC channels to myocardial ischemia/reperfusion and cellular hypoxia/reoxygenation injuries. *Proc. Natl, Acad. Sci. U.S.A.* 114, E4582–E4591. doi: 10.1073/pnas.1621384114

Heiser, J. H., Schuwald, A. M., Sillani, G., Ye, L., Muller, W. E., and Leuner, K. (2013). TRPC6 channel-mediated neurite outgrowth in PC12 cells and hippocampal neurons involves activation of RAS/MEK/ERK, PI3K, and CAMKIV signaling. *J. Neurochem.* 127, 303–313. doi: 10.1111/jnc.12376

Hirschler-Laszkiewicz, I., Tong, Q., Waybill, K., Conrad, K., Keefer, K., Zhang, W., et al. (2011). The transient receptor potential (TRP) channel TRPC3 TRP domain and AMP-activated protein kinase binding site are required for TRPC3 activation by erythropoietin. *J. Biol. Chem.* 286, 30636–30646. doi: 10.1074/jbc.M111.238360

Hofmann, T., Obukhov, A. G., Schaefer, M., Harteneck, C., Gudermann, T., and Schultz, G. (1999). Direct activation of human TRPC6 and TRPC3 channels by diacylglycerol. *Nature* 397, 259–263. doi: 10.1038/16711

Hong, C., Seo, H., Kwak, M., Jeon, J., Jang, J., Jeong, E. M., et al. (2015). Increased TRPC5 glutathionylation contributes to striatal neuron loss in Huntington's disease. *Brain* 138, 3030–3047. doi: 10.1093/brain/awv188

Huang, W. C., Young, J. S., and Glitsch, M. D. (2007). Changes in TRPC channel expression during postnatal development of cerebellar neurons. *Cell Calcium* 42, 1–10. doi: 10.1016/j.ceca.2006.11.002

Islam, Z., Nagampalli, R. S. K., Fatima, M. T., and Ashraf, G. M. (2018). New paradigm in ankyrin repeats: beyond protein-protein interaction module. *Int. J. Biol. Macromol.* 109, 1164–1173. doi: 10.1016/j.ijbiomac.2017.11.101

Jia, Y., Zhou, J., Tai, Y., and Wang, Y. (2007). TRPC channels promote cerebellar granule neuron survival. *Nat. Neurosci.* 10, 559–567. doi: 10.1038/nn1870

Jiang, Z., Yue, W. W. S., Chen, L., Sheng, Y., and Yau, K. W. (2018). Cyclic-nucleotide- and HCN-channel-mediated phototransduction in intrinsically photosensitive retinal ganglion cells. *Cell* 175, 652–664.e12. doi: 10.1016/j.cell.2018.08.055

Kaneko, Y., and Szallasi, A. (2014). Transient receptor potential (TRP) channels: a clinical perspective. *Br. J. Pharmacol.* 171, 2474–2507. doi: 10.1111/bph.12414

Khoshnam, S. E., Winlow, W., Farzaneh, M., Farbood, Y., and Moghaddam, H. F. (2017). Pathogenic mechanisms following ischemic stroke. *Neurol. Sci.* 38, 1167–1186. doi: 10.1007/s10072-017-2938-1

Lai, T. W., Shyu, W. C., and Wang, Y. T. (2011). Stroke intervention pathways: NMDA receptors and beyond. *Trends Mol. Med.* 17, 266–275. doi: 10.1016/j.molmed.2010.12.008

Lee, J., Kim, B. H., Yu, K. S., Kim, H. S., Kim, J. D., Cho, J. Y., et al. (2017). A first-in-human, double-blind, placebo-controlled, randomized, dose escalation study of

DWP05195, a novel TRPV1 antagonist, in healthy volunteers. *Drug Des. Dev. Ther.* 11, 1301–1313. doi: 10.2147/dddt.S128727

Lepage, P. K., Lussier, M. P., McDuff, F. O., Lavigne, P., and Boulay, G. (2009). The self-association of two N-terminal interaction domains plays an important role in the tetramerization of TRPC4. *Cell Calcium* 45, 251–259. doi: 10.1016/j.ceca.2008.11.002

Leuner, K., Kazanski, V., Muller, M., Essin, K., Henke, B., Gollasch, M., et al. (2007). Hyperforin–a key constituent of St. John's wort specifically activates TRPC6 channels. *FASEB J.* 21, 4101–4111. doi: 10.1096/fj.07-8110com

Leuner, K., Li, W., Amaral, M. D., Rudolph, S., Calfa, G., Schuwald, A. M., et al. (2013). Hyperforin modulates dendritic spine morphology in hippocampal pyramidal neurons by activating Ca^{2+} -permeable TRPC6 channels. *Hippocampus* 23, 40–52. doi: 10.1002/hipo.22052

Li, H., Huang, J., Du, W., Jia, C., Yao, H., and Wang, Y. (2012). TRPC6 inhibited NMDA receptor activities and protected neurons from ischemic excitotoxicity. *J. Neurochem.* 123, 1010–1018. doi: 10.1111/jnc.12045

Li, J., Zhang, X., Song, X., Liu, R., Zhang, J., and Li, Z. (2019). The structure of TRPC ion channels. *Cell Calcium* 80, 25–28. doi: 10.1016/j.ceca.2019.03.005

Li, M., Liu, E., Zhou, Q., Li, S., Wang, X., Liu, Y., et al. (2018). TRPC1 null exacerbates memory deficit and apoptosis induced by amyloid-beta. *J. Alzheimers Dis.* 63, 761–772. doi: 10.3233/jad-180077

Li, W., Yang, F., Gao, J., Tang, Y., Wang, J., and Pan, Y. (2019). Over-expression of TRPC6 via CRISPR based synergistic activation mediator in BMSCs ameliorates brain injury in a rat model of cerebral ischemia/reperfusion. *Neuroscience* 415, 147–160. doi: 10.1016/j.neuroscience.2019.06.041

Li, Y., Jia, Y. C., Cui, K., Li, N., Zheng, Z. Y., Wang, Y. Z., et al. (2005). Essential role of TRPC channels in the guidance of nerve growth cones by brain-derived neurotrophic factor. *Nature* 434, 894–898. doi: 10.1038/nature03477

Liedtke, W., Choe, Y., Marti-Renom, M. A., Bell, A. M., Denis, C. S., Sali, A., et al. (2000). Vanilloid receptor-related osmotically activated channel (VR-OAC), a candidate vertebrate osmoreceptor. *Cell* 103, 525–535. doi: 10.1016/s0092-8674(00)00143-4

Lin, Y., Chen, F., Zhang, J., Wang, T., Wei, X., Wu, J., et al. (2013a). Neuroprotective effect of resveratrol on ischemia/reperfusion injury in rats through TRPC6/CREB pathways. *J. Mol. Neurosci.* 50, 504–513. doi: 10.1007/s12031-013-9977-8

Liu, Y., Liu, C., Qin, X., Zhu, M., and Yang, Z. (2015). The change of spatial cognition ability in depression rat model and the possible association with down-regulated protein expression of TRPC6. *Behav. Brain Res.* 294, 186–193. doi: 10.1016/j.bbr.2015.07.062

Lin, Y., Zhang, J. C., Fu, J., Chen, F., Wang, J., Wu, Z. L., et al. (2013b). Hyperforin attenuates brain damage induced by transient middle cerebral artery occlusion (MCAO) in rats via inhibition of TRPC6 channels degradation. *J. Cereb. Blood Flow Metab.* 33, 253–262. doi: 10.1038/jcbfm.2012.164

Louhivuori, L. M., Jansson, L., Nordstrom, T., Bart, G., Nasman, J., and Akerman, K. E. (2010). Selective interference with TRPC3/6 channels disrupts OX1 receptor signalling via NCX and reveals a distinct calcium influx pathway. *Cell Calcium* 48, 114–123. doi: 10.1016/j.ceca.2010.07.005

Lussier, M. P., Lepage, P. K., Bousquet, S. M., and Boulay, G. (2008). RNF24, a new TRPC interacting protein, causes the intracellular retention of TRPC. *Cell Calcium* 43, 432–443. doi: 10.1016/j.ceca.2007.07.009

Manitpisitkul, P., Shalayda, K., Russell, L., Sanga, P., Solanki, B., Caruso, J., et al. (2018). Pharmacokinetics and Safety of Mavatrep (JNJ-39439335), a TRPV1 antagonist in healthy japanese and caucasian men: a double-blind, randomized, placebo-controlled, sequential-group phase 1 study. *Clin. Pharmacol. Drug Dev.* 7, 712–726. doi: 10.1002/cpdd.413

Massart, J., and Zierath, J. R. (2019). Role of diacylglycerol kinases in glucose and energy homeostasis. *Trends Endocrinol. Metab.* 30, 603–617. doi: 10.1016/j.tem.2019.06.003

Minke, B. (1977). Drosophila mutant with a transducer defect. *Biophys. Struct. Mech.* 3, 59–64. doi: 10.1007/bf00536455

Montell, C. (2001). Physiology, phylogeny, and functions of the TRP superfamily of cation channels. *Sciences STKE* 2001:re1. doi: 10.1126/stke.2001.90.re1

Montell, C., Jones, K., Hafen, E., and Rubin, G. (1985). Rescue of the Drosophila phototransduction mutation trp by germline transformation. *Science* 230, 1040–1043. doi: 10.1126/science.3933112

Moqrich, A., Hwang, S. W., Earley, T. J., Petrus, M. J., Murray, A. N., Spencer, K. S., et al. (2005). Impaired thermosensation in mice lacking TRPV3, a heat and camphor sensor in the skin. *Science* 307, 1468–1472. doi: 10.1126/science.1108609

Moran, M. M. (2018). TRP channels as potential drug targets. *Annu. Rev. Pharmacol. Toxicol.* 58, 309–330. doi: 10.1146/annurev-pharmtox-010617-052832

Narayanan, K. L., Irmady, K., Subramaniam, S., Unsicker, K., and von Bohlen und Halbach, O. (2008). Evidence that TRPC1 is involved in hippocampal glutamate-induced cell death. *Neurosci. Lett.* 446, 117–122. doi: 10.1016/j.neulet.2008.09.034

Nilius, B., Owsianik, G., Voets, T., and Peters, J. A. (2007). Transient receptor potential cation channels in disease. *Physiol. Rev.* 87, 165–217. doi: 10.1152/physrev.00021.2006

Owsianik, G., Talavera, K., Voets, T., and Nilius, B. (2006). Permeation and selectivity of TRP channels. *Annu. Rev. Physiol.* 68, 685–717. doi: 10.1146/annurev.physiol.68.040204.101406

Pharmaceuticals, G. (2014). *Glenmark's TRPA1 Antagonist 'GRC 17536' Shows Positive Data in a Proof of Concept Study.* Available online at: https://www.prnewswire.com/news-releases/glenmarks-trpa1-antagonist-grc-17536-shows-positive-data-in-a-proof-of-concept-study-275445961.html (accessed October 25, 2019).

Pharmaceuticals, G. (2018). *Glenmark Pharma Completes 'GRC 15300' Phase-I Clinical Trials.* Available online at: http://www.thehindubusinessline.com/companies/glenmark-pharma-completes-grc15300-phasei-clinical-trials/article2292593.ece (accessed October 25, 2019).

Popugaeva, E., Chernyuk, D., Zhang, H., Postnikova, T. Y., Pats, K., Fedorova, E., et al. (2019). Derivatives of Piperazines as potential therapeutic agents for Alzheimer's disease. *Mol. Pharmacol.* 95, 337–348. doi: 10.1124/mol.118.114348

Qu, Z., Wang, Y., Li, X., Wu, L., and Wang, Y. (2017). TRPC6 expression in neurons is differentially regulated by NR2A- and NR2B-containing NMDA receptors. *J. Neurochem.* 143, 282–293. doi: 10.1111/jnc.14215

Quick, K., Zhao, J., Eijkelkamp, N., Linley, J. E., Rugiero, F., Cox, J. J., et al. (2012). TRPC3 and TRPC6 are essential for normal mechanotransduction in subsets of sensory neurons and cochlear hair cells. *Open Biol.* 2:120068. doi: 10.1098/rsob.120068

Ramirez, G. A., Coletto, L. A., Sciorati, C., Bozzolo, E. P., Manunta, P., Rovere-Querini, P., et al. (2018). Ion channels and transporters in inflammation: special focus on TRP channels and TRPC6. *Cells* 7:E70. doi: 10.3390/cells7070070

Riccio, A., Li, Y., Moon, J., Kim, K. S., Smith, K. S., Rudolph, U., et al. (2009). Essential role for TRPC5 in amygdala function and fear-related behavior. *Cell* 137, 761–772. doi: 10.1016/j.cell.2009.03.039

Riccio, A., Medhurst, A. D., Mattei, C., Kelsell, R. E., Calver, A. R., Randall, A. D., et al. (2002). mRNA distribution analysis of human TRPC family in CNS and peripheral tissues. *Brain Res.* 109, 95–104. doi: 10.1016/s0169-328x(02)00527-2

Schindl, R., Frischauf, I., Kahr, H., Fritsch, R., Krenn, M., Derndl, A., et al. (2008). The first ankyrin-like repeat is the minimum indispensable key structure for functional assembly of homo- and heteromeric TRPC4/TRPC5 channels. *Cell Calcium* 43, 260–269. doi: 10.1016/j.ceca.2007.05.015

Sell, T. S., Belkacemi, T., Flockerzi, V., and Beck, A. (2014). Protonophore properties of hyperforin are essential for its pharmacological activity. *Sci. Rep.* 4:7500. doi: 10.1038/srep07500

Shen, H., Pan, J., Pan, L., and Zhang, N. (2013). TRPC6 inhibited NMDA current in cultured hippocampal neurons. *Neuromol. Med.* 15, 389–395. doi: 10.1007/s12017-013-8226-1

Strotmann, R., Harteneck, C., Nunnenmacher, K., Schultz, G., and Plant, T. D. (2000). OTRPC4, a nonselective cation channel that confers sensitivity to extracellular osmolarity. *Nat. Cell Biol.* 2, 695–702. doi: 10.1038/35036318

Sun, P., Liu, D. Z., Jickling, G. C., Sharp, F. R., and Yin, K. J. (2018). MicroRNA-based therapeutics in central nervous system injuries. *J. Cereb. Blood Flow Metab.* 38, 1125–1148. doi: 10.1177/0271678x18773871

Szallasi, A., Cruz, F., and Geppetti, P. (2006). TRPV1: a therapeutic target for novel analgesic drugs? *Trends Mol. Med.* 12, 545–554. doi: 10.1016/j.molmed.2006.09.001

Szydlowska, K., and Tymianski, M. (2010). Calcium, ischemia and excitotoxicity. *Cell Calcium* 47, 122–129. doi: 10.1016/j.ceca.2010.01.003

Tai, Y., Feng, S., Du, W., and Wang, Y. (2009). Functional roles of TRPC channels in the developing brain. *Pflugers Arch.* 458, 283–289. doi: 10.1007/s00424-008-0618-y

Tai, Y., Feng, S., Ge, R., Du, W., Zhang, X., He, Z., et al. (2008). TRPC6 channels promote dendritic growth via the CaMKIV-CREB pathway. *J. Cell Sci.* 121, 2301–2307. doi: 10.1242/jcs.026906

Tang, Q., Guo, W., Zheng, L., Wu, J. X., Liu, M., Zhou, X., et al. (2018). Structure of the receptor-activated human TRPC6 and TRPC3 ion channels. *Cell Res.* 28, 746–755. doi: 10.1038/s41422-018-0038-2

Van Gerven, L., Alpizar, Y. A., Steelant, B., Callebaut, I., Kortekaas Krohn, I., Wouters, M., et al. (2017). Enhanced chemosensory sensitivity in patients with idiopathic rhinitis and its reversal by nasal capsaicin treatment. *J. Allergy Clin. Immunol.* 140, 437–446.e2. doi: 10.1016/j.jaci.2017.03.014

Venkat, P., Chen, J., and Chopp, M. (2018a). Exosome-mediated amplification of endogenous brain repair mechanisms and brain and systemic organ interaction in modulating neurological outcome after stroke. *J. Cereb. Blood Flow Metab.* 38, 2165–2178. doi: 10.1177/0271678x18782789

Venkat, P., Shen, Y., Chopp, M., and Chen, J. (2018b). Cell-based and pharmacological neurorestorative therapies for ischemic stroke. *Neuropharmacology* 134, 310–322. doi: 10.1016/j.neuropharm.2017.08.036

Venkatachalam, K., and Montell, C. (2007). TRP channels. *Annu. Rev. Biochem.* 76, 387–417. doi: 10.1146/annurev.biochem.75.103004.142819

Voets, T., Vriens, J., and Vennekens, R. (2019). Targeting TRP channels - valuable alternatives to combat pain, lower urinary tract disorders, and type 2 diabetes? *Trends Pharmacol. Sci.* 40, 669–683. doi: 10.1016/j.tips.2019.07.004

Wang, H., Cheng, X., Tian, J., Xiao, Y., Tian, T., Xu, F., et al. (2020). TRPC channels: structure, function, regulation and recent advances in small molecular probes. *Pharmacol. Ther.* doi: 10.1016/j.pharmthera.2020.107497 [Epub ahead of print].

Wang, J., Lu, R., Yang, J., Li, H., He, Z., Jing, N., et al. (2015). TRPC6 specifically interacts with APP to inhibit its cleavage by gamma-secretase and reduce Abeta production. *Nat. Commun.* 6:8876. doi: 10.1038/ncomms 9876

Wang, J., Sun, R., Li, Z., and Pan, Y. (2019). Combined bone marrow stromal cells and oxiracetam treatments ameliorates acute cerebral ischemia/reperfusion injury through TRPC6. *Acta Biochim. Biophys. Sin.* 51, 767–777. doi: 10.1093/abbs/gmz059

Weissmann, N., Sydykov, A., Kalwa, H., Storch, U., Fuchs, B., Mederos y Schnitzler, M., et al. (2012). Activation of TRPC6 channels is essential for lung ischaemia-reperfusion induced oedema in mice. *Nat. Commun.* 3:649. doi: 10.1038/ncomms1660

Winn, M. P., Conlon, P. J., Lynn, K. L., Farrington, M. K., Creazzo, T., Hawkins, A. F., et al. (2005). A mutation in the TRPC6 cation channel causes familial focal segmental glomerulosclerosis. *Science* 308, 1801–1804. doi: 10.1126/science.1106215

Woo, J. S., Lee, K. J., Huang, M., Cho, C. H., and Lee, E. H. (2014). Heteromeric TRPC3 with TRPC1 formed via its ankyrin repeats regulates the resting cytosolic Ca^{2+} levels in skeletal muscle. *Biochem. Biophys. Res. Commun.* 446, 454–459. doi: 10.1016/j.bbrc.2014.02.127

Wouters, M. M., Balemans, D., Van Wanrooy, S., Dooley, J., Cibert-Goton, V., Alpizar, Y. A., et al. (2016). Histamine receptor H1-mediated sensitization of TRPV1 mediates visceral hypersensitivity and symptoms in patients with irritable bowel syndrome. *Gastroenterology* 150, 875–887.e9. doi: 10.1053/j.gastro.2015.12.034

Wu, J., Ryskamp, D., Birnbaumer, L., and Bezprozvanny, I. (2018). Inhibition of TRPC1-dependent store-operated calcium entry improves synaptic stability and motor performance in a mouse model of Huntington's disease. *J. Huntingtons Dis.* 7, 35–50. doi: 10.3233/jhd-170266

Wu, J., Shih, H. P., Vigont, V., Hrdlicka, L., Diggins, L., Singh, C., et al. (2011). Neuronal store-operated calcium entry pathway as a novel therapeutic target for Huntington's disease treatment. *Chem. Biol.* 18, 777–793. doi: 10.1016/j.chembiol.2011.04.012

Wu, Q. J., and Tymianski, M. (2018). Targeting NMDA receptors in stroke: new hope in neuroprotection. *Mol. Brain* 11:15. doi: 10.1186/s13041-018-0357-8

Wu, Q. Y., Sun, M. R., Wu, C. L., Li, Y., Du, J. J., Zeng, J. Y., et al. (2015). Activation of calcium-sensing receptor increases TRPC3/6 expression in T lymphocyte in sepsis. *Mol. Immunol.* 64, 18–25. doi: 10.1016/j.molimm.2014.10.018

Xu, H., Ramsey, I. S., Kotecha, S. A., Moran, M. M., Chong, J. A., Lawson, D., et al. (2002). TRPV3 is a calcium-permeable temperature-sensitive cation channel. *Nature* 418, 181–186. doi: 10.1038/nature00882

Xu, N., Meng, H., Liu, T., Feng, Y., Qi, Y., and Wang, H. (2018). TRPC1 deficiency exacerbates cerebral ischemia/reperfusion-induced neurological injury by potentiating Nox4-derived reactive oxygen species generation. *Cell. Physiol. Biochem.* 51, 1723–1738. doi: 10.1159/000495676

Yang, L. P., Jiang, F. J., Wu, G. S., Deng, K., Wen, M., Zhou, X., et al. (2015). Acute treatment with a novel TRPC4/C5 channel inhibitor produces antidepressant and anxiolytic-like effects in mice. *PLoS One* 10:e0136255. doi: 10.1371/journal.pone.0136255

Yang, X. W., Grossman, R. B., and Xu, G. (2018). Research progress of polycyclic polyprenylated acylphloroglucinols. *Chem. Rev.* 118, 3508–3558. doi: 10.1021/acs.chemrev.7b00551

Yang, Z., Zhu, L., Li, F., Wang, J., Wan, H., and Pan, Y. (2014). Bone marrow stromal cells as a therapeutic treatment for ischemic stroke. *Neurosci. Bull.* 30, 524–534. doi: 10.1007/s12264-013-1431-y

Yao, C., Zhang, J., Chen, F., and Lin, Y. (2013). Neuroprotectin D1 attenuates brain damage induced by transient middle cerebral artery occlusion in rats through TRPC6/CREB pathways. *Mol. Med. Rep.* 8, 543–550. doi: 10.3892/mmr.2013.1543

Yao, C., Zhang, J., Liu, G., Chen, F., and Lin, Y. (2014). Neuroprotection by (-)-epigallocatechin-3-gallate in a rat model of stroke is mediated through inhibition of endoplasmic reticulum stress. *Mol. Med. Rep.* 9, 69–76. doi: 10.3892/mmr.2013.1778

Yu, Y., Sweeney, M., Zhang, S., Platoshyn, O., Landsberg, J., Rothman, A., et al. (2003). PDGF stimulates pulmonary vascular smooth muscle cell proliferation by upregulating TRPC6 expression. *Am. J. Physiol. Cell Physiol.* 284, C316–C330. doi: 10.1152/ajpcell.00125.2002

Zhang, J., Mao, X., Zhou, T., Cheng, X., and Lin, Y. (2014). IL-17A contributes to brain ischemia reperfusion injury through calpain-TRPC6 pathway in mice. *Neuroscience* 274, 419–428. doi: 10.1016/j.neuroscience.2014.06.001

Zhou, J., Du, W., Zhou, K., Tai, Y., Yao, H., Jia, Y., et al. (2008). Critical role of TRPC6 channels in the formation of excitatory synapses. *Nat. Neurosci.* 11, 741–743. doi: 10.1038/nn.2127

Zhou, Y., Castonguay, P., Sidhom, E. H., Clark, A. R., Dvela-Levitt, M., Kim, S., et al. (2017). A small-molecule inhibitor of TRPC5 ion channels suppresses progressive kidney disease in animal models. *Science* 358, 1332–1336. doi: 10.1126/science.aal4178

16

TRP Channels Role in Pain Associated with Neurodegenerative Diseases

Milena Duitama†, Viviana Vargas-López†, Zulma Casas, Sonia L. Albarracin, Jhon-Jairo Sutachan and Yolima P. Torres‡*

Departamento de Nutrición y Bioquímica, Pontificia Universidad Javeriana, Bogotá, Colombia

***Correspondence:**
Yolima P. Torres
yolima.torres@javeriana.edu.co*

† These authors have contributed equally to this work

Transient receptor potential (TRP) are cation channels expressed in both non-excitable and excitable cells from diverse tissues, including heart, lung, and brain. The TRP channel family includes 28 isoforms activated by physical and chemical stimuli, such as temperature, pH, osmotic pressure, and noxious stimuli. Recently, it has been shown that TRP channels are also directly or indirectly activated by reactive oxygen species. Oxidative stress plays an essential role in neurodegenerative disorders, such as Alzheimer's and Parkinson's diseases, and TRP channels are involved in the progression of those diseases by mechanisms involving changes in the crosstalk between Ca^{2+} regulation, oxidative stress, and production of inflammatory mediators. TRP channels involved in nociception include members of the TRPV, TRPM, TRPA, and TRPC subfamilies that transduce physical and chemical noxious stimuli. It has also been reported that pain is a complex issue in patients with Alzheimer's and Parkinson's diseases, and adequate management of pain in those conditions is still in discussion. TRPV1 has a role in neuroinflammation, a critical mechanism involved in neurodegeneration. Therefore, some studies have considered TRPV1 as a target for both pain treatment and neurodegenerative disorders. Thus, this review aimed to describe the TRP-dependent mechanism that can mediate pain sensation in neurodegenerative diseases and the therapeutic approach available to palliate pain and neurodegenerative symptoms throughout the regulation of these channels.

Keywords: pain, Alzheimer's disease, Parkinson's disease, TRP channels, neurodegeneration

Transient receptor potential (TRP) proteins constitute a group of non-selective cation channels (Gees et al., 2010) found in most cell membranes, except in the nuclear and mitochondrial membranes. TRPs are expressed in plasma membrane and help to modulate the driving force for the influx of Na^{+}, K^{+}, Ca^{2+}, and Mg^{2+} ions, and trace metal ions (Nilius and Owsianik, 2011), while in specific organelles, such as the cilium and lysosomes, they regulate organelle and cellular activity (Moran, 2018). Numerous excitable and non-excitable tissues express TRPs, where they are involved in sensory signal transduction (nociception, taste, pressure, temperature, vision, and pheromone signaling), as well as homeostatic regulation (muscle contraction, vessel relaxation, and cell proliferation) (Gees et al., 2010). In the central nervous system (CNS), several TRP channels are expressed in both neurons and glia, fulfilling critical roles in neurogenesis, structural/functional plasticity, and cell homeostasis (Nilius, 2012; Vennekens et al., 2012; Katz et al., 2017).

It has been described that diverse ion channels expressed in the brain's cells, including TRPs, are involved in the progression of neurodegenerative diseases such as Parkinson's and Alzheimer's. Also, several members of TRPs subfamilies are highly expressed in neurons and microglia mediating neuropathic pain (Haraguchi et al., 2012). TRP channels are part of cellular pathways related to the synthesis of many inflammatory mediators associated with neuroprotection/neurotoxicity, where they contribute to intracellular calcium regulation and signaling and painful stimuli transduction (Ji and Suter, 2007; Miyake et al., 2014; Lee and Kim, 2017). Therefore, TRP channels became of interest as promising targets for the treatment of both neurodegenerative diseases and pain.

In this review, we summarize the evidence of the role of TRP channels in the progression of neurodegenerative diseases such as Alzheimer's and Parkinson's diseases. Also, we discussed the possible involvement of TRP channels in pain associated with these neurodegenerative diseases and the use of TRP channels as possible pharmacological targets for pain treatment in patients with neurodegenerative diseases. A better understanding of the molecular mechanisms involved in neurodegeneration and pain is necessary to prevent and treat neurodegeneration and chronic pain.

TRPs STRUCTURE AND EXPRESSION

TRP multigene superfamily is formed by 28 members that encode integral membrane proteins that function as cation channels (Vennekens et al., 2012). TRP channels have some structural similarity, sharing as common a three-dimensional structure with six transmembrane segments (S1 through S6), two variable cytoplasmic domains (N- and C terminal), and small loop forming the channel pore between S5 and S6 segments (Catterall and Swanson, 2015). The distinguishing features between TRP channel subfamilies have been reported in the N- and C-terminal cytosolic domains, which contain residues and regulatory motifs unique for each family (Gaudet, 2008).

Unlike other cation-selective channel families, TRPs are classified by primary amino acid sequence rather than selectivity, ligand function, mechanisms of regulation, or sequence homology (Moran et al., 2004; Wu et al., 2010). TRP channels are divided into seven subfamilies: TRPC (Canonical), TRPV (Vanilloid), TRPA (Ankyrin), and TRPM (Melastatin), TRPP (Polycystic), and TRPML (Mucolipin). The seventh family, the no mechanoreceptor potential C channels (NOMPC or TRPN), is not found in mammals (Skryma et al., 2011). Alternatively, based on their sequence and topological features, TRP genes superfamilies are divided into Group 1 (TRPC, TRPV, TRPM, TRPA, and TRPN), and Group 2 (TRPP and TRPML). TRP subunits, in the same or different subfamilies, form functional homomeric or heteromeric ion channels with distinct biophysical and regulatory properties (Hellwig et al., 2005; Cheng, 2018). Heteromultimerization among mammalian TRP subunits have been observed for the TRPC, TRPV, TRPM, and TRPP families, displaying distinctive features (Hellwig et al., 2005; Cheng, 2018). For instance, formation of heteromeric complexes TRPC1/3, TRPC1/4, TRPC1/5, TRPC3/4, TRPC4/5 showed novel non-selective cationic channels with a voltage dependence or dynamic gating (Cheng et al., 2010; Kim et al., 2014; Woo et al., 2014). Also, TRPV1/3, TRPV5/6, TRPM6/TRPM7 or TRPML1/2 channels form heteromeric channels with intermediate conductance levels and gating kinetic properties (Cheng et al., 2007; Ma et al., 2011; Zhang et al., 2014; Goldenberg et al., 2015; Kim et al., 2016). Heteromerization within the mammalian TRP channel superfamily has also been observed. For instance, heteromeric TRPP2/TRPC1 and TRPP2/TRPV4 channels exhibit new receptor-operated property implicated in mechanosensation or thermosensitive roles (Du et al., 2014), and TRPC1/TRPC6/TRPV4 may mediate mechanical hyperalgesia and primary afferent nociceptor sensitization (Cheng, 2018).

The first TRP subfamily characterized was the canonical TRPC. The seven members of this subfamily are divided into four groups according to their sequence homology into Group I (TRPC1), group II (TRPC2), group III (TRPC3, TRPC6, TRPC7), and group IV (TRPC4 and TRPC5) (Nilius and Flockerzi, 2014). TRPC channels at the N-terminal domain show ankyrin repeats (3–4), a coiled-coil region, and a caveolin binding region. Meanwhile, the cytoplasmic C-terminal domain contains the TRP motif EWKFAR, a highly conserved proline-rich motif, and a region to interact with the IP_3 receptor as well with calmodulin (calmodulin/IP_3 receptor-binding region) (Putney et al., 2004). All TRPC are non-selective cation channels permeable to Ca^{2+} (Bon and Beech, 2013) linked to cellular processes such as cell division, differentiation, apoptosis, transduction of external stimuli, and refill of intracellular Ca^{2+} stores. In addition, they act amplifying receptor-activated Ca^{2+} signaling *via* interaction with second messengers (Numaga-Tomita et al., 2019). TRPC channels are widely distributed in cells of different tissues, including brain, heart, smooth muscle, liver, testis, ovaries, salivary glands (Beech et al., 2003), endothelium, kidneys (Freichel et al., 2005), and adrenal glands (Philipp et al., 2000). For instance, TRPC4/5 mRNA has been found in cortico-limbic brain regions, like the hippocampus and prefrontal cortex of adult rats (Fowler et al., 2007). TRPC channels are involved in diverse neuronal functions *via* receptor-mediated regulation by neurotrophic factors or neuropeptides, and cation influx through TRPCs control cellular functions and neuronal activity by regulating the membrane potential (Katz et al., 2017).

The TRPV subfamily is made up of six members, which are classified into four groups according to their homology: TRPV1/TRPV2, TRPV3, TRPV4, and TRPV5/TRPV6 (Smith et al., 2002; Xu et al., 2002; Nilius and Owsianik, 2011). TRPV channels were named after the discovery that its founding member (TRPV1) was activated by the vanilloid capsaicin, the compound responsible for a hot spicy taste (Szallasi and Blumberg, 1999). TRPV channels form homo- or hetero-tetramers, highly calcium selective, and mostly located on the plasma membrane. Each monomeric subunit typically contains three to five N-terminal ankyrin repeats and a TRP box at their C terminal. To this date, the most studied member of the

TRP family is the TRPV1 receptor. TRPV1, TRPV2, TRPV3, and TRPV4 are moderately Ca^{2+} permeable, while TRPV5 and TRPV6 are highly selective Ca^{2+} channels and strictly regulated by $[Ca^{2+}]i$ (Gees et al., 2010). It is known that TRPV members have different gating properties, as studies using wild type and knockout mice models revealed that although TRPV2–6 channels share high sequence similarities with TRPV1, and they do not respond to temperature stimuli (Samanta et al., 2018). Furthermore, TRPV2 and TRPV4, unlike to other members of the family, are not sensitive to capsaicin (Caterina et al., 1999). TRPV1 channel is a homo-tetramer in which each monomer contains six ankyrin repeats in the N-terminal domain. The ion-conducting pore is formed by the transmembrane segments S5 and S6 and the pore-forming P loop and is similar to voltage-gated Na^+ and K^+ channels (Samanta et al., 2018). TRPV1 channels were first described in pain-sensitive neurons in dorsal root ganglia (DRG) and trigeminal ganglion neurons (Gees et al., 2010). Specifically, they are localized in peripheral small unmyelinated C- fibers, where they act as polymodal integrators of noxious stimuli in skin, muscles, joints, and internal organs (Samanta et al., 2018); also, TRPV2-4 channels are expressed in DRG neurons. TRPV3 is found in the brain, tongue, testis (Xu et al., 2002), skin, keratinocytes, and in cells surrounding hair follicles (Mandadi et al., 2009), while TRPV4 is expressed in non-neuronal cells like insulin-secreting β-cells, keratinocytes, smooth muscle cells, and different epithelial and bone cell types (Nilius et al., 2008).

The TRPA subfamily is constituted exclusively by the mammalian TRPA1 channel, first identified as an ankyrin-like transmembrane protein sharing similarities with other TRP channel subfamilies (Jaquemar et al., 1999). TRPA1 is a non-selective cation channel formed by homo- or hetero-tetramer subunits. The structure of human TRPA1 (hTRPA1) was determined by cryo-electron microscopy and shares a common structure with other TRP channels (Paulsen et al., 2015). TRPA1 has calcium-binding domains located in the C-terminal (Meents et al., 2019), 16 ankyrin repeat sequences in the N-terminal domain (Meents et al., 2017; Samanta et al., 2018), a putative selectivity filter located at the entrance of the pore, and a voltage sensor in the C-terminal (Meents et al., 2019). These domains allow TRPA1 channels to interact with other proteins, form molecular springs, and have better elasticity. This channel is expressed throughout the body, including the brain, heart, small intestine, lung, bladder, joints, and skeletal muscles (Kono et al., 2013). TRPA1 is highly expressed in DRG and trigeminal ganglia neurons (Takahashi et al., 2008) and acts as a mechanosensor in peripheral sensory pathways and the inner ear (Brierley et al., 2011).

TRPM channel subfamily consists of eight members grouped in four pairs: TRPM1 and TRPM3; TRPM2 and TRPM8; TRPM4 and TRPM5; and TRPM6 and TRPM7 (Fleig and Penner, 2004). All TRPM family members share common structural characteristics with other TRP channels (Fujiwara and Minor, 2008); however, they have a large cytosolic domain of between 732 and 1,611 amino acids for each subunit, which makes them the largest members of the TRP superfamily (Huang et al., 2020). Furthermore, unlike the TRPC, TRPV, and TRPA subfamilies, TRPM have a unique N-terminal (TRPM homology domain) without ankyrin repeats implicated in the channel assembly and trafficking (Kraft and Harteneck, 2005). Within subfamily members, the C-terminal section of TRPM channels is particularly variable, with TRPM2, TRPM6, and TRPM7, including active enzymatic domains (Samanta et al., 2018). TRPM2 has a nucleoside diphosphate pyrophosphatase domain (Chubanov et al., 2004) that specifically binds and hydrolyzes to ADP-ribose, while TRPM6 and TRPM7 contain α-kinase domains (Nadler et al., 2001; Drennan and Ryazanov, 2004). TRPMs are widely expressed in different tissues and organs; for instance, TRPM 2, 3, 4, 5, 6, and 7 are expressed in the CNS and periphery nervous system (PNS) (Mickle et al., 2015). Also, TRPM4, TRPM5, and TRPM8 are preferentially expressed in the prostate, while TRPM4, TRPM5, and TRPM6 are expressed in the intestine, and TRPM7 in heart, pituitary, bone, and adipose tissue (Bernardini et al., 2015). By contrast, TRPM1 is expressed by melanocytes and in malignant melanoma cells (Mickle et al., 2015).

As mentioned before, several members of the TRPC, TRPV, TRPM, and TRPA families are expressed in neurons and glial cells in the CNS and PNS (**Figure 1**; Riccio et al., 2002; Moran et al., 2004; Abel and Zukin, 2008; Harteneck and Leuner, 2014; Zhang and Liao, 2015; Echeverry et al., 2016; Belrose and Jackson, 2018). Evidence has shown that TRPs in the CNS have critical roles in modulating growth cone guidance, synaptogenesis, synaptic plasticity, and in the development of several neurodegenerative diseases (Nilius, 2012; Vennekens et al., 2012; Katz et al., 2017). Notably, even when the role of TRPs in nociception in the PNS has been extensively described, their role in the CNS is almost unknown, and it has only recently gained attention.

ACTIVATION MECHANISMS OF TRPs

TRP channels display a wide variety of activation mechanisms, which include physical stimuli, ligand binding, second messengers, and reactive oxygen and nitrogen species (Vennekens et al., 2012).

TRPC channels are modulated by a diverse group of second-messengers lipids that either regulate the channel activity or its insertion into the plasma membrane (Nilius and Szallasi, 2014). TRPCs activation mechanism converges various types of intracellular stimuli, including phospholipase C (PLC), protein kinase C (PKC) activity, diacylglycerol (DAG), intracellular calcium, and phosphatidylinositol 4,5-bisphosphate (PIP_2) levels to modulate membrane potential and calcium input (Ramsey et al., 2006). Due to the flexible role of TRPC3 channel in calcium signaling and functional coupling with metabotropic receptors involving the PLC pathway in DRGs, as well as its regulation by pro-inflammatory molecules inducing channel sensitization (Séguéla et al., 2014), it has been of interest as a potential target for the management of chronic pain. Although most TRPCs are activated through PLC, which is a downstream effector of growth factors and neurotrophins, For instance, TRPC3, 6, and 7 are activated primarily by Gq/11 proteins, which are

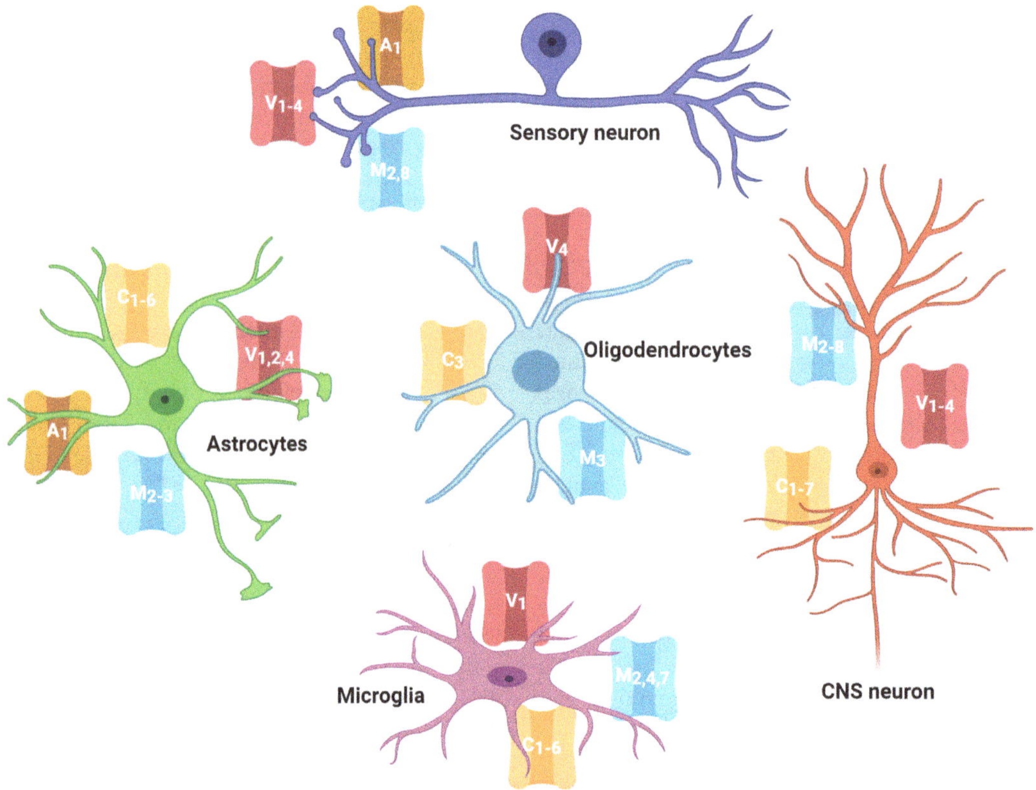

FIGURE 1 | TRP channels expressed in the nervous system cells. Several members of the TRPC, TRPV, TRPM, and TRPA families are highly expressed in cells of the central and peripheral nervous system (neurons, astrocytes, oligodendrocytes, and microglia). TRP families are represented by capital letters as follow, C, TRPC; M, TRPM; V, TRPV; A, TRPA. Numbers indicates specific members of each family.

coupled downstream PLC-β; nevertheless, the $G\alpha_{i/o}$ family are the dominant activators for TRPC4 and 5 (Nilius and Szallasi, 2014), which effectors of the PLC pathway are critical for the activation of TRPC channels remains a matter of debate, however, it is thought that specific TRPC channels may use different signaling effectors of this pathway (Putney, 2005). In this vein, it has been described that TRPC activation is dependent on recognition and lipid signals, and for instance, TRPC1, 2, 4, and 5 are activated by several DAGs (Lucas et al., 2003).

Besides lipid signaling, oxidative metabolism has a pivotal role in regulating TRPC channels activity (Kitajima et al., 2011) since they can be modulated by the production of reactive oxidative species (ROS) and reactive nitrogen species (RNS). TRPC channels can be considered redox-sensitive proteins that are targeted by ROS (Kim et al., 2013), and specifically, it has been reported that TRPC3 and TRPC4 are directly activated in response to oxidative stress (Aarts and Tymianski, 2005; Miller, 2006). It has been described that redox sensed by TRPC channels let the system indirectly to transduce lipid accumulation produced by the PIP_2/DAG pathway (Malczyk et al., 2016), and the redox modifications of the lipid membrane environment that surrounds the channel (Poteser et al., 2006). For instance, TRPC3 activation by 1-oleoyl-2-acetyl-sn-glycerol (OAG) or mechanical stretch has shown to induce ROS production in rat neonatal cardiomyocytes (Kitajima et al., 2011). Additionally, it has been described in human embryonic kidney (HEK) cells that nitric oxide (NO) activates TRPC5 channels through mechanisms that require oxidation of extracellular cysteines in response to the NO donor S-nitroso-N-acetyl-DL-penicillamine (Yoshida et al., 2006). Also, intracellular oxidation regulates TRPC5 activation by glutathionylation, nitrosylation, and hydroxylation reactions, respectively, in Cys176 and Cys178 in contact with the intracellular redox environment, resulting in a sustained increase in $[Ca^{2+}]$i and consequent cellular toxicity and neurodegeneration (Hong et al., 2015). In addition, oxidative metabolism also regulates the expression of TRPC channels (Song et al., 2011). Together ROS generation and Ca^{2+} signaling through TRPC channels modulate cellular processes that allow physiological and pathological responses in several organs (Malczyk et al., 2016) including kidney (Kim et al., 2013), brain (Hong et al., 2015), and the immune system (López-Requena et al., 2019). These factors have been associated in the pathogenesis of several chronic neurological disorders, including Alzheimer's disease (AD) and Parkinson's disease (PD), since ROS could activate cell death processes directly, through protein oxidation, lipids, and acting as second messengers in the cell death process (Gopalakrishna and Jaken, 2000; Nakamura and Lipton, 2009).

TRPV channels are activated by chemical ligands, such as capsaicin or cannabinoids, but also by noxious heat (>43°C), low pH (<6) (Caterina et al., 1997; Tominaga et al., 1998) and voltage changes inducing depolarization (Cao, 2020). TRPVs are also activated by lipid signaling (Cortright and Szallasi, 2004; Jung et al., 2004), and eicosanoids, signaling molecules produced by the enzymatic or non-enzymatic oxidation of arachidonic acid or other similar polyunsaturated fatty acids (Hwang et al., 2000). Specifically, TRPV1 activation can be achieved, regulated, and enhanced by several inflammatory molecules throughout metabolites downstream of G-protein coupled, such as PIP_2 (Bhave et al., 2002), IP_3 and DAG (Burgess et al., 1989), protein kinases such as PKA (Vlachová et al., 2003), PKC (Bhave et al., 2002; Varga et al., 2006), Ca^{2+}/calmodulin-dependent protein kinase II (CaMKII) (Jin et al., 2004; Rosenbaum et al., 2004), and arachidonic acid metabolites like 12-HPETE (Shin et al., 2002).

It has been described that DRG neurons express TRPV1 to transduce and modulate pain stimuli in response to ligands and temperature (Caterina et al., 1997; Basbaum et al., 2009). Furthermore, it has also been shown that Bradykinin can regulate nociceptors such as TRPV1 activity, an inflammatory response mediator, that simultaneously stimulates the synthesis of PLC and its downstream targets (PIP_3 and DAG), and arachidonic acid that further enhance cell excitation (Suh and Oh, 2005). During the inflammatory response, other pro-inflammatory mediators such as prostaglandins and sympathetic amines, sensitize nociceptors, including TRPV1, boosting pain sensation, or hyperalgesia (Zarpelon et al., 2013). A relationship between cytokines and oxidative stress has been found in hyperalgesia. For instance, NADPH oxidase leads to the production of superoxide anion by the TNF-α-induced NF-kB activation and consequentially causes overexpression of pro-inflammatory cytokines such as IL-1β (Possebon et al., 2014). Also, TNF-α and IL-1β activate cyclooxygenase-2 to produce prostanoids, which sensitize nociceptors, causing hyperalgesia (Verri et al., 2006).

TRPA1 channels have a wide range of natural and synthetic ligands (reactive electrophilic agonists) that induce channel gating by covalently bound to cysteine and lysine residues within the N-terminal and transmembrane domains, or promote the formation of C422–C622 disulfide bonds (Kimura, 2015). Also, polyunsaturated fatty acids (Viana, 2016), temperature (17–40°C) (Laursen et al., 2014; Moparthi et al., 2016) and changes in pH can activate TRPA1channels (Fujita et al., 2008; De La Roche et al., 2013; Zimova et al., 2018). De La Roche et al. (2013) reported activation of TRPA1, expressed in HEK 293T cells, with solutions above pH 5.4. However, it has been shown that in a Ca^{2+} dependent manner, pH between 7.4 and 8.5, also activates mouse TRPA1 channels heterologous expressed in HEK 293 cells (Fujita et al., 2008). Although the mechanism of how Ca^{2+} can modulate the sensitivity of the channel to more basic pH is still elusive, it has been shown that Ca^{2+} potentiates the activation and desensitization states of TRPA1 channels (Zimova et al., 2018). TRPA1 is a sensor for chemical irritants and a major contributor to chemo-nociception that is closely associated with TRPV1 channels, in terms of both expression and function (reviewed in Wang et al., 2019). Similarly to TRPV1, allogenic activators of TRPA1 channels are released from inflammatory environments or tissue injury sites to activate the channel (Chen and Hackos, 2015). For example, several lipid peroxidation products, oxidized lipids, and activators of the inflammasome, stimulate TRPA1 channels by an indirect mechanism involving H_2O_2 production (Trevisan et al., 2014). Additionally, endogenous lipidergic activators like nitrated fatty acids, produced by inflammatory processes, covalently bind to activate TRPA1 channels (Brewster et al., 2015).

TRPM activation mechanisms vary greatly among subfamily members, however, more than half of the members are sensitive to a wide range of temperatures, from cold to hot. For instance, TRPM4 and TRPM8 are activated by temperatures below 15 and 26°C, respectively (Talavera et al., 2005; Yao et al., 2011), while TRPM5 and TRPM2 are activated by temperatures above 35°C (Togashi et al., 2006). TRPM3 is the only member of this family that is activated by harmful heat, around 52°C in peripheral sensory neurons (Vriens et al., 2011). Some channels in this subfamily also respond to redox status, intracellular calcium, low temperatures, or ligands such as menthol. For instance, TRPM2 play a role in the transduction of oxidative stress stimuli (Oancea et al., 2011). In cortical neurons, TRPM2 channels are involved in the cytotoxic influx of Ca^{2+} that is induced by reactive oxygen species such as H_20_2 (Kaneko et al., 2006). TRPM2 also activated by-products of nucleotides metabolisms like ADP-ribose (ADPR) and nicotinamide adenine dinucleotide (NAD) (Nadler et al., 2001; Hara et al., 2002; Kraft and Harteneck, 2005). It is not clear whether ROS directly or indirectly activates TRPM2 downstream of ADPR or NAD, however, recent evidence shows that oxidative stress triggers the production of ADPR mitochondrial that is released to the cytosol to activate TRPM2 (Perraud et al., 2005). It has been also described that H_2O_2 production after DNA damage, especially during certain phases of the cell cycle, induces an accumulation of 2′-deoxy-ATP mediated by an increase in NAD synthesis and a decrease in reserves of cellular ATP (Fliegert et al., 2017). The increased ratio of 2′-deoxy-ATP to ATP facilitates the synthesis of 2′-deoxy-NAD and subsequent hydrolysis to 2′-deoxy-ADPR. It is known that increasing amounts of cellular 2′-deoxy-ADPR mediates TRPM2 activation with similar potency but greater efficacy than ADPR, making it a TRPM2 super-antagonist (Fliegert et al., 2017). These findings are in congruence with the suggestions that TRPM2 activation under an oxidative environment could be related to pathological cell death in neurodegenerative diseases (Xie et al., 2010). TRPM4 and TRPM5 channels are activated by Ca^{2+}, but they are not calcium-permeable (Oancea et al., 2011). The sensitivity of TRPM4 to intracellular Ca^{2+} is controlled by multiple signaling events, including ATP, PKC-dependent phosphorylation, calmodulin (CaM) binding, and membrane potential (Nilius et al., 2005). PIP_2, Ca^{2+}, and the voltage regulate the sensitivity of these channels, however, an increase in temperature in the range of 15 to 35°C further displaces the dependence of the voltage toward more negative potentials (Talavera et al., 2005). TRPM7 is also regulated by ROS and Ca^{2+} entry. Ca^{2+} has been considered as a relevant factor for the strong and lasting activation of TRPM7 in conditions of anoxia, oxidative stress, and metabolic imbalance, which could suggest mechanisms in which TRPM7 is involved and could induce even cell death (Aarts et al., 2003).

The PLC pathway, mediated by increased in intracellular calcium concentration, is an important mechanism involved in the modulation of some members of the TRPM family involved in depletion of PIP_2 and the desensitization of TRPM4, TRPM5, TRPM7, and TRPM8 channels. Specifically, for TRPM4 it has been reported to cause a shift to the left of its voltage dependence and increase its sensitivity to Ca^{2+} 100 times (Owsianik et al., 2006). TRPM8 activation is inhibited by Gq-coupled receptors that mediate PLC activation, however, depletion of Ca^{2+} store activates chemical signaling through lysophospholipids (LPLs), enhancing TRPM8 activity (Vanden Abeele et al., 2006). Also, exogenous PIP_2 (Liu and Qin, 2005), cold, or menthol (Rohács et al., 2005) activates TRPM8.

TRP CHANNELS AND NEURODEGENERATIVE DISEASES

Neuronal cell death rarely occurs in healthy brains, however, it can be triggered by internal/external factors in most neurodegenerative diseases (NDDs), where neurons initially lose their ability to maintain homeostasis due to changes in neuronal morphology, function, and viability (Dugger and Dickson, 2017; Chi et al., 2018). NDDs are categorized by their clinical features, anatomical structures affected, or molecular abnormalities (Kovacs, 2016). Although different in etiology, NDDs share common features, including mitochondria dysfunction, impaired energy metabolism, abnormal voltage-dependent anion channel activation, DNA damage, pro-inflammatory cytokines production, and disruption of cellular and axonal transport (Dugger and Dickson, 2017; Chi et al., 2018).

In the elderly, neurodegenerative diseases are a common and growing cause of mortality and morbidity, being AD and PD the most studied (Rahimi and Kovacs, 2014). AD is the most common form of dementia and makes up to 60–80% of all dementia cases worldwide, affecting an estimated 34 million people globally (Erkkinen et al., 2018). Meanwhile, PD affects 0.2 people per 100 of the population (independently of age), and almost 1–3% of the population older than 60 years (Tysnes and Storstein, 2017). Patients with AD or PD present learning and memory impairments, poor communication skills, irritability, symptoms of anxiety/depression, and progressive motor dysfunction (Batista and Pereira, 2016), and 40–85% of them suffer from painful conditions (Jost and Buhmann, 2019). Although the mechanisms that lead to these painful conditions are not fully understood, it is thought that neuropathological changes that occur in people with AD and PD dementia could alter pain perception (Van Kooten et al., 2016).

Calcium concentration level in neurons is exquisitely controlled to maintain cell homeostasis and to prevent neurodegeneration. The machinery that regulates intracellular Ca^{2+} levels is complex and includes several voltage-dependent plasma membrane calcium-conducting channels, glutamate receptors such as N-methyl-D-aspartate receptors and α-amino-3-hydroxy-5-methyl-4-isoxazolepropionic acid receptor, calcium release activated channels, and TRPCs. In addition, calcium flow from the endoplasmatic reticulum (ER) is highly regulated by Ryanodine receptors, Inositol trisphosphate receptor, calcium-dependent kinases, and phosphatases (Brini et al., 2014). Alterations in Ca^{2+} homeostasis have been related to the appearance and progression of several NDDs, including AD and PD (Marambaud et al., 2009; Nevzati et al., 2014). Indeed, it has been reported that exposure to either Aβ peptides (Li et al., 2009) or α-synuclein oligomers (Danzer et al., 2007) induces neuronal death by activating Ca^{2+}dependent signaling pathways and metabolic derangements (Arundine and Tymianski, 2003), most likely by increasing mitochondrial Ca^{2+} levels and the release of proapoptotic factors (Orrenius et al., 2003; Beech, 2005

In physiological conditions, activation of G-coupled receptors at the plasma membrane induces the release of Ca^{2+} from the ER, which in turn stimuli the influx of extracellular Ca^{2+} through a diversity of plasma membrane channels. This process is known as store-operated Ca^{2+} entry (SOCE) (Putney, 1986). SOCE calcium fluxes are mediated by calcium selective ion channels ORAI (calcium release-activated calcium channel proteins) (Kraft, 2015) that allow the calcium release-activated calcium current (I_{CRAC}) and store-operated calcium current (I_{SOC}) mediated by relatively selective Ca^{2+} to non-selective cation channels, such as TRPC1/4/5 (Parekh and Putney, 2005; Yuan et al., 2007). It has been suggested that Orai binds to TRPC1 and the stromal interaction molecule 1 (STIM1) during SOCE activation, enhancing calcium currents (Liao et al., 2008; Zhang et al., 2016). In this regard, TRPCs play a role in $[Ca^{2+}]i$ regulation by modulating SOCE (Minke and Cook, 2002), which joint to other TRPs, such as TRPC3, TRPC4, TRPM2, and TRPM7, respond to oxidative stress (Selvaraj et al., 2012), and may contribute to neurodegeneration (**Figure 2**). Given the expression of TRP channels in brain regions damaged during the development of PD and AD, and their role in Ca^{2+} homeostasis and ROS/RNS sense, they are now considered key players in neuronal degeneration and potentially on altered pain perception (**Figure 3**) (Bernd and Appendino, 2007; Nilius and Flockerzi, 2014; Rojo et al., 2014).

TRPs IN PARKINSON'S DISEASE

PD is characterized by a marked loss of dopaminergic neurons (DNs) in substantia nigra (SN) (Cacabelos, 2017). Although the mechanism by which these neurons degenerate is not well known, mitochondrial dysfunction, oxidative stress, inflammation, altered calcium homeostasis, NO synthesis, protein aggregation, excitotoxicity, and glutathione (GSH) depletion (Mandel et al., 2003), and activation of microglia-mediated by glucocorticoid receptors (GR) (Maatouk et al., 2018), are related to degeneration of DNs (Channels, 2017). Considering that oxidative stress and changes in Ca^{2+} homeostasis are involved in PD, it has been suggested that TRP channels could mediate some of the mechanisms that lead to the development of the disease.

Kim et al. (2005) showed that capsaicin, a TRPV1 agonist, elicits cell death of mesencephalic DNs. Additionally, it has been reported that TRPV1 activation triggers Ca^{2+}-dependent

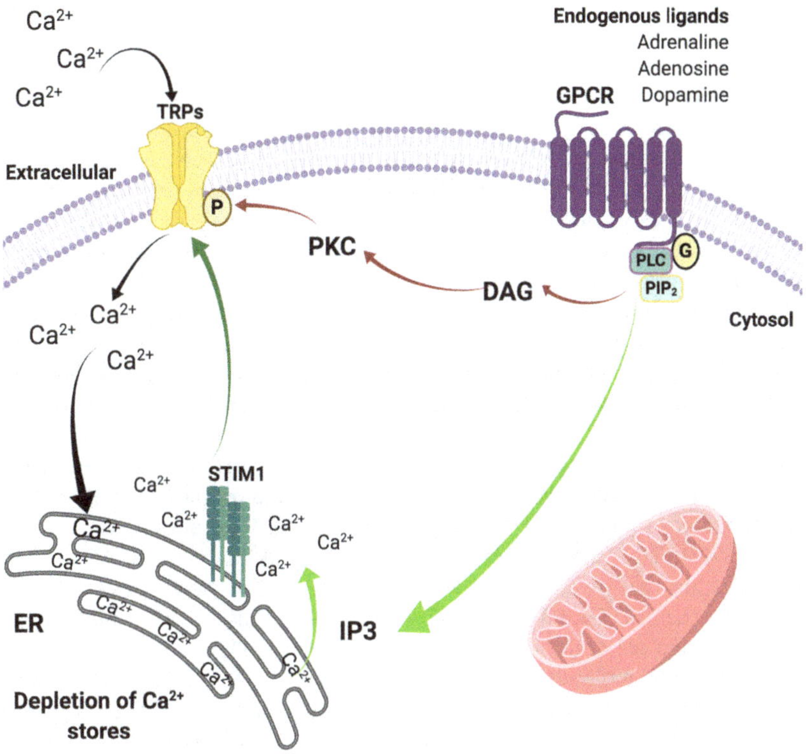

FIGURE 2 | SOCE through TRP channels. Activation of G-protein coupled receptors activates the phospholipase C pathway that induces the hydrolysis of PIP_2 to DAG (red arrows) that actives PKC, which in turn phosphorylates TRP channels. In parallel, the generation of IP_3 (green arrows) promotes the release of Ca^{2+} from the ER. The depletion of intracellular Ca^{2+} stores from the ER is sensed by STIM1, which also activates Ca^{2+} channels in the plasma membrane such as TRPs (dark green arrow), allowing the entry of Ca^{2+} from the extracellular medium to the cytosol (black arrows) to refill de ER deposits.

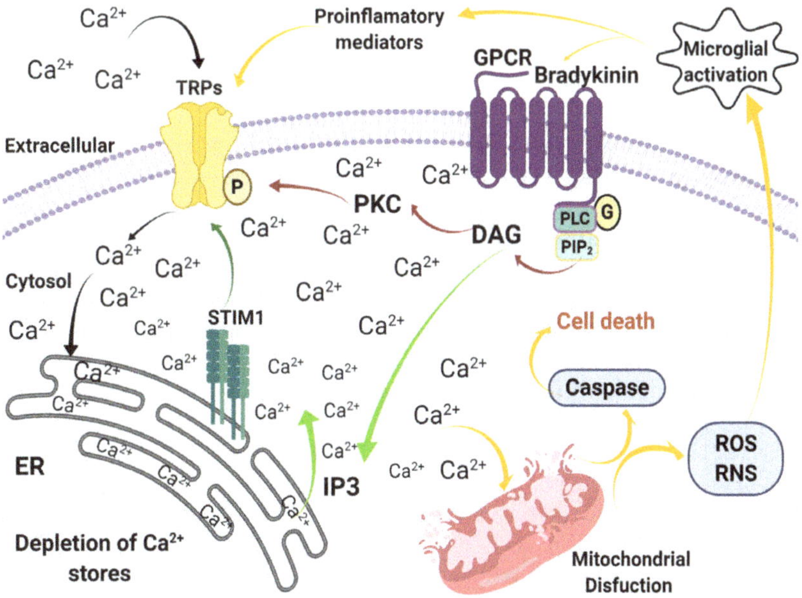

FIGURE 3 | Alterations in calcium homeostasis mediated by SOCE during inflammation and oxidative stress. Activation of G-coupled receptors by pro-inflammatory mediators, such as bradykinin, induces the release of Ca^{2+} from the ER stores through the PLC pathway (green arrows), followed by an influx of Ca^{2+} through Ca^{2+} permeable channels such as TRPs (black arrows). The increase $[Ca^{2+}]i$ then induces mitochondrial dysfunction that leads to caspase activation, ROS and RNS production, microglia activation, and production of pro-inflammatory mediators (yellow arrows).

cell death (Kim et al., 2006) and NADPH-oxidase-mediated production of ROS in microglia (Shirakawa and Kaneko, 2018), suggesting that a similar mechanism could operate in death of DNs in PD. For instance, TRPV1 antagonists such as capsazepine and iodo-resiniferatoxin inhibit DNs death *in vivo* and *in vitro* (Kim et al., 2005). Mechanistically, it is thought that TRPV1 activation induces an increase in [Ca^{2+}]i that impairs mitochondrial function, induces cytochrome release, and caspase-3 cleavage. Consequently, activation of TRPV1 channels contributes to dopaminergic neuron damage *via* Ca^{2+} signaling and mitochondrial disruption (Kim et al., 2005). Although the nature of the endogenous ligands that induce the activation of TRPV1 in PD has not been elucidated, these channels are endogenously activated by anandamide, an endocannabinoid, which is increased in untreated PD patients (Pisani et al., 2010).

In contrast to the toxic role of TRPV1 activation on DNs, TRPC1 has been suggested as a protector and critical mediator of DNs survival (Sun et al., 2012). DNs are characterized by a pacemaker activity that is thought to be dependent on the activation of the Ca^{2+} channel $Ca_V1.3$ and Na^+ channels. Interestingly, Cav1.3-mediated cell death is prevented by translocation of stromal interacting molecule-1 (STIM1) induced by Ca^{2+}depletion of ER, allowing it to interact with and activate calcium permeable channels like TRPC1 to refill the ER Ca^{2+} store (Soboloff et al., 2012; Kraft, 2015). That process protects DNs against the Cav1.3-mediated cell death. Neurotoxins that mimic PD symptoms, such as 1-methyl-4-phenyl-1, 2, 3, 6-tetrahydropyridine (MPTP), increase the activity of the Cav1.3 channel by downregulating the expression of TRPC1, which lead to a decrease in SOCE and the release of Ca^{2+} from ER to the cytosol in DNs and mesenchymal stem cells (Sun et al., 2018). It has been described that MPP^+ (1-methyl-4-phenylpyridinium), a toxic metabolite product of enzymatic activity of MAO-B on MPTP, kills DNs in SN (Choi et al., 2015). In this vein, it has been shown that Cav1.3 silencing or TRPC1 overexpression decreases caspase 3 and inhibits MPP^+-induced cell death. Therefore, TRPC1 expression facilitates STIM1-Cav1.3 interaction, and it is essential for the survival of DNs in PD (Sun et al., 2017). Moreover, Chen et al. (2013) found that the downregulation of Homer 1 protein inhibited the generation of ROS induced by MPP^+ in DNs, without affecting the activity of endogenous antioxidant enzymes; this inhibition was further potentiated by BAPTA-AM. Exposure of DNs to MPP^+ induces a rapid increase in cytosolic Ca^{2+} concentrations after its release from the ER, an effect that was prevented in DNs with low Homer1 expression (Chen et al., 2013).

Beyond its role in DNs-induced cell death, MPP^+ can directly activate microglia and promote the production of several pro-inflammatory mediators and iNOS (Kim et al., 2018; Lee et al., 2019). Once microglia are activated, the release of pro-inflammatory microglial cytokines and chemokines induce the death of dopaminergic (DA) neurons, evidencing the vulnerability of these neurons to glia-mediated neurotoxicity. In the MPTP model, M1 microglia have been associated with dopamine neurodegeneration by the induction of microglial NOS and NADPH oxidase (NOX) (Appel et al., 2015). Mizoguchi et al. found that brain derived neurotrophic factor (BDNF) induces a sustained elevation of [Ca^{2+}]i through the overregulation of TRPC3, which is also crucial for the suppression of NO induced by BDNF-activated microglia. This signaling pathway has been linked to the inflammatory response that mediates DA death in PD (Mizoguchi et al., 2014).

Furthermore, Parkinsonian disorders are often associated with changes in the frequency and firing mode of GABAergic neurons (Zhou et al., 2008). In SN and Globus Pallidus internus, GABAergic neurons project and regulate the firing pattern of thalamic nuclei, superior colliculus, and brainstem motor nuclei, regulating the smoothness and coordination of movements (Zhou et al., 2008). TRPC3 channels selectively expressed in the SN GABA projection neurons regulate the firing pattern of these neurons. The expression of TRPC3 in SN maintains a constant influx of Na^+ that generates a tonic depolarized potential that contributes to the high frequency and regularity pattern of firing of these neurons (Zhou et al., 2008). However, it has been described that ROS-induced increased TRPC3 activity could lead to a more depolarized potential in GABAergic projecting neurons, contributing to the unbalance of disinhibition and inhibition cycles observed in PD (Zhou et al., 2008).

TRPM7, a Zn^{2+}, Ca^{2+}, and Mg^{2+} permeable channel, has been associated with NDDs given its regulation by intracellular Mg^{2+} levels and ROS (Nadler et al., 2001; Sun et al., 2015). PD animal models have shown that Mg^{2+} deficits increase the vulnerability of DNs to MPTP neurotoxicity (Muroyama et al., 2009). Furthermore, Mg^{2+}supplementation inhibits the toxicity of (methyl-4-phenylpyridium ion) by decreasing the death of DNs and maintaining the length of their neurites. These results are in agreement with the observation that TRPM7 is significantly decreased in the SN of PD patients and that long-term Mg^{2+} deficiencies significantly decrease the number of DNs in SN (Oyanagi et al., 2006). These results suggest that DNs utilize TRPM7 channels to regulate Mg^{2+} levels, and that loss of TRPM7 channel function may be involved in the development of PD (Landman et al., 2006).

It has been reported that PD patients have significantly elevated cortisol levels compared to control subjects of the same age (Bellomo et al., 1991; Ros-Bernal et al., 2011). Interestingly, expression of TRPM6 and TRPM7 can be regulated by glucocorticoids (GCs) in a tissue-dependent manner (Cuffe et al., 2015). In the brain, GC signaling is mediated by GRs well as by mineralocorticoid receptors expressed in neurons and glia (Sierra et al., 2008). A large number of studies indicate that activation of GRs by GC promotes inflammatory response (Bhattacharyya et al., 2010), particularly in microglia (Maatouk et al., 2018). For instance, inflammation caused by a low dose of Lipopolysaccharides (LPS) directly administrated in substantia nigra causes a specific loss of dopaminergic neurons (Castaño et al., 2002). Interestingly, pre-treatment with a low dose of dexamethasone (DXM, 1 mg/Kg) diminished nigrostriatal dopaminergic neurons damage in mice treated with 1-methyl-4-phenyl-1,2,3,6-tetrahydropiridine (MPTP, 40 mg/Kg), while a high dose of DXM (10 mg/Kg) further aggravate loss of dopaminergic neurons (Kurkowska-Jastrzębska et al., 2004). However, physiological levels of GC and functional response of GRs are necessary to prevent neurodegeneration; indeed, it has been reported that in the absence of GR, microglia-induced dopaminergic neuronal loss (Barcia et al., 2011).

TRPs IN ALZHEIMER DISEASE

Altered Ca^{2+} homeostasis has been considered one critical factor regulating neuronal death in AD (Small, 2009). For instance, mutations in presenilins, catalytic subunits of the gamma-secretase, have been linked to Ca^{2+} signaling dysregulation, proteolytic processing of amyloid precursor protein (APP), and thereby increasing production of Aβ peptide (Guo et al., 1997, 1999; Schneider et al., 2001; Banerjee and Hasan, 2005). Aggregation of the Aβ peptide may induce the release of Ca^{2+} stored in the ER, resulting in an overload of cytosolic Ca^{2+}. In response to the rise in $[Ca^{2+}]$i, endogenous levels of GSH are reduced, leading to a ROS accumulation within cells (Ferreiro et al., 2008). In addition, the deposition of Aβ also induces microglial activation (Seabrook et al., 2006) and the release of pro-inflammatory cytokines, initiating pro-inflammatory signaling pathways that subsequently contributes to neuronal damage and death (Wang et al., 2015). Pro-inflammatory cytokines also sensitized TRPV1 channels expressed in a variety of cells, such as microglia, astrocytes, pericytes, and neurons (Tóth et al., 2005), suggesting that these channels contribute to AD-related neuroinflammatory processes. Inhibition of TRPV1 dependent generation of ROS significantly diminishes the detrimental effect of activated microglia and the inflammatory response elicited by astrocytes upon stimulation with the Aβ peptide (Harada and Okajima, 2006; Benito et al., 2012). However, capsaicin activation of TRPV1 protects the hippocampus function by rescuing the effect of Aβ peptide on the hippocampal gamma oscillations (Balleza-Tapia et al., 2018). These differences compared to the response of TRPV1 after activation by capsaicin, could be accounted for by experimental conditions, likely related to β-amyloid concentrations used in both studies (Balleza-Tapia et al., 2018). Purely fibrillary beta-amyloid preparations have been reported to be more toxic in some experimental models (Kurudenkandy et al., 2014; Cohen et al., 2015), and this possibly induces pathological activation of inflammatory mechanisms, mediated by TRPV1 in primary astrocyte culture (Devesa et al., 2011; Tsuji and Aono, 2012).

In the brain, TRPA1 channels play an essential role in their development and function of non-neuronal cells, such as astrocytes (Shigetomi et al., 2012, 2013). Although AD is a complex disease in which several mechanisms may act, recent studies have evaluated the role of Ca^{2+} related signaling pathways in the etiology and development of the disease (Yamamoto et al., 2007; Takada et al., 2013). Lee et al. (2016) demonstrated *in vitro* that Aβ triggers a TRPA1-dependent Ca^{2+} influx and astrocytic activation. Additionally, ablation of TRPA1 in APP/PS1 transgenic mice slowed the progression of AD and improved learning and memory performance, and reduced Aβ plaques and cytokines (Lee et al., 2016). These results have been further supported by TRPA1 expression in HEK cells, where Aβ is also capable of inducing TRPA1 dependent Ca^{2+} signaling, that activate transcription factors such as NF-κB and NFAT and promote expression of pro-inflammatory cytokines (Lee et al., 2016).

Interestingly, loss-of-function or pharmacological inhibition of TRPM2 channels prevents microglial activation and TNF-α production induced by a wide range of Aβ42 concentrations (10–300 nM), proving a novel role of TRPM2 in microglial activation triggered by Aβ42 peptides (Alawieyah et al., 2018). Likewise, Ostapchenko et al. (2015) demonstrated that TRPM2 ablation in AD models decreases microglial activation, improves the expression of synaptic markers and reduces the deficits in memory observed in aging animals (Ostapchenko et al., 2015). Furthermore, it has been shown that TRPM2 endogenous expression in rat striatum neurons and activation by Aβ and oxidative stress is enough to drive cell death, suggesting that TRPM2 is an active transducer of ROS signaling that may contribute to neuronal death in AD (Fonfria et al., 2005). At a cellular level, ROS levels are regulated by a complex mechanism that involves antioxidant enzymes and small-molecule antioxidants such as GSH (Geon et al., 2015). GSH levels tend to be lower with age and have been considered as markers of cognitive impairment severity (McCaddon et al., 2003). Interestingly, in neuronal cultures that recapitulate aging, GSH supplementation significantly decreases TRPM2 expression and activity (Sita et al., 2018). Therefore, downregulation of the antioxidant defense plus the Aβ-induced production of ROS and cytokines in AD can lead to the activation of several TRP channels that can increase $[Ca^{2+}]$i, leading to excitotoxicity and apoptosis (Park et al., 2014).

Although some advances have made in understanding the role of TRP channels in neurodegenerative diseases, we are still far from having an integrated comprehension of the role of these channels in the etiology and development of these diseases. For instance, more studies are needed to unveil how all these channels work together either to degenerate or protect neurons in PD and AD.

TRPs INVOLVEMENT IN PAIN, ALZHEIMER'S, AND PARKINSON'S DISEASES

During the past decade it has been an increasing awareness of pain and pain management as important issues to address in the elderly (Ali et al., 2018) and patients with neurodegenerative diseases (Cravello et al., 2019). Pain symptoms in NDD patients include sleep disorders, musculoskeletal problems, reduced mobility, falls, malnutrition, cognitive impairment, increased drugs use, diminished social behavior, anhedonia, and depression (Cravello et al., 2019). Prevalence of painful symptoms in patients with AD range from 38 to 75%, and from 40 to 86% in PD (Batista and Pereira, 2016; Van Kooten et al., 2016; de Tommaso et al., 2017; Cravello et al., 2019).

Even when PD was previously considered as a purely motor disorder, now it is known that non-motor symptoms, including pain, occur throughout the course of the disease and significantly affect the quality of life (Jost and Buhmann, 2019).

Some nociceptive pain associated with PD is a secondary consequence of the motor impairment (abnormal muscular tone, spasms, rigidity, reduced active mobility, osteoarticular problems, and local inflammation), however, as many as 43% of Parkinson patients exhibits characteristics typical of neuropathic dysfunction (burning, tingling, formicating, decreased nocifensive flexion reflex, and lowered cold threshold) (Reichling and Levine, 2011; Skogar and Lokk, 2016; de Tommaso et al., 2017). Neuropathic pain has been recently studied in a model of nigro-estriatal pathway lesion, which induces allodynia and hyperalgesia in rats (Romero-Sánchez et al., 2019).

Similarly, it has been described that pain is more prevalent in AD patients, and that intensity of pain is also positively correlated with dementia severity (Cao et al., 2019). Typical cognitive impairment observed in AD also affect the assessment of a painful experience and the ability to describe it (Cravello et al., 2019). It has been reported that neural circuits mediating pain perception and its behavioral expression may be hyperactive or underactive in AD: Specifically, altered pain response seems to depend on the extension of the brain tissue damage, stage of the disease, and type of pain (acute stimuli or chronic medical conditions) (Monroe et al., 2012).

Recently, neuropathological changes occurring during the progress of dementias are being considered as possible causes of pain perception alterations (Cravello et al., 2019), and it has been suggested that primary neuropathic pain is not a simple consequence of nervous system deterioration but instead the result of the very same cellular processes that underlie neurodegenerative diseases (Reichling and Levine, 2011; Cravello et al., 2019). The neuropathological changes that occur in AD affect structures comprised in CNS processing affective-motivational (hippocampus, entorhinal cortex, cingulate gyrus, hippocampus, amygdala), cognitive-evaluative (prefrontal cortices), and sensory-discriminative (somatosensory cortex) aspects of pain (Monroe et al., 2012; Achterberg et al., 2013; Dugger and Dickson, 2017). Similarly, in PD, insufficient input from dopaminergic neurons to basal ganglia and motor and prefrontal cortices results in enhanced inhibitory inputs, which leads not only to body movement-related symptoms but also cognitive and emotional symptoms associated to altered pain perception (Chi et al., 2018).

Figure 4 shows brain's structures involved in pain perception, which include the prefrontal cortex, hippocampus, amygdala, entorhinal cortex, anterior cingulate cortex, basal ganglia, thalamus, insula, and sensory cortex (Fenton et al., 2015; Mano and Seymour, 2015; Cao et al., 2019), and TRP channels expressed in each one of these structures (Kauer and Gibson, 2009; Harteneck and Leuner, 2014; Nilius and Szallasi, 2015; Frias and Merighi, 2016; Katz et al., 2017). As described before, TRP channels have an unique role in nociceptive, neuropathic, and inflammatory pain as diverse members of their families are involved in pain pathways (Hung and Tan, 2018). For instance, members of TRPA, TRPV, and TRPM subfamilies have high expression levels in neurons mediating neuropathic pain (Naziroğlu, 2012). Interestingly, members of the TRPC and TRPM families are expressed in SN, basal ganglia, and hippocampus, brain structures that exhibit significant loss of neurons at the initial stages of the development of AD or PD, respectively. The specific role of TRPs on NDD-related pain symptoms have not been thoroughly studied. However, several lines of evidence indicate a relationship between pain, neurodegeneration and TRPs, particularly related to inflammation.

At the molecular level, it has been proposed that pain-related to NDDs is associated, not only to loss of selected neuronal population but to microglial activation, that response

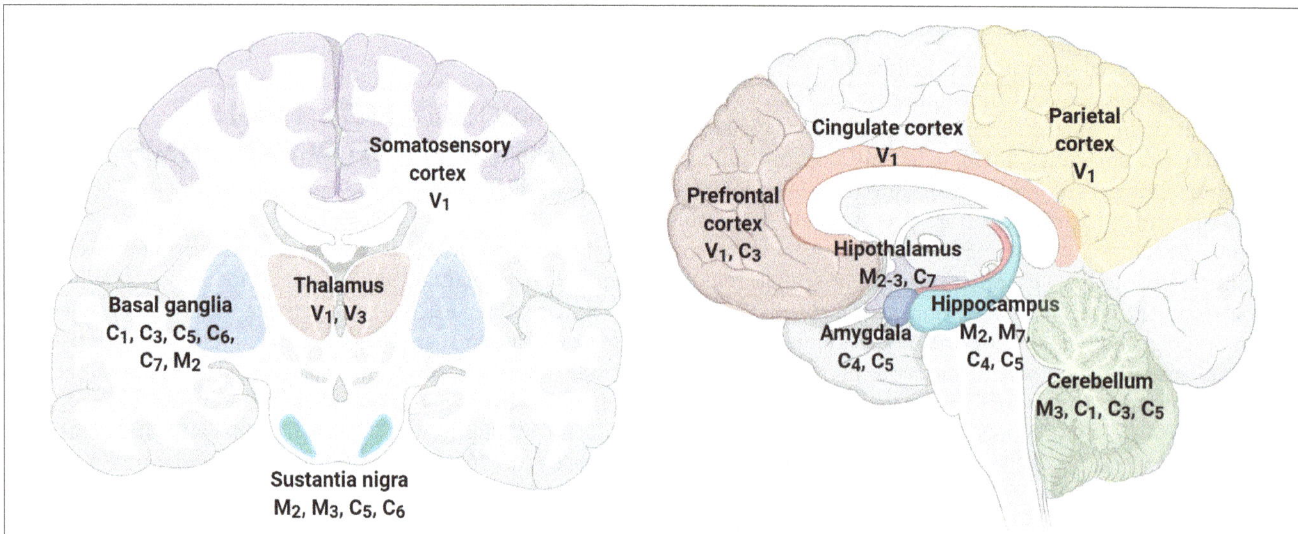

FIGURE 4 | TRP channels are expressed in brain structures involved in pain perception. Pain processing includes cortical (prefrontal, parietal, somatosensory, and cingulate), limbic (amygdala, hippocampus, thalamus, hypothalamus), and movement-related structures (Basal Ganglia, Substantia Nigra, and Cerebellum) that express several members of the TRP channels. TRP families are represented by capital letters as follow, C, TRPC; M, TRPM; V, TRPV; A, TRPA. Numbers indicates specific members of each family.

to noxious stimuli realizing inflammatory mediators such as pro-inflammatory cytokines, interleukins, and tumor necrosis factor alpha (TNFα) (Carniglia et al., 2017). Notably, chronic pain (inflammatory or neuropathic pain) related to neurodegeneration is also accompanied by neuroimmune activation and an escalated response that impairs homeostatic balance since anti-inflammatory mediators are not released, inducing further tissue damage, neuroinflammation, and neurodegeneration (Carniglia et al., 2017; Salter and Stevens, 2017; Inoue and Tsuda, 2018). The role of glial cells in the initiation, sensitization, and maintenance of chronic pain has been studied during the past two decades (Cravello et al., 2019), and it has been found that neuromodulators produced by microglia can rapidly alter synaptic plasticity, a driving force for the pathogenesis of pain after tissue or nerve injury (Chen et al., 2018).

During inflammatory pain, inflammatory molecules can change the TRP threshold activation, inducing mechanical allodynia, thermal hyperalgesia, and spontaneous pain. TRPV1, TRPA1, and TRPM2 channels have been intensely studied in pain sensation because they participate in the cellular signaling mechanism through which injury produces pain hypersensitivity. These channels can be activated by thermal stimuli and endogenous molecules derived from the inflammation process (Ma and Quirion, 2007; Hung and Tan, 2018). After an injury, inflammatory molecules such as eicosanoids, neuropeptides, and cytokines decrease the thresholds of sensory neurons, inducing sensitization in TRPV1 (Julius, 2013). As TRPA1 is highly regulated by oxidative stress and is targeted by different reactive species, so that they are activated during inflammatory progression, where ROS produced after tissue injury induces superoxidation of membrane phospholipids and activation of the channel (Julius, 2013; Mori et al., 2016; De Logu et al., 2017; Hung and Tan, 2018). The role of TRPM2 in pain generation is through their activation by reactive nitrogen species (Kaneko et al., 2006). Similar to TRPV1, TRPM2 suffers sensitization by H_2O_2 that lowered the temperature of activation (Kashio et al., 2012). Interestingly, it has been described that chronic pain is a risk factor to develop memory impairment, dementia, and other neuropsychiatric conditions (Moriarty and Finn, 2014; Whitlock et al., 2017).

TRP channels expressed in sensory neurons have an essential function in pain and inflammation transduction (Fernandes et al., 2012; Smani et al., 2015). Similarly, it has been reported that microglial TRP channels have a significant role in pain modulation as well as in AD and PD (Cravello et al., 2019) by regulating the levels of ROS, pro-inflammatory cytokines, and the homeostasis of Ca^{2+}. All these processes are connected with microglial activation, which is a cellular process proposed as a central player in both pain and neurodegenerative diseases (Miyake et al., 2014; Echeverry et al., 2016). For example, during inflammation, an upregulation of TRPM2 channels in microglia leads to an exacerbated inflammatory response mediated by ROS. This mechanism has been proposed as one of the primary inductors of inflammation and neuropathic pain (Haraguchi et al., 2012). However, It has also been shown that TRPV1 channels protect mesencephalic DA neurons by inhibiting microglia-originated oxidative stress, suggesting that TRPV1 channels may be novel targets for regulating the oxidative stress-mediated neurodegeneration observed in PD (Park et al., 2012).

TRP-dependent microglial activation involves the influx of Ca^{2+} and the activation of Ca^{2+} -mediated signaling pathways that induce the synthesis of pro-inflammatory molecules, including interleukins (IL-1β and IL-12), chemokines, prostaglandins (PGs), TNF-α, ROS, and NO. These molecules promote an exacerbated inflammatory response by the recruitment of other immune cells that conduce to neuronal damage. However, when the injurious stimuli are controlled, the inflammatory response is diminished by cytokines with anti-inflammatory activity such as transforming growth factor (TGF-β) and IL-10 by microglia. Therefore, the imbalance of microglial activation could exacerbate the pro-inflammatory response, leading to neuronal degeneration and cell death in AD and PD, and neuropathic and inflammatory pain (Suter et al., 2007; Ji et al., 2013; Beggs and Salter, 2016; Carniglia et al., 2017).

Some kinases have a described role in pain. It was reported that extracellular signal-regulated kinases 1/2 and 5 (ERK1/2 and ERK5) are expressed in microglia, and their phosphorylation is induced during neuropathic pain (Tatsumi et al., 2015; Carniglia et al., 2017). Furthermore, it was observed that neuropathic pain induced by nerve injury, promoted the phosphorylation of p38 mitogen-activated protein kinase (MAPK) in spinal microglia. p38 MAPK is activated by multiple microglial receptors, inflammatory cytokines, membrane depolarization, and Ca^{2+} influx. This pathway regulates pro-inflammatory signaling networks as well as the production of diverse inflammatory molecules associated with pain facilitation, including the cytokines TNF-α and IL-1β (Ji and Suter, 2007; Lee and Kim, 2017). Moreover, it was confirmed that the inhibition of p38 MAPK decreases the release of pro-inflammatory cytokines, inducing relieve of mechanical allodynia in diverse models of neuropathic and inflammatory pain (Jin et al., 2003; Lee and Kim, 2017; Inoue and Tsuda, 2018). Interestingly, in addition to their role in pain, the p38 MAPK pathway has also been involved in the cellular mechanisms that regulate neurodegeneration (Lee and Kim, 2017; Kheiri et al., 2019). Activated p38 MAPK was observed in peripheral blood leukocytes and neuronal cells, as well as in postmortem brain from patients with AD (Sun et al., 2003; Kheiri et al., 2019).

p38 MAPK role in AD has been associated with both Tau protein and Aβ peptide, which are essential players in AD pathologies. For instance, Aβ peptide promotes the activation of p38 MAPK, which in turn, phosphorylates Tau protein in neuronal cells (Lee and Kim, 2017). In this vein, it has been described that Aβ peptides suppress nociception and inflammatory pain in APP overexpressing CRND8 transgenic mice (Shukla et al., 2013); this finding is in accordance with the finding that mice treated with a single intracerebroventricular injection of Aβ fragment (1–40) (400 pmol/mice) displayed increased pain tolerance (Pamplona et al., 2010). However, pain sensitivity could be altered in a more complex form since i.c.v. Aβ treated mice also display anxiogenic-like and depressive-like states, which are related to alterations in cognitive/emotional components of pain processing (Pamplona et al., 2010). Also, it has been described that Tau depletion, *in-vivo* studies, negatively affects the main systems conveying nociceptive information to the CNS (Sotiropoulos et al., 2014). Tau-null (Tau−/−) mice display reduced C-fiber density and Aδ-fiber hypomyelination followed by diminished conduction properties sciatic nerves and decreased nociception but increased excitability of second-order spinal cord nociceptive neurons, resulting in heightened pain-like behaviors (Sotiropoulos et al., 2014; Lopes et al., 2016). These findings suggest that APP and Aβ peptides and Tau protein could affect in a complex way pain perception in AD patients.

Several reports also suggest that p38 MAPK is also involved in PD. It is proposed that oxidative stress in dopaminergic neurons prompted the activation of the p38 MAPK and c-Jun N-terminal kinase (JNK) signaling pathways that have linked to neuronal apoptosis in several models of PD (Oh et al., 2011; Sabens Liedhegner et al., 2011; Bohush et al., 2018). p38-MAPK activation has also been reported to contribute to mitophagy, a fundamental mechanism underlying α-synuclein accumulation associated with PD (Cheng et al., 2018).

TRP channels function has been related to p38 MAPK pathway activity. It has been reported that phosphorylated p38 MAPK stimulated by noxious cold colocalized in neurons that express TRPA1 channels (Mizushima et al., 2006). Additionally, stimulation of microglia with lipopolysaccharide and interferon γ (LPS/IFN γ) promoted the activation of TRPM2 channels and Ca^{2+} dependent signaling pathways, and the increase in p38 MAPK signaling (Miyake et al., 2014). Interestingly, the use of TRPM2 inhibitors inhibited the extracellular Ca^{2+} influx, affecting the activation of the p38 MAPK pathway. Similar results have been observed in TRPM2-KO microglia, where NO release was attenuated (Haraguchi et al., 2012). It is suggested that TRPM2 recruits the p38 MAPK pathways for NO production induced by LPS/INFγ. Furthermore, phosphorylation of p38 MAPK was abolished in TRPM2-knockout microglia, indicating that this process is selectively dependent on TRPM2 signaling. Similarly, lisophosphatidylcholine (LPC), an endogenous inflammatory phospholipid that induces TRPM2 translocation to the plasma membrane, also promotes Ca^{2+} influx and microglia activation. It has been demonstrated that LPC increases phosphorylation of p38 MAPK in microglia, which was eliminated in TRPM2-KO. From these results, it is feasible to propose TRPM2 channels as potential therapeutic targets to inhibit excessive microglial activation, neuroinflammation, and, therefore, pain through modulation of p38 MAPK phosphorylation (Miyake et al., 2014; Jeong et al., 2017; Shirakawa and Kaneko, 2018).

Considering that the p38 MAPK pathway is a central player in neurodegeneration and pain, several recent studies have been focused in search of p38 MAPK activity modulators, and some molecules have shown anti-inflammatory activity (Jeong et al., 2017; Kheiri et al., 2019). However, cross-reactivity with other kinases and the appearance of cardiovascular, psychiatric, and hepatic side effects have halted the use of these molecules, suggesting that it is necessary to study further the mechanism by which p38 MAPK could be modulated to avoid the adverse side effects observed (Ji and Suter, 2007; Kheiri et al., 2019).

In addition to the regulation of p38 MAPK phosphorylation in microglia, TRP channels also play a role in the generation of peripheral pain through oxidative stress. Oxidative stress-mediated by lipid peroxidation has been observed in both neurological and peripheral pain. It has been proposed that selenium could act as neuroprotector through a mechanism that involves TRP channels inhibition, which in turn, induces modulation of ROS overproduction and Ca^{2+} influx (Nazıroğlu et al., 2020). Selenium is an inhibitor of TRPM2 channels, which reduces oxidative stress in the cytosol (Zeng et al., 2012). Besides TRPM2, selenium also acts as TRPA1 and TRPV1 inhibitor, suggesting that selenium could be used as a modulator of neuropathic pain through TRP channel modulation (Nazıroğlu et al., 2020).

Despite high rates of painful comorbidities, lower use of analgesics among individuals with dementia has been reported (Van Kooten et al., 2016). Detriment in pain management seems to occur in part due to challenging pain assessment in patients with compromised cognition and impaired communication skills, as well as barriers to analgesics (Shen et al., 2018).

Currently, several families of agents have been of clinical utility to treat pain. The most common analgesic drug prescribed for mild to moderate pain is paracetamol (also known as acetaminophen); however, for peripheral or central neuropathic pain, this analgesic drug has poor effectiveness. Opioids, anticonvulsants, nonsteroidal anti-inflammatory drugs (NSAIDs), topical medications, and more recently, third-generation antidepressants have been used to treat pain related to nerve injury (Lynch and Watson, 2006; Yaksh et al., 2015). However, important drugs safety and side effects limit their use; this is particularly important in the case of opioids, which are the most effective pain killers but have high potential to induce addiction and may cause sedation and respiratory depression (Moran and Szallasi, 2018). Clinical daily work shows that the use of painkillers, opioids, antidepressants, or anticonvulsive drugs are often not sufficient to treat pain in neurodegenerative diseases, so it has been suggested that in selected individuals, refractory to conventional treatment of pain, cannabinoid management could be attempted (Jost and Buhmann, 2019). It has been recently shown that cannabinoids provide promising multitarget approach for the treatment of pain and neurodegeneration since they regulate the activity of TRP channels, which are considered non-cannonical endocannabionoid receptors. In this vein, it has been shown that cannabidiol, cannabinol, cannabigerol, or cannabidiolic acid binds TRPs, including TRPV1-4, TRPA1, and TRPM8 (Shirakawa and Kaneko, 2018; Muller et al., 2019; Starkus et al., 2019).

Since TRPs are involved in the progression of neurodegenerative diseases and have a role in pain, they are remarkable potential targets for the treatment of both pain and neurodegenerations (Zündorf and Reiser, 2011; Naziroğlu,

2012; Maiese, 2017; Echeverry et al., 2016; Belrose and Jackson, 2018). Recent evidence regarding the involvement of TRP channels in several diseases has led to the identification of TRP channels as potential drug targets to manage pain. For instance, capsaicin, an agonist of TRPV1, has been used in clinical trials to control neuropathic pain conditions (Kiani et al., 2015; Derry et al., 2017), however, its use would be limited by two major adverse effects of TRPV1 channel agonists/antagonists: (a) dysregulation of body temperature, and (b) long-lasting compromise of temperature sensation leading to burning injuries. Agents targeting TRPM8, TRPV2, TRPV3, TRPV4, and TRPA1 have also been tested with mixed results. Interestingly, in animal models, TRPA1 deletion or inhibition reduces pain associated with inflammation, as well as inflammation *per se* (Moilanen et al., 2015, 2016; Horváth et al., 2016). A role for TRPA1 channels in neurogenic inflammation has been suggested (Moran and Szallasi, 2018); indeed, a Phase 2 clinical trial has have reported that the Glenmark's GRC 17536 TRPA1 channel antagonist significantly reduce pain scores in a pre-specified subset of patients with painful diabetic neuropathy and intact sensory responses without notable side effects (Moran and Szallasi, 2018). Recently, TRPM2 inhibitors have been proposed as a potential candidate to treat neurodegeneration and pain, and several novel molecules targeting TRPM2 (8Br-ADPR, 8-Ph-2'-deoxy-ADPR and novel ADPR analogs capable of selectively inhibiting TRPM2) appear as potential candidates to develop novel therapeutic agents (Belrose and Jackson, 2018). Notably, a cell-permeable peptide tat-M2NX that inhibits TRPM2 provides protection from ischemic stroke in adult mice decreases infarct volume with a clinically relevant therapeutic window (when provided either prior to the infarct or 3 h following the insult) (Shimizu et al., 2016).

Since TRP channels are involved in numerous physiological processes, attention should be paid to potential side effects of drugs able to block TRP channels their function. Concerns predominantly relate to the roles of TRP channels in temperature sensation and regulation, immune function, and insulin release (Belrose and Jackson, 2018). Ultimately, assessment of the risk-benefit profile of TRPs as therapeutic targets will require the development of specific compounds with favorable pharmacokinetic and pharmacodynamic properties and identification of specific patient populations that would benefit the most (Belrose and Jackson, 2018). In this vein, it would be worth testing selective drugs targeting TRPs to manage neurodegeneration and treat associated symptoms such as pain and cognitive/motor dysfunction. The evidence suggests that the effectiveness of pharmacological agents regulating TRP channel activity to treat neuropathological processes and pain deserves further research. Evaluation of the risks and benefits of TRPs' use as therapeutic targets will need the development of compounds with favorable pharmacological properties and identification of specific patient populations that would benefit the most. In this regard, it would be worthy of testing selective drugs targeting TRPs to manage neurodegeneration and treat associated symptoms, such as pain and cognitive/motor dysfunctions. Furthermore, given that TRPs are involved in the progression of neurodegenerative diseases and have a role in pain, it is feasible to propose that these channels could act as central players that connect both processes, making TRP channels potential targets to treat pain in NDDs patients (Zündorf and Reiser, 2011; Naziroğlu, 2012; Echeverry et al., 2016; Maiese, 2017). Direct evidence describing the role of TRPs on pain related to NDDs development is still required, however, indirect evidence suggests that this subject deserves further research and supposes and interesting field of research.

AUTHOR CONTRIBUTIONS

MD, VV-L, ZC, SA, J-JS, and YT wrote the manuscript. All authors contributed to the article and approved the submitted version.

ACKNOWLEDGMENTS

VV-L received a postdoctoral fellowship from Departamento Administrativo de Ciencia, Tecnología e Innovación-COLCIENCIAS (contract #80740-574-2019) and Pontificia Universidad Javeriana (ID 8869). Figures were created with BioRender.

REFERENCES

Aarts, M., Iihara, K., Wei, W. L., Xiong, Z. G., Arundine, M., Cerwinski, W., et al. (2003). A key role for TRPM7 channels in anoxic neuronal death. *Cell* 115, 863–877. doi: 10.1016/S0092-8674(03)01017-1

Aarts, M. M., and Tymianski, M. (2005). TRPMs and neuronal cell death. *Pflugers Arch. Eur. J. Physiol.* 451, 243–249. doi: 10.1007/s00424-005-1439-x

Abel, T., and Zukin, R. S. (2008). Epigenetic targets of HDAC inhibition in neurodegenerative and psychiatric disorders. *Curr. Opin. Pharmacol.* 8, 57–64. doi: 10.1016/j.coph.2007.12.002

Achterberg, W. P., Pieper, M. J. C., van Dalen-Kok, A. H., de Waal, M. W. M., Husebo, B. S., Lautenbacher, S., et al. (2013). Pain management in patients with dementia. *Clin. Interv. Aging* 8, 1471–1482. doi: 10.2147/CIA.S36739

Alawieyah, S. S. M., Sim, J. A., Neubrand, V. E., and Jiang, L. H. (2018). A critical role of TRPM2 channel in Aβ42-induced microglial activation and generation of tumor necrosis factor-α. *Glia* 66, 562–575. doi: 10.1002/glia.23265

Ali, A., Arif, A. W., Bhan, C., Kumar, D., Malik, M. B., Sayyed, Z., et al. (2018). Managing chronic pain in the elderly: an overview of the recent therapeutic advancements. *Cureus* 10:e3293. doi: 10.7759/cureus.3293

Appel, S. H., Beers, D. R., and Zhao, W. (2015). "Role of inflammation in neurodegenerative diseases," in *Neurobiology of Brain Disorders: Biological Basis of Neurological and Psychiatric Disorders*, eds M. J. Zigmond, J. Coyle, and L. Rowland (Amsterdam: Elsevier Inc), 380–395. doi: 10.1016/B978-0-12-398270-4.00025-2

Arundine, M., and Tymianski, M. (2003). Molecular mechanisms of calcium-dependent neurodegeneration in excitotoxicity. *Cell Calcium* 34, 325–337. doi: 10.1016/S0143-4160(03)00141-6

Balleza-Tapia, H., Crux, S., Andrade-Talavera, Y., Dolz-Gaiton, P., Papadia, D., Chen, G., et al. (2018). TrpV1 receptor activation rescues neuronal function and network gamma oscillations from Aβ-induced impairment in mouse hippocampus in vitro. *eLife* 7:e37703. doi: 10.7554/eLife.37703

Banerjee, S., and Hasan, G. (2005). The InsP3 receptor: its role in neuronal physiology and neurodegeneration. *Bioessays* 27, 1035–1047. doi: 10.1002/bies.20298

Barcia, C., Ros, C. M., Annese, V., Gómez, A., Ros-Bernal, F., Aguado-Year, C., et al. (2011). IFN-γ signaling, with the synergistic contribution of TNF-α, mediates cell specific microglial and astroglial activation in experimental models of Parkinson's disease. *Cell Death Dis.* 2:e142. doi: 10.1038/cddis.2011.17

Basbaum, A. I., Bautista, D. M., Scherrer, G., and Julius, D. (2009). Cellular and molecular mechanisms of pain. *Cell* 139, 267–284. doi: 10.1016/j.cell.2009.09.028

Batista, P., and Pereira, A. (2016). Quality of life in patients with neurodegenerative diseases. *J. Neurol. Neurosci.* 7:7. doi: 10.21767/2171-6625.100074

Beech, D. J. (2005). TRPC1: store-operated channel and more. *Pflugers Arch. Eur. J. Physiol.* 451, 53–60. doi: 10.1007/s00424-005-1441-3

Beech, D. J., Xu, S. Z., McHugh, D., and Flemming, R. (2003). TRPC1 store-operated cationic channel subunit. *Cell Calcium* 33, 433–440. doi: 10.1016/S0143-4160(03)00054-X

Beggs, S., and Salter, M. W. (2016). SnapShot: microglia in disease. *Cell* 165, 1294–1294.e1. doi: 10.1016/j.cell.2016.05.036

Bellomo, G., Santambrogio, L., Fiacconi, M., Scarponi, A. M., and Ciuffetti, G. (1991). Plasma profiles of adrenocorticotropic hormone, cortisol, growth hormone and prolactin in patients with untreated Parkinson's disease. *J. Neurol.* 238, 19–22. doi: 10.1007/BF00319704

Belrose, J. C., and Jackson, M. F. (2018). TRPM2: a candidate therapeutic target for treating neurological diseases. *Acta Pharmacol. Sin.* 39, 722–732. doi: 10.1038/aps.2018.31

Benito, C., Tolõn, R. M., Castillo, A. I., Ruiz-Valdepeñas, L., Martínez-Orgado, J. A., Fernández-Sánchez, F. J., et al. (2012). β-Amyloid exacerbates inflammation in astrocytes lacking fatty acid amide hydrolase through a mechanism involving PPAR-α, PPAR-γ and TRPV1, but not CB1 or CB2 receptors. *Br. J. Pharmacol.* 166, 1474–1489. doi: 10.1111/j.1476-5381.2012.01889.x

Bernardini, M., Fiorio Pla, A., Prevarskaya, N., and Gkika, D. (2015). Human transient receptor potential (TRP) channels expression profiling in carcinogenesis. *Int. J. Dev. Biol.* 59, 399–406. doi: 10.1387/ijdb.150232dg

Bernd, N., and Appendino, G. (2007). Spices: the savory and beneficial science of pungency. *Rev. Physiol. Biochem. Pharmacol.* 159, 1–77. doi: 10.1007/112

Bhattacharyya, S., Ratajczak, C. K., Vogt, S. K., Kelley, C., Colonna, M., Schreiber, R. D., et al. (2010). TAK1 targeting by glucocorticoids determines JNK and IκB regulation in toll-like receptor-stimulated macrophages. *Blood* 115, 1921–1931. doi: 10.1182/blood-2009-06-224782

Bhave, G., Zhu, W., Wang, H., Brasier, D. J., Oxford, G. S., and Gereau, R. W. IV (2002). cAMP-dependent protein kinase regulates desensitization of the capsaicin receptor (VR1) by direct phosphorylation. *Neuron* 35, 721–731. doi: 10.1016/S0896-6273(02)00802-4

Bohush, A., Niewiadomska, G., and Filipek, A. (2018). Role of mitogen activated protein kinase signaling in Parkinson's disease. *Int. J. Mol. Sci.* 19:2973. doi: 10.3390/ijms19102973

Bon, R. S., and Beech, D. J. (2013). In pursuit of small molecule chemistry for calcium-permeable non-selective TRPC channels - Mirage or pot of gold? *Br. J. Pharmacol.* 170, 459–474. doi: 10.1111/bph.12274

Brewster, M. S. J., Gaudet, R., and Biology, C. (2015). Workings revealed by electron cryomicroscopy. *Bioassays* 37, 1184–1192. doi: 10.1002/bies.201500085.How

Brierley, S. M., Castro, J., Harrington, A. M., Hughes, P. A., Page, A. J., Rychkov, G. Y., et al. (2011). TRPA1 contributes to specific mechanically activated currents and sensory neuron mechanical hypersensitivity. *J. Physiol.* 589, 3575–3593. doi: 10.1113/jphysiol.2011.206789

Brini, M., Calì, T., Ottolini, D., and Carafoli, E. (2014). Neuronal calcium signaling: function and dysfunction. *Cell. Mol. Life Sci.* 71, 2787–2814. doi: 10.1007/s00018-013-1550-7

Burgess, G. M., Mullaney, I., McNeill, M., Dunn, P. M., and Rang, H. P. (1989). Second messengers involved in the mechanism of action of bradykinin in sensory neurons in culture. *J. Neurosci.* 9, 3314–3325. doi: 10.1523/jneurosci.09-09-03314.1989

Cacabelos, R. (2017). Parkinson's disease: from pathogenesis to pharmacogenomics. *Int. J. Mol. Sci.* 18:551. doi: 10.3390/ijms18030551

Cao, E. (2020). Structural mechanisms of transient receptor potential ion channels. *J. Gen. Physiol.* 152:e201811998. doi: 10.1085/jgp.201811998

Cao, S., Fisher, D. W., Yu, T., and Dong, H. (2019). The link between chronic pain and Alzheimer's disease. *J. Neuroinflammation* 16:204. doi: 10.1186/s12974-019-1608-z

Carniglia, L., Ramírez, D., Durand, D., Saba, J., Turati, J., Caruso, C., et al. (2017). Neuropeptides and microglial activation in inflammation, pain, and neurodegenerative diseases. *Mediators Inflamm.* 2017:5048616. doi: 10.1155/2017/5048616

Castaño, A., Herrera, A. J., Cano, J., and Machado, A. (2002). Lipopolysaccharide intranigral injection induces inflammatory reaction and damage in nigrostriatal dopaminergic system. *J. Neurochem.* 70, 1584–1592. doi: 10.1046/j.1471-4159.1998.70041584.x

Caterina, M. J., Rosen, T. A., Tominaga, M., Brake, A. J., and Julius, D. (1999). A capsaicin-receptor homologue with a high threshold for noxious heat. *Nature* 398, 436–441. doi: 10.1038/18906

Caterina, M. J., Schumacher, M. A., Tominaga, M., Rosen, T. A., Levine, J. D., and Julius, D. (1997). The capsaicin receptor: a heat-activated ion channel in the pain pathway. *Nature* 389, 816–824. doi: 10.1038/39807

Catterall, W. A., and Swanson, T. M. (2015). Structural basis for pharmacology of voltage-gated sodium and calcium channels. *Mol. Pharmacol.* 88, 141–150. doi: 10.1124/mol.114.097659

Channels, T. (2017). *Transient Receptor Potential Canonical Channels and Brain Diseases*. Berlin: Springer. doi: 10.1007/978-94-024-1088-4

Chen, G., Zhang, Y. Q., Qadri, Y. J., Serhan, C. N., and Ji, R. R. (2018). Microglia in pain: detrimental and protective roles in pathogenesis and resolution of pain. *Neuron* 100, 1292–1311. doi: 10.1016/j.neuron.2018.11.009

Chen, J., and Hackos, D. H. (2015). TRPA1 as a drug target - Promise and challenges. *Naunyn. Schmiedebergs. Arch. Pharmacol.* 388, 451–463. doi: 10.1007/s00210-015-1088-3

Chen, T., Yang, Y. F., Luo, P., Liu, W., Dai, S. H., Zheng, X. R., et al. (2013). Homer1 knockdown protects dopamine neurons through regulating calcium homeostasis in an in vitro model of Parkinson's disease. *Cell. Signal.* 25, 2863–2870. doi: 10.1016/j.cellsig.2013.09.004

Cheng, J., Lu, Q., Song, L., and Ho, M. S. (2018). α-Synuclein trafficking in Parkinson's disease: insights from fly and mouse models. *ASN Neuro* 10:1759091418812587. doi: 10.1177/1759091418812587

Cheng, W. (2018). "TRP ion channels: from distribution to assembly," in *Ion Channels in Health and Sickness*, ed. K. F. Shad (Rijeka: InTech). doi: 10.5772/intechopen.76479

Cheng, W., Sun, C., and Zheng, J. (2010). Heteromerization of TRP channel subunits: extending functional diversity. *Protein Cell* 1, 802–810. doi: 10.1007/s13238-010-0108-9

Cheng, W., Yang, F., Takanishi, C. L., and Zheng, J. (2007). Thermosensitive TRPV channel subunits coassemble into heteromeric channels with intermediate conductance and gating properties. *J. Gen. Physiol.* 129, 191–207. doi: 10.1085/jgp.200709731

Chi, H., Chang, H. Y., and Sang, T. K. (2018). Neuronal cell death mechanisms in major neurodegenerative diseases. *Int. J. Mol. Sci.* 19:3082. doi: 10.3390/ijms19103082

Choi, S. J., Panhelainen, A., Schmitz, Y., Larsen, K. E., Kanter, E., Wu, M., et al. (2015). Changes in neuronal dopamine homeostasis following 1-methyl-4-phenylpyridinium (MPP+) exposure. *J. Biol. Chem.* 290, 6799–6809. doi: 10.1074/jbc.M114.631556

Chubanov, V., Waldegger, S., Mederos, Y., Schnitzler, M., Vitzthum, H., Sassen, M. C., et al. (2004). Disruption of TRPM6/TRPM7 complex formation by a mutation in the TRPM6 gene causes hypomagnesemia with secondary hypocalcemia. *Proc. Natl. Acad. Sci. U.S.A.* 101, 2894–2899. doi: 10.1073/pnas.0305252101

Cohen, M. L., Kim, C., Haldiman, T., ElHag, M., Mehndiratta, P., Pichet, T., et al. (2015). Rapidly progressive Alzheimer's disease features distinct structures of amyloid-β. *Brain* 138, 1009–1022. doi: 10.1093/brain/awv006

Cortright, D. W., and Szallasi, A. (2004). Biochemical pharmacology of the vanilloid receptor TRPV1: an update. *Eur. J. Biochem.* 271, 1814–1819. doi: 10.1111/j.1432-1033.2004.04082.x

Cravello, L., Di Santo, S., Varrassi, G., Benincasa, D., Marchettini, P., de Tommaso, M., et al. (2019). Chronic pain in the elderly with cognitive decline: a narrative review. *Pain Ther.* 8, 53–65. doi: 10.1007/s40122-019-0111-7

Cuffe, J. S. M., Steane, S., Moritz, K. M., and Paravicini, T. M. (2015). Differential mRNA expression and glucocorticoid-mediated regulation of TRPM6 and TRPM7 in the heart and kidney throughout murine pregnancy and development. *PLoS One* 10:e0117978. doi: 10.1371/journal.pone.0117978

Danzer, K. M., Haasen, D., Karow, A. R., Moussaud, S., Habeck, M., Giese, A., et al. (2007). Different species of α-synuclein oligomers induce calcium influx and seeding. *J. Neurosci.* 27, 9220–9232. doi: 10.1523/JNEUROSCI.2617-07.2007

De La Roche, J., Eberhardt, M. J., Klinger, A. B., Stanslowsky, N., Wegner, F., Koppert, W., et al. (2013). The molecular basis for species-specific activation of human TRPA1 protein by protons involves poorly conserved residues within transmembrane domains 5 and 6. *J. Biol. Chem.* 288, 20280–20292. doi: 10.1074/jbc.M113.479337

De Logu, F., Nassini, R., Materazzi, S., Carvalho Gonçalves, M., Nosi, D., Rossi Degl'Innocenti, D., et al. (2017). Schwann cell TRPA1 mediates neuroinflammation that sustains macrophage-dependent neuropathic pain in mice. *Nat. Commun.* 8:1887. doi: 10.1038/s41467-017-01739-2

de Tommaso, M., Kunz, M., and Valeriani, M. (2017). Therapeutic approach to pain in neurodegenerative diseases: current evidence and perspectives. *Expert Rev. Neurother.* 17, 143–153. doi: 10.1080/14737175.2016.1210512

Derry, S., Rice, A. S. C. S., Cole, P., Tan, T., and Moore, R. A. (2017). *Topical Capsaicin (high concentration) for Chronic Neuropathic Pain in Adults.* Chichester: John Wiley and Sons Ltd. doi: 10.1002/14651858.CD007393.pub4

Devesa, I., Planells-Cases, R., Fernández-Ballester, G., González-Ros, J. M., Ferrer-Montiel, A., and Fernández-Carvajal, A. (2011). Role of the transient receptor potential vanilloid 1 in inflammation and sepsis. *J. Inflamm. Res.* 4, 67–81. doi: 10.2147/JIR.S12978

Drennan, D., and Ryazanov, A. G. (2004). Alpha-kinases: analysis of the family and comparison with conventional protein kinases. *Prog. Biophys. Mol. Biol.* 85, 1–32. doi: 10.1016/S0079-6107(03)00060-9

Du, J., Ma, X., Shen, B., Huang, Y., Birnbaumer, L., and Yao, X. (2014). TRPV4, TRPC1, and TRPP2 assemble to form a flow-sensitive heteromeric channel. *FASEB J.* 28, 4677–4685. doi: 10.1096/fj.14-251652

Dugger, B. N., and Dickson, D. W. (2017). Pathology of neurodegenerative diseases. *Cold Spring Harb. Perspect. Biol.* 9:a028035. doi: 10.1101/cshperspect.a028035

Echeverry, S., Rodriguez, M. J., and Torres, Y. P. (2016). Transient receptor potential channels in microglia: roles in physiology and disease. *Neurotox. Res.* 30, 467–478. doi: 10.1007/s12640-016-9632-6

Erkkinen, M. G., Kim, M. O., and Geschwind, M. D. (2018). Clinical neurology and epidemiology of the major neurodegenerative diseases. *Cold Spring Harb. Perspect. Biol.* 10:a033118. doi: 10.1101/cshperspect.a033118

Fenton, B. W., Shih, E., and Zolton, J. (2015). The neurobiology of pain perception in normal and persistent pain. *Pain Manag.* 5, 297–317. doi: 10.2217/pmt.15.27

Fernandes, E. S., Fernandes, M. A., and Keeble, J. E. (2012). The functions of TRPA1 and TRPV1: moving away from sensory nerves. *Br. J. Pharmacol.* 166, 510–521. doi: 10.1111/j.1476-5381.2012.01851.x

Ferreiro, E., Oliveira, C. R., and Pereira, C. M. F. (2008). The release of calcium from the endoplasmic reticulum induced by amyloid-beta and prion peptides activates the mitochondrial apoptotic pathway. *Neurobiol. Dis.* 30, 331–342. doi: 10.1016/j.nbd.2008.02.003

Fleig, A., and Penner, R. (2004). The TRPM ion channel subfamily: molecular, biophysical and functional features. *Trends Pharmacol. Sci.* 25, 633–639. doi: 10.1016/j.tips.2004.10.004

Fliegert, R., Bauche, A., Wolf Pérez, A. M., Watt, J. M., Rozewitz, M. D., Winzer, R., et al. (2017). 2′-Deoxyadenosine 5′-diphosphoribose is an endogenous TRPM2 superagonist. *Nat. Chem. Biol.* 13, 1036–1044. doi: 10.1038/nchembio.2415

Fonfria, E., Marshall, I. C. B., Boyfield, I., Skaper, S. D., Hughes, J. P., Owen, D. E., et al. (2005). Amyloid β-peptide(1-42) and hydrogen peroxide-induced toxicity are mediated by TRPM2 in rat primary striatal cultures. *J. Neurochem.* 95, 715–723. doi: 10.1111/j.1471-4159.2005.03396.x

Fowler, M. A., Sidiropoulou, K., Ozkan, E. D., Phillips, C. W., and Cooper, D. C. (2007). Corticolimbic expression of TRPC4 and TRPC5 channels in the rodent brain. *PLoS One* 2:e573. doi: 10.1371/journal.pone.0000573

Freichel, M., Vennekens, R., Olausson, J., Stolz, S., Philipp, S. E., Weißgerber, P., et al. (2005). Functional role of TRPC proteins in native systems: implications from knockout and knock-down studies. *J. Physiol.* 567, 59–66. doi: 10.1113/jphysiol.2005.092999

Frias, B., and Merighi, A. (2016). Capsaicin, nociception and pain. *Molecules* 21:797. doi: 10.3390/molecules21060797

Fujita, F., Uchida, K., Moriyama, T., Shima, A., Shibasaki, K., Inada, H., et al. (2008). Intracellular alkalization causes pain sensation through activation of TRPA1 in mice. *J. Clin. Invest.* 118, 4049–4057. doi: 10.1172/JCI35957

Fujiwara, Y., and Minor, D. L. (2008). X-ray crystal structure of a TRPM assembly domain reveals an antiparallel four-stranded coiled-coil. *J. Mol. Biol.* 383, 854–870. doi: 10.1016/j.jmb.2008.08.059

Gaudet, R. (2008). TRP channels entering the structural era. *J. Physiol.* 586, 3565–3575. doi: 10.1113/jphysiol.2008.155812

Gees, M., Colsoul, B., and Nilius, B. (2010). The role of transient receptor potential cation channels in Ca2+ signaling. *Cold Spring Harb. Perspect. Biol.* 2:a003962. doi: 10.1101/cshperspect.a003962

Geon, H. K., Kim, J. E., Rhie, S. J., and Yoon, S. (2015). The role for oxidative stress in neurodegenerative diseases. *Exp. Neurol.* 24, 325–340. doi: 10.5607/en.2015.24.4.325

Goldenberg, N. M., Wang, L., Ranke, H., Liedtke, W., Tabuchi, A., and Kuebler, W. M. (2015). TRPV4 is required for hypoxic pulmonary vasoconstriction. *Anesthesiology* 122, 1338–1348. doi: 10.1097/ALN.0000000000000647

Gopalakrishna, R., and Jaken, S. (2000). Protein kinase C signaling and oxidative stress. *Free Radic. Biol. Med.* 28, 1349–1361. doi: 10.1016/S0891-5849(00)00221-5

Guo, Q., Fu, W., Sopher, B. L., Miller, M. W., Ware, C. B., Martin, G. M., et al. (1999). Increased vulnerability of hippocampal neurons to excitotoxic necrosis in presenilin-1 mutant knock-in mice. *Nat. Med.* 5, 101–106. doi: 10.1038/4789

Guo, Q., Furukawa, K., Sopher, B. L., Pham, D. G., Xie, J., Robinson, N., et al. (1997). Alzheimer's PS-1 mutation perturbs calcium homeostasis and sensitizes PC12 cells to death induced by amyloid β-peptide. *Neuroreport* 8, 379–383. doi: 10.1097/00001756-199612200-00074

Hara, Y., Wakamori, M., Ishii, M., Maeno, E., Nishida, M., Yoshida, T., et al. (2002). LTRPC2 Ca2+-Permeable channel activated by changes in redox status confers susceptibility to cell death. *Mol. Cell* 9, 163–173. doi: 10.1016/S1097-2765(01)00438-5

Harada, N., and Okajima, K. (2006). Regulation of inflammatory responses by sensory neurons: molecular mechanism(s) and possible therapeutic applications. *Curr. Med. Chem.* 13, 2241–2251. doi: 10.2174/092986706777935131

Haraguchi, K., Kawamoto, A., Isami, K., Maeda, S., Kusano, A., Asakura, K., et al. (2012). TRPM2 contributes to inflammatory and neuropathic pain through the aggravation of pronociceptive inflammatory responses in mice. *J. Neurosci.* 32, 3931–3941. doi: 10.1523/JNEUROSCI.4703-11.2012

Harteneck, C., and Leuner, K. (2014). "TRP channels in neuronal and glial signal transduction," in *Neurochemistry*, ed. T. Heinbockel (Rijeka: InTech). doi: 10.5772/58232

Hellwig, N., Albrecht, N., Harteneck, C., Schultz, G., and Schaefer, M. (2005). Homo- and heteromeric assembly of TRPV channel subunits. *J. Cell Sci.* 118, 917–928. doi: 10.1242/jcs.01675

Hong, C., Seo, H., Kwak, M., Jeon, J., Jang, J., Jeong, E. M., et al. (2015). Increased TRPC5 glutathionylation contributes to striatal neuron loss in Huntington's disease. *Brain* 138, 3030–3047. doi: 10.1093/brain/awv188

Horváth, Á., Tékus, V., Boros, M., Pozsgai, G., Botz, B., Borbély, É., et al. (2016). Transient receptor potential ankyrin 1 (TRPA1) receptor is involved in chronic arthritis: *in vivo* study using TRPA1-deficient mice. *Arthritis Res. Ther.* 18:6. doi: 10.1186/s13075-015-0904-y

Huang, Y., Fliegert, R., Guse, A. H., Lü, W., and Du, J. (2020). A structural overview of the ion channels of the TRPM family. *Cell Calcium* 85:102111. doi: 10.1016/j.ceca.2019.102111

Hung, C. Y., and Tan, C. H. (2018). TRP channels in nociception and pathological pain. *Adv. Exp. Med. Biol.* 1099, 13–27. doi: 10.1007/978-981-13-1756-9_2

Hwang, I., Harper, J. F., Liang, F., and Sze, H. (2000). Calmodulin activation of an endoplasmic reticulum-located calcium pump involves an interaction with the N-terminal autoinhibitory domain. *Plant Physiol.* 122, 157–167. doi: 10.1104/pp.122.1.157

Inoue, K., and Tsuda, M. (2018). Microglia in neuropathic pain: cellular and molecular mechanisms and therapeutic potential. *Nat. Rev. Neurosci.* 19, 138–152. doi: 10.1038/nrn.2018.2

Jaquemar, D., Schenker, T., and Trueb, B. (1999). An ankyrin-like protein with transmembrane domains is specifically lost after oncogenic transformation of human fibroblasts. *J. Biol. Chem.* 274, 7325–7333. doi: 10.1074/jbc.274.11.7325

Jeong, H., Kim, Y. H., Lee, Y., Jung, S. J., and Oh, S. B. (2017). TRPM2 contributes to LPC-induced intracellular Ca2+ influx and microglial activation. *Biochem. Biophys. Res. Commun.* 485, 301–306. doi: 10.1016/j.bbrc.2017.02.087

Ji, R. R., Berta, T., and Nedergaard, M. (2013). Glia and pain: Is chronic pain a gliopathy? *Pain* 154, S10–S28. doi: 10.1016/j.pain.2013.06.022

Ji, R. R., and Suter, M. R. (2007). p38 MAPK, microglial signaling, and neuropathic pain. *Mol. Pain* 3:33. doi: 10.1186/1744-8069-3-33

Jin, S. X., Zhuang, Z. Y., Woolf, C. J., and Ji, R. R. (2003). p38 mitogen-activated protein kinase is activated after a spinal nerve ligation in spinal cord microglia and dorsal root ganglion neurons and contributes to the generation of neuropathic pain. *J. Neurosci.* 23, 4017–4022. doi: 10.1523/jneurosci.23-10-04017.2003

Jin, X., Morsy, N., Winston, J., Pasricha, P. J., Garrett, K., and Akbarali, H. I. (2004). Modulation of TRPV1 by nonreceptor tyrosine kinase, c-Src kinase. *Am. J. Physiol. Cell Physiol.* 287, 558–563. doi: 10.1152/ajpcell.00113.2004

Jost, W. H., and Buhmann, C. (2019). The challenge of pain in the pharmacological management of Parkinson's disease. *Expert Opin. Pharmacother.* 20, 1847–1854. doi: 10.1080/14656566.2019.1639672

Julius, D. (2013). TRP Channels and Pain. *Annu. Rev. Cell Dev. Biol.* 29, 355–384. doi: 10.1146/annurev-cellbio-101011-155833

Jung, J., Shin, J. S., Lee, S. Y., Hwang, S. W., Koo, J., Cho, H., et al. (2004). Phosphorylation of Vanilloid Receptor 1 by Ca 2+/Calmodulin-dependent Kinase II Regulates Its Vanilloid Binding. *J. Biol. Chem.* 279, 7048–7054. doi: 10.1074/jbc.M311448200

Kaneko, S., Kawakami, S., Hara, Y., Wakamori, M., Itoh, E., Minami, T., et al. (2006). A critical role of TRPM2 in neuronal cell death by hydrogen peroxide. *J. Pharmacol. Sci.* 101, 66–76. doi: 10.1254/jphs.FP0060128

Kashio, M., Sokabe, T., Shintaku, K., Uematsu, T., Fukuta, N., Kobayashi, N., et al. (2012). Redox signal-mediated sensitization of transient receptor potential melastatin 2 (TRPM2) to temperature affects macrophage functions. *Proc. Natl. Acad. Sci. U.S.A.* 109, 6745–6750. doi: 10.1073/pnas.1114193109

Katz, B., Payne, R., and Minke, B. (2017). "TRP channels in vision," in *Neurobiology of TRP Channels*, ed. T. L. R. Emir (Boca Raton, FL: CRC Press), 27–63. doi: 10.4324/9781315152837

Kauer, J. A., and Gibson, H. E. (2009). Hot flash: TRPV channels in the brain. *Trends Neurosci.* 32, 215–224. doi: 10.1016/j.tins.2008.12.006

Kheiri, G., Dolatshahi, M., Rahmani, F., and Rezaei, N. (2019). Role of p38/MAPKs in Alzheimer's disease: implications for amyloid beta toxicity targeted therapy. *Rev. Neurosci.* 30, 9–30. doi: 10.1515/revneuro-2018-0008

Kiani, J., Sajedi, F., Nasrollahi, S. A., and Esna-Ashari, F. (2015). A randomized clinical trial of efficacy and safety of the topical clonidine and capsaicin in the treatment of painful diabetic neuropathy. *J. Res. Med. Sci.* 20, 359–363.

Kim, E. Y., Anderson, M., Wilson, C., Hagmann, H., Benzing, T., and Dryer, S. E. (2013). NOX2 interacts with podocyte TRPC6 channels and contributes to their activation by diacylglycerol: essential role of podocin in formation of this complex. *Am. J. Physiol. Cell Physiol.* 305, 960–971. doi: 10.1152/ajpcell.00191.2013

Kim, J., Kwak, M., Jeon, J. P., Myeong, J., Wie, J., Hong, C., et al. (2014). Isoform- and receptor-specific channel property of canonical transient receptor potential (TRPC)1/4 channels. *Pflugers Arch. Eur. J. Physiol.* 466, 491–504. doi: 10.1007/s00424-013-1332-y

Kim, K. I., Chung, Y. C., and Jin, B. K. (2018). Norfluoxetine prevents degeneration of dopamine neurons by inhibiting microglia-derived oxidative stress in an MPTP Mouse model of Parkinson's disease. *Mediators Inflamm.* 2018:4591289. doi: 10.1155/2018/4591289

Kim, S., Barry, D. M., Liu, X. Y., Yin, S., Munanairi, A., Meng, Q. T., et al. (2016). Facilitation of TRPV4 by TRPV1 is required for itch transmission in some sensory neuron populations. *Sci. Signal.* 9:ra71. doi: 10.1126/scisignal.aaf1047

Kim, S. R., Lee, D. Y., Chung, E. S., Oh, U. T., Kim, S. U., and Jin, B. K. (2005). Transient receptor potential vanilloid subtype 1 mediates cell death of mesencephalic dopaminergic neurons *in vivo* and *in vitro*. *J. Neurosci.* 25, 662–671. doi: 10.1523/JNEUROSCI.4166-04.2005

Kim, S. U. S. R., Kim, S. U. S. R., Oh, U., and Jin, B. K. (2006). Transient receptor potential vanilloid subtype 1 mediates microglial cell death *in vivo* and in vitro via Ca 2+ -mediated mitochondrial damage and cytochrome c release. *J. Immunol.* 177, 4322–4329. doi: 10.4049/jimmunol.177.7.4322

Kimura, H. (2015). Signaling molecules: hydrogen sulfide and polysulfide. *Antioxid. Redox Signal.* 22, 362–376. doi: 10.1089/ars.2014.5869

Kitajima, N., Watanabe, K., Morimoto, S., Sato, Y., Kiyonaka, S., Hoshijima, M., et al. (2011). TRPC3-mediated Ca2+ influx contributes to Rac1-mediated production of reactive oxygen species in MLP-deficient mouse hearts. *Biochem. Biophys. Res. Commun.* 409, 108–113. doi: 10.1016/j.bbrc.2011.04.124

Kono, T., Kaneko, A., Omiya, Y., Ohbuchi, K., Ohno, N., and Yamamoto, M. (2013). Epithelial transient receptor potential ankyrin 1 (TRPA1)-dependent adrenomedullin upregulates blood flow in rat small intestine. *Am. J. Physiol. Gastrointest. Liver Physiol.* 304, 428–436. doi: 10.1152/ajpgi.00356.2012

Kovacs, G. G. (2016). Molecular pathological classification of neurodegenerative diseases: turning towards precision medicine. *Int. J. Mol. Sci.* 17:189. doi: 10.3390/ijms17020189

Kraft, R. (2015). STIM and ORAI proteins in the nervous system. *Channels* 9, 245–252. doi: 10.1080/19336950.2015.1071747

Kraft, R., and Harteneck, C. (2005). The mammalian melastatin-related transient receptor potential cation channels: an overview. *Pflugers Arch. Eur. J. Physiol.* 451, 204–211. doi: 10.1007/s00424-005-1428-0

Kurkowska-Jastrzębska, I., Litwin, T., Joniec, I., Ciesielska, A., Przybyłkowski, A., Członkowski, A., et al. (2004). Dexamethasone protects against dopaminergic neurons damage in a mouse model of Parkinson's disease. *Int. Immunopharmacol* 4, 1307–1318. doi: 10.1016/j.intimp.2004.05.006

Kurudenkandy, F. R., Zilberter, M., Biverstål, H., Presto, J., Honcharenko, D., Strömberg, R., et al. (2014). Amyloid-β-induced action potential desynchronization and degradation of hippocampal gamma oscillations is prevented by interference with peptide conformation change and aggregation. *J. Neurosci.* 34, 11416–11425. doi: 10.1523/JNEUROSCI.1195-14.2014

Landman, N., Jeong, S. Y., Shin, S. Y., Voronov, S. V., Serban, G., Kang, M. S., et al. (2006). Presenilin mutations linked to familial Alzheimer's disease cause an imbalance in phosphatidylinositol 4,5-bisphosphate metabolism. *Proc. Natl. Acad. Sci. U.S.A.* 103, 19524–19529. doi: 10.1073/pnas.0604954103

Laursen, W. J., Bagriantsev, S. N., and Gracheva, E. O. (2014). TRPA1 channels: chemical and temperature sensitivity. *Curr. Top. Membr.* 74, 89–112. doi: 10.1016/B978-0-12-800181-3.00004-X

Lee, E., Hwang, I., Park, S., Hong, S., Hwang, B., Cho, Y., et al. (2019). MPTP-driven NLRP3 inflammasome activation in microglia plays a central role in dopaminergic neurodegeneration. *Cell Death Differ.* 26, 213–228. doi: 10.1038/s41418-018-0124-5

Lee, J. K., and Kim, N. J. (2017). Recent advances in the inhibition of p38 MAPK as a potential strategy for the treatment of Alzheimer's disease. *Molecules* 22:1287. doi: 10.3390/molecules22081287

Lee, K. I., Lee, H., Lin, H. C., Tsay, H. J., Tsai, F. C., Shyue, S. K., et al. (2016). Role of transient receptor potential ankyrin 1 channels in Alzheimer's disease. *J. Neuroinflammation* 13:92. doi: 10.1186/s12974-016-0557-z

Li, L. M., Liu, Q. H., Qiao, J. T., and Zhang, C. (2009). Aβ31-35-induced neuronal apoptosis is mediated by JNK-dependent extrinsic apoptosis pathway. *Neurosci. Bull.* 25, 361–366. doi: 10.1007/s12264-009-0629-5

Liao, Y., Erxleben, C., Abramowitz, J., Flockerzi, V., Zhu, M. X., and Armstrong, D. L. (2008). STIM1 suggest a STIM-regulated heteromeric Orai / TRPC model for SOCE / Icrac channels. *Proc. Natl. Acad. Sci. U.S.A.* 105, 2895–2900. doi: 10.1073/pnas.0712288105

Liu, B., and Qin, F. (2005). Functional control of cold- and menthol-sensitive TRPM8 ion channels by phosphatidylinositol 4,5-bisphosphate. *J. Neurosci.* 25, 1674–1681. doi: 10.1523/JNEUROSCI.3632-04.2005

Lopes, S., Lopes, A., Pinto, V., Guimarães, M. R., Sardinha, V. M., Duarte-Silva, S., et al. (2016). Absence of Tau triggers age-dependent sciatic nerve morphofunctional deficits and motor impairment. *Aging Cell* 15, 208–216. doi: 10.1111/acel.12391

López-Requena, A., Boonen, B., Van Gerven, L., Hellings, P. W., Alpizar, Y. A., and Talavera, K. (2019). "Roles of neuronal TRP channels in neuroimmune interactions," in *Neurobiology of TRP Channels*, 2nd Edn, ed. T. L. R. Emir (Boca Raton, FL: CRC Press), 277–294. doi: 10.4324/9781315152837-15

Lucas, P., Ukhanov, K., Leinders-Zufall, T., and Zufall, F. (2003). A diacylglycerol-gated cation channel in vomeronasal neuron dendrites is impaired in TRPC2 mutant mice: Mechanism of pheromone transduction. *Neuron* 40, 551–561. doi: 10.1016/S0896-6273(03)00675-5

Lynch, M. E., and Watson, C. P. N. (2006). The pharmacotherapy of chronic pain: a review. *Pain Res. Manag.* 11, 11–38. doi: 10.1155/2006/642568

Ma, W., and Quirion, R. (2007). Inflammatory mediators modulating the transient receptor potential vanilloid 1 receptor: therapeutic targets to treat inflammatory and neuropathic pain. *Expert Opin. Ther. Targets* 11, 307–320. doi: 10.1517/14728222.11.3.307

Ma, X., Cheng, K. T., Wong, C. O., O'Neil, R. G., Birnbaumer, L., Ambudkar, I. S., et al. (2011). Heteromeric TRPV4-C1 channels contribute to store-operated Ca2+ entry in vascular endothelial cells. *Cell Calcium* 50, 502–509. doi: 10.1016/j.ceca.2011.08.006

Maatouk, L., Compagnion, A. C., Sauvage, M. C., Bemelmans, A. P., Leclere-Turbant, S., Cirotteau, V., et al. (2018). TLR9 activation via microglial glucocorticoid receptors contributes to degeneration of midbrain dopamine neurons. *Nat. Commun.* 9:2450. doi: 10.1038/s41467-018-04569-y

Maiese, K. (2017). Warming up to new possibilities with the capsaicin receptor TRPV1: mTOR, AMPK, and Erythropoietin. *Curr. Neurovasc. Res.* 14, 184–189. doi: 10.2174/1567202614666170313105337

Malczyk, M., Veith, C., Schermuly, R. T., Gudermann, T., Dietrich, A., Sommer, N., et al. (2016). NADPH oxidases—do they play a role in TRPC regulation under hypoxia? *Pflugers Arch. Eur. J. Physiol.* 468, 23–41. doi: 10.1007/s00424-015-1731-3

Mandadi, S., Sokabe, T., Shibasaki, K., Katanosaka, K., Mizuno, A., Moqrich, A., et al. (2009). TRPV3 in keratinocytes transmits temperature information to sensory neurons via ATP. *Pflugers Arch. Eur. J. Physiol.* 458, 1093–1102. doi: 10.1007/s00424-009-0703-x

Mandel, S., Grünblatt, E., Riederer, P., Gerlach, M., Levites, Y., and Youdim, M. B. H. (2003). Neuroprotective strategies in Parkinson's disease: an update on progress. *CNS Drugs* 17, 729–762. doi: 10.2165/00023210-200317100-00004

Mano, H., and Seymour, B. (2015). Pain: A distributed brain information network? *PLoS Biol* 13:e1002037. doi: 10.1371/journal.pbio.1002037

Marambaud, P., Dreses-Werringloer, U., and Vingtdeux, V. (2009). Calcium signaling in neurodegeneration. *Mol. Neurodegener.* 4:20. doi: 10.1186/1750-1326-4-20

McCaddon, A., Hudson, P., Hill, D., Barber, J., Lloyd, A., Davies, G., et al. (2003). Alzheimer's disease and total plasma aminothiols. *Biol. Psychiatry* 53, 254–260. doi: 10.1016/s0006-3223(02)01451-8

Meents, J. E., Ciotu, C. I., and Fischer, M. J. M. (2019). Trpa1: a molecular view. *J. Neurophysiol.* 121, 427–443. doi: 10.1152/jn.00524.2018

Meents, J. E., Fischer, M. J. M., and McNaughton, P. A. (2017). Sensitization of TRPA1 by Protein Kinase A. *PLoS One* 12:e0170097. doi: 10.1371/journal.pone.0170097

Mickle, A. D., Shepherd, A. J., and Mohapatra, D. P. (2015). Sensory TRP channels: the key transducers of nociception and pain. *Prog. Mol. Biol. Transl. Sci.* 131, 73–118. doi: 10.1016/bs.pmbts.2015.01.002

Miller, B. A. (2006). The role of TRP channels in oxidative stress-induced cell death. *J. Membr. Biol.* 209, 31–41. doi: 10.1007/s00232-005-0839-3

Minke, B., and Cook, B. (2002). TRP channel proteins and signal transduction. *Physiol. Rev.* 82, 429–472. doi: 10.1152/physrev.00001.2002

Miyake, T., Shirakawa, H., Kusano, A., Sakimoto, S., Konno, M., Nakagawa, T., et al. (2014). TRPM2 contributes to LPS/IFNγ-induced production of nitric oxide via the p38/JNK pathway in microglia. *Biochem. Biophys. Res. Commun.* 444, 212–217. doi: 10.1016/j.bbrc.2014.01.022

Mizoguchi, Y., Kato, T. A., Seki, Y., Ohgidani, M., Sagata, N., Horikawa, H., et al. (2014). Brain-derived neurotrophic factor (BDNF) induces sustained intracellular Ca2+ elevation through the up-regulation of surface transient receptor potential 3 (TRPC3) channels in rodent microglia. *J. Biol. Chem.* 289, 18549–18555. doi: 10.1074/jbc.M114.555334

Mizushima, T., Obata, K., Katsura, H., Yamanaka, H., Kobayashi, K., Dai, Y., et al. (2006). Noxious cold stimulation induces mitogen-activated protein kinase activation in transient receptor potential (TRP) channels TRPA1- and TRPM8-containing small sensory neurons. *Neuroscience* 140, 1337–1348. doi: 10.1016/j.neuroscience.2006.03.024

Moilanen, L. J., Hämäläinen, M., Lehtimäki, L., Nieminen, R. M., Muraki, K., and Moilanen, E. (2016). Pinosylvin Inhibits TRPA1-induced calcium influx *in vitro* and TRPA1-mediated acute paw inflammation *in vivo*. *Basic Clin. Pharmacol. Toxicol.* 118, 238–242. doi: 10.1111/bcpt.12485

Moilanen, L. J., Hämäläinen, M., Nummenmaa, E., Ilmarinen, P., Vuolteenaho, K., Nieminen, R. M., et al. (2015). Monosodium iodoacetate-induced inflammation and joint pain are reduced in TRPA1 deficient mice - potential role of TRPA1 in osteoarthritis. *Osteoarthr. Cartil.* 23, 2017–2026. doi: 10.1016/j.joca.2015.09.008

Monroe, T. B., Gore, J. C., Chen, L. M., Mion, L. C., and Cowan, R. L. (2012). Pain in people with Alzheimer disease: potential applications for psychophysical and neurophysiological research. *J. Geriatr. Psychiatry Neurol.* 25, 240–255. doi: 10.1177/0891988712466457

Moparthi, L., Kichko, T. I., Eberhardt, M., Högestätt, E. D., Kjellbom, P., Johanson, U., et al. (2016). Human TRPA1 is a heat sensor displaying intrinsic U-shaped thermosensitivity. *Sci. Rep.* 6:28763. doi: 10.1038/srep28763

Moran, M. M. (2018). TRP channels as potential drug targets. *Annu. Rev. Pharmacol. Toxicol.* 58, 309–330. doi: 10.1146/annurev-pharmtox-010617-052832

Moran, M. M., and Szallasi, A. (2018). Targeting nociceptive transient receptor potential channels to treat chronic pain: current state of the field. *Br. J. Pharmacol.* 175, 2185–2203. doi: 10.1111/bph.14044

Moran, M. M., Xu, H., and Clapham, D. E. (2004). TRP ion channels in the nervous system. *Curr. Opin. Neurobiol.* 14, 362–369. doi: 10.1016/j.conb.2004.05.003

Mori, Y., Takahashi, N., Polat, O. K., Kurokawa, T., Takeda, N., and Inoue, M. (2016). Redox-sensitive transient receptor potential channels in oxygen sensing and adaptation. *Pflugers Arch. Eur. J. Physiol.* 468, 85–97. doi: 10.1007/s00424-015-1716-2

Moriarty, O., and Finn, D. P. (2014). Cognition and pain. *Curr. Opin. Support. Palliat. Care* 8, 130–136. doi: 10.1097/SPC.0000000000000054

Muller, C., Morales, P., and Reggio, P. H. (2019). Cannabinoid ligands targeting TRP channels. *Front. Mol. Neurosci.* 11:487. doi: 10.3389/fnmol.2018.00487

Muroyama, A., Inaka, M., Matsushima, H., Sugino, H., Marunaka, Y., and Mitsumoto, Y. (2009). Enhanced susceptibility to MPTP neurotoxicity in magnesium-deficient C57BL/6N mice. *Neurosci. Res.* 63, 72–75. doi: 10.1016/j.neures.2008.09.009

Nadler, M. J. S., Hermosura, M. C., Inabe, K., Perraud, A. L., Zhu, Q., Stokes, A. J., et al. (2001). LTRPC7 is a Mg·ATP-regulated divalent cation channel required for cell viability. *Nature* 411, 590–595. doi: 10.1038/35079092

Nakamura, T., and Lipton, S. A. (2009). Cell death: protein misfolding and neurodegenerative diseases. *Apoptosis* 14, 455–468. doi: 10.1007/s10495-008-0301-y

Nazıroğlu, M., Öz, A., and Yıldızhan, K. (2020). Selenium and neurological diseases: focus on peripheral pain and TRP channels. *Curr. Neuropharmacol.* 18, 501–517. doi: 10.2174/1570159x18666200106152631

Naziroğlu, M. (2012). Molecular role of catalase on oxidative stress-induced Ca2 signaling and TRP cation channel activation in nervous system. *J. Recept. Signal Transduct.* 32, 134–141. doi: 10.3109/10799893.2012.672994

Nevzati, E., Schatlo, B., Fathi, A.-R., Fandino, J., and Muroi, C. (2014). Intraoperative visualization of bilateral thrombosis in the posterior inferior cerebellar artery apparent in the telovelomedullary segment. *Case Rep. Neurol. Med.* 2014:247652. doi: 10.1155/2014/247652

Nilius, B. (2012). Transient receptor potential (TRP) channels in the brain: the good and the ugly. *Eur. Rev.* 20, 343–355. doi: 10.1017/S1062798711000597

Nilius, B., and Flockerzi, V. (2014). Handbook of experimental pharmacology–mammalian transient receptor potential (TRP) cation channels. *Handb. Exp. Pharmacol.* 223, 1119–1142. doi: 10.1007/978-3-319-05161-1

Nilius, B., and Owsianik, G. (2011). The transient receptor potential family of ion channels. *Genome Biol.* 12:218. doi: 10.1186/gb-2011-12-3-218

Nilius, B., and Szallasi, A. (2014). Transient receptor potential channels as drug targets: from the science of basic research to the art of medicine. *Pharmacol. Rev.* 66, 676–814. doi: 10.1124/pr.113.008268

Nilius, B., and Szallasi, A. (2015). "Are brain TRPs viable targets for curing neurodegenerative disorders and improving mental health?" in *TRP Channels as Therapeutic Targets: From Basic Science to Clinical Use*, ed. A. Szallasi (Amsterdam: Elsevier Inc), 419–456. doi: 10.1016/B978-0-12-420024-1.00023-0

Nilius, B., Talavera, K., Owsianik, G., Prenen, J., Droogmans, G., and Voets, T. (2005). Gating of TRP channels: A voltage connection? *J. Physiol.* 567, 35–44. doi: 10.1113/jphysiol.2005.088377

Nilius, B., Vennekens, R., and Owsianik, G. (2008). Vanilloid transient receptor potential cation channels: an overview. *Curr. Pharm. Des.* 14, 18–31. doi: 10.2174/138161208783330763

Numaga-Tomita, T., Oda, S., Nishiyama, K., Tanaka, T., Nishimura, A., and Nishida, M. (2019). TRPC channels in exercise-mimetic therapy. *Pflugers Arch. Eur. J. Physiol.* 471, 507–517. doi: 10.1007/s00424-018-2211-3

Oancea, E., Wicks, N. L., and Gene, M. (2011). "TRPM7, the Mg2+ Inhibited Channel and Kinase," in *Advances in Experimental Medicine and Biology*, ed. M. Islam (Dordrecht: Springer), 135–145. doi: 10.1007/978-94-007-0265-3

Oh, C. K., Han, B. S., Choi, W. S., Youdim, M. B. H., and Oh, Y. J. (2011). Translocation and oligomerization of Bax is regulated independently by activation of p38 MAPK and caspase-2 during MN9D dopaminergic neurodegeneration. *Apoptosis* 16, 1087–1100. doi: 10.1007/s10495-011-0627-8

Orrenius, S., Zhivotovsky, B., and Nicotera, P. (2003). Regulation of cell death: the calcium-apoptosis link. *Nat. Rev. Mol. Cell Biol.* 4, 552–565. doi: 10.1038/nrm1150

Ostapchenko, V. G., Chen, M., Guzman, M. S., Xie, Y. F., Lavine, N., Fan, J., et al. (2015). The transient receptor potential melastatin 2 (TRPM2) channel contributes to β-amyloid oligomer-related neurotoxicity and memory impairment. *J. Neurosci.* 35, 15157–15169. doi: 10.1523/JNEUROSCI.4081-14.2015

Owsianik, G., Talavera, K., Voets, T., and Nilius, B. (2006). Permeation and selectivity of trp channels. *Annu. Rev. Physiol.* 68, 685–717. doi: 10.1146/annurev.physiol.68.040204.101406

Oyanagi, K., Kawakami, E., Kikuchi-Horie, K., Ohara, K., Ogata, K., Takahama, S., et al. (2006). Magnesium deficiency over generations in rats with special references to the pathogenesis of the parkinsonism-dementia complex and amyotrophic lateral sclerosis of Guam. *Neuropathology* 26, 115–128. doi: 10.1111/j.1440-1789.2006.00672.x

Pamplona, F. A., Pandolfo, P., Duarte, F. S., Takahashi, R. N., and Prediger, R. D. S. (2010). Altered emotionality leads to increased pain tolerance in amyloid β (Aβ1-40) peptide-treated mice. *Behav. Brain Res.* 212, 96–102. doi: 10.1016/j.bbr.2010.03.052

Parekh, A. B., and Putney, J. W. (2005). Store-operated calcium channels. *Physiol. Rev.* 85, 757–810. doi: 10.1152/physrev.00057.2003

Park, E. S., Kim, S. R., and Jin, B. K. (2012). Transient receptor potential vanilloid subtype 1 contributes to mesencephalic dopaminergic neuronal survival by inhibiting microglia-originated oxidative stress. *Brain Res. Bull.* 89, 92–96. doi: 10.1016/j.brainresbull.2012.07.001

Park, L., Wang, G., Moore, J., Girouard, H., Zhou, P., Anrather, J., et al. (2014). The key role of transient receptor potential melastatin-2 channels in amyloid-β-induced neurovascular dysfunction. *Nat. Commun.* 5:5318. doi: 10.1038/ncomms6318

Paulsen, C. E., Armache, J. P., Gao, Y., Cheng, Y., and Julius, D. (2015). Structure of the TRPA1 ion channel suggests regulatory mechanisms. *Nature* 520, 511–517. doi: 10.1038/nature14367

Perraud, A. L., Takanishi, C. L., Shen, B., Kang, S., Smith, M. K., Schmitz, C., et al. (2005). Accumulation of free ADP-ribose from mitochondria mediates oxidative stress-induced gating of TRPM2 cation channels. *J. Biol. Chem.* 280, 6138–6148. doi: 10.1074/jbc.M411446200

Philipp, S., Trost, C., Warnat, J., Rautmann, J., Himmerkus, N., Schroth, G., et al. (2000). TRP4 (CCE1) protein is part of native calcium release-activated Ca2+-like channels in adrenal cells. *J. Biol. Chem.* 275, 23965–23972. doi: 10.1074/jbc.M003408200

Pisani, V., Moschella, V., Bari, M., Fezza, F., Galati, S., Bernardi, G., et al. (2010). Dynamic changes of anandamide in the cerebrospinal fluid of Parkinson's disease patients. *Mov. Disord.* 25, 920–924. doi: 10.1002/mds.23014

Possebon, M. I., Mizokami, S. S., Carvalho, T. T., Zarpelon, A. C., Hohmann, M. S. N., Staurengo-ferrari, L., et al. (2014). Activation and cytokine production and activation of the NO - Cyclic. *J. Nat. Prod.* 77, 2488–2496.

Poteser, M., Graziani, A., Rosker, C., Eder, P., Derler, I., Kahr, H., et al. (2006). TRPC3 and TRPC4 associate to form a redox-sensitive cation channel: evidence for expression of native TRPC3-TRPC4 heteromeric channels in endothelial cells. *J. Biol. Chem.* 281, 13588–13595. doi: 10.1074/jbc.M512205200

Putney, J. W. (1986). A model for receptor-regulated calcium entry. *Cell Calcium* 7, 1–12. doi: 10.1016/0143-4160(86)90026-6

Putney, J. W. (2005). Physiological mechanisms of TRPC activation. *Pflugers Arch. Eur. J. Physiol.* 451, 29–34. doi: 10.1007/s00424-005-1416-4

Putney, J. W., Trebak, M., Vazquez, G., Wedel, B., and Bird, G. S. J. (2004). Signalling mechanisms for TRPC3 channels. *Novartis Found. Symp.* 258, 123–133.

Rahimi, J., and Kovacs, G. G. (2014). Prevalence of mixed pathologies in the aging brain. *Alzheimers Res. Ther.* 6:82. doi: 10.1186/s13195-014-0082-1

Ramsey, I. S., Delling, M., and Clapham, D. E. (2006). an Introduction To Trp Channels. *Annu. Rev. Physiol.* 68, 619–647. doi: 10.1146/annurev.physiol.68.040204.100431

Reichling, D. B., and Levine, J. D. (2011). Pain and death: neurodegenerative disease mechanisms in the nociceptor. *Ann. Neurol.* 69, 13–21. doi: 10.1002/ana.22351

Riccio, A., Medhurst, A. D., Mattei, C., Kelsell, R. E., Calver, A. R., Randall, A. D., et al. (2002). mRNA distribution analysis of human TRPC family in CNS and peripheral tissues. *Mol. Brain Res.* 109, 95–104. doi: 10.1016/S0169-328X(02)00527-2

Rohács, T., Lopes, C. M. B., Michailidis, I., and Logothetis, D. E. (2005). PI(4,5)P2 regulates the activation and desensitization of TRPM8 channels through the TRP domain. *Nat. Neurosci.* 8, 626–634. doi: 10.1038/nn1451

Rojo, A. I., McBean, G., Cindric, M., Egea, J., López, M. G., Rada, P., et al. (2014). Redox control of microglial function: molecular mechanisms and functional significance. *Antioxid. Redox Signal.* 21, 1766–1801. doi: 10.1089/ars.2013.5745

Romero-Sánchez, H. A., Mendieta, L., Austrich-Olivares, A. M., Garza-Mouriño, G., Benitez-Diaz Mirón, M., Coen, A., et al. (2019). Unilateral lesion of the nigroestriatal pathway with 6-OHDA induced allodynia and hyperalgesia reverted by pramipexol in rats. *Eur. J. Pharmacol.* 869:172814. doi: 10.1016/j.ejphar.2019.172814

Ros-Bernal, F., Hunot, S., Herrero, M. T., Parnadeau, S., Corvol, J. C., Lu, L., et al. (2011). Microglial glucocorticoid receptors play a pivotal role in regulating dopaminergic neurodegeneration in parkinsonism. *Proc. Natl. Acad. Sci. U.S.A.* 108, 6632–6637. doi: 10.1073/pnas.1017820108

Rosenbaum, T., Gordon-Shaag, A., Munari, M., and Gordon, S. E. (2004). Ca2+/Calmodulin modulates TRPV1 activation by capsaicin. *J. Gen. Physiol.* 123, 53–62. doi: 10.1085/jgp.200308906

Sabens Liedhegner, E. A., Steller, K. M., and Mieyal, J. J. (2011). Levodopa activates apoptosis signaling kinase 1 (ASK1) and promotes apoptosis in a neuronal model: implications for the treatment of Parkinson's disease. *Chem. Res. Toxicol.* 24, 1644–1652. doi: 10.1021/tx200082h

Salter, M. W., and Stevens, B. (2017). Microglia emerge as central players in brain disease. *Nat. Med.* 23, 1018–1027. doi: 10.1038/nm.4397

Samanta, A., Hughes, T. E. T., and Moiseenkova-Bell, V. Y. (2018). "Transient receptor potential (TRP) channels. *Subcell. Biochem.* 87, 141–165. doi: 10.1007/978-981-10-7757-9_6

Schneider, I., Reversé, D., Dewachter, I., Ris, L., Caluwaerts, N., Kuipér, C., et al. (2001). Mutant Presenilins disturb neuronal calcium homeostasis in the brain of transgenic mice, decreasing the threshold for excitotoxicity and facilitating long-term potentiation. *J. Biol. Chem.* 276, 11539–11544. doi: 10.1074/jbc.M010977200

Seabrook, T. J., Jiang, L., Maier, M., and Lemere, C. A. (2006). Minocycline affects microglia activation, Aβ deposition, and behavior in APP-tg mice. *Glia* 53, 776–782. doi: 10.1002/glia.20338

Séguéla, P., Ase, A. R., Grant, R., O'Donnell, D., and Groschner, K. (2014). Contribution of TRPC3 to store-operated calcium entry and inflammatory transductions in primary nociceptors. *Mol. Pain* 10:43. doi: 10.1186/1744-8069-10-43

Selvaraj, S., Sun, Y., and Singh, B. (2012). TRPC channels and their implications for neurological diseases. *CNS Neurol. Disord. Drug Targets* 9, 94–104. doi: 10.2174/187152710790966650

Shen, C., Zhao, X., Dwibedi, N., Wiener, R. C., Findley, P. A., and Sambamoorthi, U. (2018). Opioid use and the presence of Alzheimer's disease and related dementias among elderly Medicare beneficiaries diagnosed with chronic pain conditions. *Alzheimers Dement. Transl. Res. Clin. Interv.* 4, 661–668. doi: 10.1016/j.trci.2018.10.012

Shigetomi, E., Jackson-Weaver, O., Huckstepp, R. T., O'Dell, T. J., and Khakh, B. S. (2013). TRPA1 channels are regulators of astrocyte basal calcium levels and long-term potentiation via constitutive d-serine release. *J. Neurosci.* 33, 10143–10153. doi: 10.1523/JNEUROSCI.5779-12.2013

Shigetomi, E., Tong, X., Kwan, K. Y., Corey, D. P., and Khakh, B. S. (2012). TRPA1 channels regulate astrocyte resting calcium and inhibitory synapse efficacy through GAT-3. *Nat. Neurosci.* 15, 70–80. doi: 10.1038/nn.3000

Shimizu, T., Dietz, R. M., Cruz-Torres, I., Strnad, F., Garske, A. K., Moreno, M., et al. (2016). Extended therapeutic window of a novel peptide inhibitor of TRPM2 channels following focal cerebral ischemia. *Exp. Neurol.* 283, 151–156. doi: 10.1016/j.expneurol.2016.06.015

Shin, J., Cho, H., Hwang, S. W., Jung, J., Shin, C. Y., Lee, S. Y., et al. (2002). Bradykinin-12-lipoxygenase-VR1 signaling pathway for inflammatory hyperalgesia. *Proc. Natl. Acad. Sci. U.S.A.* 99, 10150–10155. doi: 10.1073/pnas.152002699

Shirakawa, H., and Kaneko, S. (2018). Physiological and pathophysiological roles of transient receptor potential channels in microglia-related CNS inflammatory diseases. *Biol. Pharm. Bull.* 41, 1152–1157. doi: 10.1248/bpb.b18-00319

Shukla, M., Quirion, R., and Ma, W. (2013). Reduced expression of pain mediators and pain sensitivity in amyloid precursor protein over-expressing CRND8 transgenic mice. *Neuroscience* 250, 92–101. doi: 10.1016/j.neuroscience.2013.06.064

Sierra, A., Gottfried-Blackmore, A., Milner, T. A., McEwen, B. S., and Bulloch, K. (2008). Steroid hormone receptor expression and function in microglia. *Glia* 56, 659–674. doi: 10.1002/glia.20644

Sita, G., Hrelia, P., Graziosi, A., Ravegnini, G., and Morroni, F. (2018). TRPM2 in the brain: role in health and disease. *Cells* 7:82. doi: 10.3390/cells7070082

Skogar, O., and Lokk, J. (2016). Pain management in patients with Parkinson's disease: challenges and solutions. *J. Multidiscip. Healthc.* 9, 469–479. doi: 10.2147/JMDH.S105857

Skryma, R., Prevarskaya, N., Gkika, D., and Shuba, Y. (2011). From urgency to frequency: facts and controversies of TRPs in the lower urinary tract. *Nat. Rev. Urol.* 8, 617–630. doi: 10.1038/nrurol.2011.142

Small, D. H. (2009). Dysregulation of calcium homeostasis in Alzheimer's disease. *Neurochem. Res.* 34, 1824–1829. doi: 10.1007/s11064-009-9960-5

Smani, T., Shapovalov, G., Skryma, R., Prevarskaya, N., and Rosado, J. A. (2015). Functional and physiopathological implications of TRP channels. *Biochim. Biophys. Acta* 1853, 1772–1782. doi: 10.1016/j.bbamcr.2015.04.016

Smith, G. D., Gunthorpe, M. J., Kelsell, R. E., Hayes, P. D., Reilly, P., Facer, P., et al. (2002). TRPV3 is a temperature-sensitive vanilloid receptor-like protein. *Nature* 418, 186–190. doi: 10.1038/nature00894

Soboloff, J., Rothberg, B. S., Madesh, M., and Gill, D. L. (2012). STIM proteins: dynamic calcium signal transducers. *Nat. Rev. Mol. Cell Biol.* 13, 549–565. doi: 10.1038/nrm3414

Song, M. Y., Makino, A., and Yuan, J. X. J. (2011). Role of reactive oxygen species and redox in regulating the function of transient receptor potential channels. *Antioxid. Redox Signal.* 15, 1549–1565. doi: 10.1089/ars.2010.3648

Sotiropoulos, I., Lopes, A. T., Pinto, V., Lopes, S., Carlos, S., Duarte-Silva, S., et al. (2014). Selective impact of Tau loss on nociceptive primary afferents and pain sensation. *Exp. Neurol.* 261, 486–493. doi: 10.1016/j.expneurol.2014.07.008

Starkus, J., Jansen, C., Shimoda, L. M. N., Stokes, A. J., Small-Howard, A. L., and Turner, H. (2019). Diverse TRPV1 responses to cannabinoids. *Channels* 13, 172–191. doi: 10.1080/19336950.2019.1619436

Suh, Y.-G., and Oh, U. (2005). Activation and activators of TRPV1 and their pharmaceutical implication. *Curr. Pharm. Des.* 11, 2687–2698. doi: 10.2174/1381612054546789

Sun, A., Liu, M., Nguyen, X. V., and Bing, G. (2003). p38 MAP kinase is activated at early stages in Alzheimer's disease brain. *Exp. Neurol.* 183, 394–405. doi: 10.1016/S0014-4886(03)00180-8

Sun, Y., Selvaraj, S., Pandey, S., Humphrey, K. M., Foster, J. D., Wu, M., et al. (2018). MPP+ decreases store-operated calcium entry and TRPC1 expression in Mesenchymal Stem Cell derived dopaminergic neurons. *Sci. Rep.* 8:11715. doi: 10.1038/s41598-018-29528-x

Sun, Y., Singh, B. B., Watt, J. A., Selvaraj, S., Birnbaumer, L., Lei, S., et al. (2012). Neurotoxin-induced ER stress in mouse dopaminergic neurons involves downregulation of TRPC1 and inhibition of AKT/mTOR signaling. *J. Clin. Invest.* 122, 1354–1367. doi: 10.1172/JCI61332DS1

Sun, Y., Sukumaran, P., Schaar, A., and Singh, B. B. (2015). TRPM7 and its role in neurodegenerative diseases. *Channels* 9, 253–261. doi: 10.1080/19336950.2015.1075675

Sun, Y., Zhang, H., Selvaraj, S., Sukumaran, P., Lei, S., Birnbaumer, L., et al. (2017). Inhibition of L-type Ca2+ channels by TRPC1-STIM1 complex is essential for the protection of dopaminergic neurons. *J. Neurosci.* 37, 3364–3377. doi: 10.1523/JNEUROSCI.3010-16.2017

Suter, M. R., Wen, Y. R., Decosterd, I., and Ji, R. R. (2007). Do glial cells control pain? *Neuron Glia Biol.* 3, 255–268. doi: 10.1017/S1740925X08000100

Szallasi, A., and Blumberg, P. M. (1999). Vanilloid (Capsaicin) receptors and mechanisms. *Pharmacol. Rev.* 51, 159–211.

Takada, Y., Numata, T., and Mori, Y. (2013). Targeting TRPs in neurodegenerative disorders. *Curr. Top. Med. Chem.* 13, 322–334. doi: 10.2174/1568026611313030009

Takahashi, N., Mizuno, Y., Kozai, D., Yamamoto, S., Kiyonaka, S., Shibata, T., et al. (2008). Molecular characterization of TRPA1 channel activation by cysteine-reactive inflammatory mediators. *Channels* 2, 287–298. doi: 10.4161/chan.2.4.6745

Talavera, K., Yasumatsu, K., Voets, T., Droogmans, G., Shigemura, N., Ninomiya, Y., et al. (2005). Heat activation of TRPM5 underlies thermal sensitivity of sweet taste. *Nature* 438, 1022–1025. doi: 10.1038/nature04248

Tatsumi, E., Yamanaka, H., Kobayashi, K., Yagi, H., Sakagami, M., and Noguchi, K. (2015). RhoA/ROCK pathway mediates p38 MAPK activation and morphological changes downstream of P2Y12/13 receptors in spinal microglia in neuropathic pain. *Glia* 63, 216–228. doi: 10.1002/glia.22745

Togashi, K., Hara, Y., Tominaga, T., Higashi, T., Konishi, Y., Mori, Y., et al. (2006). TRPM2 activation by cyclic ADP-ribose at body temperature is involved in insulin secretion. *EMBO J.* 25, 1804–1815. doi: 10.1038/sj.emboj.7601083

Tominaga, M., Caterina, M. J., Malmberg, A. B., Rosen, T. A., Gilbert, H., Skinner, K., et al. (1998). The cloned capsaicin receptor integrates multiple pain-producing stimuli. *Neuron* 21, 531–543. doi: 10.1016/S0896-6273(00)80564-4

Tóth, A., Boczán, J., Kedei, N., Lizanecz, E., Bagi, Z., Papp, Z., et al. (2005). Expression and distribution of vanilloid receptor 1 (TRPV1) in the adult rat brain. *Mol. Brain Res.* 135, 162–168. doi: 10.1016/j.molbrainres.2004.12.003

Trevisan, G., Hoffmeister, C., Rossato, M. F., Oliveira, S. M., Silva, M. A., Silva, C. R., et al. (2014). TRPA1 receptor stimulation by hydrogen peroxide is critical to trigger hyperalgesia and inflammation in a model of acute gout. *Free Radic. Biol. Med.* 72, 200–209. doi: 10.1016/j.freeradbiomed.2014.04.021

Tsuji, F., and Aono, H. (2012). Role of transient receptor potential vanilloid 1 in inflammation and autoimmune diseases. *Pharmaceuticals* 5, 837–852. doi: 10.3390/ph5080837

Tysnes, O. B., and Storstein, A. (2017). Epidemiology of Parkinson's disease. *J. Neural Transm.* 124, 901–905. doi: 10.1007/s00702-017-1686-y

Van Kooten, J., Binnekade, T. T., Van Der Wouden, J. C., Stek, M. L., Scherder, E. J. A., Husebø, B. S., et al. (2016). A review of pain prevalence in Alzheimer's, vascular, frontotemporal and lewy body dementias. *Dement. Geriatr. Cogn. Disord.* 41, 220–232. doi: 10.1159/000444791

Vanden Abeele, F., Zholos, A., Bidaux, G., Shuba, Y., Thebault, S., Beck, B., et al. (2006). Ca2+-independent phospholipase A2-dependent gating of TRPM8 by lysophospholipids. *J. Biol. Chem.* 281, 40174–40182. doi: 10.1074/jbc.M605779200

Varga, V., Helenius, J., Tanaka, K., Hyman, A. A., Tanaka, T. U., and Howard, J. (2006). Yeast kinesin-8 depolymerizes microtubules in a length-dependent manner. *Nat. Cell Biol.* 8, 957–962. doi: 10.1038/ncb1462

Vennekens, R., Menigoz, A., and Nilius, B. (2012). TRPs in the brain. *Rev. Physiol. Biochem. Pharmacol.* 163, 27–64. doi: 10.1007/112-2012-8

Verri, W. A., Cunha, T. M., Parada, C. A., Poole, S., Cunha, F. Q., and Ferreira, S. H. (2006). Hypernociceptive role of cytokines and chemokines: targets for analgesic drug development? *Pharmacol. Ther.* 112, 116–138. doi: 10.1016/j.pharmthera.2006.04.001

Viana, F. (2016). TRPA1 channels: molecular sentinels of cellular stress and tissue damage. *J. Physiol.* 594, 4151–4169. doi: 10.1113/JP270935

Vlachová, V., Teisinger, J., Sušánková, K., Lyfenko, A., Ettrich, R., and Vyklický, L. (2003). Functional role of C-terminal cytoplasmic tail of rat vanilloid receptor 1. *J. Neurosci.* 23, 1340–1350. doi: 10.1523/jneurosci.23-04-01340.2003

Vriens, J., Owsianik, G., Hofmann, T., Philipp, S. E., Stab, J., Chen, X., et al. (2011). TRPM3 is a nociceptor channel involved in the detection of noxious heat. *Neuron* 70, 482–494. doi: 10.1016/j.neuron.2011.02.051

Wang, W. Y., Tan, M. S., Yu, J. T., and Tan, L. (2015). Role of pro-inflammatory cytokines released from microglia in Alzheimer's disease. *Ann. Transl. Med.* 3:136. doi: 10.3978/j.issn.2305-5839.2015.03.49

Wang, X.-L., Cui, L.-W., Liu, Z., Gao, Y.-M., Wang, S., Li, H., et al. (2019). Effects of TRPA1 activation and inhibition on TRPA1 and CGRP expression in dorsal root ganglion neurons. *Neural Regen. Res.* 14, 140–148. doi: 10.4103/1673-5374.243719

Whitlock, E. L., Diaz-Ramirez, L. G., Glymour, M. M., Boscardin, W. J., Covinsky, K. E., and Smith, A. K. (2017). Association between persistent pain and memory decline and dementia in a longitudinal cohort of elders. *JAMA Intern. Med.* 177, 1146–1153. doi: 10.1001/jamainternmed.2017.1622

Woo, J. S., Lee, K. J., Huang, M., Cho, C. H., and Lee, E. H. (2014). Heteromeric TRPC3 with TRPC1 formed via its ankyrin repeats regulates the resting cytosolic Ca2+ levels in skeletal muscle. *Biochem. Biophys. Res. Commun.* 446, 454–459. doi: 10.1016/j.bbrc.2014.02.127

Wu, L., Sweet, T., and Clapham, D. E. (2010). Current progress in the mammalian TRP ion channel family. *Pharmocol. Rev.* 62, 381–404. doi: 10.1124/pr.110.002725.Abbreviations

Xie, Y. F., MacDonald, J. F., and Jackson, M. F. (2010). TRPM2, calcium and neurodegenerative diseases. *Int. J. Physiol. Pathophysiol. Pharmacol.* 2, 95–103.

Xu, H., Ramsey, I. S., Kotecha, S. A., Moran, M. M., Chong, J. A., Lawson, D., et al. (2002). TRPV3 is a calcium-permeable temperature-sensitive cation channel. *Nature* 418, 181–186. doi: 10.1038/nature00882

Yaksh, T., Woller, S., Ramachandran, R., and Sorkin, L. (2015). The search for novel analgesics: targets and mechanisms. *F1000Prime Rep.* 7:56. doi: 10.12703/p7-56

Yamamoto, S., Wajima, T., Hara, Y., Nishida, M., and Mori, Y. (2007). Transient receptor potential channels in Alzheimer's disease. *Biochim. Biophys. Acta* 1772, 958–967. doi: 10.1016/j.bbadis.2007.03.006

Yao, J., Liu, B., and Qin, F. (2011). Modular thermal sensors in temperature-gated transient receptor potential (TRP) channels. *Proc. Natl. Acad. Sci. U.S.A.* 108, 11109–11114. doi: 10.1073/pnas.1105196108

Yoshida, T., Inoue, R., Morii, T., Takahashi, N., Yamamoto, S., Hara, Y., et al. (2006). Nitric oxide activates TRP channels by cysteine S-nitrosylation. *Nat. Chem. Biol.* 2, 596–607. doi: 10.1038/nchembio821

Yuan, J. P., Zeng, W., Huang, G. N., Worley, P. F., and Muallem, S. (2007). STIM1 heteromultimerizes TRPC channels to determine their function as store-operated channels. *Nat. Cell Biol.* 9, 636–645. doi: 10.1038/ncb1590

Zarpelon, A. C., Cunha, T. M., Alves-Filho, J. C., Pinto, L. G., Ferreira, S. H., McInnes, I. B., et al. (2013). IL-33/ST2 signalling contributes to carrageenin-induced innate inflammation and inflammatory pain: Role of cytokines, endothelin-1 and prostaglandin E 2. *Br. J. Pharmacol.* 169, 90–101. doi: 10.1111/bph.12110

Zeng, B., Chen, G. L., and Xu, S. Z. (2012). Divalent copper is a potent extracellular blocker for TRPM2 channel. *Biochem. Biophys. Res. Commun.* 424, 279–284. doi: 10.1016/j.bbrc.2012.06.107

Zhang, E., and Liao, P. (2015). Brain transient receptor potential channels and stroke. *J. Neurosci. Res.* 93, 1165–1183. doi: 10.1002/jnr.23529

Zhang, H., Sun, S., Wu, L., Pchitskaya, E., Zakharova, O., Tacer, K. F., et al. (2016). Store-operated calcium channel complex in postsynaptic spines: a new therapeutic target for Alzheimer's disease treatment. *J. Neurosci.* 36, 11837–11850. doi: 10.1523/JNEUROSCI.1188-16.2016

Zhang, Z., Yu, H., Huang, J., Faouzi, M., Schmitz, C., Penner, R., et al. (2014). The TRPM6 kinase domain determines the Mg ATP sensitivity of TRPM7/M6 heteromeric ion channels. *J. Biol. Chem.* 289, 5217–5227. doi: 10.1074/jbc.M113.512285

Zhou, F. W., Matta, S. G., and Zhou, F. M. (2008). Constitutively active TRPC3 channels regulate basal ganglia output neurons. *J. Neurosci.* 28, 473–482. doi: 10.1523/JNEUROSCI.3978-07.2008

Zimova, M., Hackländer, K., Good, J. M., Melo-Ferreira, J., Alves, P. C., and Mills, L. S. (2018). Function and underlying mechanisms of seasonal colour moulting in mammals and birds: what keeps them changing in a warming world? *Biol. Rev.* 93, 1478–1498. doi: 10.1111/brv.12405

Zündorf, G., and Reiser, G. (2011). Calcium dysregulation and homeostasis of neural calcium in the molecular mechanisms of neurodegenerative diseases provide multiple targets for neuroprotection. *Antioxid. Redox Signal.* 14, 1275–1288. doi: 10.1089/ars.2010.3359

Permissions

All chapters in this book were first published by Frontiers; hereby published with permission under the Creative Commons Attribution License or equivalent. Every chapter published in this book has been scrutinized by our experts. Their significance has been extensively debated. The topics covered herein carry significant findings which will fuel the growth of the discipline. They may even be implemented as practical applications or may be referred to as a beginning point for another development.

The contributors of this book come from diverse backgrounds, making this book a truly international effort. This book will bring forth new frontiers with its revolutionizing research information and detailed analysis of the nascent developments around the world.

We would like to thank all the contributing authors for lending their expertise to make the book truly unique. They have played a crucial role in the development of this book. Without their invaluable contributions this book wouldn't have been possible. They have made vital efforts to compile up to date information on the varied aspects of this subject to make this book a valuable addition to the collection of many professionals and students.

This book was conceptualized with the vision of imparting up-to-date information and advanced data in this field. To ensure the same, a matchless editorial board was set up. Every individual on the board went through rigorous rounds of assessment to prove their worth. After which they invested a large part of their time researching and compiling the most relevant data for our readers.

The editorial board has been involved in producing this book since its inception. They have spent rigorous hours researching and exploring the diverse topics which have resulted in the successful publishing of this book. They have passed on their knowledge of decades through this book. To expedite this challenging task, the publisher supported the team at every step. A small team of assistant editors was also appointed to further simplify the editing procedure and attain best results for the readers.

Apart from the editorial board, the designing team has also invested a significant amount of their time in understanding the subject and creating the most relevant covers. They scrutinized every image to scout for the most suitable representation of the subject and create an appropriate cover for the book.

The publishing team has been an ardent support to the editorial, designing and production team. Their endless efforts to recruit the best for this project, has resulted in the accomplishment of this book. They are a veteran in the field of academics and their pool of knowledge is as vast as their experience in printing. Their expertise and guidance has proved useful at every step. Their uncompromising quality standards have made this book an exceptional effort. Their encouragement from time to time has been an inspiration for everyone.

The publisher and the editorial board hope that this book will prove to be a valuable piece of knowledge for researchers, students, practitioners and scholars across the globe.

List of Contributors

Bhupesh Vaidya and Shyam Sunder Sharma
Department of Pharmacology and Toxicology, National Institute of Pharmaceutical Education and Research (NIPER), Mohali, India

Akito Nakao, Yoshihiro Matsunaga and Katsumi Hayashida
Laboratory of Molecular Biology, Department of Synthetic Chemistry and Biological Chemistry, Graduate School of Engineering, Kyoto University, Kyoto, Japan

Nobuaki Takahashi
The Hakubi Center for Advanced Research, Kyoto University, Kyoto, Japan

Julia Hermann and Melanie Bender
Institute of Pharmacology, Heidelberg University, Heidelberg, Germany

Dagmar Schumacher, Vladimir Kuryshev, Marc Freichel and Volodymyr Tsvilovskyy
Institute of Pharmacology, Heidelberg University, Heidelberg, Germany
DZHK (German Centre for Cardiovascular Research), Partner Site Heidelberg/Mannheim, Heidelberg, Germany

Marcel S. Woo and Artem Shaposhnykov
Institut für Neuroimmunologie und Multiple Sklerose, Universitätsklinikum Hamburg-Eppendorf, Hamburg, Germany

Chris Meier
Organic Chemistry, Department of Chemistry, University of Hamburg, Hamburg, Germany

Andreas H. Guse
The Calcium Signaling Group, Department of Biochemistry and Molecular Cell Biology, University Medical Center Hamburg-Eppendorf, Hamburg, Germany

Sina C. Rosenkranz, Vanessa Vieira, Karsten Heidermann, Benjamin Schattling and Manuel A. Friese
Institut für Neuroimmunologie und Multiple Sklerose, Universitätsklinikum Hamburg-Eppendorf, Hamburg, Germany

Katharina Held
Laboratory of Endometrium, Endometriosis and Reproductive Medicine, Department of Development and Regeneration, KU Leuven, Leuven, Belgium
Laboratory of Ion Channel Research, Department of Cellular and Molecular Medicine and VIB-KU Leuven Center for Brain and Disease Research, KU Leuven, Leuven, Belgium

Balázs István Tóth
Laboratory of Cellular and Molecular Physiology, Department of Physiology, Faculty of Medicine, University of Debrecen, Debrecen, Hungary

Sung-Min Hwang
Gachon Pain Center, Department of Physiology, Gachon University College of Medicine, Incheon, South Korea

Ji Yeon Lee
Gil Medical Center, Department of Anesthesiology and Pain Medicine, Gachon University, Incheon, South Korea

Jueun Roh, Eun Jin Go, Yong Ho Kim and Chul-Kyu Park
Gachon Pain Center and Department of Physiology, College of Medicine, Gachon University, Incheon, South Korea

Giorgia Chinigò
Laboratory of Cell Physiology, Department of Life Sciences, Univ. Lille, Inserm, U1003 - PHYCEL, University of Lille, Lille, France
Laboratory of Cellular and Molecular Angiogenesis, Department of Life Sciences and Systems Biology, University of Torino, Turin, Italy

Hélène Castel and Oana Chever
UNIROUEN, Inserm U1239, DC2N, Normandie Université, Rouen, France
Institute for Research and Innovation in Biomedicine, Rouen, France

Dimitra Gkika
CNRS, Inserm, CHU Lille, Centre Oscar Lambret, UMR 9020-UMR 1277-Canther-Cancer Heterogeneity, Plasticity and Resistance to Therapies, University of Lille, Lille, France
Institut Universitaire de France, Paris, France

Boris Lavanderos, Ian Silva, Pablo Cruz, Octavio Orellana-Serradell and María Paz Saldías
Program of Cellular and Molecular Biology, Institute of Biomedical Sciences, Faculty of Medicine, Universidad de Chile, Santiago, Chile
Millennium Nucleus of Ion Channel-Associated Diseases (MiNICAD), Santiago, Chile

Oscar Cerda
Program of Cellular and Molecular Biology, Institute of Biomedical Sciences, Faculty of Medicine, Universidad de Chile, Santiago, Chile
Millennium Nucleus of Ion Channel-Associated Diseases (MiNICAD), Santiago, Chile
The Wound Repair, Treatment and Health (WoRTH) Initiative, Santiago, Chile

Meera Manchanda, Emma Leishman, Kishan Sangani, Ali Alamri and Heather B. Bradshaw
Bradshaw Laboratory of Lipid Neuroscience, Indiana University Bloomington, Bloomington, IN, United States

Oliver Schnapauff and Mathias Gelderblom
Klinik und Poliklinik für Neurologie, Universitätsklinikum Hamburg-Eppendorf, Hamburg, Germany

Lisa Epping and Sven G. Meuth
Klinik für Neurologie mit Institut für Translationale Neurologie, Universität Münster, Münster, Germany

Wolfgang Liedtke
Departments of Neurology, Anesthesiology and Neurobiology, Duke University Medical Center, Durham, NC, United States

Huilong Luo
Faculté de Pharmacie, Inserm, UMRS-1144, Optimisation Thérapeutique en Neuropsychopharmacologie, Université de Paris, Paris, France
Department of Chemical and Biological Engineering, University of Wisconsin-Madison, Madison, WI, United States

Bruno Saubamea, Stéphanie Chasseigneaux, Véronique Cochois, Maria Smirnova and Catarina Chaves
Faculté de Pharmacie, Inserm, UMRS-1144, Optimisation Thérapeutique en Neuropsychopharmacologie, Université de Paris, Paris, France

Fabienne Glacial and Nicolas Perrière
BrainPlotting, Paris, France

Salvatore Cisternino
Faculté de Pharmacie, Inserm, UMRS-1144, Optimisation Thérapeutique en Neuropsychopharmacologie, Université de Paris, Paris, France
Service Pharmacie, Assistance Publique Hôpitaux de Paris (AP-HP), Hôpital Universitaire Necker - Enfants Malades, Paris, France

Xavier Declèves
Faculté de Pharmacie, Inserm, UMRS-1144, Optimisation Thérapeutique en Neuropsychopharmacologie, Université de Paris, Paris, France
Biologie du médicament et toxicologie, Assistance Publique Hôpitaux de Paris (AP-HP), Hôpital Universitaire Cochin, Paris, France

Lu Liu, Manli Chen, Yueying Zheng and Shengmei Zhu
Department of Anesthesiology, The First Affiliated Hospital, College of Medicine, Zhejiang University, Hangzhou, China

Kun Lin, Xuwu Xiang and Jing Yang
Department of Anesthesiology, The First Affiliated Hospital, Zhejiang University School of Medicine, Hangzhou, China

Xiaoxing Xiong
Department of Anesthesiology, The First Affiliated Hospital, College of Medicine, Zhejiang University, Hangzhou, China
Central Laboratory, Renmin Hospital of Wuhan University, Wuhan, China

Kihwan Lee
Gachon Pain Center and Department of Physiology, Gachon University College of Medicine, Incheon, South Korea

Youn Yi Jo
Department of Anesthesiology and Pain Medicine, Gil Medical Center, Gachon University, Incheon, South Korea

Gehoon Chung
Department of Oral Physiology and Program in Neurobiology, School of Dentistry, Seoul National University, Seoul, South Korea

Jung Hoon Jung
Program in Neurosciences and Mental Health, The Hospital for Sick Children, Toronto, ON, Canada

Jaepyo Jeon, Jin-Bin Tian and Michael X. Zhu
Department of Integrative Biology and Pharmacology, McGovern Medical School, The University of Texas Health Science Center at Houston, Houston, TX, United States

Fan Bu, Guanghua Sun, Shun-Ming Ting, Jun Li and Jaroslaw Aronowski
Department of Neurology, McGovern Medical School, The University of Texas Health Science Center at Houston, Houston, TX, United States

Lutz Birnbaumer
Institute for Biomedical Research (BIOMED UCACONICET), Buenos Aires, Argentina
School of Medical Sciences, Catholic University of Argentina (UCA), Buenos Aires, Argentina
Neurobiology Laboratory, National Institute of Environmental Health Sciences, Durham, NC, United States

Lijuan Gu
Central Laboratory, Renmin Hospital of Wuhan University, Wuhan, China

Milena Duitama, Viviana Vargas-López, Zulma Casas, Sonia L. Albarracin, Jhon-Jairo Sutachan and Yolima P. Torres
Departamento de Nutrición y Bioquímica, Pontificia Universidad Javeriana, Bogotá, Colombia

Index

N

O

P

R

S

T

www.ingramcontent.com/pod-product-compliance
Lightning Source LLC
LaVergne TN
LVHW082150200926
848484LV00008B/2134